AUTOIMMUNE DISORDERS – PATHOGENETIC ASPECTS

Edited by **Clio P. Mavragani**

Autoimmune Disorders – Pathogenetic Aspects
Edited by Clio P. Mavragani

Published by InTech
Janeza Trdine 9, 51000 Rijeka, Croatia

Publishing Process Manager Alenka Urbancic

Technical Editor Teodora Smiljanic

Cover Designer InTech Design Team

Additional hard copies can be obtained from orders@intechopen.com

Autoimmune Disorders – Pathogenetic Aspects, Edited by Clio P. Mavragani
p. cm.
ISBN 978-953-307-643-0

For EU product safety concerns:
IN TECH d.o.o., Prolaz Marije Krucifikse Kozulić 3, 51000 Rijeka, Croatia,
info@intechopen.com or visit our website at intechopen.com.

Meet the editor

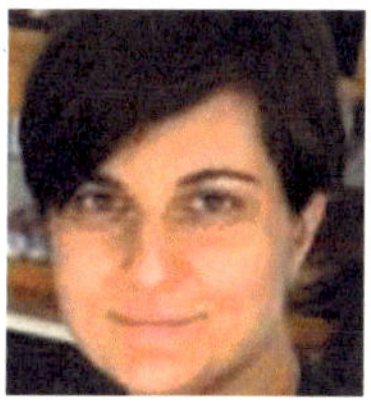

Dr. Mavragani received her MD and PhD degrees, both with honors, from the National University of Athens, Greece. She also received a Diploma Degree in Internal Medicine from Imperial College, University of London with distinction. She was trained in Rheumatology at the Department of Pathophysiology, University of Athens under the mentorship of Professor HM Moutsopoulos). Following her clinical fellowship, she joined the lab of Peggy Crow at Hospital for Special Surgery in New York as a recipient of S. Niarchos Foundation International Exchange Fellowship. Her research focuses on the activation of type I IFN system in systemic autoimmune disorders, including Sjogren's syndrome and systemic lupus erythematosus, the interactions between TNF and IFNs pathways, as well as the potential role of type I interferons as biomarkers of response in patients with rheumatoid arthritis receiving anti-TNF therapies.

Contents

Preface

The term "Autoimmune disorders" refers to a heterogeneous and multifaceted group of diseases which can affect virtually any organ system of the human body. They all arise from a misdirected attack of the organism's immune defenses against "self molecules" initially designed to protect them, resulting in chronic inflammation, autoantibody formation and tissue damage. They can be divided into systemic (response against ubiquitous self antigens) and organ-specific (against specific organs).

Despite the unprecedented progress in the field of autoimmunity, the initial triggers for the aberrant immune reaction against "self" still remain to be defined. The interplay of environmental triggers, and an appropriate genetic makeup seem to be the prevailing belief for the pathogenesis of autoimmunity with many questions still unanswered. Furthermore, the contribution of autoimmune mechanisms in the generation of co-morbid conditions mainly manifested as cardiovascular burden or malignant transformation is currently a focus of intensive research.

The present edition entitled "Autoimmune disorders - Pathogenetic aspects" aims to present the current available evidence of etiopathogenetic insights of both systemic and organ specific autoimmune disorders, the crossover interactions among autoimmunity, cardiovascular morbidity and malignancy, as well as novel findings in the exciting fields of osteoimmunology and immunology of pregnancy.

We hope that this edition will provide a comprehensive overview of the recent advances in the field of autoimmunity, and at the same time foster further research efforts which will ultimately translate into better patient outcomes.

Clio P. Mavragani, MD
Department of Experimental Physiology,
School of Medicine,
University of Athens,
Greece

Part 1

Pathogenesis of Systemic Autoimmune Disorders: Genetic and Enviromental Contributors

1

Autoimmune Diseases: The Role of Environment and Gene Interactions

Wellington K. Ayensu[1,3], Emmanuel O. Keku[2], Raphael D. Isokpehi[1,3], Ibrahim O. Farah[1], Chris A. Arthur[4] and Sophia S. Leggett[4]
[1]*College of Science, Engineering & Technology, Jackson State University, Jackson,*
[2]*Department of Public Health and Preventive Medicine, School of Medicine, St. George's University, St. George, Grenada,*
[3]*Bioinformatics Section; Jackson State University, Jackson,*
[4]*School of Health Sciences, College of Public Service, Jackson State University, Jackson,*
[1,3,4]*USA*
[2]*West Indies*

1. Introduction

Data from epidemiological studies indicate global increase in the incidence and prevalence of numerous autoimmune diseases (AD) as seen in the United States (Jacobson et al.1997). According to estimate from the US National Institute of Health (NIH) the prevalence of AD is in the range of 23.5 billion. From 1996 to date at least 237,203 cases per year of AD are diagnosed in the US; and of this, 42,137 are new cases of primary glomerulonephritis, multiple sclerosis, polymyositis/dermatomyositis and systemic lupus erythematosus (SLE). Early in 1996 alone 6,722,573 women and 1,789,273 men suffered from varieties of diseases that had components of autoimmunity. Currently up to 150 autoimmune based diseases have been identified and approximately 40 more are awaiting confirmation. Similarly the incidence of several autoallergic diseases, type 1 insulin dependent diabetes mellitus (IDDM), rheumatoid arthritis, and Graves' disease, hyperthyroidism included are on the increase. Of the 1.2 million new cases of AD diagnosed every 5 years, at least one or more cases will include these autoimmune disease components. (Jacobson et al.1997)

The global incidence and prevalence for each AD is currently lacking and that calls for improvement on data collection and reporting. Nearly 10% of developed world's population suffer from AD and contribute significantly to chronic diseases and mortality. Women are three times more likely to be at risk than men in acquiring these diseases with non-Caucasians at higher risk. We are also seeing global prevalence of allergic respiratory diseases on the increase for the past 20-30 years. Over 15 million people in US suffer from asthma alone; approximately 50 million are diagnosed with some form of allergic diseases (Smith et al, 1997). Presently the direct annual health care cost for AD in US is in excess of $100 billion US dollars as compared to $57 billion for cancer. Hospitalization alone takes over half the cost of the direct expenditures. Almost 20% of the population classified as 'high-cost patients' consume more than 80% of the resources. Consequently the cost to public health from clinical management of these conditions is on the increase. All indications point to future better management of asthmatics through research and interventional efforts directed at communities, hospitalizations and high-cost patients in order to decrease health care resource use and provide cost savings. This calls for rigorous investigations into the role of environmental xenobiotics/substances and/or pollutants that are risk factors in the development of autoimmune diseases. In this chapter we intend to survey the public health concerns imposed by pollutants of the air, water and the food chain with concentration on typical examples of the effects of mercury on health to demonstrate the likelihood of dangers imposed through environmental and genetic disturbances in health.

2. Environmental chemicals and autoimmune diseases

Many scientists concur that several species within mammals to amphibians, birds, reptiles, and fish so far under monitoring systems are close to total extinction; well over 30,000 plant and animal species are estimated to be lost each year, a morbidity rate generally agreed to be much faster than at any time. Loss of species seems to be explained in most cases through the global weather changes as well as pollutional activities of man. But industrial activities seem to play major role in this problem; the latest data emanating from the industrial front estimate that at least 85,000 possible pollutants are currently being released into the environment through industrial activities alone http://www.epa.gov/glnpo/lmmb/substs.html (FDA/EPA).

2.1 Chemicals and substances of public health concern

These pollutants cover the heavy metals like thallium, aluminium, cadmium, lead, gold and mercury as well as pesticides, herbicides, preservatives, dyes, plastics, bisphenol A and rubber products. The Environmental Working Group indicated from studies in 2005 that a cocktail of 287 pollutants are measured in new born US fetal cord blood (http://www.ewg.org/reports/bodyburden2/execsumm.php). Perfluorooctanoic acid (*PFOA or* C8), and perfluorooctanoate, a synthetic but stable perfluorinated carboxylic acid and fluorosurfactant PFOA's were included in the findings as well as pesticides, dioxins, flame retardants. Recently another concern has been brought to the limelight by the internal Florida Department of Environmental Protection (DEP) Workgroup. It is stated that the current update of the American Chemical Society's Abstract Service reveals that as of August 2007 over 98% of the commercially available compounds are not under regulatory practices as they should be. This amounts to about 15 million out of over 32 million substances commonly referred to as Emerging Substances of Concern, or ESOC that have been registered for regulation (Chemical Abstract Service [CAS] website): http://www.cas.org/cgi-bin/cas/regreport.pl.
Much uncertainty surrounds the outcome from releases of these substances into the environment. No information about the pharmacokinetics or pharmacodynamics interactions among life forms on these substances are available. No available information on transport and toxicological effects are on record. Within two years between 2005 and 2007 over 5 million new chemicals have been reported to be registered and 5 million more chemicals became commercially available. Currently CAS informs that within each week more than 50 new substances or additions to existing substances to the database is the norm; http://www.cas.org/index.html. Apparently the ratio of unregulated to regulated chemicals keeps growing exponentially. The ESOC chemicals fall under various categories of organic groups encompassing from flame retardants (PBDEs), pharmaceuticals to endocrine-modulating chemicals (EMCs), nanoparticles to biological metabolites as well as newly discovered Industrial chemicals and toxins. They are constantly being discharged into

the environment where they find their way into our water bodies posing an unknown level of risk to life forms including humans, animals, and plants.

Regulatory Agencies are therefore challenged to find answers to solve what may be an unknown outcome of these ESOC substances being continually released into the biosphere. In the absence of detail knowledge on the environmental outcome and without effective regulation no useful assessment can be made on the environmental risk posed. Thus vast majority of ESOC substances have to be non-traditionally managed by other means such as prevention and effects-based environmental assessment methods. That effort is even more tasking and presents difficulties in monitoring the trends of the etiology of diseases now becoming prevalent in the environment under such practices. ESOC substances are now recognized to be of global concern; among these are included polybromina -teddiphenyl ethers (PBDEs), perfluorooctanoic acid (PFOA), siloxanes, perfluorooctanesulfonate (PFOS) and hexa- bromocyclododecanes (HBCDs). PBDEs and HBCDs come under flame-retardant chemicals that are moderately long-lived and volatile; readily released to the atmosphere because they do not strongly bind to substrates. Once in the atmosphere they are globally transported and readily bioaccumulate in biological tissues.

2.1.1 Nanoparticles

Human activities now have added sources of environmental contaminants. Human-originated nanomaterials are naturally man-made structures that differ in size range from 1 to 100 nanometers (nm). They are commonly used in drug delivery nanotherapeutic pharmaceuticals, cosmetics, personal care products, energy storage products, fabrics, lubricants and equipments like golf balls. The use of nanomaterials has been on the increase and now it is ubiquitous. Their minuscule sizes allow traversing not only biological membranes but also the blood/brain barrier (BBB) and display physical and chemical properties different from parental compounds. Examples are gold or silver metals known to be inducers of autoimmunity but also possess magnetic properties.

The intrinsic stereospecificity of these substances allow these molecules to play significant toxicological role in the environment (Donaldson et al 2004) and are therefore of public health concern. Carbon black displays enhanced severe effect than titanium dioxide (Renwick et al 2004), while the nanoparticle sizes of both chemicals are inducers of increased lung inflammation and destruction of the epithelial linings than their larger size. Adsorptions onto the surface of nanoparticles may play synergistic role in the reactivity; in vitro studies with fractions of diesel exhaust particles showed effects on cells (Xia et al 2004). Atmospheric nanoparticles may be complex enough to form interactions with organics and metals capable of higher levels of toxicity; metallic iron potentiates the effect of carbon black nanoparticles resulting in enhanced reactivity displayed as oxidative stress (Wilson et al 2002). Conversely other combinations with pullulan (polysaccharide polymer of maltotriose units, also known as α-1,4- ;α-1,6-glucan) and dextran tend to reduce toxicity of the respective nanoparticles (Gupta and Gupta 2005, Berry et al 2003).

Some nanoscale materials may be catalytic or behave as semiconductors, properties that can only increase the likelihood that nanomaterial could produce unanticipated toxicological effects. Nonbiodegradable ceramics, metals and metal oxides within nanomaterials are quite environmentally stable and persistent (EPA, 2007) and therefore undergo bioaccumulation in the food chain (Biswas and Wu, 2005). They are currently implicated in the induction of acute and chronic biological toxicity (Oberdörster, 2004a and 2004b; Lovern and Klaper, 2005; Lam et al., 2004; Shvedovaet al., 2005; Fortner et al., 2005) of unknown physiological mechanisms and hence consequences.

2.1.2 Particulate matter

Nanoparticles compare with particle pollution or particulate matter (PM), a group of complex mixture of extremely small air-borne particles and liquid droplets in air suspensions. There are a number of components covering acids (nitrates and sulfates, organic chemicals, metals, soil or dust and sulfates, organic chemicals, metals, soil or dust or mold spores). Particles less than 10 micrometers in diameter (PM_{10}) pose an even worse health concern because of their inhalation properties that allow for accumulation in the respiratory system; they are found in all types of combustion (motor vehicles, power plants, wood burning, etc.) and some industrial processes. Severe health risks are posed among fine particles less than 2.5 micrometers in diameter ($PM_{2.5}$). Fine particles easily lodge and penetrate deeply into the bronchial tree and into the deepest alveolar areas of the lung upon inhalation. Coarse particles measuring between 2.5 and 10 micrometers are derived from crushing or grinding operations, and dust from paved or unpaved roads.

Properties of PM link them to a variety of significant health problems starting from offensive asthma to early mortality of exposed patients who suffer from cardiac and bronchial diseases. Exposures to PM result in high rate of respiratory symptoms involving irritation of the airways, coughing, or difficulty breathing, decline in lung functions, aggravated asthma, and development of chronic bronchitis, irregular heartbeat and nonfatal heart attacks. Individuals with a variety of health issues particularly those with prior heart or lung diseases tend to suffer premature deaths on exposure to PM. Children and older adults are the most likely to be affected by particle pollution exposure but healthy individuals are found to experience temporary symptoms from exposure to elevated levels www.epa.gov/asthma; and plays esthetic role by significantly effecting visibility impairment in the nation's cities and national parks. To protect public health and welfare, EPA has continually issued National Ambient Air Quality Standards (NAAQS) since 1971 for six criteria pollutants among which are particulate matter and Sulfur Dioxide (SO_2), Ozone (O_3), Nitrogen Dioxide (NO_2), Lead (Pb), and Carbon Monoxide (CO). The NAAQS from EPA has undergone revisions in 1987 and 1997 and again in September 2006 and it is helpful to familiarize oneself; there is an urgent need for studies to unravel the pharmacokinetics and pharmacodynamics of these particles to help disclose the role played in disease pathogenesis especially concerning the autoimmune state- asthma being one of the priorities.

3. Autoimmune diseases: etiologies and mechanisms

All indications show that tissue burdens of PBDE in life forms including humans are doubling in every two to five years. Human breast milk has been found to contain as much as 419 ng/g lipid weight of PBDE (Schecter et al., 2003). The question then arises whether these molecules contribute to what we measure in the increases in the incidence of ADs. These substances are known to interfere with the reproductive and developmental stages of mammals as well as in birds and invertebrates (McKernan *et al.*, 2006, Wollenberger 2005); they are carcinogenic, endocrine-modulating, and have neurotoxicological effects (Birnbaum, 2005). Autoimmune diseases present a major affront to the health of Americans as well as of global concern. Vast arrays of diseases come under auto-allergic/-immunity; these cover maladies that may present as localized to be organ specific or systemically distributed to the extremities to involve all organ systems typically noted in systemic lupus erythematosus (SLE). In health the Immune System guards us against invasion of foreign substances including harmful bacteria, viruses, and parasites quite well without any perturbation. At times, however this machinery loses control and begins to attack even the self itself. Hypersensitivity responses resulting from direct attack of body components by antibodies or immune cells instead of attacking foreign substances alone generally come under autoimmunity or autoallergic responses. Autoimmune state becomes apparent with rise of demonstrable presence of autoantibodies or complexes of these with body substances or the presence of cells, T lymphocytes that attack self-constituents. Minor and harmless autoimmune states exist in normal persons in general; it is part component of the defense system as envisaged by Jerne's hypothesis (<http://www.enotes.com/microbiology encyclopedia/). In the disease state, however, autoimmunity becomes defined when the benign state results rather in pathology; it sets in motion homeostatic deterioration. The process is dependent on both genetic influences and environmental triggers.

For the past decades it has been conclusively demonstrated that alleles of the major histocompatibility complex (*MHC*) contribute to the susceptibility to autoimmunity but relatively recently there is an unparalleled discovery of novel genes in molecular pathways implicated in autoimmunity. Some of the variants identified clearly participate in the modulation of T-lymphocyte (T-cell) activation and do contribute to many different forms of human autoimmunity. Other genes tend to have restricted roles, with susceptibility apparently confined to one autoimmune condition or to a specific ethnic group. To gain insight into the initiation mechanisms of autoimmune diseases requires identification of the genetic determinants underlying disease pathogenesis and this implicates new biochemical pathways. The Autoimmune state may be either the direct originator of disease itself or arise as a secondary disease from perturbations from other chronic diseases. Direct autoimmune states are phenotypically demonstrated in patients that have antibodies in the active disease phase: examples are represented by idiopathic thrombocytopenia (ITP), Grave's disease and myasthenia gravis, pemphigus vulgaris and bullous pemphigoid, diseases that can be transferred among species through antibody transfers.

Disease transfer through T lymphocytes exchanges have not conclusively been demonstrated to lead to pathology but with the aid of cytokines may rather alleviate or exacerbate disease state. Indirect cause of autoimmunity has been defined by Rose and Bona, 1993 as when disease can be induced in an animal model. SLE is well represented by several genetically determined mouse models which, while not exactly clinical replica of the human disease do very closely replicate pathological and serological characteristics clinically seen to occur. Hashimoto's thyroiditis and multiple sclerosis can be reproduced by immunizing animals with an antigen analogous to the putative autoantigen of the human disease. Absence of direct and indirect evidence with markers describing the state of autoimmunity become circumstantial: positive family histories for disease, presence of certain MHC class II alleles are examples.

Currently it takes a great effort to assess accurately the initiation levels of these diseases in humans; the very initiating factors are difficult to focus on and in which stage/s or area of the metabolic processes gets initially disturbed becomes challenging to screen and allow for therapeutic management. Majority of ADs such as multiple sclerosis (MS), insulin-dependent diabetes mellitus (IDDM), rheumatoid arthritis (RA), systemic lupus erythematosus (SLE), and thyroiditis one finds representative spectrum of autoimmune diseases that appear to have etiological background in dysregulated immune system. Enough supporting evidence exist to confirm the autoimmune nature of many of these disorders but still it is gravely challenging to decipher their precise etiology and/or the initiating factors. Of late a small fraction of the T cells, the regulatory T cells are among the focal area of studies and have become recognized as particularly crucial for control of autoreactive immune responses. Normally the processing of a self antigen by the antigen presenting cells (APC) allow binding of processed antigenic fragments to the MHC molecules within the APC followed by display of these MHC-peptide complexes on APC's membrane surface for presentation to the appropriate T cells; this eventually terminates in activation of antigen-specific T cells. These T cells are then capable of attacking the self tissues expressing that particular self antigen. The process is believed to be the critical steps in the initiation of anti-self T cell responses.

Genome wide studies indicate that costimulatory signals examplified by CTLA4 or PD1 and the modulators of T-cell receptor signaling (LYP, encoded by *PTPN22*), somehow must be confirmatory key checkpoint for human autoimmunity as happens in the T-cell during the period of T-cell receptor training to eliminate self-antigen carrying T cells in the thymus. This notion of the crypticity of self antigenic determinants (Sercarz et al., 1993; Moudgil and Sercarz, 2005) takes strength from the premise that rely on potentially immunogenic regions (determinants/epitopes) within a self antigen that are processed and presented by the MHC molecule to T cells at different levels of immunogenecity. This means that certain 'dominant self' epitopes are well processed and presented, whereas others, the (cryptic or recessive self) (Sercarz et al., 1993) ones are poorly or never processed and presented. Thus this type of staging of determinants (dominance/crypticity) in turn plays a critical role in thymus gradation of the T cell repertoire: the T cells specific for dominant self epitopes are tolerized with ease while those purportly aimed at cryptic self epitopes evade tolerance induction and become part of the mature T cell repertoire (Gammon and Sercarz, 1989; Cibotti et al., 1992; Sinha et al., 2004).

T cells that evade tolerance induction are capable of being activated in the periphery under certain stressful inflammatory circumstances such as occur during infection; this has the consequence of enhanced processing and presentation of once latent (cryptic) determinants (Lehmann et al., 1992; Lanzavecchia, 1995). These activated T cells at times are capable of escaping appropriate constraint from regulatory T cells and permitted to execute their effector function of initiating autoimmune damage. The unveiling of previously cryptic determinants leading to activation of self-reactive T cells that escaped tolerance induction during thymic selection, owing to the crypticity of self determinants is considered a primary cornerstone of a theory of autoimmunity (Moudgil and Sercarz, 2005). The idea of determinant hierarchy provides a vital link between the thymic selection of potentially autoreactive T cells and the subsequent activation of these T cells in the periphery under conditions that facilitate the revelation of previously cryptic determinants. Peripheral ongoing immune tolerance of the mature immune system also attracts attention as another source of autoimmune initiation. This idea is supported by variations seen in the expressions of "self-antigen" in the thymus (e.g., insulin in T1D); in this instance T-cells are selected for survival according to the affinity of their cell surface receptors for self-antigen. This may represent a major key step in the genesis of autoimmune disease.

Other means of autoimmune genesis stem from APCs. These cells play crucial role in antigen processing and presentation to the T-helper (Th) cells. Dendritic cells for example are key cells in the initiation and perpetuation of immune responses. Highly polymorphic genes within the *MHC*, with links to autoimmune inductions, encode proteins to which antigens bind and presented directly to T-cells by APCs. Another source of autoimmune initiation focus on the cell surface marker CD4-positive Th cells; they are the conductors of the adaptive immune response and many genes with an established role in autoimmune disease have their expression in this cell type.

Autoimmune diseases present specific issues that need attention. Drugs used to manage known chronic and acute diseases are implicated in triggering and are therefore thought to be indirect causes of various autoimmune diseases following administration. Many of the prescription drugs commonly used for highly prevalent diseases come under this category: these inexhaustively include drugs like Alferon N, Allopurinol, Atenolol, Atorvastatin, captopril, Penicillin, Carbamazepine, chlorpromazine, Chlorthalidone, cimetidine, Ethosuximide, gold salts, griseofulvin, Hydralazine, Interleukins, Infergen, Interferons, Interferon Alfa, Hydrochlorothiazide, Intron A, Isoniazid, Levodopa, Lithium, Lovastatin, Mesantoin, Methimazole, Methyldopa, Methylsergide, Metoprolol, Minocycline, Minoxidil, Ophthalmic timolol, Nitrofurantoin, Oral contraceptives, Quinidine, Phenytoin, PegIntron, P-aminobenzoic, Penicillamine, Perphenazine, Trimethadione, Pravostatin, Phenylbutazone, Procainamide, Valproic acid, Propylthiouracil, Simvastatin, sulfasalazine, sulfonamides, streptomycin, Sulfonamide antimicrobials, Tetracyclines, Tiotropium Bromide inhaler and Tumor Necrosis factor.

The concern here can well be summarized with the incidence and/or prevalence of asthma, one of the most common chronic diseases of childhood estimated to affect 6 million children. More than 22 million Americans are diagnosed with asthma, and approximately 50 million of individuals are diagnosed with some form of allergic diseases. Presently in US the annual direct health care cost for AD in general is in excess of $100 billion US dollars as compared to $57 billion for cancer. Hospitalization alone takes over half the cost of the direct expenditures. "High- cost patients" that form about 20% of the population spend more than 80% of the resources. As a result, the cost to public health from clinical management of these conditions is on the increase.

4. Global problems associated with asthma and COPD

Epidemiological data following the natural history of asthma reveal that in 1999 mortality rates from the disease declined in comparison to previous years. This was followed by a surge in recent decades in asthma prevalence also in the United States and other Western countries; data suggest this trend may also be reaching a plateau. The general trend of global asthma incidence is rising worldwide but looking at US data we see increased morbidity and mortality from asthma from 1980s -1990s with plateau in the 1990s. This finding is the reverse of what was seen in the 1978-1980 where an increase in mortality due to asthma was measured: from 1990-1999 mortality declined. Commencing from 1995 the rate of outpatient visits for asthma increased; whereas the rates of hospital admissions declined *from 19.5 per 10,000* of the population in 1995 to *15.7 in 1998* attributed to enhanced rates of dispensed steroid prescriptions for inhaled medications. This finding has been interpreted as due to the improved treatment of asthma responsible for these favorable developments.

The implication, if it holds supports explanations of certain changes in environmental chemicals releases. Recent increases in asthmatic conditions in the population may be linked to many causes the cardinal one being the amount and types of substances that are being released increasingly into the biosphere. Releases of substances most of which have an unknown effect and still others closely linked to inductions of asthmatic features in the ever increasing population with genetic predispositions present ominous threat to the very survival of several species including man himself.

Exposures to environmental factors early on in childhood play significant role in the risk in developing asthma. Clinicians have known for quite a while that asthma is not a single disease. Risk to asthma stems from early environmental factors as well as the presence of susceptibility genes; subsequent disease induction and progression from inflammation as well as response to therapeutic agents plays big roles in disease etiology. It is a typical consequence of environmentally induced autoallergic disease known to be heterogeneous (Asosingh et al 2007, Dompeling et al, 2000, Dweik et al, 2001, Kharitonov and Barnes, 2001, Weiss, 2002, Pascual and Peters 2005, Salvato, 2001, Wu et al, 2000) existing in many forms. The immunologic profile of the asthmatic airways presents as proliferation and activation of helper T lymphocytes (CD4+) of the subtype T_H2 responsible for the allergic inflammation in atopic asthmatics. Upon stimulation these cells release a number of cytokines covering IL-4, agent for IgE synthesis, IL-5, essential for eosinophils' maturation, and IL-3 and granulocyte-macrophage colony-stimulating factor, GMCSF (Bolland and Ravetch 2000, Candore et al, 2002, Lang et al, 2010, Pollard et al 1997).

In allergic as well as nonallergic individuals we observe populations of eosinophils in the airways with increased levels in asthmatics with allergies http://www. clevelandclinicmeded .com/ medical pubs/disease management/allergy/ bronchial-asthma/that have higher rates of asthmatic attacks. These cells serve as the source of mediators that exert damaging effects on the airways. Ultimately, mediators lead to degranulation of effector/proinflammatory cells in the airways that release other mediators and oxidants, a common final pathway that culminates in chronic injury and inflammation commonly seen in asthma. Chronicity of the asthmatic condition has been confirmed by several parameters. Low pH and high output of reactive oxygen and nitrogen species (ROS) during asthmatic exacerbations are specific biomarkers in expired air reflecting altered airway redox problems (Clynes et al, 1988, Comhair et al, 2000, De Raeve et al, 1997, Dweik et al 2001). Superoxide, hydrogen peroxide, and hydroxyl radicals are among ROS agents that are responsible for the inflammatory changes in the asthmatic airway (Candore et al 2002, Bolland and Ravetch 2000, Pollard et al, 1997). These ROS originate from the lungs of asthmatic patients induced by activated inflammatory cells (ie, eosinophils, alveolar macrophages, and neutrophils) (Holgate et al, 2000).

Pathogenicity in asthma in particular is portrayed by overall interactions between neural mechanisms, inflammatory cell mediators such as leukotrienes and prostaglandins, and intrinsic abnormalities of the arachidonic acid pathway and smooth muscle; all these cells play significant roles in the initial as well as disease progression. Inflammation is the most likely etiological basis of airway hyperreactivity and variable airflow obstruction.

Asthma usually persists into later childhood and adulthood from early childhood in the presence of the appropriate genetic background. Tolerance to allergens is a normal security that prevents such responses, but the specific immunological events that mediate tolerance in this setting are still under scrutiny. Despite the explosion of information about asthma, the nature of the basic pathogenesis has not been established. However, asthma clearly does not result from a single genetic abnormality, but is rather a complex multigenic disease with a strong environmental contribution. For example, asthmatic children and adults sensitive to inhalant allergens such as dust mites, mold spores, cat dander, etc portray such reactions right from childhood compared with adult-onset asthmatics. Local epithelial environment within the connective tissue is believed to be actively involved in regulation of events and the relation between the airway epithelium and the subepithelial mesenchyme is proposed to be a key determinant in the concept of *airway remodeling* (Davies et al, 2003; Weiss, 2002; Li and Wilson 1997, Pascual and Peters, 2005, Salvato 2001). Difficulties and/or problems underlying diagnosis and classification of these diseases are simply due to the fact that most of the ADs become apparent only at variable phases of several chronic stages of organic ailments. Some ADs present as auto allergies covering several fields of diseases: the incidence of several of these diseases is also on the increase and covers type 1 insulin dependent diabetes mellitus (IDDM), rheumatoid arthritis, and Graves' disease, hyperthyroidism included. There is scarcity of information on the global incidence and prevalence for each AD. Some autoimmune/allergic diseases (AD) can be seen in cases of chronic obstructive pulmonary diseases (COPD). As such the incidence of these disorders has not been well defined. However, sharp global increases in the prevalence have been observed in the United States.

Etiological initiators of and pathogenesis of most ADs are obscure; they are presumed to be numerous with cigarette smoking a typical COPD-associated. Cigarette smoking is clearly the major risk factor for COPD but exposures to other noxious substances including dusts and chemicals found under occupational settings are known to contribute to the development of the disease (Pauwels et al, 2001).The attributable fraction contributing to COPD cases caused by occupational exposures is estimated to be in the range of less than 15% to as high as 31% among those who never smoked (Hnizdo et al, 2004). We find that minority groups have been historically overexposed to hazardous industrial substances and are candidates with increased risk for work-related airflow obstruction putting them highly in the AD group as well; making it necessary to improve on data collection and reporting. Estimation shows, however that nearly 10% of developed world's population suffer from AD and contribute significantly to chronic diseases and mortality. Women are three times more likely at risk than men in acquiring these diseases with non-Caucasians in the higher risk groups. The global prevalence of allergic respiratory diseases including COPD has been also on the increase for the past 20-30 years.

5. Mercury as environmental inducer of autoimmunity

Psychoneuroimmunological studies demonstrate in various ways that homeostatic regulation of the internal milieu links the soma with the neural pathways; stressors effects relate the two in bidirectional pathways. Current Naturopathic Medical view of diseases also links the involvement of the genes to autoimmune proneness. In this wise the authors concentrate on the metal mercury as a representative highly reactive toxic agent within the body as a means of gaining an insight into the problem of etiologies of autoimmune diseases. Mercury has a high affinity binding to *sulfhydryl* as well as to *hydroxyl, carboxyl,* and *phosphoryl* functional groups very commonly displayed on macromolecules, proteins and the genetic materials. It is widely distributed as an environmental and industrial pollutant. No known beneficial metabolomic effect is assigned to mercury in the physiology of humans, yet a 70 kg man is loaded with an equivalent of 13mg mercury (Pier, 1975) distributed in the skin, nails, hair, and kidneys. The net outcome of exposure to mercury is dose-dependent and at low concentrations mercury is the agent for the induction of several diseases that affect most systems of the body.

The central nervous system (CNS), the brain and the kidneys suffer most where Mercury Induced Autoimmunity (MeIA) can be particularly threatening in onset and severe among especially non-Caucasians that manifest *defined* major histocompatibility complex (MHC) haplotypes. Several data confirm that mercury is also associated with polyclonal cell stimulation. Mercury Induced Autoimmunity (MeIA) engages helper T lymphocytes in the induction of disease process in responder animals (Jiang YG, Möller G 1995, Horwitz and Stohl, 1993; Puck JM, Sneller MC. 1997) and in humans (Liossis et al 1996). It is suggested there is a genetic basis for airway hyperresponsiveness with linkage to chromosomes 5q, 11q (Li and

Wilson1997) and 12q24 in Hispanic subgroups (Salvato 2001). While MeIA is well characterized into different arrays of disease susceptibility in animal studies (De Raeve et al 1997) and in humans (Holgate et al, 2000, Li and Wilson 1997,) the role of mercury in the pathogenesis of autoallergic/immune syndromes like asthma and SLE is not well characterized.

Our Microarray data resulting from low doses (1-3 μg/mL) exposures of human cell lines to mercury indicate differential expressions of several genes located on many human chromosomes. Most genes affected were expressed more than twice the control level; several genes were also down-regulated with mercury treatment. We found close to a total of two hundred highly up-regulated genes with greater than a two-fold change difference ($p \leq 0.002$) in the lowest mercury concentration (1μg/mL); 12 genes were moderately over-expressed with an increase of more than one fold ($p \leq 0.005$); and a total of more than two thousand genes were down-regulated albeit most repressions were not statistically significant ($p>0.05$) according to the Wilcoxon's Signed Rank test. Only forty of these genes were down regulated to statistically significant levels at $p \leq 0.05$ according to the Welch's ANOVA/- Welch's test. Clear distinctions were seen in the gene expression profiles of the experimental versus controls. Affected genes distributed among almost all of human chromosomes with higher than normal effects on genes associated with chromosomes 1-10, 12, 14-18, 20 (sex-determining region Y), 21 (splicing factor and ATP-binding), X (including BCL-co-repressor). Genes affected include potassium voltage-gated channel–subfamily H member 2 (KCNH2), stress responses, G-protein signal transduction, putative MAPK activating protein (PM20, PM21), *ras* homolog gene family, cytokine receptor activity and polymerase (DNA directed), regulatory subunit (50kDa), leptin receptor involved in hematopoietin/interferon-class (D200-domain), and thymidine kinase 2, mitochondrial TK2 (HGNC) and related genes. Closely associated genes on a chromosome tend to be influenced for expression perhaps due to the availability of close and adjacent *phosphorylation* receptors found by bioinformatics tools.

Identified genes of interest that were over- or under-expressed operate in several pathways including principally the immune and cell cycle (cyclin-dependent kinases) pathways, apoptosis, and cytokine expressions (Figs 1-3) as well as the TGF-beta and the GABA, NMDA receptor subtypes. We have since confirmed that mercury has significant effect on GABA receptors in microarray experimentations in murine cell lines (unpublished data). Our lab results reinforce the capability of mercury exerting significant influence in most metabolic processes probably generating ROS (Kavuru et al 1998; Lang 2000, 2006, Montuschi and Barnes 2002, Wu et al 2000) that participate in the degree of disease outcome of the autoallergic/asthmatic syndromes. The auto allergic phase is the body's adverse response to the onslaught resulting in signs and symptoms invariably difficult to definitively differentially diagnose early on in disease. Estimates from the National Institute of Health (NIH) data indicate that in US alone the prevalence of AD to be about 23.5 billion (Jacobson et al, 1997); in 1996 approximately 1 in 31(3.13%) or 8.5 million people were afflicted with one form or other of AD. Since then at least 237,203 cases of AD are diagnosed annually; of this 42,137 are new cases of primary glomerulonephritis, multiple sclerosis, polymyositis/ dermatomyositis and systemic lupus erythematosus (SLE). Of the total 6,722,573 are women and 1,789,273 men suffering from varieties of diseases that had autoimmune components (Jacobson et al, 1997, Smith et al, 1997). Currently almost 100 types of AD have been identified and approximately 40 more autoimmune-based diseases are awaiting clarification and confirmation.

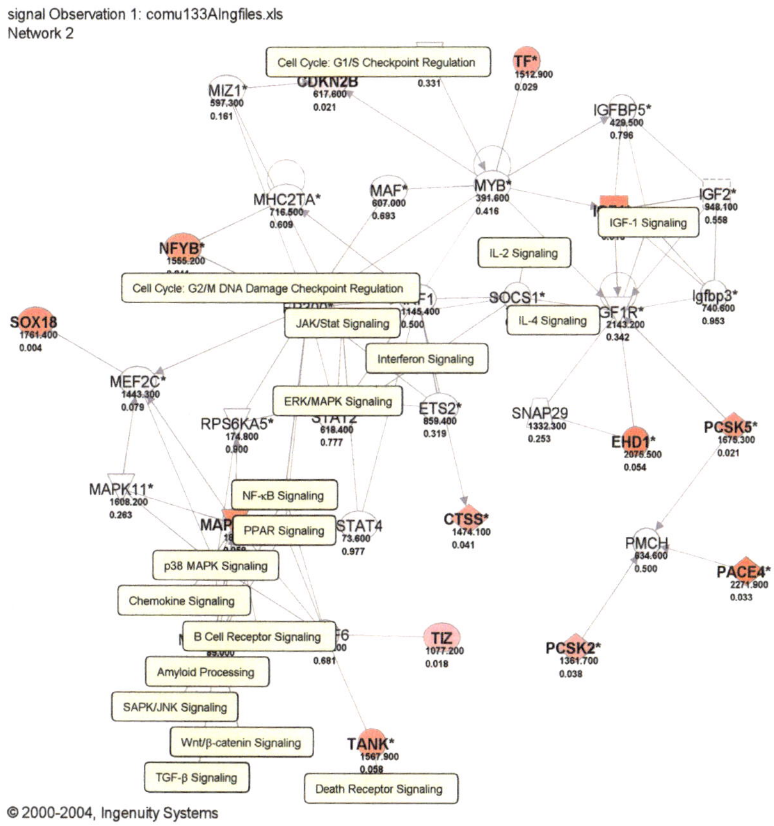

Fig. 1. Results: HepG2 Genes affected by Mercury exposure

5.1 Mercury toxicity: evidence for autoimmunity and neural problems

Mercury (Hg) has long been recognized as a neurotoxicant; however, many experiments with murine models have conclusively implicated this heavy metal as inducer of autoallergies as well as immunotoxicant. In particular Hg has consistently been shown to induce autoimmune disease in susceptible animals with phenotypic consequence of autoantibodies overproduction and pathophysiological signs of lupus-like diseases. This finding has been endorsed by epidemiological studies demonstrating links between occupational Hg exposure and lupus. Mercury rather may interact with triggering events, such as genetic predisposition, exposure to antigens, or infection, to exacerbate disease. Non mercury-susceptible mice that are exposed to mercury do succumb to mercury-induced autoimmune disease (MeIA) with very low doses and short term exposures of inorganic Hg (20-200 μg/kg) exacerbates disease and accelerates mortality in the graft versus host disease model of chronic lupus in C57Bl/6 x DBA/2 mice.

Furthermore, low dose Hg exposure increases the severity and prevalence of experimental autoimmune myocarditis (induced by immunization with cardiac myosin peptide in adjuvant) in A/J mice. Immunosuppression as well as immuno-stimulatory signals results from exposure to the metal in many species humans and rodents included (Pollard et al., 1999). MeIA is prominent among some genetically predisposed individuals that carry syntenic genes as haplotypes in linkage disequilibrium. Some of these individuals are

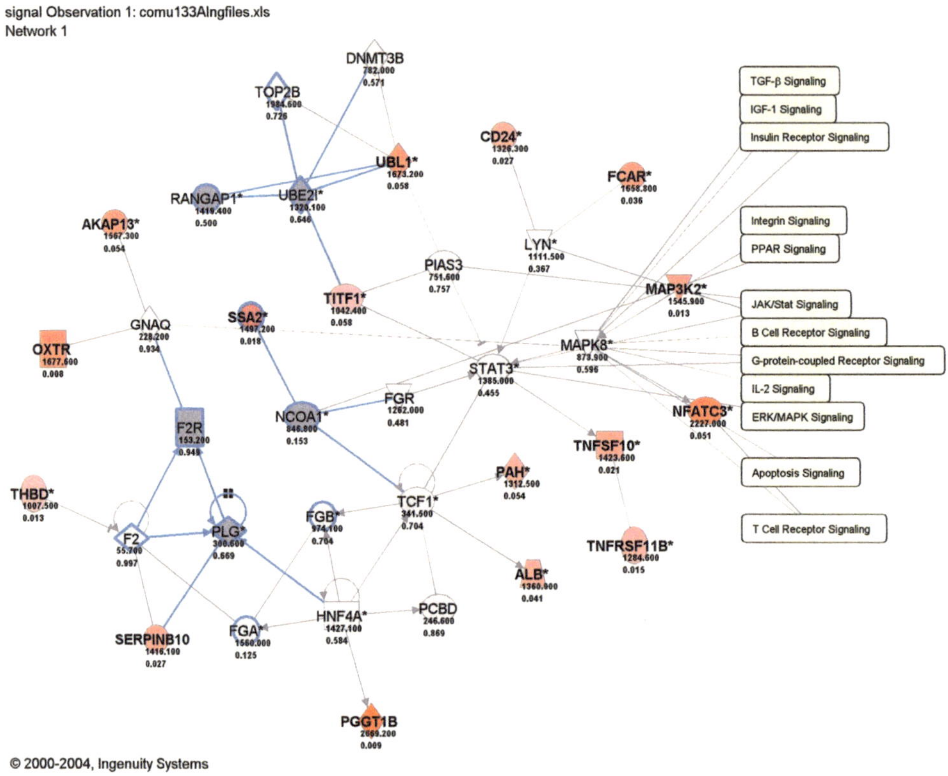

Fig. 2. Results: HepG2 Genes affected by Mercury exposure

genetically prone to develop spontaneous autoimmune diseases. The etiology and pathogenicity of these, mostly systenic, autoimmune states have been difficult to trace. Immunological findings support the notion that the origins of majority of these idiopathic autoimmune diseases can be traced to environmental contaminants of the biosphere with xenobiotic compounds like silver, gold and mercury strongly implicated. *Exposure* to low levels of mercury (<40µg/kg body weight) in susceptible persons may be unsafe; predisposed individuals develop all types of AD typically systemic lupus erythematosus (SLE). Evidence is derived not only from experiments of nature as happened in Miamata in Japan but also from many strains of inbred mice described below. These strains of animals do develop lupus-like disease that imitate closely a simplified version of human systemic lupus erythematous (SLE), with the production of autoantibodies and the subsequent development of immune-complex mediated glomerulonephritis (Theofilopoulos et al., 1985).

The general consensus is that the dose of mercury, duration of exposure as well as the genetic background of the exposed animal (Hanley et al., 2002; Hultman et al., 1992, 1993; Jiang and Möller, 1995; Kono et al., 1998; Pollard et al., 2002) contributes to disease outcome. The H-2 haplotype plays important role in the specificity of resulting autoantibody as well as susceptibility to immune complex generation; but there is a role for involvement of non-MHC genes in MeIA susceptibility also. Acute renal tubular lesions and immunosuppression follow exposure to large doses, whereas chronic administration of smaller doses of mercury leads to the development of SLE (Bariety et al., 1971; Kasturi et al., 1995; Roman-Franco et al., 1978). Mercury-induced autoimmunity shares the same pathogenicity and clinical

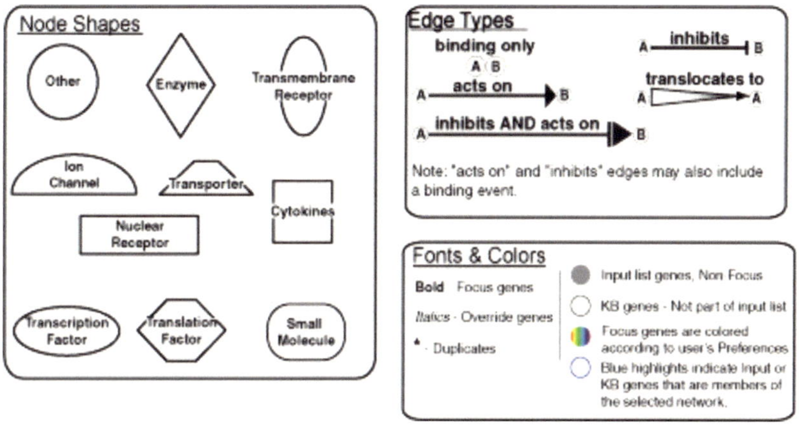

Fig. 3. Key for Both Figs 1 and 2

manifestations seen in patients suffering from clinically diagnosed systemic lupus erythematosus (SLE) (Dubey et al., 1991; Hirsch et al., 1982; Mathieson et al., 1992); the symptomatology is also the same (Biancone et al., 1996; Jiang and Möller, 1995; Kono et al., 1998) with very minor differences.

In humans most of the genes participating in immunity are located on the major histocompatibility complex (MHC) on chromosome 6 with its equivalent on the H-2 region on chromosome 17 in mice. The complexity of the interactions leading to disease state are reflected in the arrays of disease manifestations. Various susceptibility modes are demonstrated by different combinations of gene haplotypes in different strains of animals. BALB/c mice of *H-2*^{d} haplotype are highly susceptible to MeIA phenotypically demonstrated as lymphoproliferation without accompanying immune-complex glomerulonephritis (ICGN) (Jiang and Möller, 1995). Mice with *B10.D2* haplotype specificity are capable of lymphoproliferation but with less severe ICGN than BALB/c mice on exposure to mercury. The *H-2*^{d} haplotype *DBA/2* strain of mice is however, resistant to both lymphoproliferation and ICGN (Hultman et al., 1992; Jiang and Möller, 1995; Kono et al., 1998; Takeuchi et al., 1995). *RT-1*^{n} rats are susceptible, whereas *RT-1*^{1} haplotypes are resistant (Eneström and Hultman, 1995; Sapin et al., 1984). An *H-2*^{s} haplotype carrying A.SW mice and others show high susceptibility to Hg-induced autoantibodies, whereas *C57BL/6* strains (*H-2*^{b}) are less susceptible. DBA/2 mice strains bearing *H-2*^{d} haplotypes are not responsive while *H-2*^{k}-bearing mice show intermediate susceptibility (Dubey et al., 1991; Hultman et al., 1993; Jiang and Möller, 1995; Kono et al., 1998).

Most SLE susceptibility loci have been mapped in New Zealand hybrid models; at least 12 of them are located outside the H-1, the murine major histocompatibility complex, H-2. Three regions commonly noted by linkage studies in New Zealand models are found on murine chromosomes 1, 4, and 7 (Drake 1995, Kono et al., 1994, Morel et al., 1994); these have equivalent syntenies in human loci (Duits et al., 1995; Moser et al., 1998; Salmon et al., 1996) that seem to be *ethnically* distinct (Duits et al., 1995: Salmon et al., 1996). Another region along both *H-2 class II* and *TNF-_* gene polymorphisms have been described to act as H-2-linked predisposing genetic elements for the development of SLE; a very strong evidence suggests the contribution of *TNF-* polymorphism that may be the modulator of the initial steps of disease development (The *Wbw2* locus (telomeric to H-2)) which was not linked with autoantibody production might play a role in determining lupus susceptibility; this reaffirms the clustering of functionally related H-2 and non-H-2 genes in the H-2 region on chromosome 17 to be active players in the induction of SLE, a typical example of AD usually quoted. Genetic variants do exist in autoimmune susceptibility that may be a basis for health disparity among races and forewarns that in dealing with xenobiotics like mercury, susceptibility among different racial groups may exhibit differences enough to be taken into account in therapeutic managements.

It has been determined that mercury is immunologically processed uniquely in disease pathogenesis. The process involves the antinuclear autoantibody, (AnoA Abs) response directed against fibrillarin. The AnoA Abs response directed against fibrillarin is one of the most representative manifestations of MeIA that is linked to *H-2ˢ* (Hanley et al., 2002; Hultman et al., 1992; Hultman et al., 1993; Pollard et al., 2002) and, more specifically, to the class *II I-Aˢ* molecule, by analysis of H-2 congenic mice (Pollard et al., 2002) and is described below. The discovery of potential SLE inducibility on mercury exposure in humans offers the opportunity for comparison with data from murine models of SLE. This means that identification of potential SLE susceptibility loci in humans offers the chance to compare data from murine models of SLE induced by xenobiotics such as mercury.

Mercury-induced cell death (MeICD) is processed through proteolytic breakdown of fibrillarin, a 34kDa MWt macrophage degradable protein component of small nucleolarribonucleoprotein particles (snRNPs); the generation of a unique (19kDa) proteolytic fragment required no pre-interaction between mercury and fibrillarin (Pollard et al, 1997, 2002).

MeICD was associated with a novel protease transiently synthesized and that stimulate *self-reactivity* quite differently from that elicited by full-length protein. Above all *xenobiotic-induced autoimmunity characterized by autoantibody responses against native self-Ag did not require pre-interaction between xenobiotic and Ag*. The genetically restricted anti-fibrillarin autoantibody response of MeIA was not found directed against a fibrillarin-Hg complex as expected of MHC-dependent antigen processing although a metal-protein interaction occurred (Pollard et al., 1997, 2002). This finding endorses a longstanding belief that SLE-prone patients could generate self-autoantibodies spontaneously even without any physical presence of observable inducers of auto-antigens. Cell demise through MeICD was found to be mediated through both nonapoptotic and apoptotic protease activities but the processing pathway of fibrillarin was different enough to suggest the action of different *proteases* (Casiano et al., 1996; Pollard et al., 1997, 2002). It was surmised that the cleavage patterns for a number of auto-antigens must differ between non-apoptosis ($HgCl_2$, heat, ethanol) and apoptosis (anti-Fas) induced cell death (Casiola-Rosen et al., 1995; Pollard et al., 1997). Apparently an MHC-restricted autoantibody response and interaction with $HgCl_2$ are characteristics that differentiate fibrillarin as an autoantigen in $HgCl_2$-induced autoimmunity. The observation that specific cleavage fragments of fibrillarin result from $HgCl_2$ induced death and not other forms of cell death means that *novel* cleavage fragments probably act as *autoimmunogens*. Besides other effects of mercury on the immune system including specific cytokine requirements (Gillespie et al., 1995; Ochel et al., 1991; Van Vliet et al., 1993), inhibition of Fas-mediated cell death are possible means of terminating self-tolerance leading to the equivalent of the SLE state (Whitekus et al., 1999).

As detected in Asthmatic states MeIA is one of the autoimmune models in which T_H1/T_H2 imbalance play critical roles (Biancone et al., 1996; Dubey et al., 1991; Hirsch et al., 1982; Jiang and Möller, 1995; Mirtcheva et al., 1989; Sapin et al., 1984). Although the mechanism by which mercury modifies the immune system is obscure, cationic mercury has a high affinity for *sulfhydryl* groups as the principal site for binding and also has a substantial affinity for *amines, phosphoryl, carboxyl, and hydroxyl groups* (ATSDR, 1999). Mercury is capable of linking with macromolecules including the genetic materials and proteins to form complexes that can activate the immune system. Some of the modified proteins may have epitopes closely resembling self-immunogens (*cryptic antigens*) easily leading to autoimmune disorders in predisposed individuals (Pollard et al., 1997, 2002; Takeuchi et al., 1995). The activation of $CD4^+$ and $CD8^+$ T cells requires a prior induction of antigen presenting cells (APC) (Jiang and Möller, 1995). Mercury binds to molecules on accessory APC cells and transforms molecules on these cells to superantigens capable of activating T cells with a particular set of Vβ Ag-binding receptors (Jiang and Möller, 1995). The mechanism of MeIA can therefore be differentiated from mechanisms induced by polyclonal cell-activators (PCA) such as pokeweed mitogen, PWM. These PCA do not require helper T cells assistance in antibody/cellular inductions.

The presence or absence of IFN-γ on the responder or the non-responder T_H1/T_H2 cell types respectively is thought to be prerequisite in the response to or failure of response respectively (Kono et al., 1998). The balance between the T_H1/T_H2-type responses does not contribute directly to autoimmune susceptibility. Rather IFN-γ has been found to be necessary for the activation of the immune system to respond to poor epitopes, including both self and non-self Ags leading to humoral and cellular auto responses. Dose differentials of IFN-γ appear to directly contribute to disease proneness. High dose immunization with Ag and a strong adjuvant tend to override the IFN-γ requirement (Ferber et al., 1996; Jones et al., 1997). Similarly, a strong genetic predisposition may decrease the threshold for susceptibility enough to overcome the IFN-γ requirement (Abbas et al., 1996). Susceptibility to autoimmune diseases therefore is generally considered a multi-process with many stages or focal barriers evidenced by clinical observations in SLE patients (Andre et al., 1996; Hultgren et al., 1996; Manoury-Schwartz et al., 1997; Vermeire et al., 1997). Lupus is therefore not inherited as a simple Mendelian trait but inherited as a multifactorial and complex trait.

Latest information confirms that the steps to disease state are characterized by unknown, but a large number of susceptibility alleles that give rise to quantitative phenotypic effects. Dose effect allows each of the susceptibility alleles to have partial contribution to probability of increased disease severity. Still nongenetic factors do contribute to disease susceptibility. Recent linkage analyses have revealed over 100 large genomic regions, each represented as a quantitative trait locus (QTL)http://www.discoverymedicine.com/tag/quantitative-trait-locus/ that are associated with increased susceptibility to lupus in mice (Kono et al., 2006) and at least 8 validated QTLs in families of lupus patients (Tsao, 2003) that partially overlap with the mouse QTLs. Some of the genes contribute to the murine lupus QTLs and participate in human SLE. Analysis of these genes is providing insight into pathogenesis of human SLE. Use has been made of linkage analyses on some model murine species that spontaneously get the lupus; these have involved analyses using 129, MRL-*Fas^lpr^*, BXSB.*Yaa*, and the F_1 hybrid between NZB and NZW (BWF1) and their recombinant inbred derivatives, NZM2410 and NZM2328.

Statistically significant associations between over 100 genomic regions and a lupus-related phenotype covering most commonly lupus nephritis or anti-nuclear autoantibody (ANA) synthesis have been analyzed. Through substitution techniques whereby for example a QTL located in a lupus susceptible strain was replaced with the corresponding genomic interval from a resistant strain only 35 of the 100 genomic regions have been so far confirmed (Morel, 2010). Substitution of the *Adnz1* region (in NZM.C57Lc4 congenic strain) in lupus-prone NZM2328 mice with the appropriate genomic interval from a non-autoimmune genome led to the predicted and expected milder form of glomerulonephritis (Waters et al., 2004). Conversely when the susceptible QTL was bred into a non-autoimmune genome such as B6.NZM2410.*Sle1* mice, which carry the NZM2410-derived*Sle1* QTL that showed the strongest association with lupus nephritis, produced the expected high levels of ANA (Mohan et al., 1998). The implication was that none of the susceptibility loci was sufficient for the induction of full-blown lupus pathology; each of these loci directed the expression of typical phenotypes such as ANA or increased lymphocyte activation (Morel et al., 1997). Therefore each of these component phenotypes itself has an independent genetic basis, at least in the mouse.

In human SLE, risk haplotypes of some of the susceptibility genes such as *STAT4* (Sigurdsson et al., 2008) or *IRF7/PHRF1* (Salloum et al., 2010) correspond to production of specific autoantibody profiles, suggesting that, as in mice, component phenotypes have unique genetic basis also. Confounders make the human analyses harder and difficult to explore due to the unavoidable co-expressivity of all other susceptibility alleles. Intersections of gene-function properties have been identified among the 35 validated murine susceptibility loci. High overlaps have been detected on chromosomes 1, 4, 7, and 13; longer areas are seen on chromosome 1; where 16 independent loci have been identified in 6 strains. The overlap is very conspicuous in the telomeric portion of chromosome 1 with its equivalent region localized in the human *1q23-42* site, a region identified to have many known linkages to human SLE (Tsao, 2003). These results tend to imply that at least some lupus-prone genes are shared among lupus-prone mouse strains and humans as well in that region.

Characterization of the original QTLs lupus congenic strains corresponded to a cluster of susceptibility loci best demonstrated for *Sle1*: this corresponds to at least 7 independent loci. Phenotypic expressions of *Sle1*, ANA synthesis have been linked with 3 independent sub-loci, *Sle1a, Sle1b,* and *Sle1c* (Morel et al., 2001). Further studies demonstrated that ANA production was feasible by the way of various distinct paths in each of these 3 sub loci. *Sle1a* regulates inducement of activated, nucleosome-reactive $CD4^+$ T cells and inhibits the number of $CD4^+$ $Foxp3^+$ http://www.discoverymedicine.com/tag/foxp3/regulatory T cells (Chen et al., 2005a; Cuda et al., 2007) with contribution from two independent sub-loci within *Sle1a, Sle1a1* and *Sle1a2* (Cuda et al., 2010). Findings indicate *Sle1b* function to regulate tolerance in immature B cells (Kumar et al., 2006; Wandstrat et al., 2004). *Sle1c,* with its two subloci, *Sle1c1* affects germinal center B-cell responses, and *Sle1c2,* that induces appearance of autoreactive $CD4^+$ T cells respectively (Boackle et al., 2001; Chen et al., 2005b). *Sle1d,* sandwiched between*Sle1b* and *Sle1c2,* enhances the severity of glomerulonephritis when mice carrying this allele are crossed with NZW mice (Morel et al., 2001). Also interlocked between *Sle1a* and *Sle1b* is the *Fcgr2b* the presence of which reduces expression on germinal-center B cells and plasma cells (Rahman et al., 2007): a phenotype known to have links with lupus patients (Mackay et al., 2006). The obvious deduction is that other lupus-prone strains may express identical state of genetic complexity in that region and at other loci and therefore is an avenue of either common or strain-specific genes, possible determinant of individual gene level and hence probable disparity among races.

Synergistic interactions between specific loci were also found to be linked with co-expressivity found in *Sle1* and *Yaa* on a B6 background that led to severe lupus nephritis (Croker et al., 2003); the co-expression of either *Sle2* or *Sle3* with *Yaa* achieved only the phenotypes of either parent strains. In humans genetic interactions have been harder to identify for SLE (Harley et al., 2009) partly due to the extreme genetic diversity co-segregating with any gene or locus of interest. Additive effects have, however, been identified between risk variants of*STAT4* and *IRF5* (Abelson et al., 2009; Sigurdsson et al., 2008), suggestive of specific genetic interactions in human SLE. The co-expression of *Sle1, Sle2,* and *Sle3* on a B6 background has been seen to give rise to fully penetrant lupus nephritis (Morel et al., 2000).

A clear demonstration of mercury's possible influence on several metabolic pathways is seen in the number of possible pathways affected Figures 1-3: red coloration indicates upregulated genes and blue coloration indicates inhibition of gene expression on exposure to mercury. Mercury exposure leads to effects on several of biochemical pathways involving products of genes in cell cycle signaling: G2/M checkpoint regulation, TGF-β, IGF-1, insulin receptor activity, chemokine, Wint/ β-catenin, integrin, PPAR, SAPK/JNK, JAK/Stat, B and T cell receptor, G-protein-coupled receptor, IL-2, ERK/MAPK, death receptor signaling such as apoptosis, NF-κB, cell cycle and above all immune responses regulated by most of these genes. Pathways indicated are examples of mercury's potential to affect susceptible individuals that carry MHC haplotype combinations and who are prone to develop not only autoimmune and/or cancerous diseases but risk factors for obesity and other chronic associated diseases yet to be evaluated through mercury toxicity.

Our studies confirm that several genes in haplotype combinations are subjected to pronounced changes on exposure to environmental mercury. Among these genes we mention the transforming factor beta (TGF-β) superfamily of cytokines. This group of family genes is associated with regulating the cell cycle essentially for maintenance of normal immunological homeostasis and lymphocyte proliferation. Proteins synthesized from these genes play important roles in regulating essential cellular functions such as differentiation and apoptosis. TGF-β superfamily of cytokines is over expressed on mercury exposure. Some cells, lymphocytes among them are known to respond to TGF-β by undergoing apoptosis. Apoptosis may lead up to accumulation of self-antigens within a localized part of the body and break the body's immunological tolerance to give rise to the autoimmune state. The mechanisms regulating this process are yet to be clarified. Over expression of TGF-β cytokines induced by mercury may lead to transcription of Smad6 and Smad7; these molecules act as inhibitors of TG apoptosis is necessary for maintenance of tolerance. Failure to eliminate immature B cells has the consequence of autoimmune diseases and cancer development. Several aberrant functions associated with many pathways involving the cell cycle and the immune responses are therefore possible through intoxication with mercury. Such wide effects of mercury translate to risk associations when disease susceptibility is our prime concern. This means that it is only at the right genetic combinations and the appropriate line-up of associated genes that disease susceptibility ensues. That goes to argue for severity of disease as well. Mercury-exposed individuals carrying the appropriate allelic-combinations located on specific haplotypes are prone to develop autoimmune diseases.

Not only do some metals induce autoimmunity but can also affect the nervous system when present during fetal development. Mercury readily crosses the human placenta and accumulates in fetal tissue during gestation (David et al., 1972). Mercury can concentrate in umbilical cord blood significantly more than in the maternal blood (Sakamoto et al., 2004). This could affect various developmental processes (Clarkson, 1997; Hassett-Sipple et al., 1997; Pendergrass et al., 1997) leading to behavioral dysfunctions associated with autism (Bernard et al., 2001) and others. Arrhythmias and cardiomyopathies have also been associated with mercury toxicity. Mercury intoxication can result in mental retardation, cerebral palsy, seizures and ultimately death (WHO, 1990). For the early protection of children, it becomes necessary to come up with reliable and relevant tools that identify chemicals with developmental neurotoxicity potential. Once identified, these neurotoxicants need to come under regulatory practices in order to restrict their use and to control exposure as, for example in the case of lead (Silbergeld, 1997).

5.2 Spontaneous lupus: who are at risk

To date genetic mappings endorse genetic susceptibility to autoimmunity and confirms it to be highly associated with individuals with certain combinations of genes in MHC-haplotype linkages: *Fasl* (CD95/L), *Sap* (serum amyloid P-component), *Fcγr2b* (FcγRIIB), *Cr2* (CD21/CD35) and *Ptprc* (CD45) amongst them. Deficiency in individuals of Fcer1g (FcRγ-chain) results in resistance to autoimmunity. These genes are not by any means exhaustive. As mentioned above gene type and dosage seem to determine severity of autoimmune diseases. This indicates that susceptibility and/or initiation factors operate via multiple pathways subjected to regulatory or focal checkpoints that finally give rise to the pathological state. The situation is exemplified by SLE, type 1 diabetes, IDDM and RA patients. In genetically predisposed patients the synthesis of autoantibodies and/or the generation of cellular attack of self-antigens may follow different pathways. Such mechanisms are known to be influenced by gene dosage and contributions from *ethnic* and environmental background. Clinical management or treatment schedules need to vary accordingly.

Thus lupus susceptibility genes are now of deep interest to immunologists/allergists and are being identified in the mouse and their contribution to the disease state is being actively sought through analysis of rare or common variants. Discoveries of the roles of the susceptible lupus genes mainly in the mouse have given insights and critical lead to links with human SLE disease patterns. However the molecular mechanisms by which they contribute to autoimmune pathogenesis are yet to be clearly defined. The multifactorial complex nature of lupus disease susceptibility is currently thought to operate via a combination of common genetic variants that result in small phenotypic effects; rare variants end in large phenotypic effects (Cirulli et al., 2010). So far identified common variants in lupus susceptibility genes include the PTPN22 or *IRF5* among others. Genome wide Association studies (GWAS) and analysis also reveals scarce variants such as C4 and TREX (Graham et al., 2009). Rare *SIAE* variants responsible for the loss-of-function have been linked with autoreactive B cells (Surolia et al., 2010); the *lpr* and *gld* in humans represented in lupus-prone murine strains lead to a functional decline in CD95 or C95L, respectively (Cohen et al., 1992); the *Yaa* mutation, an equivalent of a *Tlr7* gene duplication (Pisitkun et al., 2006), and a mutation in the Coronin A1 gene in the B6.Fas^{lpr}/Scr strain that regulates CD4^{+} T cell activation (Haraldsson et al., 2008) have all been located.

The murine equivalent of humans common variant genes have now been identified for SLE. NZB and NZW allele of *Fcgr2b* encode a negative regulator of B-cell signaling and predicates an autoimmune phenotype (Rahman et al., 2007; Xiu et al., 2002). Studies currently endorse links between *FCGR2B* variants and human SLE (Lee et al., 2009). *Cr2* polymorphism that function to encode the complement receptor type 2, a B-cell co-receptor known to contribute to the *Sle1c1* phenotypes (Boackle et al., 2001; Chen et al., 2005b). SLE patients do carry a common *CR2* haplotype more frequently than in healthy controls; and follicular dendritic cells (FDC) express a novel CR2 splice variants of SLE patients (Douglas et al., 2009; Wu et al., 2007). *Sle1b* corresponds to polymorphisms in four signaling lymphocytic activation molecule (SLAM) family member genes (Wandstrat et al., 2004), including *Ly108* directly implicated in the regulation of B-cell tolerance (Kumar et al., 2006). Variants of *SLAMF3* (*LY9*) and *SLAMF4* (*CD244*) have also been linked with human SLE (Graham et al., 2008; Suzuki et al., 2008). For the *Sle1* sub-loci, *Sle1a.1* corresponds to the expression of a novel splice isoform of the *Pbx1* gene that is associated with increased CD4^{+} T cell activation in both mice and humans (Cuda et al.,2007, 2010). Searches are still going on to reveal the mechanisms linking *Pbx1* expression and T cell phenotypes. Complex phenotypic expressions are associated with *Sle3* locus that includes myeloid cell-induced $CD4^+$ T-cell activation (Zhu et al., 2005) and mild glomerulonephritis (Mohan et al., 1999). Kallikrein (*Klk*) polymorphic genes, serine esterases that regulate a wide spectrum of biological functions in the kidney including inflammation, apoptosis, redox balance, fibrosis, and local blood pressure located in the *Sle3* interval have been linked with increased susceptibility to nephritis in SLE mice and SLE patients (Liu et al., 2009).

To date close to 22 identified and validated loci with confirmed associations with SLE susceptibility (Graham et al., 2009) have been mentioned in the literature. These loci are placed in one of four groups on the basis of mouse characteristics (Morel, 2010). Group one genes are thought to be directly implicated in lupus pathogenesis through their capacity to either induce or modulate disease in the mouse. A representative one is *STAT4*, a transcription factor linked with signal transduction of the IL-12 and IL-23 receptors that has a critical role in regulating the effector functions of helper T cells (Korman et al., 2008). In addition, *Stat4* deficiency modifies disease severity in the NZM lupus models (Jacob et al., 2003; Xu et al., 2006). The *IRF5* whose risk alleles are associated with an increased production of interferon alpha (IFNα) in SLE patients (Niewold et al., 2008) is a puzzling piece. In two different murine models (Richez et al., 2010; Savitsky et al., 2010) *IRF5* however, failed to establish a link between IRF5 and IFNα, pointing instead to a transcriptional control of the IgG2a locus. It is still not clarified if these discrepancies reflect species-specific functions of IRF5 or whether the association between *IRF5* polymorphisms and IFNα production does not involve a direct mechanistic link between the two genes. The second group covers GWAS-identified SLE susceptibility genes with known functions in the murine immune system but without current established link with lupus pathogenesis in man. For example, tumor necrosis factor alpha-induced protein 3 (TNFAIP3) and its binding partner TNFAIP3-interacting protein 1 (TNIP1) are negative regulators of nuclear factor κB signaling and tumor necrosis factor (TNF)-mediated apoptosis (Vereecke et al., 2009).

These findings imply that overexpression of TNFAIP3 would inhibit pathogenesis in lupus-prone mice; its deficiency would exacerbate disease. Newly discovered genes without a known function are placed in the third category of genes associated with SLE in GWAS. The *JAZF1* in this group has now been associated with multiple human phenotypes (Gateva et al., 2009) still awaiting detailed basic functions workout. *FCGR2A* belongs to the fourth group of genes and is associated with SLE risk in GWAS but has no equivalent ancestral gene in the mouse, and therefore cannot yield information for human SLE analysis.

6. Conclusions

The Biosphere is gradually being overwhelmed with several substances from industrial and other activities that has direct role in changes in the incidence and prevalent measures in various diseases. Among these diseases the autoimmune state seems to be a major avenue that impacts and disrupts the homeostatic mechanisms. Autoimmune diseases like asthma are excellent representation of environmental problems acting as indicators of atmospheric as well as the air, the soil and water bodies that are affected by pollutional activities. Thus rises in the incidence and the prevalence of AD within the communities count as direct role of the environmental pollution affecting the gene pool and becomes public health concern. It is important to follow the effects of these substances and the pathways of disease pathogenesis. Currently GWAS is becoming a powerful tool or vehicle that is helping in the understanding the functional roles of the polymorphic alleles particularly those alleles prevailing across ethnic groups. Analyses of population differences in autoimmune state is a first and important step *in* unraveling the complexity of these genes affected by environmental pollutants represented by mercury. It is common knowledge now that environmental contaminants through the food chains occur; pesticides are found in fruits, vegetables and cereals of European origin estimated to contain about 300 biocides in food products (Commission of the European Communities, 2007, Suñol, 2009), also seen in the urine in majority of US population (Mage *et al.*, 2004); and human adipose tissue, serum, and placenta in agricultural areas (López-Espinosa *et al.*, 2007).

Studies in the laboratory reveal increasing concern as to whether pesticides currently used can cause neurodevelopmental toxicity (Bjorling-Poulsen *et al.*, 2008). Similar concerns go for several substances released into the environment. Regulatory checks help to determine the role they play in diseases seen in the population. We are at a time that full-genome association analyses can produce equivocal array of data, some of which are likely to provide vital new biological insights into autoimmunity that may hold the key to novel therapies. The state of the matter is that susceptibility alleles of autoimmune diseases are now believed to fall into two general groups: (1) those genes that confer susceptibility to multiple autoimmune phenotypes (*CTLA4, TPN22, PDCD1, FCRL3*); and (2) those that confer tissue specificity to autoimmunity (*INS* in T1D, *PADI4* in RA). Of note also is that allelic diversity within the *MHC* is also a major determinant of tissue specificity. Having a clear understanding of the genetic basis of autoimmunity and the application of this knowledge to appropriate clinical therapies may provide clinical social medicine benefits in several ways. It may be possible to have early diagnostic tools to detect high risk individuals at the highest genetic risk in prospective longitudinal studies aimed at defining the role of manageable/preventable environmental influences on disease. Also the identification of genetically susceptible individuals will enable targeting of preventive therapy once it becomes available at or evasion of detrimental environmental influences. It may also be helpful to align genetic profiles with prognosis as seen in degrees of disease severity in SLE, RA, IDDM etc or response to specific therapies so that more appropriate or aggressive treatments can be selectively targeted. This will particularly be of unimaginable use in health disparity studies.

7. Acknowledgments

This work was supported in part by the Mississippi IDeA Network for Biomedical Excellence, (NIH-NCRR-P20RR0 16476); Arkansas IDeA Network for Biomedical Excellence (NIH-NCRR-P20RR016460); Research Centers in Minority Institutions (RCMI)—Center for Environmental Health at Jackson State University (NIH-NCRR G12RR013459); Pittsburgh Supercomputing Centre's National Resource for Biomedical Supercomputing (T36GM095335); and National Center for Integrative Biomedical Informatics, University of Michigan (NIH-U54DA021519).

Disclaimer: The views and conclusions contained in this document are those of the authors and should not be interpreted as necessarily representing the official policies, either expressed or implied, of the funding agencies.

8. References

Abbas, A.; Murphy, K, & Sher, A. (1996). Functional diversity of helper T lymphocytes. *Nature* 383:787-796.

Abelson, A.; Gado-Vega, A, Kozyrev, S, Sanchez, E, Velazquez-Cruz, R, Eriksson, N, Wojcik, J, Reddy, L, Lima, G, D'Alfonso, S, Migliaresi, S, Baca, V, Orozco, L, Witte, T, Ortego-Centeno, N, Abderrahim, H, Pons-Estel, B, Gutierrez, C, Suarez, A, Gonzalez-Escribano, M, & et al (2009). STAT4 associates with systemic lupus erythematosus through two independent effects that correlate with gene expression and act additively withIRF5 to increase risk. *Ann Rheum Dis* 68:1746-53.

Andre, I.; Gonzalez, A, Wang B, Katz, J, Benoist, C, & Mathis D. (1996). Checkpoints in the progression of autoimmune disease: lessons from diabetes models. *Proc Natl Acad Sci USA* 93:2260- 2274.

Asosingh, K.; Swaidani, S, Aronica, M , & Erzurum, S, (2007)Th1- and Th2-dependent endothelial progenitor cell recruitment and angiogenic switch in asthma. *J Immunol,* 178: 6482-6494.

ATSDR, (1999). Toxicological Profile for Mercury: TP-93/10. Agency for Toxic Substances and Disease Registry. Centers for Disease Control, Atlanta, Georgia.

Bariety, J.; Druet, P, Laliberte, F, & Sapin, C. (1971) Glomerulonephritis with γ and β1C globulin deposits induced in the rat with mercuric chloride. *Am. J. Pathol.* 65, 293.

Bernard, S.; Enayati A, Redwood, L, Roger, H, & Binstock T, (2001) Autism: A novel form of mercury poisoning. *Med.Hypotheses* 56: 462-471.

Berry, C.; Adam, S, & Curtis, (2003) Functionalisation of magnetic nanoparticles for applications in biomedicine, *J. Phys. D: Appl. Phys* 36 R198 doi: 10.1088/0022-3727/36/13/203 Journal of Physics D: Applied Physics

Biancone L.; Andres, G, Ahn, H, Lim, A, Dai, C, Noelle, R, Yagita, H, De Martino C, & Stamenkovic, I, (1996) Distinct regulatory roles of lymphocyte costimulatory pathways on T helper type-2 mediated autoimmune disease *J. Exp Med* 183 (4), 1473-1481

Birnbaum, L. (2005). PBDEs: Toxicology update. In: *Proceedings of the 2005 National Forum on Contaminants in Fish, Section III: Presentations,* September 18–21, Baltimore, Maryland: *U.S. Environmental Protection Agency.* EPA-823-R-05-006. Available: http://epa.gov/waterscience/fish/forum/2005/proceedings2005.pdf)

Biswas, P, & Wu, C,(2005)Nanoparticles and the Environment – A Critical Review Paper, *J. Air Waste Ma.,* 55, 708-746.

Bjorling-Poulsen, M.; Andersen, H, & Grandjean P. (2008),Potential developmental neurotoxicity of pesticides used in Europe. *Environ. Health, 7:50-72.*

Boackle, S.; Holers, V, Chen X, Szakonyi, G, Karp, D, Wakeland, E, & Morel, L, (2001) Cr2, a candidate gene in the murine Sle1c lupus susceptibility locus, encodes a dysfunctional protein. *Immunity* 15: 775-85.

Bolland, S & Ravetch, J. (2000). Spontaneous autoimmune disease in Fc(γ)RIIB-deficient mice results strain-specific epistasis. *Immunity* 13:277-289.

Candore G.; Lio, D, Colonna-Romano, G, &Caruso, C. (2002) Pathogenesis of autoimmune diseases associated with 8.1 ancestral haplotype: effect of multiple gene interactions. *Autoimmun Rev,* 1, 313-317.

Casiano, C.; Martin, S, Green, & Tan, E. (1996). Selective cleavage of nuclear autoantigens during CD95 (Fas/Apo-1)- mediated T cell apoptosis. Journal of Experimental Medicine 184, 765-770.

Casciola-Rosen, L, Anhalt, G, & Rosen, A. (1995). DNA-dependent protein kinase is one of a subset of autoantigens specifically cleaved early during apoptosis. *J Exp Med* 182, 1625-1634.

Chen, Y.; Cuda, C, & Morel L. (2005a), Genetic determination of T cell help in loss of tolerance to nuclear antigens. *J Immunol* 174:7692-702.

Chen,Y.; Perry, D, Boackle, S, Sobel E, Molina, H, Croker, B, & Morel L. (2005b) Several genes contribute to the production of autoreactive B and T cells in the murine lupus susceptibility locus Sle1c. *J Immunol*175:1080-9.

Cibotti, R.; Kanellopoulos, J, Cabaniols, J, Halle-Panenko, O, Kosmatopoulos, K, Sercarz, E, &Kourilsky, P. Tolerance to a self-protein involves its immunodominant but does not involve its subdominant determinants. *Proceedings of the National Academy of Sciences USA* 89(1):416-420, 1992.

Clarkson, T (1997). The toxicology of mercury. Crit Rev Clin Lab Sci 34:369-403 Clynes, R.; Dumitru, C, & Ravetch, J. (1988). Uncoupling of immune complex formation and kidney damage in autoimmune glomerulonephritis. *Science* 279:1052-1063.deficiency of Fcer1g (FcRγ-chain) ends up in resistance to autoimmunity.

Comhair, S, Bhathena, P, Dweik, R, Kayuru, M, & Erzurum, S. (2000) Rapid loss of superoxide dismutase activity during antigen-induced asthmatic response. *Lancet* 355-624

Commission of the European Communities. (2007). Commission Staff Working Document: Monitoring of Pesticide Residues in Products of Plant Origin in the European Union, Norway, Iceland and Liechtenstein. 2005. SEC 1411.

Croker, B.; Gilkeson, G, & Morel, L (2003). Genetic interactions between susceptibility loci reveal epistatic pathogenic networks in murine lupus. *Genes Immun* 4:575-85.

Cuda C.; Wan, S, Sobel, E, Croker, B, & Morel L. (2007). Murine lupus susceptibility locus Sle1a controlsregulatory T cell number and function through multiple mechanisms. *J Immunol* 179:7439-47.

Cuda, C.; Zeumer, L, Sobel, E, Croker, B, Morel, L. (2010) Murine lupus susceptibility locus Sle1a requires the expression of two subloci to induce inflammatory T cells. *Genes Immun*, epub, May 6.

David, O.; Clark, J, & Voeller, K. (1972) *Lead* and hyperactivity. *Lancet.* 2:900-903. MedlineWeb of Science

De Raeve.; Thunnissen, F, Guo, F, Lewis, M, Kavuru, M, Secic, M, Thamassen, M, & Erzurum, S (1997). Decreased superoxide dismutase activity in asthmatic airway epithelium: correction by inhaled corticosteroid in vivo. *Am J Physiol.* 272: L148-L154.

Dompeling E.; Jobsis, R , & van Schayck, O. (2000) Siblings, day-care attendance, and the risk of asthma and wheezing.*N Engl J Med.* 343:(26) 1967-1968.

Donaldson, K.; Stone, V, Tran, C, Kreyling, W, & Borm, P, (2004). Nanotoxicology. *Occup Environ Med* 61:727-728

Douglas, K.; Windels, D, Zhao, J, Gadeliya, A, Wu, H, Kaufman, K, Harley, J, Merrill, J, Kimberly, R,Alarcon, G, Brown, E, Edberg, J, Ramsey-Goldman, R, Petri, M, Reveille, J, Vila, L, Gaffney P,James, J, Moser K, Alarcon-Riquelme, M, & et al.

(2009). Complement receptor 2 polymorphisms associated with systemic lupus erythematosus modulate alternative splicing. *Genes Immun* 10:457-69.

Drake, C..; Rozzo, S, Hischfeld, H, Smarnworawong, N, Palmer, E, & Kotzin, B (1995). Analysis of the New Zealand Black contribution to lupus-like renal disease: multiple genes that operate in a threshold manner. *J. Immunol.* 154, 2441-7.

Dubey, C.; Bellon, B, Hirsch, F, Kuhn, J, Vial M, Goldman M, & Druet, P. (1991), Increased expression of class II major histocompatibility complex molecules on B cells in rats susceptible or resistant to HgCl2-induced autoimmunity. Clin Exp Immunol. Oct;86 (1):118-23.PMID:1914225 PMCID: PMC1554158

Duits, A.; Bootsma, H, Derksen, R, Spronk, P, Kater, L, Kallenberg, C, Capel P, Westerdaal, N, Spierenburg, G, & Gmelig-Meyling, F. (1995). Skewed distribution of IgG Fc receptor IIa (CD32) polymorphism is associated with renal disease in systemic lupus erythematosus patients. Arthritis Rheum.Dec; 38(12):1832-6.

Dweik, R.; Comhair, S, Gaston, B, Thunnissen, F, Farver, C, Thomassen, M, Kavuru, M, Hammel, J, Abu-Soud, H, & Erzurum, S. (2001). Nitric oxide chemical events in the human airway during the immediate and late antigen induced asthmatic response. *Proc Natl Acad Sci USA*. 2001;98:2622- 2627.

Economic Costs of Asthma (1997) *Am. J. Respir. Crit. Care Med.*, 156(3), 787-793.

Eneström S, & Hultman P (1995) Does amalgam affect the immune system? A controversial issue. *Int Arch Allergy Immunol*. Mar, 106(3):180-203.

EPA's (2007) Report on the Environment: Science Report (SAB Review Draft) *The EPA's* 2007 Report on the Environment:

Fortner, J.; Lyon D, Sayes, C, Boyd, A, Falkner, J, Hotze, E, Alemany, L, Tao, Y, Guo, W, Gateva K, Sandling, V, Hom, J, Taylor G, Chung, S, Sun, X, Ortmann, W, Kosoy, R, Ferreira, R, Nordmark, G, Gunnarsson, I, Svenungsson, E, Padyukov, L, Sturfelt, G, Jonsen, A, Bengtsson, A, Rantapaa-Dahlqvist S, Baechler, E,

Brown, E, Alarcon, G, & et al.(2009) A large-scale replication study identifies TNIP1, PRDM1, JAZF1, UHRF1BP1 and IL10 as risk loci for systemic lupus erythematosus.*Nat Genet* 41:1228-33.

Fortner, J.; Lyon, D, Sayes, C, Boyd, A, Falkner, J, Hotze, E, Alemany, L, Tao, Y, Guo, W, Ausman, K, Colven, V, & Hughes J. (2005). C60 in Water: Nanocrystal Formation and Microbial Response *Environ. Sci. Technol.*, 39 (11), pp 4307–4316

Gammon, G.; & Sercarz, E (1989). How some T cells escape tolerance induction. *Nature* 342(6246):183-185.

Gateva ,V.; Sandling, J, Hom, G, Taylor, K, Chung, S, Sun, X, Ortmann, W, Kosoy, R, Ferreira, R, Nordmark G, Gun- narsson I, Svenungsson E, Padyukov L, Sturfelt G, Jonsen A, Bengtsson AA, Ranta- paa-Dahlqvist S, Baechler EC, Brown EE, Alarcon GS, et al (2009). A large-scale replication study identifies TNIP1, PRDM1, JAZF1, UHRF1BP1 and IL10 as risk loci for systemic lupus erythematosus. *Nat Genet* 41:1228-33.

Gillespie, K.; Qasim, F, Tibbatts, L, Thiru, S, Oliveira, D, & Mathieson, P. (1995) Interleukin-4 gene expression in mercury-induced autoimmunity. Scand J Immunol. Mar; 41(3):268-72. PMID:7871386

Graham, D.; Vyse, T, Fortin, P, Montpetit, A, Cai, Y, Lim, S, McKenzie, T, Farwell, L, Rhodes, B, Chad, L, Hudson, T, Sharpe, A, Terhorst, C, Greenwood, C, Wither, J, & Rioux, J. (2008) CNIOSGES Investig- ators. Association of LY9 in UK and Canadian SLE families. *Genes Immun* 9:93-102.

Graham, R.; Hom, G, Ortmann, W, & Behrens, T. (2009) Review of recent genome-wide association scans in lupus. *J Intern Med* 265:680-8, 2009.

Gupta, A; and Gupta, M. (2005) Review: Synthesis and surface engineering of iron oxide nanoparticles for biomedical applications, BiomaterialsVolume 26, Issue 18, Pages 3995-4021.

Hanley, A.; Karter, A, Festa, A, D'Agostino, R, Wagenknecht, L, Savage, P, Tracy, R, Saad, M, & Haffner, S. (2002) Factor analysis of metabolic syndrome using directly measured insulin sensitivity: The Insulin Resistance Atherosclero- sis Study.Diabetes.Aug;51(8):2642-7.PMID:12145182

Haraldsson, M, Louis-Dit-Sully, C, Lawson, B, Sternik, G, Santiago-Raber, M, Gascoigne, N, Theofilopoulos, A, & Kono, D (2008) The lupus-related Lmb3 locus contains a disease-suppressing Coronin-1A gene mutation. *Immunity* 28:40-51.

Harley, I, Kaufman, K, Langefeld, C, Harley, J, Kelly, J. (2009). Genetic susceptibility to SLE: new insights from fine mapping and genome-wide association studies. *Nat Rev Genet* 10:285-90.

Hassett-Sipple, B.; Swartout, J, Schoeny, R, Mahaffey, K, & Rice, G. (1997) Mercury Study Report to Congress Volume V: health Effects of Mercury and Mercury Compounds. United States Environmental Protection Agency. EPA-452/R-97-007

Hirsch, F.; Couderc, J, Sapin, C, Fournie, G & Druet, P (1982). Polyclonal effects of HgCl2 in the rat: its possible role in an experimental and immune disease. *Eur. J. Immunol.* 12, 620.

Hirsch, F.; Kuhn, J, Ventura, M, Vial, M-C, Fournie, G, & Druet, P. (1986). Autoimmunity induced by $HgCl_2$ in Brown Norway rats I. Production of monoclonal antibodies. *J. Immunol.* 36, 3272-3276.

Hnizdo, E, Sullivan, P, Bang, K, & et al, (2004). Airflow obstruction attributable to work in industry and occupation among US race/ethnic groups: a study of NHANES III data. *Am J Ind Med* 46:126–35

Holgate, S.; Davies, D, Lackie, P, Wilson S. & et al (2000). Epithelial-mesenchymal interactions in the pathogenesis of asthma. J Allergy Clin Immunol. 2000; 105: 193-204.

Horwitz, D. & Stohl W. (1993). Abnormalities in T lymphocytes. In Dubois Lupus Erythematosus. Wallace DJ and Hahn BH, eds. Lea & Febiger, Philad4elphia. 83-86.

http://www.cas.org/cgi-bin/cas/regreport.pl.

http://www.cas.org/index.html.

http://www. clevelandclinicmeded.com/

http://www.discoverymedicine.com/tag/foxp3/

http://www.discoverymedicine.com/tag/quantitative-trait-locus/

http://www.enotes.com/microbiology -encyclopedia/

www.epa.gov/asthma

(http://www.ewg.org/reports/bodyburden2/execsumm.php).

http://www.epa.gov/glnpo/lmmb/substs.html(FDA/EPA)
http://www.discoverymedicine.com/tag/major-histocompatibility-complex/
http://www.discoverymedicine.com/category/medical-specialties/immunology/autoimmunity-immunology-medical-specialties/
http://www.discoverymedicine.com/tag/autoimmunity/
http://www.discoverymedicine.com/category/medical-specialties/neurology/multiple-sclerosis/
http://www.discoverymedicine.com/category/medical-specialties/endocrinology/diabetes/
http://www.discoverymedicine.com/tag/iddm/
http://www.discoverymedicine.com/category/medical-specialties/rheumatology/rheumatoid-arthritis/
http://www.discoverymedicine.com/category/medical-specialties/rheumatology/systemic-lupus-erythematosus/
http://www.discoverymedicine.com/category/species-and-cell-types/human/immune-system/lymphocyte/tcell/

Hultgren, S,Jones, C, & Normark, S. (1996). Bacterial adhesins and their assembly. In Neidhardt,F.C. (ed.), *Escherichia coli and Salmonella; Cellular and Molecular Biology*. ASM Press, Washington, DC, pp. 2730–2756.

Hultman, P.; Bell, L, Enestrom, S, & Pollard, K. (1992). Murine susceptibility to mercury. I. Autoantibody profiles and systemic immune deposits in inbred, congenic and intra-H-2 recombinant strains. *Clin Immunol Immuno-Pathol* 65:98-108.

Hultman, P.; Bell, L, Enestrom, S, & Pollard, K. (1993). Murine susceptibility to mercury. II. Autoantibody profiles and renal immune deposits in hybrid, backcross, and H-2d congenic mice. Clin Immunol Immunopathol 68:9-20.

Jacob, C.; Zang, S, Li, L, Ciobanu, V, Quismorio, F, Mizutani, A, Satoh, M, & Koss, M. (2003) Pivotal role of Stat4 and Stat6 in the pathogenesis of the lupus-like disease in the New Zealand mixed 2328 mice. *J Immunol* 171:1564-71, 2003.

Jacobson, D.; Gange, S, Rose, N, & Graham, N. (1997) Epidemiology and estimated population burden of selected autoimmune diseases in the United States. *Clin Immunol Immunopath* , 84, 223- 243.

Jiang, Y. & Möller, G. (1995) In vitro effects of $HgCl_2$ on murine lymphocytes. I. Preferable activation of $CD4^+$ T cells in a responder strain. *J Immunol* 154: 3138-3146.

Jones, P.;Osborn, T, & Briffa, K. (1997). Estimating sampling errors in large-scale temperature averages. *Journal of Climate* 10:2548-2568.

Kasturi,L.; Eshleman, J, Wunner, W, & Shakin-Eshleman, S. (1995) The hydroxy amino acid in an Asn-X-Ser/Thr seq-uon can influence N-linked core glycosylation efficiency and the level of expression of a cell surface glycoprotein. *J. Biol. Chem.*, 270, 14756–14761

Kavuru, M.; Dweik, R & Thomassen, M. (1999) Role of bronchoscopy in asthma research. Clin Chest Med. 1999; 20:(1) 153-189.

Kavuru, M.; Lang, D, & Erzurum, S (2005) Asthma The Cleveland Clinic Disease Management Project, Allergy & Immunology.

Kharitonov, S, & Barnes, P (2001) Exhaled markers of pulmonary disease. *Am J Respir Crit Care Med.* 1693-1722. Kono, Y., Yoshinaga, M., Oku, S., Nomura, Y., Nakamura, M. and Aihoshi, S. (1994) Effect of obesity on echocardio-graphic parameters in children. *International Journal of Cardiology 446*, 7-13.

Kono, D.; Balomenos, D, Pearson, D, Park, M, Gildebrandt, B, Hultman, P, Pollard, K. (1998).The prototypic TH2 auto immunity induced by mercury is dependent on IFN- γ and not T_H1/T_H2 imbalance. *J Immunol. 161*:234-240.

Kono, D. & Theofilopoulos, A. (2006). Genetics of SLE in mice. *Springer Semin Immunopathol* 28:83-96.

Korman, B.; Kastner, D, Gregersen, P, & Remmers E. (2008). STAT4: genetics, mechanisms, and implications for auto-immunity. Curr Allergy Asthma Rep. Sep;8(5):398-403.PMID:18682104[PubMed indexed for MEDLINE] PMCID: PMC2562257

Kumar, K.; Li, L, Yan, M, Bhaskarabhatla, M, Mobley, A, Nguyen, C, Mooney, J, Schatzle, J, Wakeland,E, & Mohan, C. (2006). Regulation of B cell tolerance by the lupus susceptibility gene Ly108.*Science* 312:1665-9.

Lam, C.; James J, McCluskey, R & Hunter R (2004). Pulmonary toxicity of single-walled carbon nanotubes in mice 7 and 90 days after intratracheal instillation. *Toxicol. Sci.* 77:126-134.

Lang, D. (2000). Anti-leukotriene agents and aspirin-sensitive asthma—Are we removing the second bassoonist or skating to where the puck is gonna be?. *Ann Allergy Asthma Immunol,* 85: 5-8.

Lang, D. (2006). The long acting beta agonist controversy: A critical examination of the evidence. Cleve *Clin J Med;* 73 973-992.

Lang, S.; Butterfield, D, Schulted, M, Kelley, D, & Lilley, M, (2010). Elevated concentrations of formate, acetate and dissolved organic carbon found at the Lost City hydrothermal field Geochimica et Cosmochimica Acta 74, 941–952

Lanzavecchia, A(1995). How can cryptic epitopes trigger autoimmunity? *Journal of Experimental Medicine* 181(6): 1945 -1948.

Lehmann PV, Forsthuber T, Miller A, Sercarz EE. Spreading of T-cell autoimmunity to cryptic determinants of an autoantigen. *Nature* 358(6382):155-, 1992.

Lee, Y.; Ji, J, & Song, G, (2009) Fcγ receptor IIB and IIIB polymorphisms and susceptibility to systemic lupus erythe-matosus and lupus nephritis: a meta-analysis. Lupus 18:727-34.

Li, X.; & Wilson, J. (1997). Increased vascularity of the bronchial mucosa in mild asthma. Am J Respir Crit Care Med. 156: 229-233.

Liossis S-NC.; Kovacs, B, Dennis, G, Kammer, G. & Tsokos G. (1996). B cells from patients with systemic lupus eryth-ematosus display abnormal antigen receptor-mediated signal transduction events. J Clin Invest 98:2549-2557.

Liu, K.; Li, Q, gado-Vega, A, Abelson, A, Sanchez, E, Kelly, A, Li, L, Liu, Y, Zhou, J, Yan, M, Ye, Q, Liu, S, Xie, C, Zhou, X, Chung, S, Pons-Estel, B, Witte, T, de Ramon, E, Bae, S, Barizzone, N, & et al.(2009) Kallikrein genes are associated with lupus and glomerular basement membrane-specific antibody-induced nephritis in mice and humans. *J Clin Invest* 119:911-23.

Lopez-Espinosa, M.; Granada, A, Carreno, J, Salvatierra, M, Olea-Serrano, F, & Olea, N. (2007). Organochlorine pesticides in placentas from Southern Spain and some related factors. *Placenta.* Jul;28(7):631-8. Epub 2006 Nov 15. PMID:17109956 [PubMed - indexed for MEDLINE]

Lovern, S.; & Klaper R. (2005). Impact of titanium dioxide and carbon nanoparticles on Daphnia magna. Society of Environmental Toxicology and Chemistry, Midwest Regional Chapter Annual Meeting. Abstract.

Mackay, M.; Stanevsky, A, Wang, T, Aranow, C, Li, M, Koenig, S, & Ravetch, J, (2006) Diamond B. Selective dysregulation of the FcγIIB receptor on memory B cells in SLE. *J Exp Med* 203:2157-64.

Mage, D.; Allen, R, Gondy, G, Smith, W, Barr, D & Needham, L.(2004). Estimating pesticide dose from urinary pesticide concentration data by creatinine correction in Third National Health and Nutrition Examination Survey (NHANES- III). *J Expo Anal Environ Epidemiol.* Nov;14(6):457-65.

Manoury-Schwartz, B.; Chiocchia, G, Bessis, N, Abehsira-Amar, O, Batteux, F, Muller, S, Huang, S, Boissier, M, & Fournier C. (1997). High susceptibility to collagen-induced arthritis in mice lacking IFN-γ receptors. *J Immunol* 158:5501- 5506.

Mathieson, P.; Thiru, & D, Oliveira, D. (1992). Mercuric chloride-treated Brown Norway rats develop widespread tissue injury including necrotizing vasculitis. *Lab Invest* 67:121-132.

McKernan, M.; Rattner, B, Ackerson, B, Barton, M, Schoen, K, Hale R. & Ottinger, M. (2006). Comparative toxicity of polybrominated flame retardants in avian embryos. Poster at (2006) Society of Environmental Toxicology and Chemistry Meeting.

Mirtcheva, J.; Pfeiffer, C, De Bruijn, J, Jacquesmart, F, & Gleichmann, E. (1989).Immunological alterations inducible by mercury compounds. III. H-2A acts as an immune response and H-2^e as an immune "suppression" locus for $HgCl_2$-induced antinuclear autoantibodies. *Eur J Immunol* 19:2257- 2268.

Mohan, C.; Alas, E, Morel, L, Yang, P, Wakeland, E, (1998). Genetic dissection of SLE pathogenesis - Sle1 on murine chromosome 1 leads to a selective loss of tolerance to H2A/H2B/DNA subnucleosomes. *J Clin Invest* 10 11362-72.

Mohan, C.; Yu, Y, Morel, L, Yang, P & Wakeland, E. (1999). Genetic dissection of Sle pathogenesis: Sle3 on murine chromosome 7 impacts T cell activation, differentiation, and cell death. *J Immunol* 162:6492-502.

Monroe, R. & Halvorsen S. (2006). Mercury abolishes neurotrophic factor-stimulated Jak-STAT signaling in nerve cells by oxidativestress. Toxicological Sciences 94, 129-138.

Montuschi, P. & Barnes, P. (2002). Exhaled leukotrienes and prostaglandins. *J Allergy Clin Immunol.* 109: 615-620.

Morel, L.; Rudofsky, U, Longmate, U, Schiffenbauer, J, & Wakeland, E. (1994). Polygenic control of susceptibility to murine systemic lupus erythematosus. *Immunity* 1:219.

Morel, L.; Mohan, C, Yu, Y, Croker, B, Tian, N, Deng, A, & Wakeland, E (1997). Functional dissection of systemic lupus erythematosus using congenic mouse strains. *J Immunol* 158:6019-28.

Morel, L.; Croker, B, Blenman, K, Mohan, C, Huang G, Gilkeson, G, & Wakeland, E. (2000) Genetic reconstitution of systemic lupus erythematosus immunopathology with polycongenic murine strains. *Proc Natl Acad Sci USA* 97:6670-5.

Moser, K.; Neas, B, Salmon, J, Yu, H, Gray-McGuire, C, Asundi, N, Bruner, G, Fox, J, Kelly, J, Henshall, S, Basino, D, Dietz, M, Hogue, R, Koelsch, G, Nightingale, L, Shaver, T, Abdou, N, Albert, D, Carson, C, Petri, M, Tread- well, E, James, J, & Harley, J. (1998). Genome scan of human systemic lupus erythematosus: evidence for linkage on chromosome 1q in African-American pedigrees. *Proc Natl Acad Sci USA* 95(25):14869-14874.

Morel, L.; Blenman, K, Croker, B, & Wakeland, E. (2001). The major murine systemic lupus erythematosus susceptibi-lity locus, Sle1, is a cluster of functionally related genes. *Proc Natl Acad Sci U S A* 98:1787-92.

Morel, L. (2010) Genetics of SLE: Evidence from mouse models. *Nat Rev Rheumatol* 6:348-57.

Moudgil, K.; & Sercarz, E. (2005). Understanding crypticity is the key to revealing the pathogenesis of autoimmunity. *Trends in Immunology* 26(7):355-359, 2005.

Niewold, T.; Kelly, J, Flesch, M, Espinoza, L, Harley, J, & Crow, M. (2008). Association of the IRF5 risk haplotype with high serum interferon-alpha activity in systemic lupus erythematosus patients. *Arthritis Rheum* 58:2481-7.

Oberdörster. E. (2004). Manufactured Nanomaterials (Fullerenes, C_{60}) Induce Oxidative Stress in the Brain of Juvenile Largemouth Bass. *Environ Health Perspect* 112:1058-1062.

Oberdörster, G.; Sharp, Z, Atudorei, V, Elder, A, Gelein, R, & et al. (2004). Translocation of inhaled ultrafine particles to the brain. *Inhal Toxicol* 46:437–445.

Oberdorster, E. (2004b). Toxicity of nC60 fullerenes to tow aquatic species: Daphnia and largemouth bass. American Chemical Society, Anaheim, California. March 27–April 2004. Abstract IEC21.

Ochel, M.; Vohr, H, Pfeiffer, C, & Gleichman, E (1991). IL-4 is required for the IgE and IgG1 increase and IgG1 auto-antibody formation in mice treated with mercuric chloride. J Immunol. May 1;146(9):3006-11.

Pascual, R. & Peters, S. (2005) airway remodeling contributes to the progressive loss of lung function in asthma: an overview. *J Allergy Clin Immunol.* 116: 477-486.

Patrick, L. (2002). Mercury toxicity and antioxidants: Part 1: Role of glutathione and alpha-lipoic acid in the treatment of mercury toxicity. *Altern. Med. Rev.* 7, 456–471.

Pauwels, R.; Buist, A, Calverley, P, & et al. (2001). Global strategy for the diagnosis, management, and prevention of chronic obstructive pulmonary disease. NHLBI/WHO Global Initiative for Chronic Obstructive Lung Disease (GOLD) Workshop summary. *Am J Respir Crit Care Med* 163: 1256–76

Pendergrass, J.; Haley, B, Vimy, M, Winfield, S, Lorscheider, F, (1997) Mercury vapor inhalation inhibits binding of GTP to tubulin in rat brain: similarity to a molecular lesion in Alzheimer diseased brain. *Neurotoxicology* 18:315-324.

Pier, S. M. (1975). The role of heavy metals in human health. *Texas Rep Biol Med. 33*(1), 85-106.

Pisitkun, P.; Deane, J, Difilippantonio, M, Tarasenko, T, Satterthwaite, A, & Bolland, S. (2006) Autoreactive B cell responses to RNA-related antigens due to TLR7 gene duplication. *Science* 312:1669-72.

Pollard, K, Lee, D, Casiano, C, Blüthner, M, Johnson, M, & Tan EM. (1997). The autoimmunity-inducing xenobiotic mercury interacts with the autoantigen fibrillarin and modifies its molecular and antigenic properties. *J Immunol* 158:3521-3528.

Pollard, K.; Pearson, D, Hultman, P, Hildebrandt, B, & Kono, D. (1999). Lupus-prone mice as models to study xenobiotic-induced acceleration of systemic autoimmunity. *Environ Health Perspect* 107(5):729-735.

Pollard, K, Pearson, L, Blüthner, M, Tan, E. (2002). Proteolytic cleavage of a self-antigen following xenobiotic-induced cell death produces a fragment with novel immunogenic properties. *J Immunol* 165(4):2263-2270.

Puck, J. & Sneller, M. (1997). ALPS: an autoimmune human lymphoproliferative syndrome associated with abnormal lymphocyte apoptosis. *Semin Immunol* 9:77-81.

Rahman, Z.; Niu, H, Perry, D, Wakeland, E, Manser, T, & Morel, L (2007). Expression of the autoimmune Fcgr2b NZW allele fails to be upregulated in germinal center B cells and is associated with increased IgG production *Genes Immun* 8:604-12.

Renwick, L.; Brown, D, Clouter, A, & Donaldson, K. (2004). Increased inflammation and altered macrophage chemo-tactic responses caused by two ultrafine particle types. *Occup Environ Med* 61:442 447 doi:10. 1136/ oem. 2003 .00 8227

Richez, C.; Yasuda, K, Bonegio, R, Watkins, A, Aprahamian, T, Busto, P, Richards, R, Liu, C, Cheung, R, Utz, P, Marshak-Rothstein, A, & Rifkin, I, (2010). IFN regulatory factor 5 is required for disease development in the FcγRIIB-/-Yaa and FcγRIIB-/- mouse models of systemic lupus erythematosus. *J Immunol*184:796-806.

Roman-Franco, A.; Turiello, M, Albini, B, Ossi, E, Milgrom, F, & Andres, G. (1978). Anti-basement membrane anti-bodies and antigen-antibody complexes in rabbits injected with mercuric chloride. *Clin Immunol Immun- opathol* 9:464-472.

Rose, N. & Bona, C. (1993). Defining criteria for autoimmune disease (Witebsky's postulate revisited). Immunol Today, 14(9), 426-430.

Sakamoto, M.; Kubota, M, Liu, X, Murata, K, Nakai, K, & Satoh, H, (2004) Maternal and fetal mercury and n-3Poly-unsaturated fatty acids as a risk and benefit of fish consumption to fetus. *Environ. Sci.Technol.* 38: 3860-63

Salloum, R.; Franek, B, Kariuki, S, Rhee, L, Mikolaitis, R, Jolly, M, Utset, T, Niewold, T (2010). Genetic variation at the IRF7/PHRF1 locus is associated with autoantibody profile and serum interferon-alpha activity in lupus patients. *Arthritis Rheum* 62:553-61.

Salmon J.; Millard S, Schachter L, Arnett F, Ginzler E, Gourley M, Ramsey-Goldman R, Peterson M & Kimberly R. (1996). FcγRIIA alleles are heritable risk factors for lupus nephritis in African -Americans. *J Clin Invest* 97: 1348-1354.

Sapin, C.; Hirsch, F, Delaporte, J, Bazin, H, & Druet, P. (1984). Polyclonal IgE increase after $HgCl_2$ injections in BN and LEW rats: a genetic analysis. Immunogenetics 20;227-234.

Salvato, G. (2001) Quantitative and morphological analysis of the vascular bed in bronchial biopsy specimens from asthmatic and non-asthmatic subjects. *Thorax*. 56: 902-906.

Savitsky, D, Yanai, H, Tamura, T, Taniguchi, T, & Honda, K. (2010). Contribution of IRF5 in B cells to the develop -ment of murine SLE-like disease through its transcriptional control of the IgG2a locus *PNAS* 107:10154-9.

Schecter, A.; Pavuk, M, Päpke, O, Ryan, J, Birnbaum, L, & Rosen, R. (2003) Polybrominated Diphenyl Ethers (PBDEs) in U.S. Mothers' Milk Polybrominated Diphenyl Ethers (PBDEs) in U.S. Mothers' Milk *Env Health Perspec- tive* 111(14) Nov.

Sercarz, E.; Lehmann, P, Ametani, A, Benichou, G, Miller, A, Moudgil, K.(1993) Dominance and crypticity of T cell antigenic determinants. *Annual Review of Immunology*11:729-766, 1993.

Shvedova, A.; Kisin, E, Mercer, R, Murray, A, Johnson, V, Potapovich, A, Yulia, Y, Gorelik. T, Arepalli, S, Schwegler -Berry, D, Hubbs, AF, Antonini, J., Evans D.E, Ku, B-Ki, Ramsey,D Maynard, A., Kagan V E., Castranova J,& Baron, P. (2005); Unusual inflammatory and fibrogenic pulmonary responses to single-walled carbon nanotubes in mice. *Am Cellular and Molecular Physiology.Lung Cell Mol. Physiol.* 289:L698-L708

Sigurdsson, S.; Nordmark, G, Garnier, S, Grundberg, E, Kwan, T, Nilsson, O, Eloranta, M, Gunnarsson, I, Svenungsson, E, Sturfelt, G, Bengtsson, A, Jonsen, A, Truedsson, L, Rantapaa-Dahlqvist, S, Eriksson, C, Alm, G, Goring, H, Pastinen, T, Syvanen, A &, et al. (2008) A risk haplotype of STAT4 for systemic lupus erythemaatosus is over-expressed, correlates with anti-dsDNA and shows additive effects with two risk alleles of IRF5. *Hum Mol Genet* 17:2868-76.

Silbergeld, E. (1997) Preventing lead poisoning in children 1997 *Annu. Rev. Public Health* 1997; 18:187-210.

Sinha P, Chi HH, Kim HR, Clausen BE, Pederson B, Sercarz EE, Forster I, Moudgil KD. Mouse lysozyme-M knockout mice reveal how the self-determinant hierarchy shapes the T cell repertoire against this circulating self antigen in wild-type mice. *Journal of Immunology* 173(3):1763-1771, 2004.

Smith, H.; Malone, C, Lawson, A, Okamoto, J, Battista, C, Saunders, B. A national estimate of the economic costs of asthma, (1997). *Am J. Respir Crit Care Med* (156): 787-793.

Smith, J.; Krishnaswamy, G, Dykes, R, Reynolds, S, & Berk, S. (1997). Clinical manifestations of IgE hypogammaglobulinemia. Ann Allergy Asthma Immunol.Mar;78(3):313-8.

Suñol, C. (2009) Use of Gene Expression of Neural Markers in Cultured Neural Cells to Identify Developmental Neurotoxicants, *Toxicological Sciences*, 113, 1-3.

Surolia, I.; Pirnie, S., Chellappa, V, Taylor, K, Cariappa, A, Moya, J, Liu, H, Bell, D, Driscoll, D, Diederichs, S, Haider, K, Netravali, I, Le, S, Elia, R, Dow, E, Lee, A, Freudenberg, J, De Jager, P, Chretien, Y, Varki, A, & et al.(2010) Functionally defective germline variants of sialic acid acetylesterase in autoimmunity. *Nature* 466:243-7.

Takeuchi, K.; Turley, S, Tan, E., Pollard, L. (1995) Analysis of the autoantibody response to fibrillarin in human disease and murine models of autoimmunity. *J. Immunol. 154,* 961-969

Theofilopoulos, A, & Dixon, F (1985). Murine models of systemic lupus erythematosus. *Adv Immunol* 37:269-379.

Tsao, B. (2003). The genetics of human systemic lupus erythematosus. Trends Immunol 24:595-602.

Van Vliet, E.; Uhrberg, M, Stein, C, & Gleichmann, E. (1993). MHC control of IL-4-dependent enhancement of B cell Ia expression and Ig class switching in mice treated with mercuric chloride. Int Arch Allergy Immunol. 1993;101(4):392-401.PMID:8102566 [PubMed - indexed for MEDLINE]

Vereecke, L.; Beyaert, R, van Loo, G.(2009) The ubiquitin-editing enzyme A20 (TNFAIP3) is a central regulator of immune pathology. Trends Immunol 30:383-91.

Vermeire, K.; Heremans, H, Vandeputte, M, Huang, S, Billiau, A, Matthys, P. (1997). Accelerated collagen-induced arthritis in IFN-γ receptor-deficient mice. J Immunol 158:5507-5513.

Wandstrat, A, Nguyen, C, Limaye, N, Chan, A, Subramanian, S, Tian, X, Yim, Y, Pertsemlidis, A, Garner, H, Morel, L, & Wakeland, E. (2004). Association of extensive polymorphisms in the SLAM/CD2 gene cluster with muri- nelupus. *Immunity* 21:769-80.

Waters, S.; McDuffie, M, Bagavant, H, Deshmukh, U, Gaskin, F, Jiang, C, Tung, K, & Fu, S. (2004). Breaking tolerance to double stranded DNA, nucleosome, and other nuclear antigens is not required for the pathogenesis of lupus glome -rulonephritis. *J Exp Med* 199:255-64, 2004.

Weiss, S. (2002) Eat dirt—The hygiene hypothesis and allergic diseases. *N Engl J Med.* 2002; 347: 930-931.

WHO, World Health Organization Geneva, (1990) Methylmercury.Environmental healthcriteria;101

Whitekus, M.; Santini, R, Rosenspire, A, McCabe, M, Jr. (1999). Protection Against CD95-Mediated Apoptosis by Inorganic Mercury in Jurkat T Cells. *The J Immunol* 162:7162-7170.

Wilson, R.; Goyal, L, Ditzel, M, Zachariou, A, Baker, D, Agapite, J, Steller, H, Meier,P, (2002). The DIAP1 RING finger mediates ubiquitination of Dronc and is indispensable for regulating apoptosis. *Nat. Cell Biol. 4(6); 445-450. (Export to RIS)* 12021771

Wollenberger, L. (March 2005). *Toxicity tests with crustaceans for detecting sublethal effects of potential endocrine disrupting chemicals.* Ph.D. thesis. Lyngby, Denmark: Environment and Resources, Technical University of Denmark. Available: http://www2.er.dtu.dk/publications/fulltext/2005/MR2005-012.pdf.

Wu, H.; Boackle, S, Hanvivadhanakul, P, Ulgiati, D, Grossman, J, Lee, Y, Shen, N, Abraham, L, Mercer, T, Park, E, Hebert, L, Rovin, B, Birmingham, D, Chang, D, Chen, C, McCurdy, D, Badsha, H, Thong, B, Chung, H, Arnett F, & et al. (2007). Association of a common complement receptor 2 haplotype with increased risk of systemic lupus erythematosus. *Proc Natl Acad Sci U S A* 104:3961-6.

Wu, W, Samoszuk, M , Comhair S. & et al (2000). Eosinophils generate brominating oxidants in allergen-induced asthma. *J Clin Invest.* 105: 1455-1463.

www.nhlbi.nih.gov/guidelines/asthma/epr3/index.htm

Xia, T.; Korge, P. Weiss, J, Li, N, Venkatesen, M, Sioutas, C, & Nel, A, (2004) Quinones and aromatic chemical compounds in particulate matter induce mitochondrial dysfunction: implications for ultrafine particle toxicity. Environ Health Perspect. Oct;112 (14):1347-58.

Xiu, Y.; Nakamura, K, Abe, M, Li, N, Wen, X, Jiang, Y, Zhang, D, Tsurui, H, Matsuoka, S, Hamano, Y, Fujii, H, Ono, M, Takaj, T, Shimokawa, T, Ra, C, Shirai, T,& Hirose, S. (2002) Transcriptional regulation of Fcgr2b gene by polymorphic promoter region and its contribution to humoral immune responses. *J Immunol*169:4340-6.

Xu, Z, Duan, B, Croker, B, & Morel L. (2006) STAT4 deficiency reduces autoantibody production and glomerulonephritis in a mouse model of lupus. *Clin Immunol* 120:189-98.

2

IRF-5 - A New Link to Autoimmune Diseases

Sujayita Roy and Paula M. Pitha
Krieger School of Arts & Sciences, Department of Biology, Johns Hopkins University
Department of Oncology, Johns Hopkins School of Medicine
United States of America

1. Introduction

Transcription factors of the interferon regulatory factor (IRF) family have a critical role in the activation of interferon (IFN) genes. All cellular IRFs share a region of homology in the amino terminus encompassing a highly conserved DNA binding motif characterized by five tryptophan repeats, but show variability in the carboxy (C-) terminal part of the IRF polypeptides. While some of these IRFs like IRF-3 and IRF-7 have a critical role in the antiviral response, the others like IRF-1, IRF-4 and IRF-8 have basic roles in the development and function of lymphoid cells. Recently, the importance of IRF-5 in the antiviral and inflammatory response *in vivo* has been clearly established, but it was also shown that this IRF has a basic function in apoptosis and B cells and macrophage differentiation. More interestingly, the role of IRF-5 pathogenicity in autoimmune diseases has been also established, as IRF-5 has been identified as one of the primary risk factors associated with Systemic Lupus Erythematosus (SLE) and other autoimmune diseases. This chapter will review the current knowledge of the mechanisms of IRF-5 activation by the TLR7 pathway and the genetic modifications of IRF-5 that may contribute to the dysregulation of the innate and adaptive immune response associated with the autoimmune disease. Furthermore we will summarize the contribution of the SLE mouse models to our understanding of the role of IRF-5 and TLR7 in the induction of the autoimmune diseases.

2. Type I IFN and SLE

Autoimmune diseases are characterized by a dysregulated expression of Type I IFN, hyper-reactivity of B cells and the production of auto-antibodies. Leukocytes from patients with different autoimmune disorders such as SLE, psoriasis, dermatomyositis and rheumatic arthritis all show overexpression of interferon-induced genes. Furthermore, clinical use of IFNα leads to development of autoimmune syndromes like type I diabetes, psoriasis and inflammatory arthritis (Gota and Calabrese 2003). Till date, it has not been determined whether the uncontrolled production of Type I IFN is a consequence of dysregulated function of the immune system or due to genetic variations of the factors involved in IFN induction or IFN signalling pathway. Type I IFNs are produced by all leucocytes in response to TLR7 or TLR9 activation and the plasmacytoid dendritic cells (pDC) are the most active producer of IFNα. pDCs represent only about 1% of the PBMCs, but they can secrete up to 10^9 IFNα molecules per cell within 12 hours (Fitzgerald-Bocarsly *et al.*, 2008).

SLE is a classical systemic autoimmune disease. The link between SLE and Type I IFN is indisputable, reviewed in (Crow 2009). The elevation of type I IFNs is the hallmark of autoimmune diseases. In SLE, there is a correlation between IFN levels and the presence of anti-ds (double-stranded) DNA antibodies and disease progression. Interferon-stimulated genes (ISG) signature is a marker for severity of the disease (Baechler *et al.*, 2003). Also the high levels of IFNα are a heritable risk for SLE (Niewold *et al.*, 2007).
Clinical findings show that elevated pDC populations along with higher IFN mRNA levels present in dermal lesions of SLE patients contribute to elevated IFN levels. (Blomberg *et al.*, 2001). pDCs also accumulate in active lupus nephritis and migrate to the glomeruli (Silvestris *et al.*, 2003). Immune complexes containing nucleic acid found in the serum from lupus patients are known to trigger a type I IFN response in pDCs (Bengtsson *et al.*, 2000). The IgG RNA/DNA complexes are internalized via receptors [fragment crystallizable gamma receptor IIa (FcγRIIa)] expressed on pDCs, and stimulate endosomic TLR7 or TLR9 followed by activation of IRF-5 and IRF-7 and IFNα production. Both TLR7 and TLR9 are expressed in pDCs. RNA-containing immune complexes signalling through TLR7 are especially efficient in inducing IFNα and there is a direct correlation between serum levels of IFNα and the presence of autoantibodies to RNA-protein complexes (Vollmer *et al.*, 2005). Autoantibodies reactive against RNA-containing autoantigens are detected in the cerebrospinal fluid of patients with cerebral lupus (Santer *et al.*, 2009). An indirect evidence for the role of IFNα in autoimmune disease is the observation showing that patients receiving anti-IFN therapy for other diseases (such as HCV-related hepatitis treated with IFNα) develop autoantibodies and SLE-like syndrome (Ho *et al.*, 2008). Another indirect observation is the induction of anti-dsDNA antibodies and full-blown SLE during a clinical anti-TNFα therapy in patients with rheumatoid arthritis (RA) (De Rycke *et al.*, 2005). *In vitro*, TNFα suppresses IFNα expression and thus suppression of TNFα in patients with arthritis, with the antibody treatment, may result in enhancement of IFNα production.

3. Induction of innate antiviral response

Almost all nucleated cells respond to viral infections by producing Type I IFNs. Type I IFNs (IFNα and IFNβ) are an essential part of the antiviral response; however, their unregulated production is associated with pathology. Virus mediated Type I IFN induction is a classical example of transcriptional regulation. Virus infection induces activation of two families of transcriptional factors, NFκB and IRF family. The IRF proteins possess a common DNA binding domain at the N terminus characterized by a helix-turn-helix motif. The motif is rich in tryptophan residues and binds the GAAA and AANNGAAA domains in the virus responsive element (VRE) of Type I IFN promoters. The C-terminal regions of IRFs are distinct and contain IRF-associated domains (IADs) which are required for protein-protein interactions: either with other IRFs or other transcriptional factors. Two members of the IRF family, IRF-3 and IRF-7 are the major players in the induction of Type I IFN (Au *et al.*, 1998; Au *et al.*, 1995; Marie *et al.*, 1998; Ronco *et al.*, 1998). In the uninfected cell, they are localized to the cytoplasm, but in response to a viral infection, they are phosphorylated and translocate to the nucleus where they associate with the co-activator CREB-binding protein and stimulate transcription of *IfnA* and *IfnB* genes. While IRF-3 alone is sufficient for induction of *IfnB* gene, IRF-7 expression is essential for expression of the entire battery of *IfnA* genes, reviewed in (Pitha and Kunzi 2007). Both IRFs can be activated by a signalling pathway that initiates upon binding of viral dsRNA to membrane Toll-like Receptors, TLR3 and TL4, or cytoplasmic receptors, Retinoic acid-Inducible Gene (RIG)-I or Melanoma Differentiation-Associated gene (MDA)-5. Recent data, however, shows that IRF-3 can be also activated by binding of the viral DNA to the cytoplasmic receptor, Absent In Melanoma (AIM)-2 (Ishikawa and Barber 2011).

4. Role of IRF-5 in the induction of an antiviral response

Another IRF, IRF-5 also stimulates Type I IFN production in infected cells. IRF-5 differs from IRF-3 and IRF-7 in activation and function. While IRF-3 and IRF-7 are induced by TLR3, TLR4 or RIG-I/MDA5 pathways, IRF-5 is activated only by TLR7 and TLR9 in a Myeloid Differentiation factor 88 (MyD88)-dependent pathway and consequently, only certain viral infections (Newcastle disease virus, NDV; VSV; and HSV) can activate IRF-5 (Barnes *et al.*, 2001). The activation of IRF-5 results in the transcription of nine differently alternatively spliced IRF-5 mRNAs, these isoforms are cell-type specific and have distinct functions (Mancl *et al.*, 2005).

Ectopic expression of IRF-5 induces several IFNα subtypes; however, the subtypes induced by IRF-5 and IRF-7 are distinct, *e.g.* IRF-7 induces mostly *IfnA1* while the major subtype induced by IRF-5 is *IfnA8* (Barnes *et al.*, 2001).

5. Downstream effectors of IFNs

The Type I IFN system is well characterized and well-studied. Type I IFNs mediate their action by engaging the ubiquitously expressed IFNα receptor (IFNAR) complex which has two units, IFNAR1 and IFNAR2, reviewed in (Uze *et al.*, 2007). On binding to their respective receptors, IFNs exert their multiple effects through receptor-mediated signalling pathways, resulting in the induction of IFN-stimulated genes (ISGs). The major signalling pathway is the JAK-STAT pathway; beginning from the Janus kinases (JAK1 and Tyk2) and followed by tyrosine phosphorylation of pre-existing signal transducer and activator of transcription (STAT). On phosphorylation, STAT1 and STAT2 assemble together, associate with interferon regulatory factor 9 (IRF-9) and form a multimeric complex (ISGF3) that translocates to the nucleus, where it interacts with interferon-responsive elements (ISRE) present in the 5′ flanking region of ISG (Improta *et al.*, 1994; Levy and Darnell 2002). While ISGF3 seems to be the main transcription factor regulating transcription of ISGs, Type I IFN also stimulates formation of STAT1 homodimers that bind to a slightly different DNA domain, the IFNγ activated site (GAS), present in the promoters of ISG that can be induced both by Type I IFN and IFNγ. The signalling by Type I IFN is not limited to the JAK-STAT pathway as this receptor can also activate both the Mitogen-Activated Protein kinase (MAPK) and Phosphoinositide 3-kinase (PI3K) pathways (Platanias 2005). Activation of IFNs through the IFNARs followed by amplification of the signal via downstream pathways results in activation of more than 300 ISGs. The function of the majority of ISGs has yet to be determined; however, the antiviral function of several of the ISG have been recently characterized, and the proteins described (Samuel 2001; Schoggins *et al.*, 2011).

Among these, ISG15 is one of the very early induced ISGs that influence a panoply of cellular functions; ISG15 is a ubiquitin homologue which is covalently attached to lysine residues (ISGylation) of the targeted proteins. Recent evidence indicates the existence of cross-talk between ubiquitinylation and ISGylation. Since ubiquitinylation is a component of many cellular and stress induced signalling pathway, ISGylation can effectively interfere with these pathways. Activation of ISGylation proceeds by similar enzymatic pathways as used for ubiquitinylation, and interestingly, all enzymes required for ISGylation are induced by IFN. Similar to ubiquitinylation, the ISGylation process is reversible and de-ISGYlating enzymes provide an additional level of control over the entire process. More than a hundred ISG15 targets have been identified, and some of these genes such as RIG-I, JAK1, Protein Kinase R (PKR) and STAT-1 are part of the IFN response system while others have different cellular functions. However, unlike the degradation-driven ubiquitinylation, ISGylation in many cases inhibits ubiquitinylation, reviewed in (Skaug and Chen 2010).

Another IFN induced gene with multiple functions is a constitutively expressed dsRNA dependent PKR whose expression is enhanced by Type I IFN. The inactive monomers of PKR are activated by viral RNA, PKR is phosphorylated and forms active dimers. Activated PKR catalyzes phosphorylation of several substrates including the α subunit of the initiation factor eIF-2 (eIF-2α) (Samuel 1993), as well as the transcription factor inhibitor IκB (Kumar *et al.*, 1994). Thus PKR affects both viral replication and many cellular functions, reviewed in (Pindel and Sadler 2011).

Other ISGs such as cytidine deaminases of the APOBEC family and adenosine deaminase ADAR1 have been recently characterized but their cellular functions are yet to be determined (Chiu and Greene 2008; George *et al.*, 2011; Schoggins *et al.*, 2011). Also interesting is a recent finding from the Rice group (Schoggins *et al.*, 2011) which shows that IRF-1, induced by both IFNγ and Type I IFN has antiviral activity against a large group of distinct viruses and that this antiviral activity is not IFN-mediated. This group also identified large number of novel antiviral ISGs and showed that a number of these proteins function at the translational level.

In addition, there are reports of host-produced antiviral micro-RNAs (miRNAs) in response to IFNs (Hansen *et al.*, 2010; Lagos *et al.*, 2010; O'Connell *et al.*, 2007; Pedersen *et al.*, 2007). Even though first identified in fishes and invertebrates, it was assumed that miRNAs were not elicited as a first line of defence in mammals. However, microarray analysis of general IFNα/β response identified a few candidate miRNAs which are increased or attenuated in response to IFNα/β. Some of these target IFNB mRNA and thus serve as negative regulators of the IFN system, while others are induced during the innate antiviral response. Therefore it seems that IFN-induced cellular miRNAs may represent fine-tuning of the IFN system.

6. Role of IRF-5 in the innate immune response

The transcription factor IRF-5 plays a key role in the innate antiviral and inflammatory response. *In vitro* studies had initially indicated that IRF-5 may be involved in the antiviral response (Barnes *et al.*, 2001), and when genetically modified *Irf-5*$^{-/-}$ mice became available, the importance of IRF-5 in the antiviral and inflammatory response *in vivo* was also demonstrated (Paun *et al.*, 2008; Takaoka *et al.*, 2005). *Irf-5*$^{-/-}$ mice exhibit high susceptibility to viral infection and show reductions in serum levels of Type I IFN as well as inflammatory cytokines such as IL-6 and TNFα. IRF-5 shows a cell type specific expression in B cells, DC, monocytes and macrophages. In contrast to IRF-3 and IRF-7, IRF-5 is activated only by TLR7 and TLR9 MyD88 dependent pathway and unlike IRF-3 and IRF-7, not by TLR3 or RIG I pathways (Schoenemeyer *et al.*, 2005). The MyD88 mediated activation of IRF-5 involves the formation of a tertiary complex consisting of MyD88 and tetramers of IRAK1, IRAK4, TRAF6 and IRF-5 and IRF-7. It was shown that both K63 ubiquitinylation by TRAF6 and phosphorylation are necessary for activation and translocation of IRF-5 to the nucleus, but the kinase that activates IRF-5 has not yet been identified (Balkhi *et al.*, 2008). Activated IRF-5 forms homodimers and heterodimers with IRF-3 and IRF-7, but while the IRF-5 synergizes with IRF-3 activation, it inhibits the transcriptional activity of IRF-7 (Barnes *et al.*, 2004). In addition to its role in the early inflammatory response, IRF-5 also has pro-apoptotic functions.

The observations discussed above show an important role for IRF-5 in the regulation of early inflammatory cytokines and chemokines' expression, as well as Type I IFN genes. The function of IRF-5 was also examined *in vivo* using the genetically modified *Irf-5*$^{-/-}$ mouse model. These mice exhibit an increased susceptibility to viral infection and reductions in serum levels of type I IFNs as well as inflammatory cytokines such as interleukin-6 and tumor necrosis factor alpha (TNFα) (Paun *et al.*, 2008; Takaoka *et al.*, 2005). Examination of the cells type in which expression of inflammatory cytokines and IFN depends on IRF-5 show that IRF-5 is required for the TLR9 mediated induction of IFN β in DC, but not in peritoneal macrophages, while the stimulation of inflammatory cytokines expression was dependent on IRF-5 in both cell types. These data indicate that the function of IRF-5 may be cell type specific.

Unexpectedly, approximately 80% of *Irf-5*$^{-/-}$ mice, (94% C57BL/6) developed an age-related splenomegaly, associated with a dramatic accumulation of $CD19^{+}B220^{-}$ B cells (Lien *et al.*, 2010). The age-related splenomegaly was dependent on genotype, and developed in mice with the mixture of 129 and C57BL/6 genotype, but did not occur in mice that were 98% of C57BL/6 background (unpublished data). Interestingly, the *Irf-5*$^{-/-}$ C57BL6 mice have attenuated responses to T-cell dependent (TD) and T-cell independent (TI) antigens (unpublished data), with a marked down-regulation of serum levels of antigen specific IgG2a and IgG2c. The Taniguchi group (Savitsky *et al.*, 2010) has shown that the down-regulation of IgG2a production occurred also in *in vitro* cultured IRF-5 knockout DC cells stimulated with CpG oligodeoxynucleotides. The synthesis of IL-6 and TNFα was also down-regulated in IRF-5 knockout B cell stimulated with TLR 9 ligand, indicating that the function of these cells is impaired (Lien *et al.*, 2010).

7. Role of IRF-5 in autoimmune diseases

The demonstration that IRF-5 is important not only for the induction of Type I IFN genes, but also for the inflammatory cytokines gave new insights into the regulation of the innate inflammatory response. However, there is also accumulating evidence that IRF-5 may play an important role in the dysregulation of the immune system leading to autoimmune diseases. Several distinctly spliced human IRF-5 isoforms (designated variants 1-10), which show cell type-specific expression and distinct cellular localization, were identified (Mancl *et al.*, 2005). The most common variations are insertions or deletions in exon 6. The majority of IRF-5 isotypes do not differ in their DNA binding sites, but differ in the interaction domain. The transcription of IRF-5 is started at one of the three different promoters. Transcript initiated at exon 1A and 1B are expressed constitutively in B cells and pDC, while transcript 1c is induced by IFN. It should be however noted that spliced variants of IRF-5 were identified only in human cells, while in inbred strains of mice, *IRF-5* encodes for a dominant unspliced transcript.

It has been known for a long time that the autoimmune disease SLE exhibits genetic predisposition, which was later mapped to a specific region on human chromosome 6. When the sequence of the human genome became available, it was found that the genomic region associated with predisposition to SLE showed the presence of several genes associated with the Type I IFN induction and signalling pathway. One of these genes is IRF-5 and a common SNP haplotype in IRF-5 (rs 2004640T) was identified in Scandinavian cohorts as a risk factor for SLE. Interestingly, the same SNP haplotype of IRF-5 has been shown later to be associated with numerous other autoimmune disorders, such as rheumatoid arthritis (RA) (Sigurdsson *et al.*, 2007) and others (Kozyrev and Alarcon-Riquelme 2007). Three specific functional alleles of IRF-5 were identified that define risk factors for SLE (Graham et al., 2006). The rs 2004640 G allele expresses isotypes initiated from exon 1A and 1C, while the rs 2004640T allele expresses transcripts from exon 1B, which provides a stronger promoter and increases the expression of IRF-5. The second SNP is the in-frame insertion- of 30 bp in exon 6 that alters the proline, glutamic acid and serine rich regions and encodes a protein that is similar to unspliced isotype IRF-5v5. The third SNP introduces a variation in the poly A termination site that makes the 3'UTR shorter which leads to an increased stability of IRF-5 mRNA (Graham *et al.*, 2006). All together, these modifications in the *IRF-5* gene result in elevated levels of IRF-5 protein which is larger than the proteins encoded by the spliced IRF- transcripts. Many additional SNPs in IRF-5 have been later identified and are reviewed in (Kozyrev and Alarcon-Riquelme 2007). The high levels of lupus associated IRF-5 expression have been detected in PBMCs of Lupus patients (Feng *et al.*, 2010). Dysregulated expression of Type I IFN is associated with SLE pathogenesis (Niewold *et al.*, 2007) and gene array analysis of PMBCs from SLE patients has revealed elevated expression of IFN-stimulated genes (Crow *et al.*, 2003). Thus, the connection between expression of specific IRF-5 haplotypes and dysregulated production of Type I IFN has been emerging. Interestingly neither IRF-3 or IRF-7 or other members of IRF family were found to be associated with predisposition to autoimmune disease. Thus IRF-5 is possibly the most important factor in the predisposition to the inflammatory diseases.

8. IRF-5 functions in uninfected cells

Another unique feature of IRF-5 is that it is also induced upon DNA damage by p53 (Mori *et al.*, 2002). This establishes the connection between IRF-5 and p53-apoptotic pathways and identifies its possible role in tumor suppression. However, IRF-5 induces apoptosis in p53 independent manner (Barnes *et al.*, 2003). *Irf-5*$^{-/-}$ Mouse Embyronic Fibroblasts (MEFs) expressing c-Ras do not undergo apoptosis even under DNA damage and can efficiently form tumors in mice. These MEFs are also resistant to viral induced apoptosis even though their IFN and cytokine profiles are normal (Yanai *et al.*, 2007). However, there are several indications that IRF-5 and p53 pro-apoptotic function are independent. Several p53 targets are activated in *Irf-5*$^{-/-}$ cells and overexpression of IRF-5 can stop the growth of B cell tumor lymphoma in the absence of p53 (Barnes *et al.*, 2003). Ectopic expression of IRF-5 induces DNA damage-induced apoptosis in p53-deficient colon cancer cells (Hu *et al.*, 2005). IRF-5 is also involved in Fas/CD95-induced apoptosis, a p53 independent phenomenon (Couzinet *et al.*, 2008). IRF-5 stimulates the cyclin-dependent kinase inhibitor p21, but it also stimulates the expression of the pro-apoptotic genes *Bak1*, *Bax*, caspase 8, and DAP kinase 2, thus indicating its ability to promote cell cycle arrest and apoptosis independently of p53 (Barnes *et al.*, 2003).

Udalova and colleagues have also identified IRF-5 as a lineage-defining factor for macrophages (Krausgruber *et al.*, 2011). Their work shows, for the first time, that IRF-5 can be both a transcription activator and repressor. Macrophages differentiate into two functionally opposite types depending on the differentiation stimulus. When bone marrow macrophages are grown with granulocyte–macrophage colony stimulating factor (GM-CSF), they differentiate into M1 type, classical pro-inflammatory macrophages which secrete cytokines like IL-12. However, when they are differentiated with M-CSF, they differentiate to the M2 type, which secretes anti-inflammatory cytokines like IL-10. The authors show that differentiation to M1 macrophages is accompanied by an increase in IRF-5 levels. Overexpression of IRF-5 in M2 macrophages forces them to express a pro-inflammatory profile of cytokines and lowers IL-10 levels, basically making the M2 macrophages functionally similar to M1. Conversely, knockdown of IRF-5 levels in M1 macrophages converts M1 macrophages to the M2 expression profile, producing high levels of IL-10 and low levels of proinflammatory cytokines. Thus IRF-5 is a determinant of macrophage plasticity. The authors also demonstrate that in macrophages, IRF-5 functions as a negative regulator of IL-10. These results open the field to many other questions such as possible cell type specificity of the suppression of IL-10 transcription, or how many other genes are negatively regulated by IRF-5. The analysis of the IRF-5 signature profile in human B cell line BJAB identifies large number of both up-regulated and down regulated genes (Barnes *et al.*, 2004).

9. Activation of IRF-5 by the TLR7 pathway

TLR7 and TLR9 recognize viral ss (single stranded)-RNA or a B form of dsDNA respectively. The recognition is dependent on endosomal internalization and acidification. The TLR7/9 signalling pathway is mediated by an adaptor molecule MyD88 (Kawai *et al.*, 1999; Muzio *et al.*, 1997). MyD88 has two domains: a C-terminal Toll/IL-1 Receptor (TIR) domain that is required for the interaction with the TLRs and an amino terminal death domain (DD) that interacts with members of the IL-1 receptor associated kinase (IRAK) family (Martin and Wesche 2002). This association between IRAK1 and MyD88 results in self-phosphorylation of IRAK-1, as well as phosphorylation by the related kinase, IRAK-4 (Cao *et al.*, 1996; Li *et al.*, 2002). After phosphorylation, IRAK1 dissociates from MyD88 and now binds to TRAF6 (TNF receptor-associated factor 6) (Burns *et al.*, 2000). TRAF6-mediated K63-linked ubiquitinylation is required for IRF-5 nuclear translocation in TLR7/9-MyD88-dependent signalling (Balkhi *et al.*, 2008). IRF-5 homo-dimerizes upon phosphorylation of serine/ threonine residues at the C-terminal end by a still undefined kinase and translocates to the nucleus (Chen *et al.*, 2008). Thus, both ubiquitinylation and phosphorylation of IRF-5 are required for nuclear translocation. IRF-5 also associates with Ikkα kinase, but that results in degradation of IRF-5-rather than activation (Balkhi *et al.*, 2010). It should be noted that TLR 7 and TL9 are the only know pathways that lead to the activation of IRF-5. Unlike IRF-3 or IRF-7, IRF-5 is not activated by TLR3 or TLR 4 via TIR-domain-containing adapter-inducing IFNβ (Trif) pathways or by the RIG-I/MAV IPS-1 pathways.

Several ligands can activate TLR7. TLR7 recognizes viral ssRNA , but IFN production can be also induced in response to imiquimod and resiquimod (Hemmi *et al.*, 2002). In addition, several other guanine nucleoside analogs are recognized exclusively via TLR7 (Lee and Kim 2007). Of physiological ligands, guanosine and uridine-rich ssRNA oligonucleotides derived from HIV-1, stimulate DCs and macrophages to secrete IFNα and other pro-inflammatory cytokines via murine TLR7 (Heil *et al.*, 2004). TLR7 also responds to ssRNA (polyU) or ssRNA derived from wild-type influenza virus (Diebold *et al.*, 2004). Since these sequences can originate from viral as well as endogenous RNA, TLR7 may be unable to discriminate between self and non-self RNA and see the self RNA as sensors of endogenous danger signals. Accordingly, small nuclear ribonucleoproteins (snRNPs), a major component of the immune complexes associated with SLE can activate human pDCs by TLR7 induced signaling pathway and stimulate production of Type I IFNs and other proinflammatory cytokines. Interestingly, the TLR7 pathway can also be activated by nuclear ribonucleoprotein complexes (Savarese *et al.*, 2006).

10. Mouse models of SLE

The mouse model of SLE provides additional information on the mechanism of SLE pathogenicity. NZB mice develop spontaneous lupus, produce autoantibodies and develop glomerulonephritis. Duplication of TLR7 and transposition of the TLR7 gene as seen in the *Yaa* mutation promotes the SLE like symptoms. The B cells of murine lupus model also show an accelerated class switching, which is controlled by the genotype (Vyse *et al.*, 1996). Our results showed that in addition to a decreased production of Type I IFN and inflammatory cytokines, *Irf-5*$^{-/-}$ mice exhibit an alteration of the B cells phenotype, associated with age related expansion of CD19^{+}B220^{-} group of B cells, decrease in plasma cells and splenomegaly (Lien *et al.*, 2010). However, the mechanism by which IRF-5 controls B cells differentiation to plasma cells is not known. *Irf-5*$^{-/-}$ mice have also decreased levels of natural antibodies and T cells dependent antigenic stimulation leads to profound decrease in serum IgG2a (Savitsky *et al.*, 2010). Finally the requirement of IRF-5 for the development of lupus like disease was demonstrated in *FcγRIIB*$^{-/-}$ mice, where IRF-5 deficiency profoundly decreased the manifestation of the disease (Richez *et al.*, 2010). Two other IRFs, IRF-4 and IRF-8 have critical functions in the B cell differentiation program. B cells development is blocked at the pre-B cells stage in IRF-4 and IRF-8 compound null mice (Lu *et al.*, 2003). IRF-4 also functions in late B cells development regulating IgG class switching and plasma cell development (Sciammas *et al.*, 2006). IRF-8 has a role in germinal centre transcription program (Lee *et al.*, 2006). Altogether, these data indicate that several members of the IRF family can affect B-cell development, however the strong genetic association between IRF-5 and autoimmune disease point out to a unique functions of IRF-5 in the immune system.

11. Induction of autoimmunity by IFNs

How the IFNs contribute to SLE and its progress remains to be fully explained. The presence of immunogenic complexes leads to dendritic cell activation and thus there is a greater antigen presentation and more IFNs are secreted. IFNα increases the expression of autoantigens such as Ro52 and also induces apoptosis via translocation of Ro52 to the nucleus (Baechler *et al.*, 2004; Bennett *et al.*, 2003). Type I IFNs also induce the maturation and activation of dendritic cells, along with upregulation of MHC Class I and II molecules (Baccala *et al.*, 2007). This promotes the development of helper T cells (Th1). In addition, Type I IFNs also enhance antibody production and class switching, decrease the selectivity of B cells for CpG-rich DNA, and permit stimulation by even non-CpG DNA and thereby promote an autoimmune response (Jego *et al.*, 2003; Le Bon *et al.*, 2006). How does IRF-5 contribute to this picture?

12. Genetic association studies and SLE

Genetic and population association studies provide a more comprehensive picture of the role of IFNs in SLE, reviewed in (Delgado-Vega *et al.*, 2010). Of the entire battery of genes identified by genome wide association studies, most of the genes are involved in innate and adaptive immune responses. These can be divided into the following groups: (1) genes implicated in processing and presentation of immune complexes, (2) genes involved in the IFN-inducing pathways, and (3) genes involved in the Type I IFN signalling pathway. Of the first group, the MHC region shows up as a prime candidate in correlation studies, but is challenging to study since the region has hundreds of potential candidate genes (Deng and Tsao 2010; Sestak *et al.*, 2011). In the IFN-inducing pathways, transcription factor IRF-5 was the first identified gene directly to be associated with increased risk of lupus (Graham *et al.*, 2006; Sigurdsson *et al.*, 2005). IRF-5 allele variants with the highest probability of being causal were identified and shown to affect IRF-5 expression. Patients with a risk haplotype of IRF-5 show higher serum IFN activity, when compared to patients lacking this risk genotype. Finally, in the IFN signalling pathway, STAT4, a downstream interacting protein of IFNAR, is also strongly associated with lupus (Kariuki *et al.*, 2009). STAT4 is associated with increased sensitivity to IFNα and the presence of anti-dsDNA autoantibodies. In addition, polymorphisms in the Janus kinase tyrosine kinase 2 (TYK2), which binds to IFNAR, and is part of the initiation of the JAK-STAT pathway, was also found to be associated with lupus and strengthen the link between IFNα expression and SLE. Several other gene products that are part of the IFN signalling pathway, such as TNFAIP3, TYK2, and TREX1, have been also associated with susceptibility to SLE (Adrianto *et al.*, 2011; Fan *et al.*, 2011; Hellquist *et al.*, 2009). Recently identified SNPs in IRF7 also seem to be associated with SLE. (Fu *et al.*, 2011). It is unlikely that the alteration of the function of a single master gene will be responsible for the pathogenesis of SLE; rather it may be combination of malfunction of several genes. Without doubt there is still the potential of finding new genes that contribute to the development of SLE.

13. IRF-5 polymorphisms and association with SLE

IRF-5 was identified as a risk factor for SLE in two very important association studies. Sigurdsson *et al.* looked at sets of lupus patients from Sweden, Finland and Iceland and analyzed 4 SNPs of IRF-5 (Sigurdsson *et al.*, 2005). Graham *et al.* (Graham *et al.*, 2007) describe two functional SNPs within the IRF-5 gene which are a risk haplotype for SLE. One SNP, rs2004640, creates a donor splice site in intron 1 of IRF-5 and the isoform expresses an alternative of untranslated exon 1B. A second SNP is located about 5 kb downstream of IRF-5 and could not be tied to functional importance but is used as a haplotype tag (Graham *et al.*, 2007). Later, several groups identified a second polymorphism that has more easily identifiable functional roles. rs10954213 alters the polyadenylation site of IRF-5 and the resultant mRNA cal be correlated to higher levels of IRF-5 seen in SLE (Sigurdsson *et al.*, 2008). The A allele of this SNP leads to a shorter and more stable mRNA. Finally, an insertion- deletion is found in the 6th exon of IRF-5 that can potentially change the protein isoforms expressed IRF-5 by 10 amino acids (Kozyrev *et al.*, 2007). The deletion results in expression of the isoforms V1 and V4, while the insertion give rise to isoforms V5 and V6. The lupus risk haplotype, TCA, includes the insertion TCA and thus individuals with lupus are expected to express the corresponding isoforms (V5 and V6). The sequence added by the insertion/deletion gives rise to a proline-rich region which can be potentially recruited for additional protein -protein interactions and/or protein stability by altering the degradation rate of the resulting protein.

Even though the genetic association of lupus and IRF-5 has been consistent, the initial studies dealt with an overwhelmingly European population and there are some suggestions that the association factors might be population specific. Studies in Asian populations have identified new susceptibility genes for lupus, while some of the previously known ones have been discounted (Kawasaki *et al.*, 2008; Li *et al.*, 2011; Shimane *et al.*, 2009; Shin *et al.*, 2008; Siu *et al.*, 2008), reviewed in (Kim *et al.*, 2009). Given that the majority of lupus patients are women, genetic imprinting remains yet an unexplored topic. However very interesting is a recent finding showing that IRF-5 is expressed at higher levels in female than in male mice and that the IRF-5 promoter is under hormonal regulation (Shen *et al.*, 2010).

14. Conclusions and future perspectives

Identification of the IRF-5 gene as a genetic risk factor for SLE helps to dissect its role in the IFNα pathway in pathogenesis of SLE. The SNP, rs10954213, that affects the levels of IRF-5 expression through increasing the stability of its mRNA, has a great impact on function and expression of protein, but has not found to be strongly associated as a risk haplotype. Thus many questions remain. Higher levels of IRF-5 might result not only in continued production of type I IFN but also of the proinflammatory cytokines. Are these cytokines responsible for the activation of the immune cells such as B cells? Hyper activation of B cells is one of the markers of SLE and the results in mice indicate that IRF-5 has an important role in cell differentiation and induction of IgG2a subtype, which is an important subtype for the induction of autoimmunity. In humans, the IgG2a isotype corresponds to IgG1, which is the dominant subclass of serum autoantibodies in SLE (Manolova *et al.*, 2002). The biological role of IRF-5 isoforms remains to be determined. Presently we do not know whether TCA haplotype IRF-5 has a distinct function from the other IRF-5 variants or whether it induces different group of the inflammatory genes or IFN A variants. It would be of great interest to learn about the roles of the IRF-5 induced genes and their variation in SLE patients. Now

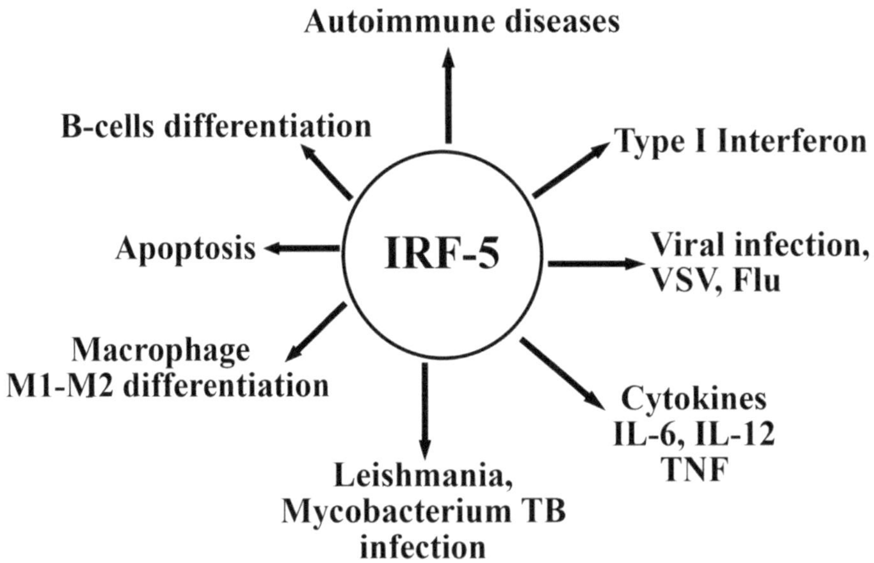

Fig. 1. Various roles of IRF-5 in immunity and autoimmune diseases.

that IRF-5 has been identified as an important factor in induction of type IFN in lupus, it will be important to determine which of the other IRF-5 regulated genes contribute to the pathogenicity of the disease. A recent observation that EBV might also be implicated in the activation of Type I IFN in SLE patients (Yadav *et al.*, 2011) might be an important link in dissecting the cross-talk between genetic predisposition or risk factors and environmental stimuli. Is there any cross talk between IRF-5 and some of the other gene products that were also identified to be associated with Lupus disease? Many of these questions remain yet to be explored to understand the impact of IRF-5 in SLE biology (Figure 1).

15. Acknowledgement

This work was supported by the NIAID grant R01 AI067632-05 to PMP.

16. References

Adrianto I, Wen F, Templeton A, Wiley G, King JB, Lessard CJ, Bates JS, Hu Y, Kelly JA, Kaufman KM, Guthridge JM, Alarcon-Riquelme ME, Anaya JM, Bae SC, Bang SY, Boackle SA, Brown EE, Petri MA, Gallant C, Ramsey-Goldman R, Reveille JD, Vila LM, Criswell LA, Edberg JC, Freedman BI, Gregersen PK, Gilkeson GS, Jacob CO, James JA, Kamen DL, Kimberly RP, Martin J, Merrill JT, Niewold TB, Park SY, Pons-Estel BA, Scofield RH, Stevens AM, Tsao BP, Vyse TJ, Langefeld CD, Harley JB, Moser KL, Webb CF, Humphrey MB, Montgomery CG, Gaffney PM. 2011. Association of a functional variant downstream of TNFAIP3 with systemic lupus erythematosus. *Nat Genet* 43(3):253-8.

Au WC, Moore PA, LaFleur DW, Tombal B, Pitha PM. 1998. Characterization of the interferon regulatory factor-7 and its potential role in the transcription activation of interferon A genes. *J Biol Chem* 273(44):29210-7.

Au WC, Moore PA, Lowther W, Juang YT, Pitha PM. 1995. Identification of a member of the interferon regulatory factor family that binds to the interferon-stimulated response element and activates expression of interferon-induced genes. *Proc Natl Acad Sci U S A* 92(25):11657-61.

Baccala R, Hoebe K, Kono DH, Beutler B, Theofilopoulos AN. 2007. TLR-dependent and TLR-independent pathways of type I interferon induction in systemic autoimmunity. *Nat Med* 13(5):543-51.

Baechler EC, Batliwalla FM, Karypis G, Gaffney PM, Moser K, Ortmann WA, Espe KJ, Balasubramanian S, Hughes KM, Chan JP, Begovich A, Chang SY, Gregersen PK, Behrens TW. 2004. Expression levels for many genes in human peripheral blood cells are highly sensitive to ex vivo incubation. *Genes Immun* 5(5):347-53.

Baechler EC, Batliwalla FM, Karypis G, Gaffney PM, Ortmann WA, Espe KJ, Shark KB, Grande WJ, Hughes KM, Kapur V, Gregersen PK, Behrens TW. 2003. Interferon-inducible gene expression signature in peripheral blood cells of patients with severe lupus. *Proc Natl Acad Sci U S A* 100(5):2610-5.

Balkhi MY, Fitzgerald KA, Pitha PM. 2008. Functional regulation of MyD88-activated interferon regulatory factor 5 by K63-linked polyubiquitination. *Mol Cell Biol* 28(24):7296-308.

Balkhi MY, Fitzgerald KA, Pitha PM. 2010. IKKalpha negatively regulates IRF-5 function in a MyD88-TRAF6 pathway. *Cell Signal* 22(1):117-27.

Barnes BJ, Kellum MJ, Pinder KE, Frisancho JA, Pitha PM. 2003. Interferon regulatory factor 5, a novel mediator of cell cycle arrest and cell death. *Cancer Res* 63(19):6424-31.

Barnes BJ, Moore PA, Pitha PM. 2001. Virus-specific activation of a novel interferon regulatory factor, IRF-5, results in the induction of distinct interferon alpha genes. *J Biol Chem* 276(26):23382-90.

Barnes BJ, Richards J, Mancl M, Hanash S, Beretta L, Pitha PM. 2004. Global and distinct targets of IRF-5 and IRF-7 during innate response to viral infection. *J Biol Chem* 279(43):45194-207.

Bengtsson AA, Sturfelt G, Truedsson L, Blomberg J, Alm G, Vallin H, Ronnblom L. 2000. Activation of type I interferon system in systemic lupus erythematosus correlates with disease activity but not with antiretroviral antibodies. *Lupus* 9(9):664-71.

Bennett L, Palucka AK, Arce E, Cantrell V, Borvak J, Banchereau J, Pascual V. 2003. Interferon and granulopoiesis signatures in systemic lupus erythematosus blood. *J Exp Med* 197(6):711-23.

Blomberg S, Eloranta ML, Cederblad B, Nordlin K, Alm GV, Ronnblom L. 2001. Presence of cutaneous interferon-alpha producing cells in patients with systemic lupus erythematosus. *Lupus* 10(7):484-90.

Burns K, Clatworthy J, Martin L, Martinon F, Plumpton C, Maschera B, Lewis A, Ray K, Tschopp J, Volpe F. 2000. Tollip, a new component of the IL-1RI pathway, links IRAK to the IL-1 receptor. *Nat Cell Biol* 2(6):346-51.

Cao Z, Henzel WJ, Gao X. 1996. IRAK: a kinase associated with the interleukin-1 receptor. *Science* 271(5252):1128-31.

Chen W, Lam SS, Srinath H, Jiang Z, Correia JJ, Schiffer CA, Fitzgerald KA, Lin K, Royer WE, Jr. 2008. Insights into interferon regulatory factor activation from the crystal structure of dimeric IRF5. *Nat Struct Mol Biol* 15(11):1213-20.

Chiu YL, Greene WC. 2008. The APOBEC3 cytidine deaminases: an innate defensive network opposing exogenous retroviruses and endogenous retroelements. *Annu Rev Immunol* 26:317-53.

Couzinet A, Tamura K, Chen HM, Nishimura K, Wang Z, Morishita Y, Takeda K, Yagita H, Yanai H, Taniguchi T, Tamura T. 2008. A cell-type-specific requirement for IFN regulatory factor 5 (IRF5) in Fas-induced apoptosis. *Proc Natl Acad Sci U S A* 105(7):2556-61.

Crow MK. 2009. Developments in the clinical understanding of lupus. *Arthritis Res Ther* 11(5):245.

Crow MK, Kirou KA, Wohlgemuth J. 2003. Microarray analysis of interferon-regulated genes in SLE. *Autoimmunity* 36(8):481-90.

De Rycke L, Baeten D, Kruithof E, Van den Bosch F, Veys EM, De Keyser F. 2005. The effect of TNFalpha blockade on the antinuclear antibody profile in patients with chronic arthritis: biological and clinical implications. *Lupus* 14(12):931-7.

Delgado-Vega AM, Alarcon-Riquelme ME, Kozyrev SV. 2010. Genetic associations in type I interferon related pathways with autoimmunity. *Arthritis Res Ther* 12 Suppl 1:S2.

Deng Y, Tsao BP. 2010. Genetic susceptibility to systemic lupus erythematosus in the genomic era. *Nat Rev Rheumatol* 6(12):683-92.

Diebold SS, Kaisho T, Hemmi H, Akira S, Reis e Sousa C. 2004. Innate antiviral responses by means of TLR7-mediated recognition of single-stranded RNA. *Science* 303(5663):1529-31.

Feng D, Stone RC, Eloranta ML, Sangster-Guity N, Nordmark G, Sigurdsson S, Wang C, Alm G, Syvanen AC, Ronnblom L, Barnes BJ. 2010. Genetic variants and disease-associated factors contribute to enhanced interferon regulatory factor 5 expression in blood cells of patients with systemic lupus erythematosus. *Arthritis Rheum* 62(2):562-73.

Fitzgerald-Bocarsly P, Dai J, Singh S. 2008. Plasmacytoid dendritic cells and type I IFN: 50 years of convergent history. *Cytokine Growth Factor Rev* 19(1):3-19.

Fu Q, Zhao J, Qian X, Wong JL, Kaufman KM, Yu CY, Mok MY, Harley JB, Guthridge JM, Song YW, Cho SK, Bae SC, Grossman JM, Hahn BH, Arnett FC, Shen N, Tsao BP. 2011. Association of a functional IRF7 variant with systemic lupus erythematosus. *Arthritis Rheum* 63(3):749-54.

George CX, Gan Z, Liu Y, Samuel CE. 2011. Adenosine deaminases acting on RNA, RNA editing, and interferon action. *J Interferon Cytokine Res* 31(1):99-117.

Gota C, Calabrese L. 2003. Induction of clinical autoimmune disease by therapeutic interferon-alpha. *Autoimmunity* 36(8):511-8.

Graham RR, Kozyrev SV, Baechler EC, Reddy MV, Plenge RM, Bauer JW, Ortmann WA, Koeuth T, Gonzalez Escribano MF, Pons-Estel B, Petri M, Daly M, Gregersen PK, Martin J, Altshuler D, Behrens TW, Alarcon-Riquelme ME. 2006. A common haplotype of interferon regulatory factor 5 (IRF5) regulates splicing and expression and is associated with increased risk of systemic lupus erythematosus. *Nat Genet* 38(5):550-5.

Graham RR, Kyogoku C, Sigurdsson S, Vlasova IA, Davies LR, Baechler EC, Plenge RM, Koeuth T, Ortmann WA, Hom G, Bauer JW, Gillett C, Burtt N, Cunninghame Graham DS, Onofrio R, Petri M, Gunnarsson I, Svenungsson E, Ronnblom L, Nordmark G, Gregersen PK, Moser K, Gaffney PM, Criswell LA, Vyse TJ, Syvanen AC, Bohjanen PR, Daly MJ, Behrens TW, Altshuler D. 2007. Three functional variants of IFN regulatory factor 5 (IRF5) define risk and protective haplotypes for human lupus. *Proc Natl Acad Sci U S A* 104(16):6758-63.

Hansen A, Henderson S, Lagos D, Nikitenko L, Coulter E, Roberts S, Gratrix F, Plaisance K, Renne R, Bower M, Kellam P, Boshoff C. 2010. KSHV-encoded miRNAs target MAF to induce endothelial cell reprogramming. *Genes Dev* 24(2):195-205.

Heil F, Hemmi H, Hochrein H, Ampenberger F, Kirschning C, Akira S, Lipford G, Wagner H, Bauer S. 2004. Species-specific recognition of single-stranded RNA via toll-like receptor 7 and 8. *Science* 303(5663):1526-9.

Hellquist A, Jarvinen TM, Koskenmies S, Zucchelli M, Orsmark-Pietras C, Berglind L, Panelius J, Hasan T, Julkunen H, D'Amato M, Saarialho-Kere U, Kere J. 2009. Evidence for genetic association and interaction between the TYK2 and IRF5 genes in systemic lupus erythematosus. *J Rheumatol* 36(8):1631-8.

Hemmi H, Kaisho T, Takeuchi O, Sato S, Sanjo H, Hoshino K, Horiuchi T, Tomizawa H, Takeda K, Akira S. 2002. Small anti-viral compounds activate immune cells via the TLR7 MyD88-dependent signaling pathway. *Nat Immunol* 3(2):196-200.

Ho V, McLean A, Terry S. 2008. Severe systemic lupus erythematosus induced by antiviral treatment for hepatitis C. *J Clin Rheumatol* 14(3):166-8.

Hu G, Mancl ME, Barnes BJ. 2005. Signaling through IFN regulatory factor-5 sensitizes p53-deficient tumors to DNA damage-induced apoptosis and cell death. *Cancer Res* 65(16):7403-12.

Improta T, Schindler C, Horvath CM, Kerr IM, Stark GR, Darnell JE, Jr. 1994. Transcription factor ISGF-3 formation requires phosphorylated Stat91 protein, but Stat113 protein is phosphorylated independently of Stat91 protein. *Proc Natl Acad Sci U S A* 91(11):4776-80.

Ishikawa H, Barber GN. 2011. The STING pathway and regulation of innate immune signaling in response to DNA pathogens. *Cell Mol Life Sci* 68(7):1157-65.

Jego G, Palucka AK, Blanck JP, Chalouni C, Pascual V, Banchereau J. 2003. Plasmacytoid dendritic cells induce plasma cell differentiation through type I interferon and interleukin 6. *Immunity* 19(2):225-34.

Kariuki SN, Kirou KA, MacDermott EJ, Barillas-Arias L, Crow MK, Niewold TB. 2009. Cutting edge: autoimmune disease risk variant of STAT4 confers increased sensitivity to IFN-alpha in lupus patients in vivo. *J Immunol* 182(1):34-8.

Kawai T, Adachi O, Ogawa T, Takeda K, Akira S. 1999. Unresponsiveness of MyD88-deficient mice to endotoxin. *Immunity* 11(1):115-22.

Kawasaki A, Kyogoku C, Ohashi J, Miyashita R, Hikami K, Kusaoi M, Tokunaga K, Takasaki Y, Hashimoto H, Behrens TW, Tsuchiya N. 2008. Association of IRF5 polymorphisms with systemic lupus erythematosus in a Japanese population: support for a crucial role of intron 1 polymorphisms. *Arthritis Rheum* 58(3):826-34.

Kim I, Kim YJ, Kim K, Kang C, Choi CB, Sung YK, Lee HS, Bae SC. 2009. Genetic studies of systemic lupus erythematosus in Asia: where are we now? *Genes Immun* 10(5):421-32.

Kozyrev SV, Alarcon-Riquelme ME. 2007. The genetics and biology of Irf5-mediated signaling in lupus. *Autoimmunity* 40(8):591-601.

Kozyrev SV, Lewen S, Reddy PM, Pons-Estel B, Witte T, Junker P, Laustrup H, Gutierrez C, Suarez A, Francisca Gonzalez-Escribano M, Martin J, Alarcon-Riquelme ME. 2007. Structural insertion/deletion variation in IRF5 is associated with a risk haplotype and defines the precise IRF5 isoforms expressed in systemic lupus erythematosus. *Arthritis Rheum* 56(4):1234-41.

Krausgruber T, Blazek K, Smallie T, Alzabin S, Lockstone H, Sahgal N, Hussell T, Feldmann M, Udalova IA. 2011. IRF5 promotes inflammatory macrophage polarization and TH1-TH17 responses. *Nat Immunol* 12(3):231-8.

Kumar A, Haque J, Lacoste J, Hiscott J, Williams BR. 1994. Double-stranded RNA-dependent protein kinase activates transcription factor NF-kappa B by phosphorylating I kappa B. *Proc Natl Acad Sci U S A* 91(14):6288-92.

Lagos D, Pollara G, Henderson S, Gratrix F, Fabani M, Milne RS, Gotch F, Boshoff C. 2010. miR-132 regulates antiviral innate immunity through suppression of the p300 transcriptional co-activator. *Nat Cell Biol* 12(5):513-9.

Le Bon A, Thompson C, Kamphuis E, Durand V, Rossmann C, Kalinke U, Tough DF. 2006. Cutting edge: enhancement of antibody responses through direct stimulation of B and T cells by type I IFN. *J Immunol* 176(4):2074-8.

Lee CH, Melchers M, Wang H, Torrey TA, Slota R, Qi CF, Kim JY, Lugar P, Kong HJ, Farrington L, van der Zouwen B, Zhou JX, Lougaris V, Lipsky PE, Grammer AC, Morse HC, 3rd. 2006. Regulation of the germinal center gene program by interferon (IFN) regulatory factor 8/IFN consensus sequence-binding protein. *J Exp Med* 203(1):63-72.

Lee MS, Kim YJ. 2007. Signaling pathways downstream of pattern-recognition receptors and their cross talk. *Annu Rev Biochem* 76:447-80.

Levy DE, Darnell JE, Jr. 2002. Stats: transcriptional control and biological impact. *Nat Rev Mol Cell Biol* 3(9):651-62.

Li P, Chang YK, Shek KW, Lau YL. 2011. Lack of association of TYK2 gene polymorphisms in chinese patients with systemic lupus erythematosus. *J Rheumatol* 38(1):177-8.

Li S, Strelow A, Fontana EJ, Wesche H. 2002. IRAK-4: a novel member of the IRAK family with the properties of an IRAK-kinase. *Proc Natl Acad Sci U S A* 99(8):5567-72.

Lien C, Fang CM, Huso D, Livak F, Lu R, Pitha PM. 2010. Critical role of IRF-5 in regulation of B-cell differentiation. *Proc Natl Acad Sci U S A* 107(10):4664-8.

Lu R, Medina KL, Lancki DW, Singh H. 2003. IRF-4,8 orchestrate the pre-B-to-B transition in lymphocyte development. *Genes Dev* 17(14):1703-8.

Mancl ME, Hu G, Sangster-Guity N, Olshalsky SL, Hoops K, Fitzgerald-Bocarsly P, Pitha PM, Pinder K, Barnes BJ. 2005. Two discrete promoters regulate the alternatively spliced human interferon regulatory factor-5 isoforms. Multiple isoforms with distinct cell type-specific expression, localization, regulation, and function. *J Biol Chem* 280(22):21078-90.

Manolova I, Dancheva M, Halacheva K. 2002. Predominance of IgG1 and IgG3 subclasses of autoantibodies to neutrophil cytoplasmic antigens in patients with systemic lupus erythematosus. *Rheumatol Int* 21(6):227-33.

Marie I, Durbin JE, Levy DEs. 1998. Differential viral induction of distinct interferon-alpha genes by positive feedback through interferon regulatory factor-7. *EMBO J.* 17(22):6660-9.

Martin MU, Wesche H. 2002. Summary and comparison of the signaling mechanisms of the Toll/interleukin-1 receptor family. *Biochim Biophys Acta* 1592(3):265-80.

Mori T, Anazawa Y, Iiizumi M, Fukuda S, Nakamura Y, Arakawa H. 2002. Identification of the interferon regulatory factor 5 gene (IRF-5) as a direct target for p53. *Oncogene* 21(18):2914-8.

Muzio M, Ni J, Feng P, Dixit VM. 1997. IRAK (Pelle) family member IRAK-2 and MyD88 as proximal mediators of IL-1 signaling. *Science* 278(5343):1612-5.

Niewold TB, Hua J, Lehman TJ, Harley JB, Crow MK. 2007. High serum IFN-alpha activity is a heritable risk factor for systemic lupus erythematosus. *Genes Immun* 8(6):492-502.

O'Connell RM, Taganov KD, Boldin MP, Cheng G, Baltimore D. 2007. MicroRNA-155 is induced during the macrophage inflammatory response. *Proc Natl Acad Sci U S A* 104(5):1604-9.

Paun A, Reinert JT, Jiang Z, Medin C, Balkhi MY, Fitzgerald KA, Pitha PM. 2008. Functional characterization of murine interferon regulatory factor 5 (IRF-5) and its role in the innate antiviral response. *J Biol Chem* 283(21):14295-308.

Pedersen IM, Cheng G, Wieland S, Volinia S, Croce CM, Chisari FV, David M. 2007. Interferon modulation of cellular microRNAs as an antiviral mechanism. *Nature* 449(7164):919-22.

Pindel A, Sadler A. 2011. The role of protein kinase R in the interferon response. *J Interferon Cytokine Res* 31(1):59-70.

Pitha PM, Kunzi MS. 2007. Type I interferon: the ever unfolding story. *Curr Top Microbiol Immunol* 316:41-70.

Platanias LC. 2005. Introduction: interferon signals: what is classical and what is nonclassical? *J Interferon Cytokine Res* 25(12):732.

Richez C, Yasuda K, Bonegio RG, Watkins AA, Aprahamian T, Busto P, Richards RJ, Liu CL, Cheung R, Utz PJ, Marshak-Rothstein A, Rifkin IR. 2010. IFN regulatory factor 5 is required for disease development in the FcgammaRIIB-/-Yaa and FcgammaRIIB-/- mouse models of systemic lupus erythematosus. *J Immunol* 184(2):796-806.

Ronco LV, Karpova AY, Vidal M, Howley PM. 1998. Human papillomavirus 16 E6 oncoprotein binds to interferon regulatory factor-3 and inhibits its transcriptional activity. *Genes Dev* 12(13):2061-72.

Samuel CE. 1993. The eIF-2 alpha protein kinases, regulators of translation in eukaryotes from yeasts to humans. *J Biol Chem* 268(11):7603-6.

Samuel CE. 2001. Antiviral actions of interferons. *Clin Microbiol Rev* 14(4):778-809, table of contents.

Santer DM, Yoshio T, Minota S, Moller T, Elkon KB. 2009. Potent induction of IFN-alpha and chemokines by autoantibodies in the cerebrospinal fluid of patients with neuropsychiatric lupus. *J Immunol* 182(2):1192-201.

Savarese E, Chae OW, Trowitzsch S, Weber G, Kastner B, Akira S, Wagner H, Schmid RM, Bauer S, Krug A. 2006. U1 small nuclear ribonucleoprotein immune complexes induce type I interferon in plasmacytoid dendritic cells through TLR7. *Blood* 107(8):3229-34.

Savitsky DA, Yanai H, Tamura T, Taniguchi T, Honda K. 2010. Contribution of IRF5 in B cells to the development of murine SLE-like disease through its transcriptional control of the IgG2a locus. *Proc Natl Acad Sci U S A* 107(22):10154-9.

Schoenemeyer A, Barnes BJ, Mancl ME, Latz E, Goutagny N, Pitha PM, Fitzgerald KA, Golenbock DT. 2005. The interferon regulatory factor, IRF5, is a central mediator of toll-like receptor 7 signaling. *J Biol Chem* 280(17):17005-12.

Schoggins JW, Wilson SJ, Panis M, Murphy MY, Jones CT, Bieniasz P, Rice CM. 2011. A diverse range of gene products are effectors of the type I interferon antiviral response. *Nature*.

Sciammas R, Shaffer AL, Schatz JH, Zhao H, Staudt LM, Singh H. 2006. Graded expression of interferon regulatory factor-4 coordinates isotype switching with plasma cell differentiation. *Immunity* 25(2):225-36.

Sestak AL, Furnrohr BG, Harley JB, Merrill JT, Namjou B. 2011. The genetics of systemic lupus erythematosus and implications for targeted therapy. *Ann Rheum Dis* 70 Suppl 1:i37-43.

Shen H, Panchanathan R, Rajavelu P, Duan X, Gould KA, Choubey D. 2010. Gender-dependent expression of murine Irf5 gene: implications for sex bias in autoimmunity. *J Mol Cell Biol* 2(5):284-90.

Shimane K, Kochi Y, Yamada R, Okada Y, Suzuki A, Miyatake A, Kubo M, Nakamura Y, Yamamoto K. 2009. A single nucleotide polymorphism in the IRF5 promoter region is associated with susceptibility to rheumatoid arthritis in the Japanese population. *Ann Rheum Dis* 68(3):377-83.

Shin HD, Kim I, Choi CB, Lee SO, Lee HW, Bae SC. 2008. Different genetic effects of interferon regulatory factor 5 (IRF5) polymorphisms on systemic lupus erythematosus in a Korean population. *J Rheumatol* 35(11):2148-51.

Sigurdsson S, Goring HH, Kristjansdottir G, Milani L, Nordmark G, Sandling JK, Eloranta ML, Feng D, Sangster-Guity N, Gunnarsson I, Svenungsson E, Sturfelt G, Jonsen A, Truedsson L, Barnes BJ, Alm G, Ronnblom L, Syvanen AC. 2008. Comprehensive evaluation of the genetic variants of interferon regulatory factor 5 (IRF5) reveals a novel 5 bp length polymorphism as strong risk factor for systemic lupus erythematosus. *Hum Mol Genet* 17(6):872-81.

Sigurdsson S, Nordmark G, Goring HH, Lindroos K, Wiman AC, Sturfelt G, Jonsen A, Rantapaa-Dahlqvist S, Moller B, Kere J, Koskenmies S, Widen E, Eloranta ML, Julkunen H, Kristjansdottir H, Steinsson K, Alm G, Ronnblom L, Syvanen AC. 2005. Polymorphisms in the tyrosine kinase 2 and interferon regulatory factor 5 genes are associated with systemic lupus erythematosus. *Am J Hum Genet* 76(3):528-37.

Sigurdsson S, Padyukov L, Kurreeman FA, Liljedahl U, Wiman AC, Alfredsson L, Toes R, Ronnelid J, Klareskog L, Huizinga TW, Alm G, Syvanen AC, Ronnblom L. 2007. Association of a haplotype in the promoter region of the interferon regulatory factor 5 gene with rheumatoid arthritis. *Arthritis Rheum* 56(7):2202-10.

Silvestris F, Tucci M, Quatraro C, Dammacco F. 2003. Recent advances in understanding the pathogenesis of anemia in multiple myeloma. *Int J Hematol* 78(2):121-5.

Siu HO, Yang W, Lau CS, Chan TM, Wong RW, Wong WH, Lau YL, Alarcon-Riquelme ME. 2008. Association of a haplotype of IRF5 gene with systemic lupus erythematosus in Chinese. *J Rheumatol* 35(2):360-2.

Skaug B, Chen ZJ. 2010. Emerging role of ISG15 in antiviral immunity. *Cell* 143(2):187-90.

Takaoka A, Yanai H, Kondo S, Duncan G, Negishi H, Mizutani T, Kano S, Honda K, Ohba Y, Mak TW, Taniguchi T. 2005. Integral role of IRF-5 in the gene induction programme activated by Toll-like receptors. *Nature* 434(7030):243-9.

Uze G, Schreiber G, Piehler J, Pellegrini S. 2007. The receptor of the type I interferon family. *Curr Top Microbiol Immunol* 316:71-95.

Vollmer J, Tluk S, Schmitz C, Hamm S, Jurk M, Forsbach A, Akira S, Kelly KM, Reeves WH, Bauer S, Krieg AM. 2005. Immune stimulation mediated by autoantigen binding sites within small nuclear RNAs involves Toll-like receptors 7 and 8. *J Exp Med* 202(11):1575-85.

Vyse TJ, Morel L, Tanner FJ, Wakeland EK, Kotzin BL. 1996. Backcross analysis of genes linked to autoantibody production in New Zealand White mice. *J Immunol* 157(6):2719-27.

Yadav P, Tran H, Ebegbe R, Gottlieb P, Wei H, Lewis RH, Mumbey-Wafula A, Kaplan A, Kholdarova E, Spatz L. 2011. Antibodies elicited in response to EBNA-1 may cross-react with dsDNA. *PLoS One* 6(1):e14488.

Yanai H, Chen HM, Inuzuka T, Kondo S, Mak TW, Takaoka A, Honda K, Taniguchi T. 2007. Role of IFN regulatory factor 5 transcription factor in antiviral immunity and tumor suppression. *Proc Natl Acad Sci U S A* 104(9):3402-7.

3

SLAM Family Receptors and Autoimmunity

Jordi Sintes, Ricardo Bastos and Pablo Engel
Immunology Unit, Department of Cell Biology, Immunology and Neurosciences, Medical School, University of Barcelona
Institut d'Investigacions Biomèdiques August Pi i Sunyer, Barcelona
Spain

1. Introduction

The immune system is responsible for the defense against a wide array of pathogens but without responding to each individual's (self) antigens. Autoimmune diseases are characterized by a loss of tolerance to self antigens that leads to the appearance of auto-reactive lymphocytes. The main factors that contribute to the development of autoimmunity are genetic susceptibility and infection. Disease susceptibility is the result of the combined action of multiple genes. It has been shown that certain gene polymorphisms can influence the establishment of self-tolerance. The human immune system is a complex machinery involving numerous proteins. Cell-surface proteins expressed by leukocytes are of particular relevance due not only to their participation in the network of interactions that regulate the innate and adaptive immune responses, but also to their potential as excellent targets for diagnostic and therapeutic interventions (Diaz-Ramos et al., 2011). These molecules deliver signals that modulate leukocyte development, activation, survival, clonal expansion, and important effector functions. Some of these cell-surface signaling molecules have the capacity to activate lymphocytes and other leukocytes, while others function as down-modulators of immune responses, playing a key role in the establishment of tolerance to self antigens. Thus, it is not surprising that many of the allelic variants associated with autoimmunity identified, to date, correspond to leukocyte cell-surface molecules (Maier & Hafler, 2009). In this review we will discuss recent observations that point to a key role of signaling lymphocyte activation molecule family (SLAMF) receptors in the development of autoimmunity.

2. Signaling lymphocyte activation molecule family of cell-surface molecules

In recent years, the SLAMF of leukocyte cell-surface molecules has been identified as a group of receptors that modulates the activation and differentiation of a wide array of cell types involved in both innate and adaptive immune responses (Calpe et al., 2008; Detre et al., 2010; Schwartzberg et al., 2009; Vinuesa et al., 2010). The SLAMF, also known as the CD150 family, consists of nine structurally related leukocyte cell-surface glycoproteins that belong to the immunoglobulin (Ig) superfamily, namely: SLAMF1 (CD150 or SLAM), SLAMF2 (CD48), SLAMF3 (CD229 or LY9), SLAMF4 (CD244 or 2B4), SLAMF5 (CD84), SLAMF6 (CD352, NTB-A or Ly108), SLAMF7 (CD319 or CRACC), SLAMF8 (CD353 or BLAME) and SLAMF9 (CD84-H1) (Table 1).

Receptor	Aliases	Expression
SLAMF1	CD150, SLAM	B, T, DC, platelet, Mϕ
SLAMF2	**CD48**	B, T, monocyte, NK, DC, pDC, granulocytes, HSC, MPP
SLAMF3	CD229, **LY9**	B, T, pDC
SLAMF4	**CD244,** 2B4	NK, CD8 and γδ T, monocyte, basophil, eosinophil, mast cell, HSC, MPP
SLAMF5	**CD84**	B, T, mast cell, platelet, monocyte, granulocytes, Mϕ, DC, pDC, HSC, MPP
SLAMF6	CD352, NTB-A (Ly108 in mice)	B, T, NK, neutrophil, pDC
SLAMF7	CD319, CRACC, CS1	B, T, NK, DC, pDC
SLAMF8	CD353, BLAME	B, DC, monocyte, Mϕ
SLAMF9	CD84-H1, SF2001	B, T, monocyte, DC

Table 1. Members of the SLAM (CD150) family. The expression data apply largely to human cells. Receptor gene name is shown in bold. B=B cells, DC=dendritic cell, pDC=plasmacytoid DC, HSC= hematopoietic stem cells, Mϕ=macrophages, MPP=multipotent hematopoietic progenitors, NK=natural killer cells, SLAMF=SLAM family, T=T cells.

2.1 Genomic organization of the SLAM locus

Seven of the genes encoding SLAMF members are clustered within a 400-500 kilobase (kb) genomic segment on human chromosome 1q23 and on mouse chromosome 1H3 (Calpe et al., 2008; Engel et al., 2003). However, genes coding CD353 and SLAMF9 (CD84-H1) are located outside of, but in close proximity to, the SLAM locus (Calpe et al., 2008; Veillette et al., 2006). This characteristic implies that those genes encoding the SLAMF members were created by successive gene duplications of a single ancestor gene, raising the possibility that numerous polymorphisms and splice variants of most of the family members have subsequently been formed in this way. The majority of such variations mainly affect their corresponding ectodomains or the length of their respective cytoplasmic tails (Calpe et al., 2008; Veillette, 2010). Human EAT-2 and mouse Eat-2a and Eat-2b genes are also located close to the *SLAM* locus. Although the SLAMF genes are equally arranged in mouse and human genomes, they differ in its orientation; the genes that in humans are closer to the centromere are situated in mice closer to the telomere.

2.2 Structural characteristics of the SLAMF glycoproteins

2.2.1 Immunoglobulin domains and ligand interaction

SLAMF receptors are composed of an extracellular ectodomain formed by two Ig-like domains; one variable (V)-like lacking disulfide bonds followed by a truncated Ig constant 2 (C2)-like domain with two intradomain disulfide bonds, with the exception of CD229 (SLAMF3), which possesses four Ig-like domains (two tandem repeats of V-Ig/C2-Ig sets). SLAMF molecules are type I transmembrane glycoproteins containing a cytoplasmic tail, with the exception of CD48, which has a glycosylphosphatidylinositol (GPI) membrane anchor (Figure 1) (Calpe et al., 2008; Engel et al., 2003; Ma et al., 2007).

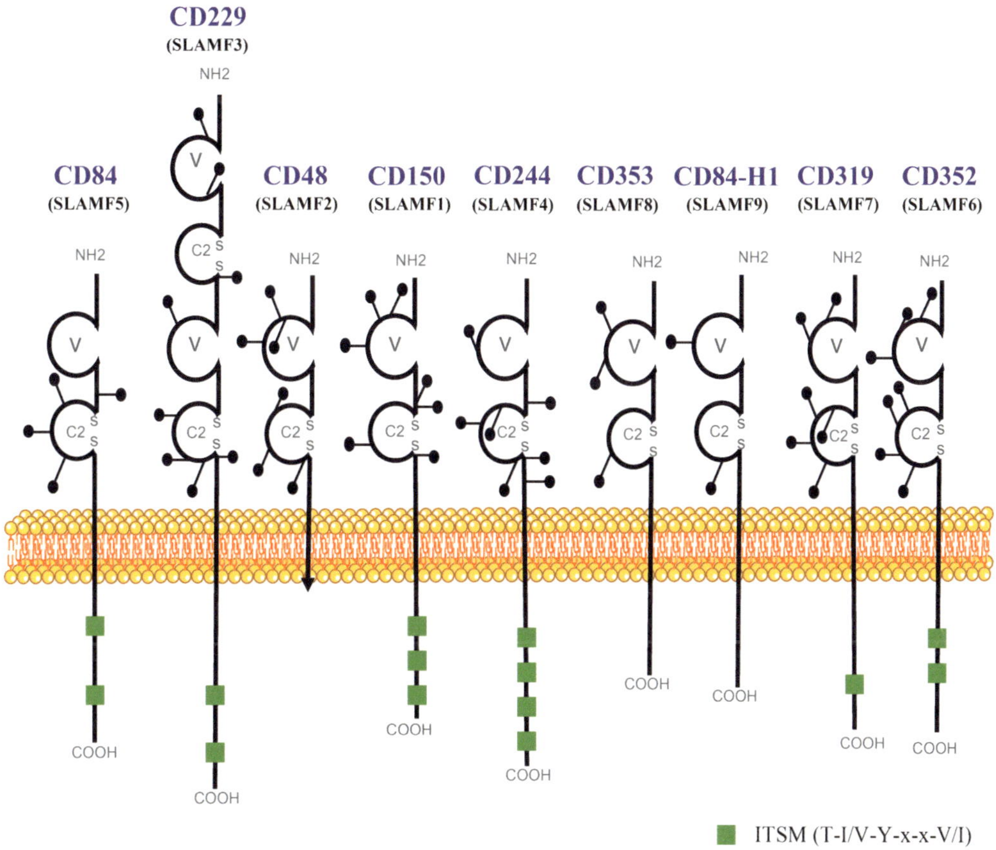

Fig. 1. Structural representation of the human SLAM family members. This structurally-related family of cell-surface receptors is composed by nine members. Their extracellular regions have two, or four in the case of CD229, Ig-like domains.

Excluding CD244, which recognizes CD48 as its ligand, SLAMF members are also characterized by acting as self-ligands through their N-terminal Ig domain (Table 2) (Engel et al., 2003). No interactions with other hematopoietic cell-surface molecules have been described, although CD150 (SLAM) has been reported to be one the major receptors for the measles virus, which accounts for its cell tropism (Tatsuo et al., 2000). Strikingly, mouse CD150 has recently been described as a microbial sensor that positively regulates bacterial killing by macrophages (Berger et al., 2010; Sintes & Engel, 2011). CD150 is able to efficiently recognize the porins OmpC and OmpF of *E. coli*'s outer membrane. Afterwards, the CD150/*E.coli* complex becomes internalized within the macrophage phagosome to govern key processes of bacterial removal machinery such as phagosome maturation and free radical species production by the NOX2 complex (Berger et al., 2010). Moreover, CD48 is known to interact with the Gram-negative lectin FimH in macrophages as well as in mast cells, although counter to CD150 functionality, FimH^{+} bacteria undergo encapsulation in caveolae rather than becoming internalized within mast cell phagosomes (Baorto et al., 1997; Shin et al., 2000). Whether other SLAMF members might function as bacterial receptors remains to be elucidated.

Receptor	Ligands	ITSMs	SAP/EAT-2 recruitment
SLAMF1	SLAMF1, measles virus, Gram-negative bacteria	2	+
SLAMF2	SLAMF4, CD2, FimH	None	-
SLAMF3	SLAMF3	H: 2 M: 1	+
SLAMF4	SLAMF2	4	+
SLAMF5	SLAMF5	2	+
SLAMF6	SLAMF6	2	+
SLAMF7	SLAMF7	H: 1 M: 0	EAT-2 (H)
SLAMF8	ND	None	-
SLAMF9	ND	None	-

Table 2. SLAM family ligands and ITSMs. H=human, ITSMs=immunoreceptor tyrosine-based binding motifs, M=mouse, ND=not determined, SLAMF=SLAM family.

2.2.2 The immunoreceptor tyrosine-based switch motif and cell signaling

Unlike other cosignaling molecules, the cytoplasmic tails of six of the SLAMF receptors ($SLAMF_{1,3\text{-}7}$) do not contain any ITAMs or ITIMs motifs, but rather possess one or more copies of a unique immunoreceptor tyrosine-based switch motif (ITSM) T-I/V-Y-x-x-V/I (where T is threonine, I is isoleucine, V is valine, Y is tyrosine and x denotes any amino acid), in addition to various tyrosine Y residues (Detre et al., 2010; Engel et al., 2003) (Figure 1 and Table 2). In the same way ITAM or ITIM becomes phosphorylated after receptor ligation, the homophilic engagement of SLAMF members triggers the phosphorylation of Y residues within the ITSM. Subsequently, ITSM serves as a docking site for intracellular adapter molecules and enzymes bearing SH2 domains such as SHP-2, SHP-1, Csk, and SHIP-1 (Mikhalap et al., 1999; Parolini et al., 2000; Tangye et al., 1999). The adapter molecules SLAM-associated protein (SAP), EWS/FLI activated transcript-2 (EAT-2) and EAT-2-related transducer (ERT), have high affinity for this unique motif (Calpe et al., 2008; Veillette et al., 2009). Importantly, the SAP-encoding gene (*SH2D1A*) is mutated in patients with X-linked lymphoproliferative disease.

SH2D1A is located on the X chromosome in humans and mice (Xq25 and XA5, respectively), which differs from SLAMF receptors and EAT-2 (Calpe et al., 2008). SAP is a small protein (15 kDa) composed of a SH2 domain followed by a 28-amino-acid tail (Figure 2). Human and mouse SAP molecules share 87% of their amino acid sequence, being highly similar in the SH2 domain. SAP is known to be expressed by NK, T cells, NKT cells, eosinophils, platelets and a subset of B cells (Engel et al., 2003). The SAP/SLAMF-receptor interaction occurs between the arginine 32 (R32), located in the SH2-domain of SAP, and the pY-containing ITSMs of SLAMF molecules. Apart from engaging these pY residues, SAP is able to specifically bind to the nonphosphorylated Y_{281} from one of the CD150 ITSMs. The high avidity shown by SAP to bind to these pY residues explain its ability to block the interaction of other SH2-containing molecules of lesser affinity to the same motif (Finerty et al., 2002; Howie et al., 2002; Lewis et al., 2001; Poy et al., 1999; Sayos et al., 1998).

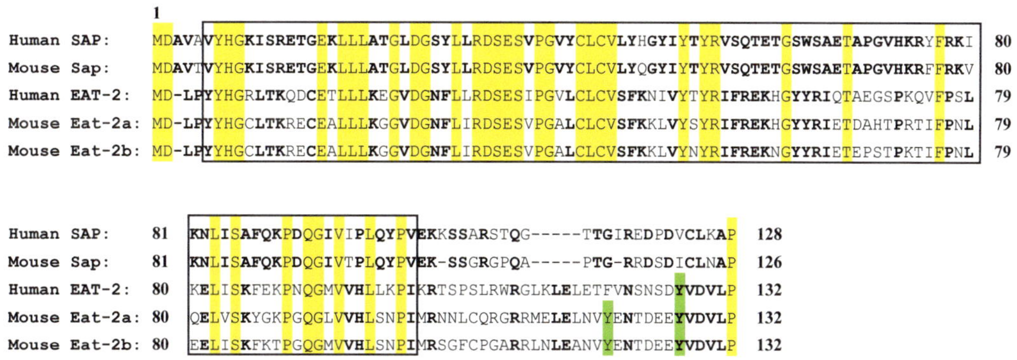

Fig. 2. Alignment of SAP and EAT-2 amino acidic sequences. The SH2 domains of SAP and EAT-2 are boxed. Conserved residues among both adaptors are highlighted in yellow, and those specifically conserved for each molecule are shown in bold. In green are the tyrosine residues present in the tail of EAT-2.

One of the particular features of SAP is that its arginine 78 (R78) interacts with the aspartic acid residue 100 (D100) of Fyn, a Src-related protein tyrosine kinase. Such association sequentially mediates Fyn recruitment to the cytoplasmic tail of the CD150 receptor and, following tyrosine phosphorylation, leads to the recruitment of SHIP, docking protein (Dok) 1, and Dok2 (Chan et al., 2003; Chen et al., 2006; Latour et al., 2001; Latour et al., 2003). Therefore, SAP has the ability to simultaneously associate with SLAMF molecules and Fyn, thus forming a trimolecular complex that also reportedly regulates the activation of Vav-1, Casitas B-lineage lymphoma (Cbl), Bcl-10, and protein kinase C-theta (PKC-θ)-mediated activation of NF-κB1 in T cells (Cannons et al., 2004; Cannons et al., 2010b; Claus et al., 2008; Zhong & Veillette, 2008). Furthermore, SAP can additionally engage Lck, which phosphorylates CD84, CD150, CD229 and CD244 (Howie et al., 2002; Martin et al., 2005; Nakajima et al., 2000; Tangye et al., 2003). The SAP-SH2 domain has also been described as interacting with the SH3 domain of PAK-interacting protein (β-PIX), a guanine nucleotide exchange factor (GEF) specific for Rac/Cdc42 GTPases (Gu et al., 2006).

Both human and murine EAT-2 genes are located at chromosome 1 (1q23 in humans and 1H3 in mice), in close proximity to SLAMF loci (Calpe et al., 2006). In contrast to human EAT-2, mouse and rat EAT-2 genes are duplicated with an identical genomic organization and encode two similar proteins, namely EAT-2A or EAT-2 and EAT-2B or ERT (Engel et al., 2003). The EAT-2B-encoding gene is a non-functional pseudo-gene in humans. In a manner similar to SAP, human and mouse EAT-2 genes encode small proteins composed of an SH2 domain followed by a short C-terminal tail, but also containing one and two tyrosines, respectively (Y_{120} and Y_{127}) (Figure 2) (Calpe et al., 2006; Roncagalli et al., 2005). EAT-2 is preferentially found not only in NK cells, but also in DC and macrophages, whereas EAT-2B is detected only in NK cells. Human EAT-2 is expressed by NK cells, activated $CD4^+$ and $CD8^+$ T cells, and γδ T lymphocytes (Calpe et al., 2006; Morra et al., 2001; Tassi & Colonna, 2005).

EAT-2 and EAT-2B can bind to the Src-like kinases Hck, Lyn, Lck, and Fgr kinases through their catalytic domains, although neither can directly bind to the SH3 domain of Fyn since both lack the R78 responsible for the association of SAP with Fyn (Calpe et al., 2006; Latour et al., 2003). Nevertheless, EAT-2 and mouse EAT-2A can couple to the SH2 domain of Fyn in NK cells when their C-terminal tyrosines undergo phosphorylation (Clarkson et al., 2007).

Another significant difference between EAT-2 and SAP is that EAT-2-mediated function has not been properly characterized. It was initially believed that these two adapter molecules played opposing roles in leukocyte activation (Ma et al., 2007). Multiple and more accurate studies have clearly confirmed that SAP is a positive regulator of lymphocyte activation, although data concerning EAT-2 activity remains controversial (Clarkson et al., 2007; Cruz-Munoz et al., 2009; Roncagalli et al., 2005; Tassi & Colonna, 2005; Wang et al., 2010b). Roncagalli *et al.* first described that, unlike SAP, EAT-2 and ERT were inhibitors of NK cell function when they became associated with CD244 (2B4) in 129*Sv* mice (Roncagalli et al., 2005). On the other hand, this same group demonstrated that mouse CD319 (SLAMF7) acts as a positive regulator of NK cell in a EAT-2A-dependent manner (Cruz-Munoz et al., 2009). Interestingly, a recent paper has shed light on the role played by EAT-2 in C57BL/6 NK cells. Wang and colleagues have shown that both, EAT-2A and ERT positively regulate mouse CD244- and CD84-specific NK cell functions (Wang et al., 2010b). The authors attribute this disparity in mouse EAT-2 functionality to the genetic background used to generate mice lacking or overexpressing EAT-2. Although there is convincing evidence, using mice with a pure genetic background, that EAT-2 acts as a positive modulator of NK cell functions, further experiments are needed to determine the mechanisms underlying EAT-2 downstream signaling.

It is important to keep in mind that SAP and EAT-2 specifically participate in the recruitment of Src-like kinases at the right time and in a precise cell compartment. In addition, since SAP and EAT-2 can bind to the same ITSM, it has been suggested that both adapter molecules may be able to compete for the same docking site. The outcome of this competition can result in the differential recruitment of intracellular kinases or phosphatases, and thus, in variations in the nature and intensity of activation and differentiation processes.

2.3 SLAMF receptors are expressed on hematopoietic cells

SLAMF receptors display a wide-ranging and differential distribution pattern among hematopoietic cells. They can be found on many immune cell types including different subsets of T and B lymphocytes, NK and NKT cells, monocytes, macrophages, DCs, pDCs, platelets, granulocytes, and hematopoietic stem and progenitor cells (Table 1) (Calpe et al., 2008; Engel et al., 2003; Ma et al., 2007). It should be noted that the analyses of SLAMF expression in mouse have thus far not been as exhaustive as in humans, and therefore some species-specific discrepancies may exist. As summarized in Table 1, their heterogeneous, but sometimes overlapping, expression patterns indicate that SLAMF members may play either redundant or specific functions in the regulation of a broad range of both innate and adaptive immune responses.

Kiel and colleagues first discovered that SLAMF receptors are selectively expressed among primitive mouse progenitors in the adult bone marrow in such a way that it is possible to highly purify HSCs using a simple combination of monoclonal antibodies (mAbs) against three of these receptors (CD150, CD244, and CD48) (Kiel et al., 2005). However, the direct combination of mAbs against SLAMF receptors is not suitable for purification of human HSCs (Sintes et al., 2008).

2.4 SLAMF receptors function as regulators of innate and adaptive immune responses

These receptors have been shown to modulate lymphocyte activation processes that are key elements in the initiation and progression of autoimmune diseases, such as the development of NKT cells, cytokine production in the thymus and periphery, NK- and CD8+ T- cell cytotoxicity, or germinal center (GC)-dependent antibody production (Figure 3 and Table 3) (Ma et al., 2007; Schwartzberg et al., 2009).

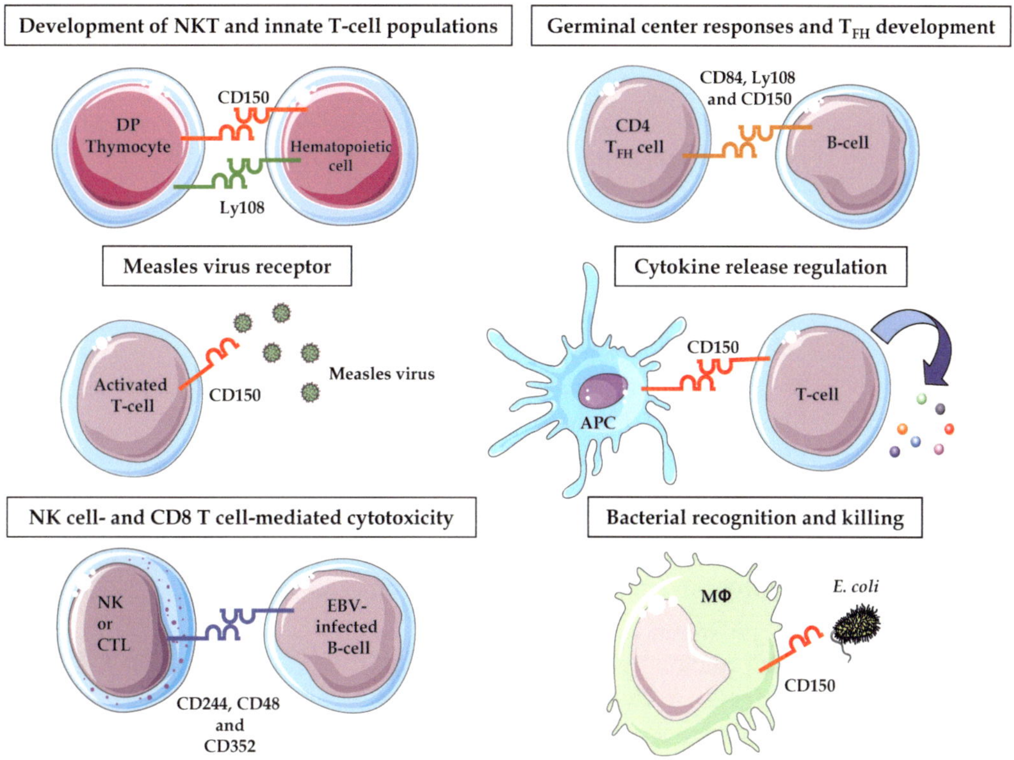

Fig. 3. SLAM family-mediated functions.

The differentiation of NKT cells and other innate-like lymphocytes appears to be triggered by SAP/Fyn signaling, which occurs when CD150 (SLAMF1) and Ly108 (SLAMF6) both present on the surface of double positive (DP) thymocytes, though not on thymic epithelial cells, homotypically engage (Griewank et al., 2007; Veillette et al., 2007). Additionally, non-obese diabetic (NOD) mice display diminished NKT cell numbers, which has been linked to a deficiency in CD150 expression during the DP thymocyte stage (Jordan et al., 2007). Supporting this concept, a recent paper has shown that impaired CD150 signaling affects the production of IL-4 and IL-10 by NOD mice NKT cells (Baev et al., 2008). Yet another recent report found that CD1d, CD150, Ly108, and SAP expression in DP thymocytes can be controlled by the transcription factor c-Myb. This regulation seems to be highly selective as other SLAMF members located in the same locus, such as SLAMF2, SLAMF3, and SLAMF5, are not affected (Hu et al., 2010). Despite this data, the generation of double or triple knock-out mice for specific SLAMF molecules would not only aid in comprehensively mapping those cell-surface molecules essential to the development of innate-like lymphocytes such as NKT cells, but would also help to precisely identify the overlapping functions of SLAMF receptors.

Although EBV is unable to infect mouse cells, several studies of SAP-deficient mice ($SAP^{-/-}$) have unraveled the various molecular and cellular mechanisms involved in the

Receptor	**Functions** (self-ligation, Ab stimulation or mutant mice)
SLAMF1	**T**: ↑ IL-4, IFN-γ secretion **Mϕ**: ↑ bacterial killing, IL-6, IL-12, TNF-α secretion **DC**: ↑ IL-8, IL-12 secretion **Platelet**: ↑ aggregates stability
SLAMF2	**T:** ↑ proliferation, IL-2 secretion **B, NK, DC:** regulates proliferation and activation
SLAMF3	**T:** ↓ IFN-γ secretion, ERK activation ↑ IL-2, IL-4 secretion and T-cell proliferation
SLAMF4	**NK, CD8 T**: ↑ cytotocicity, IFN-γ secretion **Eosinophil**: ↑ killing, cytokines, peroxidase release
SLAMF5	**T**: ↑ proliferation, IFN-γ secretion, T_{FH} function, T-B cell adhesion **Mast cell**: ↓ FcεRI-mediated signalling **Platelet**: ↑ aggregates stability
SLAMF6	**NK**: ↑ cytotoxicity, IL-8, IFN-γ, TNF-α secretion **CD8 T**: ↑ cytotoxicity, IFN-γ secretion **CD4 T**: Th1 polarized response **Neutrophil:** ↑ bacterial killing, ROS and cytokine production
SLAMF7	**B**: ↑ proliferation **NK**: ↑ cytotoxicity and killing
SLAMF8	ND
SLAMF9	ND

Table 3. Functions of SLAMF members. Ab= antibody, B=B cells, DC=dendritic cell, IFN=interferon, IL=interleukin, Mϕ=macrophages, ND=not determined, NK=natural killer cells, SLAMF=SLAM family, T=T cells, Th1=T helper 1 cell.

pathogenesis of XLP. In contrast to XLP patients, mice lacking SAP exhibit increased levels of $CD8^+$ T cell cytotoxicity compared with their wild-type (*wt*) counterparts (Chen et al., 2005; Crotty et al., 2006; Czar et al., 2001; Wu et al., 2001). After acute infection with lymphocytic choriomeningitis virus (LCMV) mice presented elevated levels of Ag-specific and IFN-γ secreting $CD8^+$ T cells. However, these mice died since were unable to resolve chronic infections (Crotty et al., 2006; Czar et al., 2001; Wu et al., 2001). Concomitantly, $SAP^{-/-}$ mice can also present compromised antibody responses to viruses such as murine γ-herpesvirus-68 (MHV-68) and influenza, as well as to parasites like *Toxoplasma gondii* and *Leishmania major* (Chen et al., 2005; Czar et al., 2001; Kamperschroer et al., 2006; Wu et al., 2001; Yin et al., 2003).

Multiple studies have clearly demonstrated the existence of a specific defect in $CD4^+$ T cell immunity. As in humans, $SAP^{-/-}$ mouse $CD4^+$ T cells are afflicted with such a defect; namely, they fail to properly differentiate into Th2 cells, subsequently presenting reduced levels of IL-4 (derived from diminished GATA-3 transcription factor levels), IL-10, and IL-

13. It has also been reported that SAP-mediated IL-4 release is dependent upon Fyn. On the other hand, Th1 cytokines such as IFN-γ typically become elevated (Cannons et al., 2004; Czar et al., 2001; Davidson et al., 2004; Wu et al., 2001). In addition, Wu *et al.* demonstrated that following infection with the parasite *L. major*, which is dependent upon Th2 cytokines to induce disease, $SAP^{-/-}$ mice became more resistant to the parasitic infections (Wu et al., 2001). XLP patients exhibit an extreme deficiency in IL-10 secretion by $CD4^{+}$ T cells, but not in either IL-4 or IFN-γ production (Ma et al., 2005). In this same study Ma *et al.* reported that upon Ag-stimulation of $CD4^{+}$ T cells, ICOS (CD278) levels are reduced in XLP patients in the same way that occurs in $SAP^{-/-}$ T cells (Cannons et al., 2006; Ma et al., 2005).

Another group of defects noted in both $SAP^{-/-}$ mice and XLP patients concern B cell-mediated responses, including the absence of GC formation and deficient humoral responses to T cell-dependent antigen following viral infection or immunization (Cannons et al., 2006; Crotty et al., 2003; Hron et al., 2004). In this regard, diminished numbers of memory B cells in the peripheral blood, as well as long-lived plasma cells, are usually observed in $SAP^{-/-}$ mice. As a consequence, low titers of serum antibodies are detected (Crotty et al., 2003; Czar et al., 2001; Ma et al., 2005; Qi et al., 2008; Yin et al., 2003). It was initially postulated that these alterations might largely stem from defects inherent to B-cell responses, even though it remains unclear whether or not B cells express SAP. However, compelling and abundant evidence indicates that the defective help provided to B cells by $SAP^{-/-}$ $CD4^{+}$ T_{FH} cells is responsible for this impaired GC formation (Cannons et al., 2006; Crotty et al., 2003; Ma et al., 2005). The help that T cells, namely T_{FH}, provide to GC B cells is widely known to be essential to the effective production of memory B cells and long lived plasma cells, as well as for successful Ig class switching and antibody affinity maturation (Vinuesa et al., 2005; Vinuesa et al., 2010). This direct role played by T cells was confirmed by adoptive transfer of *wt* $CD4^{+}$ T cells to $SAP^{-/-}$ mice, since they were able to abrogate this GC defect (Cannons et al., 2006; Crotty et al., 2003; Morra et al., 2005). Concomitantly, an excellent study from Qi and colleagues revealed that SAP deficiency selectively impairs the capacity of $CD4^{+}$ T cells to firmly interact with cognate B cells, but not with DCs (Qi et al., 2008). $SAP^{-/-}$ mice exhibit impaired recruitment and retention of T cells within the emerging GC, a defect which abrogates the GC reaction's sustainability. Along this same line of investigation, this group has recently reported that mouse CD84 and Ly108 are required for long-lasting T-cell:B-cell contact, optimal T_{FH} function, and GC formation, although to a lesser extent compared with $SAP^{-/-}$ mice (Cannons et al., 2010a). Nevertheless, how cognate T:B interactions are influenced by SLAMF/SAP-mediated signals has not been fully elucidated.

3. Role of SLAMF receptors in autoimmune disease susceptibility

Multiple cellular and molecular mechanisms are required to maintain self-tolerance, and failure at any of these checkpoints can precipitate tolerance breakdown and lead to autoimmunity. Autoimmune diseases are characterized by variable etiologies and courses of pathogenesis, principally due to the different ways tolerance breakdown occurs. A wide array of genomic association studies suggests that the heterogeneous and alternative contribution of various genetic factors determines to some extent autoimmune disease susceptibility (Vyse & Todd, 1996; Wandstrat & Wakeland, 2001). Interestingly, the functional pathways that are defective in several human and murine autoimmune conditions frequently overlap (Krishnan et al., 2006; Morel, 2010). Chromosome 1 comprises a large amount of polymorphic genes related to an assortment of autoimmune disorders such as systemic lupus erythematosus (SLE), inflammatory bowel diseases (IBD), rheumatoid arthritis (RA) or multiple sclerosis (Morel, 2010; Tsao et al., 1997; Vyse & Todd, 1996; Wandstrat et al., 2004).

3.1 SLAM locus haplotypes and polymorphisms in mice and humans systemic autoimmunity

A wide array of clinical manifestations are associated with human and mouse SLE, an autoimmune condition in which both environmental factors and a predisposing genetic background contribute to its development. This pathology is clearly marked by a humoral autoimmune component derived from the loss of tolerance to nuclear Ag due to the production of antinuclear antibodies (ANA) such as anti-chromatin and anti-ss or dsDNA. These functional abnormality result in the accumulation of immune complex deposits in the kidney that can ultimately lead to fatal nephritis (Crispin et al., 2010; Fairhurst et al., 2006; Krishnan et al., 2006). Given the important immunoregulatory functions of the SLAMF receptors described above, it is not surprising that there is increasing evidence of their contribution to autoimmune disease susceptibility, particularly for SLE, but also diabetes. In fact, two major susceptibility loci for these two diseases, *Sle1b* and *Nkt1*, correspond to the locus on chromosome 1 where the genes encoding for the SLAM receptors are located (Wang et al., 2010a). Genetic and genomic analysis of this locus has revealed a high degree of polymorphism both in mice and humans. Studies in mice have allowed the identification and characterization of two major haplotypes of this locus: the haplotype 1, represented by C57BL/6 and related strains and the haplotype 2 by BALB/c and strains of mice that develop auto-antibodies spontaneously, e.g. NZB/NZW and NZM2410 (Furukawa et al., 2010; Morel et al., 2001; Wandstrat et al., 2004; Wang et al., 2010a). The differences between these two haplotypes are mainly based on: a) genomic structural variations (for example, an increase from one to four in the number of copies of CD244); (b) nonsynonymous mutations in the ligand binding domains of CD229, CD84 and CD48; (c) changes in the levels of transcription of some SLAMF genes; (d) and changes in the expression of isoforms generated by alternative splicing of some members of the family (Wang et al., 2010a). In the complex task of studying SLE pathogenesis, the contribution of mouse models has been extremely helpful due to their ability to closely mimic human SLE (Morel, 2010). In particular, mapping analysis of the autoimmune-prone NZM2410 (NZB x NZW, F1) mouse strain, which bears all the susceptibility Sle loci (*Sle1*, *Sle2*, and *Sle3*), revealed that these animals can fully develop SLE. These loci can independently cause a loss of tolerance to chromatin, the extent of which can differ over various serological and cellular phenotypes (Morel et al., 2001). Congenic mice *(B6.Sle1b)*, derived from the mouse strains NZM2410 (NZB x NZW/F1) and C57BL/6, that contain the Sle1b locus (haplotype 2) in a haplotype 1 background produce high titers of anti-nuclear antibodies and develop lupus (Figure 4) (Morel et al., 2001; Wandstrat et al., 2004). Thus, if a gene in this region of chromosome 1 is knockout through homologous recombination in 129-derived embryonic stem cells (ES cells) and the resultant mouse is backcrossed with B6, the interpretation of the phenotype of the mutant mouse may be affected by epistatic interactions between the 129 and B6 genomes. This has been recently observed by analysing the phenotype of knockout mice of two SLAMF genes (SLAMF1 and SLAMF2), which were generated with a 129-derived ES cell line. While Slamf1$^{-/-}$ and Slamf2$^{-/-}$ mice develop features of lupus if backcrossed on to the B6 genetic background [B6.129], Slamf1$^{-/-}$ and Slamf2$^{-/-}$ mice, backcrossed on the BALB/c background [BALB/c.129], do not manifest any sign of autoimmune disease (Keszei et al., 2011a).

Genetic linkage and association studies of families containing SLE patients as well as case-control studies of populations have identified several linkage regions, including one at 1q23, which contains multiple susceptibility genes, such as those present in the SLAM locus (Tsao et al., 2002). Indeed, the 1q23 locus has been identified in several genome-wide scans in humans and it has been replicated in subsequent linkage studies that have targeted this region (Moser et al., 1998; Shai et al., 1999).

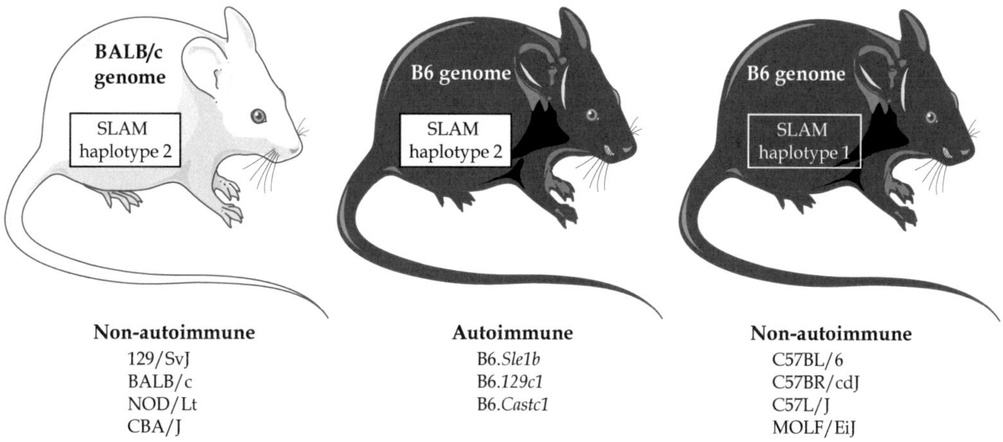

Fig. 4. SLAM haplotype 2 in the context of the B6 genome results in spontaneous autoimmunity.

Furthermore, as already mentioned, the syntenic region in mice has also been related to different mouse models of spontaneous lupus (Morel et al., 2001). Interestingly, SAP$^{-/-}$ mice (129*SvJ* background) are resistant to experimentally pristane-induced lupus. A deficiency in *Sh2d1a* abrogates the development of hypergammaglobulinemia, autoantibodies including anti-dsDNA, and renal disease (Hron et al., 2004). However, the mechanisms by which this SAP deficiency protects mice against lupus remain to be elucidated.

A family-based association study of UK and Canadian families with SLE has revealed multiple polymorphisms (SNPs) in the promoter and coding region of two members of the SLAMF, SLAMF3 (CD229) and SLAMF7 (CD319) (Cunninghame Graham et al., 2008). The authors of this study found that the strongest association was with a nonsynonymous SNP (rs509749) in exon 8 of SLAMF3 (CD229). This Val602Met change in the cytoplasmic tail lies within the consensus binding site for SAP and may therefore affect downstream signaling events of SLAMF3. The risk allele of this variant was found associated with decreased numbers of CD4^{+} naïve T cells and activated T cells and with increased numbers of CD8^{+} memory T cells. According to the authors, the skewing in the T-cell populations may indicate a state of chronic T-cell activation (Cunninghame Graham et al., 2008). Despite of these data, the association of this polymorphism with SLE has not been replicated in independent cohorts of SLE patients both of Japanese and European origin (Suarez-Gestal et al., 2009; Suzuki et al., 2008). Polymorphisms in another member of the SLAMF, namely SLAMF4 (CD244), have also been found associated with rheumatoid arthritis (RA) and SLE

(Suzuki et al., 2008). In one large-scale, case-control association study, two SNPs (rs3766379 and rs6682654) were found associated with increased susceptibility to RA in two independent cohorts from Japan. Interestingly, the genotype distribution of these SLAMF4 (CD244) SNPs in a SLE cohort was similar to that in the RA cohorts, suggesting that these polymorphisms in SLAMF4 (CD244) increase the risk for developing RA as well as SLE (Suzuki et al., 2008). In a recently published report, the SNP (rs3766379) in the SLAMF4 (CD244) gene was also found significantly associated with the susceptibility to SLE in another cohort of individuals of Japanese origin. This association was preferentially observed in subsets of SLE patients with nephritis and neuropsychiatric lupus (Ota et al., 2010). Taken together, and despite some conflicting results, these studies clearly indicate a high degree of polymorphism among the SLAMF genes and suggest the contribution of some of them in conferring susceptibility to autoimmunity. Further investigations are needed to determine the precise role and mechanism of these cell-receptors and their variants in increasing the risk to develop autoimmune diseases.

3.2 SLAMF spliced variants and their role in autoimmunity

As mentioned above, polymorphisms of the SLAMF genes also result in the differential expression of isoforms generated by alternative splicing. These variations in splice isoform expression are likely to have functional consequences and have also been implicated as candidates for other autoimmune susceptibility loci (Evsyukova et al., 2010; Gillett et al., 2009; Muschen et al., 1999; Ueda et al., 2003).

One of the strongest candidates of the SLAMF linked to lupus susceptibly in mice is Ly108 (CD352, SLAMF6). The polymorphism in Ly108 results in the expression of two alternatively spliced isoforms which differ exclusively in their cytoplasmic region (Wandstrat et al., 2004). These two isoforms, Ly108-1 and Ly108-2, are differentially expressed between normal mice and mice susceptible to lupus: whereas the expression of Ly108-1, with two domains ITSM, is increased in the B and T cells of lupus-prone mice, Ly108-2, with three motifs ITSM, is increased in these cells in normal animals (Kumar et al., 2006). The higher expression of the isoform Ly108-1 in lymphocytes of lupus-prone mice is associated with increased survival rates and ill-suited elimination of autoreactive B cells, resulting in increased autoantibody production (Kumar et al., 2006). Regardless of the fact that it bears an ITSM less than Ly108-2, Ly108-1 is more apt than Ly108-2 to trigger SAP-mediated tyrosine-phosphorylation signals, which involve Vav-1 and c-Cbl in T cells (Zhong & Veillette, 2008). Recently, Ly108 has been reported to promote long-lived stable T:B cell contacts (Cannons et al., 2010a). Since functional defects in both T and B lymphocytes are required for ANA production, it is possible that dysregulation of Ly108 isoform downstream signaling (derived from T:B engagement) might lead to disruption of peripheral tolerance and triggering of the autoimmune process in SLE. A third protein isoform, Ly108-H1, which is absent in two lupus-prone congenic animals has been recently identified (Keszei et al., 2011b). Ly108-H1 is encoded by a splice variant of Ly108 that lacks both exons 7 and 8. Transgenic mice expressing Ly108-H1 isoform present a dramatic reduction of $CD4^+$ T cell–dependent autoimmunity in congenic B6.Sle1b mice, demonstrating that an immune response–suppressing isoform of Ly108 can regulate the pathogenesis of lupus. Nonetheless, how Ly108 isoform-mediated signals are able to breach this tolerance remains to be clarified. Interestingly, SLAMF6-driven co-stimulation of human peripheral T cells is defective in SLE T cells (Chatterjee et al., 2011).

Spliced variants of SLAMF receptors have been also studied in humans. Human activated T cells express, in addition to membrane-form of SLAMF1, mRNA encoding a soluble secreted form of SLAMF1 (sSLAMF1) lacking 30 amino acids (aa) encompassing the entire 22-aa transmembrane region (Cocks et al., 1995). This soluble isoform may play a role in immunomodulation since sSLAM induces proliferation of purified B cells, but also Ig synthesis by these cells (Punnonen et al., 1997).

Most importantly, an altered expression of two SLAMF receptors in humans, SLAMF4 (CD244) and SLAMF7 (CD319), as well as a differential expression of isoforms of these molecules has been described in PBMCs from patients with SLE (Kim et al., 2010). Two different splice variants of human SLAMF4 (CD244), h2B4-A and h2B4-B, with different functional roles in human NK cells, had been previously identified by the same authors (Kumaresan & Mathew, 2000; Mathew et al., 2009). While both isoforms share the same intracellular domain, h2B4-B has five additional amino acids between the V and the C2 regions and is differentially regulated in SLE patients. In contrast, the two SLAMF7 (CD319) isoforms described, CS1-L and CS1-S, have identical extracellular domains but differ in their cytoplasmic tail. CS1-S lacks the two ITSM required for intracellular signaling and while CS1-L functions as an activating receptor, CS1-S does not show any signaling function in NK cells (Lee et al., 2004). Whereas healthy individuals express three-to sevenfold higher levels of CS1-L over CS1-S, this expression ratio is altered in SLE patients. This differential expression of both isoforms in PBMCs of SLE patients is reminiscent of Ly108 expression in lupus-prone mice (Kim et al., 2010).

Thus, an emerging concept derived from these and other studies, is that the differential expression of SLAMF receptor isoforms may contribute to susceptibility to break self-tolerance. In addition to the findings described above, cDNAs enoding SLAMF receptors that lack an extracellular domain, part of the cytoplasmic tail or the transmembrane segment, have been found in different databases (Ensemble, NCBI, EC gene). All these cDNAs, generated by alternative splicing, are mainly based on ESTs (Expressed Sequence Tags) and require experimental validation. Although it is not yet known if they are expressed as proteins, their expression would clearly have functional consequences, as it has been demonstrated in the case of Ly108 in mice. Indeed, the lack of an extracellular Ig domain can directly affect the recognition and the binding to the ligand, and changes that affect the length of the cytoplasmic tail can dramatically affect signal transduction. Preliminary data from our laboratory confirm the existence at the protein level of some of the isoforms predicted for CD84 (SLAMF5) and CD229 (SLAMF3) molecules (unpublished results). Altogether, these data suggest a critical role of aberrant expression of SLAMF spliced variants in conferring susceptibility to autoimmune diseases, in particular to SLE.

4. Conclusion

Lessons from genetic studies in mice have been key to support the hypothesis that SLAMF receptors function as disease modifiers and/or susceptibility factors of systemic autoimmunity. These studies are especially relevant since the phenotype of genetically manipulated mice is very similar to that in SLE patients, with the production of autoantibodies as well as multiorgan involvement, including severe nephritis. Although the interpretation of the phenotypes of knockout mice of the SLAMF receptors has been complicated by issues related to genetic background, all the data clearly underscore that these receptors play a critical role in the development of autoimmune diseases. An emerging concept is that aberrant alternative splicing plays an important role in the pathogenesis of autoimmune diseases. Studies reviewed in this chapter show that SLAMF isoforms expression appears to be altered in lupus patients. We believe that the study of the interplay between SLAMF isoforms in SLE patients will help identify pathways regulated during autoimmune processes, giving further insight into mechanisms underlying disease susceptibility and possible therapeutic approaches.

5. Acknowledgment

This work was supported by the Ministerio de Ciencia e Inovación [Grant SAF2009-07071]. Figures 1, 3 and 4 have been produced using Servier Medical Art (www.servier.com).

6. References

Baev, D.V., Caielli, S., Ronchi, F., et al. (2008). Impaired SLAM-SLAM homotypic interaction between invariant NKT cells and dendritic cells affects differentiation of IL-4/IL-10-secreting NKT2 cells in nonobese diabetic mice. *J Immunol.* 181, 869-877.

Baorto, D.M., Gao, Z., Malaviya, R., et al. (1997). Survival of FimH-expressing enterobacteria in macrophages relies on glycolipid traffic. *Nature.* 389, 636-639.

Berger, S.B., Romero, X., Ma, C., et al. (2010). SLAM is a microbial sensor that regulates bacterial phagosome functions in macrophages. *Nat Immunol.* 11, 920-927.

Calpe, S., Erdos, E., Liao, G., et al. (2006). Identification and characterization of two related murine genes, Eat2a and Eat2b, encoding single SH2-domain adapters. *Immunogenetics.* 58, 15-25.

Calpe, S., Wang, N., Romero, X., et al. (2008). The SLAM and SAP gene families control innate and adaptive immune responses. *Adv Immunol.* 97, 177-250.

Cannons, J.L., Qi, H., Lu, K.T., et al. (2010a). Optimal germinal center responses require a multistage T cell:B cell adhesion process involving integrins, SLAM-associated protein, and CD84. *Immunity.* 32, 253-265.

Cannons, J.L., Wu, J.Z., Gomez-Rodriguez, J., et al. (2010b). Biochemical and genetic evidence for a SAP-PKC-theta interaction contributing to IL-4 regulation. *J Immunol.* 185, 2819-2827.

Cannons, J.L., Yu, L.J., Hill, B., et al. (2004). SAP regulates T(H)2 differentiation and PKC-theta-mediated activation of NF-kappaB1. *Immunity.* 21, 693-706.

Cannons, J.L., Yu, L.J., Jankovic, D., et al. (2006). SAP regulates T cell-mediated help for humoral immunity by a mechanism distinct from cytokine regulation. *J Exp Med.* 203, 1551-1565.

Chan, B., Lanyi, A., Song, H.K., et al. (2003). SAP couples Fyn to SLAM immune receptors. *Nat Cell Biol.* 5, 155-160.

Chatterjee, M., Kis-Toth, K., Thai, T.H., et al. (2011). SLAMF6-driven co-stimulation of human peripheral T cells is defective in SLE T cells. *Autoimmunity.* 44, 211-218.

Chen, G., Tai, A.K., Lin, M., et al. (2005). Signaling lymphocyte activation molecule-associated protein is a negative regulator of the CD8 T cell response in mice. *J Immunol.* 175, 2212-2218.

Chen, R., Latour, S., Shi, X., et al. (2006). Association between SAP and FynT: Inducible SH3 domain-mediated interaction controlled by engagement of the SLAM receptor. *Mol Cell Biol*. 26, 5559-5568.

Clarkson, N.G., Simmonds, S.J., Puklavec, M.J., et al. (2007). Direct and indirect interactions of the cytoplasmic region of CD244 (2B4) in mice and humans with FYN kinase. *J Biol Chem*. 282, 25385-25394.

Claus, M., Meinke, S., Bhat, R., et al. (2008). Regulation of NK cell activity by 2B4, NTB-A and CRACC. *Front Biosci*. 13, 956-965.

Cocks, B.G., Chang, C.C., Carballido, J.M., et al. (1995). A novel receptor involved in T-cell activation. *Nature*. 376, 260-263.

Crispin, J.C., Liossis, S.N., Kis-Toth, K., et al. (2010). Pathogenesis of human systemic lupus erythematosus: recent advances. *Trends Mol Med*. 16, 47-57.

Crotty, S., Kersh, E.N., Cannons, J., et al. (2003). SAP is required for generating long-term humoral immunity. *Nature*. 421, 282-287.

Crotty, S., McCausland, M.M., Aubert, R.D., et al. (2006). Hypogammaglobulinemia and exacerbated CD8 T-cell-mediated immunopathology in SAP-deficient mice with chronic LCMV infection mimics human XLP disease. *Blood*. 108, 3085-3093.

Cruz-Munoz, M.E., Dong, Z., Shi, X., et al. (2009). Influence of CRACC, a SLAM family receptor coupled to the adaptor EAT-2, on natural killer cell function. *Nat Immunol*. 10, 297-305.

Cunninghame Graham, D.S., Vyse, T.J., Fortin, P.R., et al. (2008). Association of LY9 in UK and Canadian SLE families. *Genes Immun*. 9, 93-102.

Czar, M.J., Kersh, E.N., Mijares, L.A., Lanier, G., et al. (2001). Altered lymphocyte responses and cytokine production in mice deficient in the X-linked lymphoproliferative disease gene SH2D1A/DSHP/SAP. *Proc Natl Acad Sci U.S.A*. 98, 7449-7454.

Davidson, D., Shi, X., Zhang, S., et al. (2004). Genetic evidence linking SAP, the X-linked lymphoproliferative gene product, to Src-related kinase FynT in T(H)2 cytokine regulation. *Immunity*. 21, 707-717.

Detre, C., Keszei, M., Romero, X., et al. (2010). SLAM family receptors and the SLAM-associated protein (SAP) modulate T cell functions. *Semin Immunopathol*. 32, 157-171.

Diaz-Ramos, M.C., Engel, P. & Bastos, R. (2011). Towards a comprehensive human cell-surface immunome database. *Immunol Lett*. 134, 183-187.

Engel, P., Eck, M.J. & Terhorst, C. (2003). The SAP and SLAM families in immune responses and X-linked lymphoproliferative disease. *Nat Rev Immunol*. 3, 813-821.

Evsyukova, I., Somarelli, J.A., Gregory, S.G., et al. (2010). Alternative splicing in multiple sclerosis and other autoimmune diseases. *RNA Biol*. 7, 462-473.

Fairhurst, A.M., Wandstrat, A.E. & Wakeland, E.K. (2006). Systemic lupus erythematosus: multiple immunological phenotypes in a complex genetic disease. *Adv Immunol*. 92, 1-69.

Finerty, P.J.,Jr, Muhandiram, R. & Forman-Kay, J.D. (2002). Side-chain dynamics of the SAP SH2 domain correlate with a binding hot spot and a region with conformational plasticity. *J Mol Biol*. 322, 605-620.

Furukawa, H., Tohma, S., Kitazawa, H., et al. (2010). Role of SLAM-associated protein in the pathogenesis of autoimmune diseases and immunological disorders. *Arch Immunol Ther Exp (Warsz).* 58, 37-44.

Gillett, A., Maratou, K., Fewings, C., et al. (2009). Alternative splicing and transcriptome profiling of experimental autoimmune encephalomyelitis using genome-wide exon arrays. *PLoS One.* 4, e7773.

Griewank, K., Borowski, C., Rietdijk, S., et al. (2007). Homotypic interactions mediated by Slamf1 and Slamf6 receptors control NKT cell lineage development. *Immunity.* 27, 751-762.

Gu, C., Tangye, S.G., Sun, X., et al. (2006). The X-linked lymphoproliferative disease gene product SAP associates with PAK-interacting exchange factor and participates in T cell activation. *Proc Natl Acad Sci U.S.A.* 103, 14447-14452.

Howie, D., Simarro, M., Sayos, J., et al. (2002). Molecular dissection of the signaling and costimulatory functions of CD150 (SLAM): CD150/SAP binding and CD150-mediated costimulation. *Blood.* 99, 957-965.

Hron, J.D., Caplan, L., Gerth, A.J., et al. (2004). SH2D1A regulates T-dependent humoral autoimmunity. *J Exp Med.* 200, 261-266.

Hu, T., Simmons, A., Yuan, J., et al. (2010). The transcription factor c-Myb primes $CD4^+CD8^+$ immature thymocytes for selection into the iNKT lineage. *Nat Immunol* 11, 435-441.

Jordan, M.A., Fletcher, J.M., Pellicci, D., et al. (2007). Slamf1, the NKT cell control gene Nkt1. *J Immunol.* 178, 1618-1627.

Kamperschroer, C., Dibble, J.P., Meents, et al. (2006). SAP is required for Th cell function and for immunity to influenza. *J. Immunol.* 177, 5317-5327.

Keszei, M., Latchman, Y.E., Vanguri, V.K., et al. (2011a). Auto-antibody production and glomerulonephritis in congenic Slamf1$^{-/-}$ and Slamf2$^{-/-}$ [B6.129] but not in Slamf1$^{-/-}$ and Slamf2$^{-/-}$ [BALB/c.129] mice. *Int Immunol.* 23, 149-158.

Keszei, M., Detre, C., Rietdijk, S.T., et al. (2011b). A novel isoform of the Ly108 gene ameliorates murine lupus. *J Exp Med.* 208, 811-822.

Kiel, M.J., Yilmaz, O.H., Iwashita, T., et al. SLAM family receptors distinguish hematopoietic stem and progenitor cells and reveal endothelial niches for stem cells. *Cell.* 121, 1109-1121.

Kim, J.R., Mathew, S.O., Patel, R.K., et al. (2010). Altered expression of signalling lymphocyte activation molecule (SLAM) family receptors CS1 (CD319) and 2B4 (CD244) in patients with systemic lupus erythematosus. *Clin Exp Immunol.* 160, 348-358.

Krishnan, S., Chowdhury, B. & Tsokos, G.C. (2006). Autoimmunity in systemic lupus erythematosus: integrating genes and biology. *Semin Immunol* 18, 230-243.

Kumar, K.R., Li, L., Yan, M., et al. (2006). Regulation of B cell tolerance by the lupus susceptibility gene Ly108. *Science.* 312, 1665-1669.

Kumaresan, P.R. & Mathew, P.A. (2000). Structure of the human natural killer cell receptor 2B4 gene and identification of a novel alternative transcript. *Immunogenetics.* 51, 987-992.

Latour, S., Gish, G., Helgason, C.D., et al. (2001). Regulation of SLAM-mediated signal transduction by SAP, the X-linked lymphoproliferative gene product. *Nat Immunol* 2, 681-690.

Latour, S., Roncagalli, R., Chen, R., et al. (2003). Binding of SAP SH2 domain to FynT SH3 domain reveals a novel mechanism of receptor signalling in immune regulation. *Nat Cell Biol.* 5, 149-154.

Lee, J.K., Boles, K.S. & Mathew, P.A. (2004). Molecular and functional characterization of a CS1 (CRACC) splice variant expressed in human NK cells that does not contain immunoreceptor tyrosine-based switch motifs. *Eur J Immunol.* 34, 2791-2799.

Lewis, J., Eiben, L.J., Nelson, D.L., et al. (2001). Distinct interactions of the X-linked lymphoproliferative syndrome gene product SAP with cytoplasmic domains of members of the CD2 receptor family. *Clin Immunol.* 100, 15-23.

Ma, C.S., Hare, N.J., Nichols, et al. (2005). Impaired humoral immunity in X-linked lymphoproliferative disease is associated with defective IL-10 production by CD4+ T cells. *J Clin Invest.* 115, 1049-1059.

Ma, C.S., Nichols, K.E. & Tangye, S.G. (2007). Regulation of cellular and humoral immune responses by the SLAM and SAP families of molecules. *Annu Rev Immunol.* 25, 337-379.

Maier, L.M. & Hafler, D.A. (2009). Autoimmunity risk alleles in costimulation pathways. *Immunol Rev.* 229, 322-336.

Martin, M., Del Valle, J.M., Saborit, I. et al. (2005). Identification of Grb2 as a novel binding partner of the signaling lymphocytic activation molecule-associated protein binding receptor CD229. *J Immunol.* 174, 5977-5986.

Mathew, S.O., Rao, K.K., Kim, J.R., et al. (2009). Functional role of human NK cell receptor 2B4 (CD244) isoforms. *Eur J Immunol.* 39, 1632-1641.

Mikhalap, S.V., Shlapatska, L.M., Berdova, A.G., et al. (1999). CDw150 associates with src-homology 2-containing inositol phosphatase and modulates CD95-mediated apoptosis. *J Immunol.* 162, 5719-5727.

Morel, L. (2010). Genetics of SLE: evidence from mouse models. *Nat Rev Rheumatol.* 6, 348-357.

Morel, L., Blenman, K.R., Croker, B.P. et al. (2001). The major murine systemic lupus erythematosus susceptibility locus, Sle1, is a cluster of functionally related genes. *Proc Natl Acad. Sci U.S.A.* 98, 1787-1792.

Morra, M., Barrington, R.A., Abadia-Molina, A.C., et al. (2005). Defective B cell responses in the absence of SH2D1A. *Proc Natl Acad Sci U.S.A.* 102, 4819-4823.

Morra, M., Lu, J., Poy, F., et al. (2001). Structural basis for the interaction of the free SH2 domain EAT-2 with SLAM receptors in hematopoietic cells. *EMBO J.* 20, 5840-5852.

Moser, K.L., Neas, B.R., Salmon, J.E., et al. (1998). Genome scan of human systemic lupus erythematosus: evidence for linkage on chromosome 1q in African-American pedigrees. *Proc Natl Acad Sci U.S.A.* 95, 14869-14874.

Muschen, M., Warskulat, U., Perniok, A.,et al. (1999). Involvement of soluble CD95 in Churg-Strauss syndrome. *Am J Pathol.* 155, 915-925.

Nakajima, H., Cella, M., Bouchon, A., et al. (2000). Patients with X-linked lymphoproliferative disease have a defect in 2B4 receptor-mediated NK cell cytotoxicity. *Eur J Immunol.* 30, 3309-3318.

Ota, Y., Kawaguchi, Y., Takagi, K., et al. (2010). Single nucleotide polymorphisms of CD244 gene predispose to renal and neuropsychiatric manifestations with systemic lupus erythematosus. *Mod Rheumatol.* 20, 427-431.

Parolini, S., Bottino, C., Falco, M., et al. (2000). X-linked lymphoproliferative disease. 2B4 molecules displaying inhibitory rather than activating function are responsible for the inability of natural killer cells to kill Epstein-Barr virus-infected cells. *J Exp Med.* 192, 337-346.

Poy, F., Yaffe, M.B., Sayos, J., et al. (1999). Crystal structures of the XLP protein SAP reveal a class of SH2 domains with extended, phosphotyrosine-independent sequence recognition. *Mol Cell.* 4, 555-561.

Punnonen, J., Cocks, B.G., Carballido, J.M., et al. (1997). Soluble and membrane-bound forms of signaling lymphocytic activation molecule (SLAM) induce proliferation and Ig synthesis by activated human B lymphocytes. *J Exp Med.* 185, 993-1004.

Qi, H., Cannons, J.L., Klauschen, F., et al. (2008). SAP-controlled T-B cell interactions underlie germinal centre formation. *Nature.* 455, 764-769.

Roncagalli, R., Taylor, J.E., Zhang, et al (2005). Negative regulation of natural killer cell function by EAT-2, a SAP-related adaptor. *Nat Immunol.* 6, 1002-1010.

Sayos, J., Wu, C., Morra, M., et al. (1998). The X-linked lymphoproliferative-disease gene product SAP regulates signals induced through the co-receptor SLAM. *Nature.* 395, 462-469.

Schwartzberg, P.L., Mueller, K.L., Qi, H., et al. (2009). SLAM receptors and SAP influence lymphocyte interactions, development and function. *Nat Rev Immunol.* 9, 39-46.

Shai, R., Quismorio, F.P.,Jr, Li, L., et al. (1999). Genome-wide screen for systemic lupus erythematosus susceptibility genes in multiplex families. *Hum Mol Genet.* 8, 639-644.

Shin, J.S., Gao, Z. &Abraham, S.N. (2000). Involvement of cellular caveolae in bacterial entry into mast cells. *Science,* 289, 785-788.

Sintes, J., Romero, X., Marin, P., et al. (2008). Differential expression of CD150 (SLAM) family receptors by human hematopoietic stem and progenitor cells. *Exp Hematol.* 36, 1199-1204.

Sintes, J. & Engel, P. (2011). SLAM (CD150) is a multitasking immunoreceptor: from cosignalling to bacterial recognition. *Immunol Cell Biol.* 89, 161-163.

Suarez-Gestal, M., Calaza, M., Endreffy, E., et al. (2009). Replication of recently identified systemic lupus erythematosus genetic associations: a case-control study. *Arthritis Res Ther.* 11, R69.

Suzuki, A., Yamada, R., Kochi, Y., *et al.* (2008). Functional SNPs in CD244 increase the risk of rheumatoid arthritis in a Japanese population. *Nat Genet.* 40, 1224-1229.

Tangye, S.G., Lazetic, S., Woollatt, E., et al. (1999). Cutting edge: human 2B4, an activating NK cell receptor, recruits the protein tyrosine phosphatase SHP-2 and the adaptor signaling protein SAP. *J Immunol.* 162, 6981-6985.

Tangye, S.G., Nichols, K.E., Hare, N.J., et al. (2003). Functional requirements for interactions between CD84 and Src homology 2 domain-containing proteins and their contribution to human T cell activation. *J Immunol.* 171, 2485-2495.

Tassi, I. & Colonna, M. (2005). The cytotoxicity receptor CRACC (CS-1) recruits EAT-2 and activates the PI3K and phospholipase Cgamma signaling pathways in human NK cells. *J Immunol.* 175, 7996-8002.

Tatsuo, H., Ono, N., Tanaka, K., et al. (2000). SLAM (CDw150) is a cellular receptor for measles virus. *Nature.* 406, 893-897.

Tsao, B.P., Cantor, R.M., Grossman, J.M., et al. (2002). Linkage and interaction of loci on 1q23 and 16q12 may contribute to susceptibility to systemic lupus erythematosus. *Arthritis Rheum.* 46, 2928-2936.

Tsao, B.P., Cantor, R.M., Kalunian, K.C., et al. (1997). Evidence for linkage of a candidate chromosome 1 region to human systemic lupus erythematosus. *J Clin Invest.* 99, 725-731.

Ueda, H., Howson, J.M., Esposito, L., et al. (2003). Association of the T-cell regulatory gene CTLA4 with susceptibility to autoimmune disease. *Nature.* 423, 506-511.

Veillette, A. (2010). SLAM-family receptors: immune regulators with or without SAP-family adaptors. *Cold Spring Harb Perspect Biol.* 2, a002469.

Veillette, A., Cruz-Munoz, M.E. & Zhong, M.C. (2006). SLAM family receptors and SAP-related adaptors: matters arising. *Trends Immunol.* 27, 228-234.

Veillette, A., Dong, Z. & Latour, S. (2007). Consequence of the SLAM-SAP signaling pathway in innate-like and conventional lymphocytes. *Immunity.* 27, 698-710.

Veillette, A., Dong, Z., Perez-Quintero, L.A., et al. (2009). Importance and mechanism of 'switch' function of SAP family adapters. *Immunol Rev.* 232, 229-239.

Vinuesa, C.G., Linterman, M.A., Goodnow, C.C., et al. (2010). T cells and follicular dendritic cells in germinal center B-cell formation and selection. *Immunol Rev.* 237, 72-89.

Vinuesa, C.G., Tangye, S.G., Moser, B., et al. (2005). Follicular B helper T cells in antibody responses and autoimmunity. *Nat Rev Immunol.* 5, 853-865.

Vyse, T.J. & Todd, J.A. (1996). Genetic analysis of autoimmune disease. *Cell.* 85, 311-318.

Wandstrat, A., & Wakeland, E. (2001). The genetics of complex autoimmune diseases: non-MHC susceptibility genes. *Nat Immunol.* 2, 802-809.

Wandstrat, A.E., Nguyen, C., Limaye, N., et al. (2004). Association of extensive polymorphisms in the SLAM/CD2 gene cluster with murine lupus. *Immunity.* 21, 769-780.

Wang, A., Batteux, F. & Wakeland, E.K. (2010a). The role of SLAM/CD2 polymorphisms in systemic autoimmunity. *Curr Opin Immunol.* 22, 706-714.

Wang, N., Calpe, S., Westcott, J., et al. (2010b). Cutting Edge: The Adapters EAT-2A and -2B Are Positive Regulators of CD244- and CD84-Dependent NK Cell Functions in the C57BL/6 Mouse. *J Immunol.* 185, 5683-5687.

Wu, C., Nguyen, K.B., Pien, G.C., et al. (2001). SAP controls T cell responses to virus and terminal differentiation of TH2 cells. *Nat Immunol.* 2, 410-414.

Yin, L., Al-Alem, U., Liang, J., et al. (2003). Mice deficient in the X-linked lymphoproliferative disease gene sap exhibit increased susceptibility to murine gammaherpesvirus-68 and hypo-gammaglobulinemia. *J Med Virol.* 71, 446-455.

Zhong, M.C. & Veillette, A. (2008). Control of T lymphocyte signaling by Ly108, a signaling lymphocytic activation molecule family receptor implicated in autoimmunity. *J Biol Chem*. 283, 19255-19264.

4

HLA and Citrullinated Peptides in Rheumatoid Arthritis

Iñaki Álvarez
Immunology Unit. Department of Cell Biology, Physiology and Immunology. Institut de Biotecnologia i Biomedicina, Universitat Autònoma de Barcelona, Spain

1. Introduction

Rheumatoid arthritis (RA) is a chronic systemic inflammatory disease that mostly attacks synovial joints, although other tissues and organs can be affected. The final effect is usually the destruction of articular cartilage and ankylosis of the joints, with a prevalence of the wrist and small joints of the hand. Diagnostic criteria have recently been revised (Aletaha et al., 2010; Neogi et al., 2010). The prevalence of RA is about 1% in the total population, being women more affected than men in a ratio of approximately 2-3:1 (Alamanos & Drosos, 2005).

RA is considered an autoimmune disorder, although the etiology and pathogenesis of the disease remain unclear. A complex set of factors are involved in the onset of the disease, including genetic and environmental. The strongest genetic association is with the genes encoding major histocompatibility complex (MHC, HLA in human) class II molecules (Gregersen et al., 1987; Stastny, 1978), although other genes have been associated with RA, including *PTPN22, STAT4, TRAF1/C5,* and others.

Antibodies against the Fc fraction of IgG are found in the serum of about 80% of patients with RA. These autoantibodies are called rheumatoid factor (RF), and the consideration of RA as an autoimmune disease has largely been based on the presence of RF in the serum of patients. Nevertheless, the presence of RF is not exclusive of RA and that, together with the absence of definitive data demonstrating an arthritogenic effect of RF, suggest that these antibodies are produced as a consequence of the immune response rather than being the cause of it (Nemazee, 1985; Tarkowski et al., 1985). However, the adaptive immune response seems to play an important role in the disease as suggested by the strong association of RA with the presence of some HLA class II alleles. Autoantibodies against citrullinated proteins (ACPAs) have been described in the serum of about 50-70% of RA patients in comparison with about 2% of the healthy population (Avouac et al., 2006; Kroot et al., 2000; Nishimura et al., 2007; Schellekens et al., 2000; van Gaalen et al., 2004; Vincent et al., 2002). The presence of ACPAs is very stable during the course of the disease and is quite specific for RA. These antibodies can be detected several years before of symptomatic disease, making the presence of ACPAs a good clinical marker for RA. Patients containing ACPAs in the serum usually have a more severe disease. The presence of these antibodies correlates very well with the presence of some of the HLA-DR alleles containing the "shared epitope" (see below). All of these data have led to the postulation that there actually are two different disorders (Klareskog et al., 2008). However, the cause of the specificity of the generation of ACPAs in RA and whether the antibodies are pathogenic or secondary to the joint inflammation remain unanswered.

Many reports have been published in the last years describing some of the features of the antibodies that recognize citrullinated proteins and showing some of the proteins that are target of these autoantibodies. The generation of an effective B cell response requires the recognition by specific $CD4^+$ T cells of peptides derived of the antigen in the context of MHC class II molecules. In this chapter some of the data indicating the importance of anti-citrulline responses will be reviewed and concretely emphasize on reviewing the last reports dealing with MHC presentation and T cell responses to citrullinated peptides will be done.

2. HLA and rheumatoid arthritis

The strongest genetic association of RA susceptibility is with some specific HLA class II alleles. In Northern Europe, the strongest association is with the serotype HLA-DR4 (Jaraquemada et al., 1986; Stastny, 1978). The association is with some allelic variants of HLA-DR4, including DRB1*0401, *0404, *0405 and *0408. However, other HLA-DR4 subtypes do not confer predisposition to RA. In Southern Europe and other populations the susceptibility to RA is associated to alleles other than DR4. Thus, DRB1*0101, *0102, *1402 and *1001 have been reported with predisposition to RA (Cutbush et al., 1993; de Juan et al., 1994; Gonzalez-Escribano et al., 1999; Hameed et al., 1997; Lacki et al., 2000; Mody & Hammond, 1994; Poor et al., 2007; Salvarani et al., 1999; Sanchez et al., 1990; Yelamos et al., 1993). A major feature shared by the alleles that confer susceptibility to RA is the presence of some residues at position 67 and 70-74 of the third hypervariable region of DRB1 (Table 1). Thus, the presence of specific residues in these positions (L...(Q/R)(K/R)RAA) led to the proposal of the "shared epitope" hypothesis (Gregersen et al., 1987), in which the molecular basis for the association of some alleles with RA was restricted to this critical region in the β chain of HLA-DR molecules. The P4 residue of the peptide core directly interacts with some of the residues that are part of the shared epitope (SE). Other residues are exposed to outside the binding groove. Thus, the side chains of these amino acids could be involved in the pathogenesis of the disease by defining the peptide preference or directly interacting with the T cell receptor (TCR), influencing the T cell repertoire selection, and specific T cell activation. Alternatively, molecular mimicry of this HLA-DR region and proteins from pathogenic agents might contribute to the disease process. Other mechanisms have been proposed to explain the role that the SE plays in the disease, including direct triggering by the five-amino acid SE sequence leading to NO production (Ling et al., 2007), ability to bind to heat shock proteins (Auger et al., 1996), and the ability to present citrullinated peptides (Hill et al., 2003). A putative "protective epitope" has also been defined for the same region, with the sequence DERAA, corresponding to DRB1*0402, *1102, *1301, *1302, and *1304, and is associated with a less severe disease (van der Helm-van Mil et al., 2005).

HLA genes show strong linkage disequilibrium, so they segregate as haplotypes with a low recombination rate, specially between HLA-DR and HLA-DQ. Different data indicate that some HLA-DQ alleles that segregate with given HLA-DR alleles play an important role in RA, although these data are not totally understood. The combination of the presence of the SE-containing HLA-DR alleles and specific HLA-DQ alleles opened the possibility that peptides containing the SE can be presented to T cells in the context of specific HLA-DQ, shaping the T-cell repertoire (Salvat et al., 1994).

HLA-DRB1 allele	Amino acid residue					
	67	70	71	72	73	74
High risk						
*04:01	L	Q	K	R	A	A
*01:01	-	-	R	-	-	-
*01:02	-	-	R	-	-	-
*04:04	-	-	R	-	-	-
*04:05	-	-	R	-	-	-
*04:08	-	-	R	-	-	-
*10:01	-	R	R	-	-	-
Protection or low risk						
*04:02	I	D	E	-	-	-
*07:01	I	D	R	-	G	Q
*11:02	I	D	E	-	-	-
*13:01	I	D	E	-	-	-
*13:02	I	D	E	-	-	-
*13:04	I	D	E	-	-	-
*15:01	I	-	A	-	-	-

Table 1. Residues in the shared epitope positions in HLA-DR molecules differentially associated to RA

3. Citrullination

Citrullination is a post-translational protein modification that consists in the deimination of the positive charged amino acid arginine, generating the neutral amino acid citrulline (Figure 1). The process requires high concentrations of Ca^{2+} and is produced in inflammatory environments (Baeten et al., 2001; Chavanas et al., 2004; Vossenaar et al., 2003). Other mechanism that triggers arginine deimination is apoptosis (Baeten et al., 2001). Environmental insults such as smoking increases the expression of PAD2 and induces citrullination in the mouse (Makrygiannakis et al., 2008).

The conversion of arginine to citrulline is carried out by a family of enzymes known as peptidyl arginine deiminases (PADs) (Vossenaar et al., 2003). Five members of this family of enzymes have been described in human (PAD1, PAD2, PAD3, PAD4 and PAD6). The members or this family are differentially expressed in many cell types (including neutrophils, monocytes, and macrophages) and tissues (Migliorini et al., 2005; Nijenhuis et al., 2004; van Venrooij & Pruijn, 2000; Vossenaar et al., 2003; Wysocka et al., 2006). Thus, PAD2 and PAD4 are expressed in the synovium of patients with RA, but PAD1, PAD3 and PAD6 are not (Foulquier et al., 2007). At least some functional haplotypes of PAD4 are associated with RA (Suzuki et al., 2003). Interestingly, PAD4 is capable of self-citrullination, which can regulate its activity and control the citrullination of other proteins (Andrade et al., 2010).

Citrullinated proteins have been detected in several inflamed tissues: arthritic joins (Vossenaar et al., 2004a), brain (Nicholas & Whitaker, 2002), muscle and lymphoid organs (Makrygiannakis et al., 2006) and lungs (Bongartz et al., 2007; Klareskog et al., 2006). In addition, some proteins from the epidermis and central nervous system are constitutively citrullinated (Kubilus et al., 1979; Nicholas et al., 2003).

The function of citrullination is not totally understood, although it is important in some physiological processes such as apoptosis (Asaga et al., 1998) and cell differentiation (Senshu et al., 1996). The loss of a positive charge can produce changes in some relevant protein features. Thus, electrostatic interactions are usually important in generating and maintaining protein structures. A citrullinated protein modifies some of the interactions that stabilize the native conformation, and decreases its isoelectric point, affecting the secondary and tertiary structure, which can result in a different protein folding that may modify the function of the protein (Gyorgy et al., 2006). Regarding the specific protein functions affected by citrullination it has been reported that arginine deimination influences protein-protein interaction (Tarcsa et al., 1996), and can modulate signalling potency (Proost et al., 2008). In addition, citrullinated proteins often change their sensitivity to degradation by proteolytic enzymes (Pritzker et al., 2000).

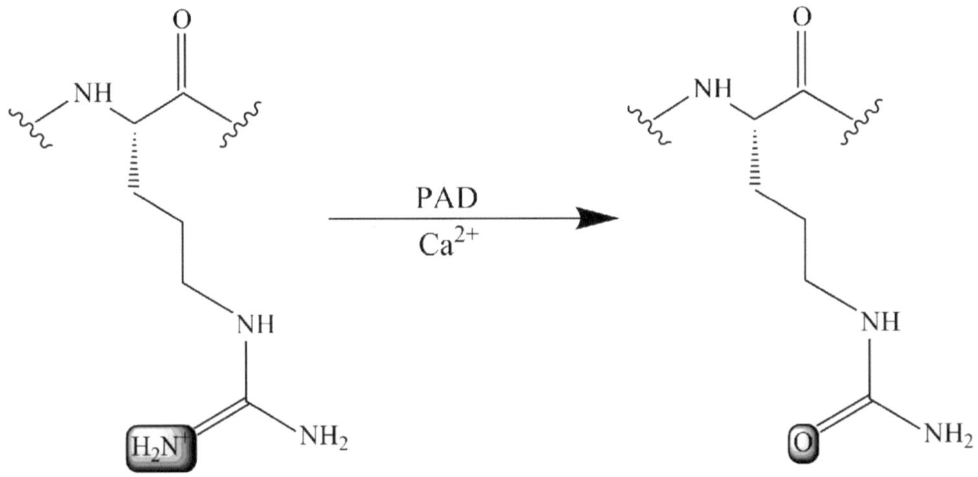

Fig. 1. **Conversion of arginine to citrulline**. The protein posttranslational modification known as citrullination consists in a deimination of arginine to citrulline. The reaction is carried out by an enzyme of the family of peptidyl arginine deiminases (PAD), and requires high concentration of Ca^{2+}. This reaction results in the loss of a positive charge in the protein.

4. Citrulline and rheumatoid arthritis

As mentioned above, the presence of citrullinated proteins is detected in the joints of patients with RA (Baeten et al., 2001), although it is not exclusive for rheumatoid synovial tissue (Vossenaar et al., 2004a). The specificity of citrullination has not been solved and several proteins have been found to be citrullinated in the synovium, including vimentin (Bang et al., 2007; Vossenaar et al., 2004b), fibrinogen (Masson-Bessiere et al., 2001), and collagen type II (Klareskog et al., 2008). The role of these modified proteins in the joints remains unknown, although some of these proteins are known targets of the autoimmune response. Thus, specific antibodies have been detected in RA patients that recognize citrullinated filaggrin (Nijenhuis et al., 2004; Schellekens et al., 1998; Sebbag et al., 1995; Simon et al., 1993), fibrinogen (Bang et al., 2007), vimentin (Burkhardt et al., 2005; Despres et al., 1994; Hayem et al., 1999; Hueber et al., 1999) and collagen type II (Burkhardt et al., 2005).

A relevant feature of ACPAs is that their presence is RA specific. Thus, in contrast with RF, patients with inflammatory diseases other than RA rarely carry ACPAs in serum. It still remains unclear why ACPAs are present in the serum of most RA patients but absent in the serum of other systemic autoinflammatory diseases.

As with RF, the generation of ACPAs in the serum of RA patients can occur several years before the onset of the disease (Aho et al., 2000; Kurki et al., 1992; Nielen et al., 2004; Rantapaa-Dahlqvist et al., 2003). The detection of these ACPAs can be used as clinical tests to predict the clinical course of the disease (Kastbom et al., 2004; Ronnelid et al., 2005). There are some clinical and genetic differences between $ACPA^{+}$ and $ACPA^{-}$ RA patients. Clinically, $ACPA^{+}$ RA patients have a more severe disease course than patients without detectable ACPAs (Forslind et al., 2004; Kastbom et al., 2004; Kroot et al., 2000; Ronnelid et al., 2005). Genetically, the detection of ACPAs in the serum of RA patients correlates very well with the presence of HLA-DR alleles containing the SE, which does not happen with RF. Some reports have shown that the presence of HLA-DRB1 alleles containing the SE is directly related and restricted to the $ACPA^{+}$ subset of RA (Huizinga et al., 2005; van der Helm-van Mil et al., 2006) and SE alleles influence both the magnitude and the specificity of this RA-specific antibody response (Verpoort et al., 2007). Other HLA-DRB1-independent genetic associations in the HLA region to ACPA positivity have been reported (Okada et al., 2009). In contrast, $ACPA^{-}$ RA is not related with the SE-carrying HLA-DRB1 alleles and it has been associated with HLA-DRB1*03 (Irigoyen et al., 2005), an DRB1 allele that does not contain the SE. Taking together, it seems clear that $ACPA^{+}$ and $ACPA^{-}$ RA do not present the same genetic background or clinical course and evidence strongly suggest that these are two different RA subsets, so they should be considered as different entities when treated.

Since ACPAs are developed before the onset of the disease and their presence predicts a more severe clinical course, this seems to indicate that the immune response against citrullinated proteins contribute to the pathogenesis of this form of RA.

5. Citrullinated peptides and HLA

The SE contains residues 70-74 of the DRβ chain, and is located in one α-helix of the binding groove. These residues are located in a position such that some of them can interact with the peptide bound to the HLA-DR molecule. Concretely, the crystal structures of HLA-DR1 and HLA-DR4 with different peptides have shown that the residues Lys71 in DRB1*0401 and Arg71 in DRB1*0101 directly interact with the amino acid located in position 4 (P4) of the peptide core bound to the binding groove of HLA-DR molecules (Dessen et al., 1997; Rosloniec et al., 2006). The binding motifs of the peptides associated to HLA-DR1 and HLA-DR4 were described years ago. More recently, our group reported an exhaustive analysis of the peptide pool associated to HLA-DR10 by mass spectrometry and identified the anchor motif of the peptide repertoire bound to this RA-associated allele (Alvarez et al., 2008). This motif was consistent with a more recent report by Kwok´s group using an approach based on binding assays (James et al., 2010). An important structural information extracted from these data is that HLA-DR molecules containing the SE do not bind peptides with basic residues in P4 position. This is due to the presence of basic residues at position 71 of the HLA-DR β chain (table 1).

Conversion of the basic amino acid arginine to the neutral citrulline produces the loss of a net positive charge on the protein or peptide that suffer this post-translational modification. Thus, citrulline is a neutral, polar, large amino acid with structural features similar to glutamine. Interestingly, peptides with arginine in P4 are poorly tolerated for the HLA-DR molecules that comprise the SE alleles (Fremont et al., 1996; Friede et al., 1996), while peptides with glutamine in P4 of the binding core have been described for DRB1*0101, DRB1*0401 and DRB1*1001 (Alvarez et al., 2008; Dengjel et al., 2005; Muntasell et al., 2004; Stern et al., 1994; Verreck et al., 1996). Basic residues, such as arginine or lysine, in P4 position of the peptide core produce electrostatic repulsion with the basic residues in position 71 of the β chain in the HLA-DR molecules that contain the SE. However, glutamine can accommodate well in the pocket and can be stabilized by hydrogen bonds with Arg71 or Lys71 in the HLA-DR β chain. Thus, positively charged amino acids (e.g., arginine) in P4 inhibit peptide binding to RA-related HLA-DR molecules containing the SE, whereas peptides with uncharged polarity (e.g., glutamine) are bound to these molecules with high affinity (Hammer et al., 1994; Hammer et al., 1995). Peptides with citrullin in P4 would interact favourably at the P4 anchoring pocket of SE-containing HLA-DR molecules. This was confirmed both for DRB1*0101, DRB1*0401 (Hill et al., 2003) and DRB1*1001 (James et al., 2010). Concretely, modified peptides derived from joint associated proteins were able to bind to RA-associated MHC molecules: the peptide spanning residues 65-77 from vimentin, vimentin (65-77) to DRB1*0101 and DRB1*0401 (Hill et al., 2003), and peptides vimentin (58-72), Fib A (737-751), Fib B (68-82) and cartilage intermediate layer protein CILP (982-996) to DRB1*1001 (James et al., 2010). These data open the possibility that in the inflamed joint, some arginines may be deiminated by activated PAD2 or PAD4 and, after protein catabolism, citrulline-containing peptides would be bound to SE HLA-DR molecules.

The peptide repertoires associated to many MHC molecules have been described, both for MHC class I and for MHC class II. However, up to now, no peptide with citrulline in P4 has been reported to be a natural ligand of any HLA-DR molecule. Some reasons make the identification of citrullinated peptides from the peptide repertoire bound to HLA-DR molecules very difficult. First, the conditions to obtain high level of protein citrullination are not totally controlled, although some protocols have been reported, as increasing intracellular calcium by the addition of ionomicine to the cell culture (Vossenaar et al., 2004c). Second and more important, after deimination induction, most of the peptides will remain containing arginine instead of citrulline, and probably, the amount of citrullinated peptides in the peptide pool will be low. Mass spectrometry analysis give information of the most abundant peptides in the MHC-associated peptide pools making complicated to find a low-abundance citrullinated peptide. An approach that could be used to solve these problems would be to enrich citrullinated peptides in the sample. Antibodies specific for citrullinated peptides can not be used because they can recognize some peptides but not others. A technique for the specific enrichment of citrulline-containing peptides has been described, based on the immobilization of a glyoxal derivative that reacts exclusively with the ureido group of the citrulline residue al low pH (Tutturen et al., 2010). The ureido group can be chemically modified by diacetyl monoxime and antipyrine (Senshu et al., 1992). The chemically modified citrulline can be detected, using a specific antibody, by Western blotting and immunohistochemistry (Makrygiannakis et al., 2008). Peptides or proteins containing the modified citrulline can also be detected by mass spectrometry (Stensland et al., 2009).

6. T cell responses to HLA-restricted citrullinated peptides

The induction of a typical humoral response that results in a production of classes of antibodies others than IgM requires the help of CD4 T cells. T cells recognize complexes formed by MHC molecules and peptides derived from antigenic proteins. In the case of ACPAs, the targets of the immune response are modified self proteins, as vimentin, fillagrin, fibrinogen and collagen type II. CD4 T cells that help in the generation of an anti-citrullinated proteins B cell response do not necessarily recognize citrullinated peptides. However, a role of T cell responses in RA is well known, which makes the identification of T cell responses against citrullinated peptides presented in the context of RA-related HLA-DR of great interest. These peptides could be citrullinated outside the binding core, in the core positions other than P4, or in P4, as discussed above.

In the last years, T cell responses to citrulline-containing peptides have been studied. First, using DR4-IE transgenic mice (expressing the chimeric molecule DR4-IE, that contains the DR4 binding groove and part of the murine class II molecule), Hill and collaborators demonstrated that deimination of arginine to citrulline significantly increased the peptide-MHC affinity when arginine was in P4 position. In addition, activated $CD4^+$ T cells were detected in these transgenic mice against a peptide spanning residues 65 to 77 of vimentin, vimentin (65-77), which had a citrulline in position 70 instead of the arginine of the unmodified protein. These results revealed that HLA-DRB1 alleles with the SE could initiate an specific autoimmune response to citrullinated self-antigens in DR4-transgenic mice (Hill et al., 2003). In this animal model, citrullinated fibrinogen induced arthritis. The disease induced in these mice was characterized by synovial hyperplasia followed by ankylosis, but lacked a large leukocyte infiltrate. Specific humoral and cellular responses to citrullinated components were observed, which were absent in wild-type mice immunized with citrullinated or unmodified fibrinogen and in transgenic mice immunized with unmodified fibrinogen (Hill et al., 2008). HLA-DRB1*0401–restricted T cell reactivity to fibrinogen (371-383) was clearly seen in transgenic mice after immunization with either citrullinated fibrinogen or unmodified fibrinogen, whereas no specific response to this peptide was detected in wild-type mice. Ten peptides derived from α, β or γ chains of human fibrinogen containing an aliphatic or aromatic residue in P1 position of the binding core and arginine or citrulline at P4 were tested to generate T cell responses. Only one citrullinated peptide, $Fib\alpha_{R84Cit}$, induced a consistent T cell response, whereas no response was seen against the corresponding arginine-containing peptide $Fib\alpha_{79\text{-}91}$. Therefore, these data confirm that a citrullinated protein can be arthritogenic when RA-associated alleles are expressed, and specific T cell responses to citrullinated peptides are part of the immune response. Citrullinated peptides-specific T cell activation plays an important role in the development and progression of arthritis in this animal model. Thus, when given prior to disease onset, treatment with CTLA-4Ig, an agent that blocks T cell costimulation, prevented T cell activation induced by citrullinated human fibrinogen. This effect was not seen with non-specific IgG1 (Yue et al.).

Other approach using the mouse model detected that a response against citrullinated peptides could be generated even when the antigen was administrated in unmodified form. Concretely, HEL was used as a model antigen, and T cells specifically reactive to citrullinated epitopes were detected among the responding repertoire to immunization with an unmodified HEL protein. In addition, antigen presenting cells (APCs), including dendritic cells and peritoneal macrophages, were able to present citrullinated peptides when provided an intact, unmodified HEL *ex vivo* (Ireland et al., 2006). Therefore, APCs were capable to capture and process the antigen, to deiminate some specific arginine residues and to present some citrullin-containing peptides to T cells in a correct way to induce an specific response against citrullinated peptides.

More than 90% of patients positive for citrullinated vimentin-specific ACPAs carry SE-containing HLA-DRB1 alleles. In a DR4-transgenic mouse model, animals were immunized with 33 citrulline-containing peptides (all possible citrullinated peptides of human vimentin) and tested for T cell reactivity. T cell responses were generated against some of these peptides restricted by HLA-DRB1*0401 (vimentin (26-44) and vimentin (415-433). Antigen presenting cells were able to generate these peptides from entire vimentin. In addition, T cell reactivity against these citrullinated peptides derived from vimentin were observed when PBMCs from ACPAs-positive, HLA-DR4-positive patients with RA were used (Feitsma et al.). These data strongly suggest the presence of HLA-DRB1*0401-restricted T cell responses against citrullinated vimentin-derived peptides in RA patients. The data do not exclude T cell responses against non-citrullinated peptides restricted by this or other HLA-DRB1 alleles, that also could facilitate a humoral response against citrullinated epitopes.

The generation of T cell responses against citrullinated peptides has also been confirmed for other autoantigens. Thus, a proliferative response was observed in more than 60% RA patients after stimulation with citrullinated aggrecan-derived peptide, aggrecan (84-103) (von Delwig et al., 2010). This response was absent in PBMCs from healthy controls, and there was no response to the unmodified aggrecan analog peptide, indicating that citrulline residue is required for T cell recognition. In addition, cytokine production was analyzed by ELISA and intracellular cytokine analysis. High levels of the proinflammatory cytokine interleukin-17 (IL-17) was produced by PBMCs from RA patients in response to stimulation with citrullinated aggrecan. This IL-17 production was absent when PBMCs from RA patients and healthy controls were stimulated with the unmodified aggrecan-derived peptide. Therefore, citrullinated aggrecan-specific T cells may play a role in the pathogenesis of RA and in the inflammatory process.

Most of the T cell responses to citrullinated peptides have been generated in models that express HLA-DRB1*0401. In addition, responses against citrullinated peptides restricted by the RA-associated, SE-containing HLA-DRB1*1001 molecule have been obtained (James et al., 2010). Authors demonstrated that HLA-DRB1*1001 can accommodate citrulline in three anchor positions, and three of the modified peptides that were evaluated developed specific $CD4^+$ T cell responses. These peptides derived from fibrinogen α, fibrinogen β and cartilage intermediate-layer protein, and these data suggest a role for these three proteins as relevant antigens in RA in HLA-DRB1*1001$^+$ patients. In addition, T cell clones specific for these sequences proliferated only in response to citrullinated peptides. One more time, these data suggest that deimination of arginine can have as a consequence the generation of new HLA-DR ligands that can be recognized by T cells as neoepitopes, and may play an important role in the initiation or progression of RA. As described recently, T cell responses to other post-translational modifications may play a similar role in generating inflammatory responses. One of this could be carbamylation of lysine to homocitrulline. Thus, mice were immunized with carbamylated peptides, which induced chemotaxis, and T and B cell responses. Mice immunized with carbamylated peptides developed erosive arthritis when citrullinated peptides were injected intra-articularly. In addition, T and B cells induced arthritis after adoptive transfer into normal recipients (Mydel et al., 2010). Therefore, the T cell response to homocitrulline-derived peptides, as well as the subsequent production of anti-homocitrulline Abs, was critical for the induction of autoimmune responses against citrulline-derived peptides which may provide a novel mechanism for the pathogenesis of arthritis.

Constitutive protein citrullination occurs in some tissues in absence of inflammation, which imply the existence of tolerance against these modified proteins. The thymus is the organ where the immunocompetent T cell repertoire is generated. During selection processes to generate central T cell tolerance, about 95-97% of the thymocytes die by apoptosis, which is an inductor of citrullination. Thus, PAD activity and arginine deimination may be active in this organ. Citrullinated peptides that bind to HLA-DR molecules in the thymus should not be able to induce an immune response in periphery. Differences in the machinery of antigen processing have been reported between thymic cells and other presenting cells. Thus, the identification and analysis of HLA-DR-associated citrullinated peptides in the thymus could reveal which peptides can generate central tolerance.

7. Conclusions

The finding that the sera of most RA patients contain antibodies specifc for citrullinated proteins opened the possibility of a new mechanism in the etiology of the disease. These antibodies are specific for RA, can be detected years before the development of the disease, and correlate with the presence of SE-containing alleles. In the last years, relevant advances on the identification of the citrullination process in the inflamed joints by PADs´activity, the presentation by RA-associated HLA-DR molecules that contain the SE, and T cell responses against citrullinated proteins have been made. Nevertheless, it remains to be defined which citrullinated peptides are really involved in the development of the disease in humans and if any of them can efficiently be presented in the context of various SE-containing HLA-DR molecules.

8. Acknowledgments

The author thanks Dr. Dolores Jaraquemada for her critical review of the manuscript.

9. References

Aho, K.;Palosuo, T.;Heliovaara, M., et al. (2000). Antifilaggrin antibodies within "normal" range predict rheumatoid arthritis in a linear fashion. *J Rheumatol,*Vol. 27 No. (12) (Dec 2000), pp. 2743-2746.

Alamanos, Y.& Drosos, A. A. (2005). Epidemiology of adult rheumatoid arthritis. *Autoimmun Rev,*Vol. 4 No. (3) (Mar 2005), pp. 130-136.

Aletaha, D.;Neogi, T.;Silman, A. J., et al. (2010). 2010 Rheumatoid arthritis classification criteria: an American College of Rheumatology/European League Against Rheumatism collaborative initiative. *Arthritis Rheum,*Vol. 62 No. (9) (Sep 2010), pp. 2569-2581.

Alvarez, I.;Collado, J.;Daura, X., et al. (2008). The rheumatoid arthritis-associated allele HLA-DR10 (DRB1*1001) shares part of its repertoire with HLA-DR1 (DRB1*0101) and HLA-DR4 (DRB*0401). *Arthritis Rheum,*Vol. 58 No. (6) (Jun 2008), pp. 1630-1639.

Andrade, F.;Darrah, E.;Gucek, M., et al. (2010). Autocitrullination of human peptidyl arginine deiminase type 4 regulates protein citrullination during cell activation. *Arthritis Rheum,*Vol. 62 No. (6) (Jan 2010), pp. 1630-1640.

Asaga, H.;Yamada, M.& Senshu, T. (1998). Selective deimination of vimentin in calcium ionophore-induced apoptosis of mouse peritoneal macrophages. *Biochem Biophys Res Commun,*Vol. 243 No. (3) (Feb 24 1998), pp. 641-646.

Auger, I.;Escola, J. M.;Gorvel, J. P., et al. (1996). HLA-DR4 and HLA-DR10 motifs that carry susceptibility to rheumatoid arthritis bind 70-kD heat shock proteins. *Nat Med,*Vol. 2 No. (3) (Mar 1996), pp. 306-310.

Avouac, J.;Gossec, L.& Dougados, M. (2006). Diagnostic and predictive value of anti-cyclic citrullinated protein antibodies in rheumatoid arthritis: a systematic literature review. *Ann Rheum Dis,*Vol. 65 No. (7) (Jul 2006), pp. 845-851.

Baeten, D.;Peene, I.;Union, A., et al. (2001). Specific presence of intracellular citrullinated proteins in rheumatoid arthritis synovium: relevance to antifilaggrin autoantibodies. *Arthritis Rheum,*Vol. 44 No. (10) (Oct 2001), pp. 2255-2262.

Bang, H.;Egerer, K.;Gauliard, A., et al. (2007). Mutation and citrullination modifies vimentin to a novel autoantigen for rheumatoid arthritis. *Arthritis Rheum,*Vol. 56 No. (8) (Aug 2007), pp. 2503-2511.

Bongartz, T.;Cantaert, T.;Atkins, S. R., et al. (2007). Citrullination in extra-articular manifestations of rheumatoid arthritis. *Rheumatology (Oxford),*Vol. 46 No. (1) (Jan 2007), pp. 70-75.

Burkhardt, H.;Sehnert, B.;Bockermann, R., et al. (2005). Humoral immune response to citrullinated collagen type II determinants in early rheumatoid arthritis. *Eur J Immunol,*Vol. 35 No. (5) (May 2005), pp. 1643-1652.

Cutbush, S.;Chikanza, I. C.;Biro, P. A., et al. (1993). Sequence-specific oligonucleotide typing in Shona patients with rheumatoid arthritis and healthy controls from Zimbabwe. *Tissue Antigens,*Vol. 41 No. (4) (Apr 1993), pp. 169-172.

Chavanas, S.;Mechin, M. C.;Takahara, H., et al. (2004). Comparative analysis of the mouse and human peptidylarginine deiminase gene clusters reveals highly conserved non-coding segments and a new human gene, PADI6. *Gene,*Vol. 330 No. (Apr 14 2004), pp. 19-27.

de Juan, M. D.;Belmonte, I.;Barado, J., et al. (1994). Differential associations of HLA-DR antigens with rheumatoid arthritis (RA) in Basques: high frequency of DR1 and DR10 and lack of association with HLA-DR4 or any of its subtypes. *Tissue Antigens,*Vol. 43 No. (5) (May 1994), pp. 320-323.

Dengjel, J.;Schoor, O.;Fischer, R., et al. (2005). Autophagy promotes MHC class II presentation of peptides from intracellular source proteins. *Proc Natl Acad Sci U S A,*Vol. 102 No. (22) (May 31 2005), pp. 7922-7927.

Despres, N.;Boire, G.;Lopez-Longo, F. J., et al. (1994). The Sa system: a novel antigen-antibody system specific for rheumatoid arthritis. *J Rheumatol,*Vol. 21 No. (6) (Jun 1994), pp. 1027-1033.

Dessen, A.;Lawrence, C. M.;Cupo, S., et al. (1997). X-ray crystal structure of HLA-DR4 (DRA*0101, DRB1*0401) complexed with a peptide from human collagen II. *Immunity,*Vol. 7 No. (4) (Oct 1997), pp. 473-481.

Feitsma, A. L.;van der Voort, E. I.;Franken, K. L., et al. Identification of citrullinated vimentin peptides as T cell epitopes in HLA-DR4-positive patients with rheumatoid arthritis. *Arthritis Rheum,*Vol. 62 No. (1) (Jan pp. 117-125.

Forslind, K.;Ahlmen, M.;Eberhardt, K., et al. (2004). Prediction of radiological outcome in early rheumatoid arthritis in clinical practice: role of antibodies to citrullinated peptides (anti-CCP). *Ann Rheum Dis,*Vol. 63 No. (9) (Sep 2004), pp. 1090-1095.

Foulquier, C.;Sebbag, M.;Clavel, C., et al. (2007). Peptidyl arginine deiminase type 2 (PAD-2) and PAD-4 but not PAD-1, PAD-3, and PAD-6 are expressed in rheumatoid arthritis synovium in close association with tissue inflammation. *Arthritis Rheum,*Vol. 56 No. (11) (Nov 2007), pp. 3541-3553.

Fremont, D. H.;Hendrickson, W. A.;Marrack, P., et al. (1996). Structures of an MHC class II molecule with covalently bound single peptides. *Science,*Vol. 272 No. (5264) (May 17 1996), pp. 1001-1004.

Friede, T.;Gnau, V.;Jung, G., et al. (1996). Natural ligand motifs of closely related HLA-DR4 molecules predict features of rheumatoid arthritis associated peptides. *Biochim Biophys Acta,*Vol. 1316 No. (2) (Jun 7 1996), pp. 85-101.

Gonzalez-Escribano, M. F.;Rodriguez, R.;Valenzuela, A., et al. (1999). Complex associations between HLA-DRB1 genes and female rheumatoid arthritis: results from a prospective study. *Hum Immunol,*Vol. 60 No. (12) (Dec 1999), pp. 1259-1265.

Gregersen, P. K.;Silver, J.& Winchester, R. J. (1987). The shared epitope hypothesis. An approach to understanding the molecular genetics of susceptibility to rheumatoid arthritis. *Arthritis Rheum,*Vol. 30 No. (11) (Nov 1987), pp. 1205-1213.

Gyorgy, B.;Toth, E.;Tarcsa, E., et al. (2006). Citrullination: a posttranslational modification in health and disease. *Int J Biochem Cell Biol,*Vol. 38 No. (10) 2006), pp. 1662-1677.

Hameed, K.;Bowman, S.;Kondeatis, E., et al. (1997). The association of HLA-DRB genes and the shared epitope with rheumatoid arthritis in Pakistan. *Br J Rheumatol,*Vol. 36 No. (11) (Nov 1997), pp. 1184-1188.

Hammer, J.;Bono, E.;Gallazzi, F., et al. (1994). Precise prediction of major histocompatibility complex class II-peptide interaction based on peptide side chain scanning. *J Exp Med,*Vol. 180 No. (6) (Dec 1 1994), pp. 2353-2358.

Hammer, J.;Gallazzi, F.;Bono, E., et al. (1995). Peptide binding specificity of HLA-DR4 molecules: correlation with rheumatoid arthritis association. *J Exp Med,*Vol. 181 No. (5) (May 1 1995), pp. 1847-1855.

Hayem, G.;Chazerain, P.;Combe, B., et al. (1999). Anti-Sa antibody is an accurate diagnostic and prognostic marker in adult rheumatoid arthritis. *J Rheumatol,*Vol. 26 No. (1) (Jan 1999), pp. 7-13.

Hill, J. A.;Southwood, S.;Sette, A., et al. (2003). Cutting edge: the conversion of arginine to citrulline allows for a high-affinity peptide interaction with the rheumatoid arthritis-associated HLA-DRB1*0401 MHC class II molecule. *J Immunol,*Vol. 171 No. (2) (Jul 15 2003), pp. 538-541.

Hill, J. A.;Bell, D. A.;Brintnell, W., et al. (2008). Arthritis induced by posttranslationally modified (citrullinated) fibrinogen in DR4-IE transgenic mice. *J Exp Med,*Vol. 205 No. (4) (Apr 14 2008), pp. 967-979.

Hueber, W.;Hassfeld, W.;Smolen, J. S., et al. (1999). Sensitivity and specificity of anti-Sa autoantibodies for rheumatoid arthritis. *Rheumatology (Oxford),*Vol. 38 No. (2) (Feb 1999), pp. 155-159.

Huizinga, T. W.;Amos, C. I.;van der Helm-van Mil, A. H., et al. (2005). Refining the complex rheumatoid arthritis phenotype based on specificity of the HLA-DRB1 shared epitope for antibodies to citrullinated proteins. *Arthritis Rheum,*Vol. 52 No. (11) (Nov 2005), pp. 3433-3438.

Ireland, J.;Herzog, J.& Unanue, E. R. (2006). Cutting edge: unique T cells that recognize citrullinated peptides are a feature of protein immunization. *J Immunol,*Vol. 177 No. (3) (Aug 1 2006), pp. 1421-1425.

Irigoyen, P.;Lee, A. T.;Wener, M. H., et al. (2005). Regulation of anti-cyclic citrullinated peptide antibodies in rheumatoid arthritis: contrasting effects of HLA-DR3 and the shared epitope alleles. *Arthritis Rheum,*Vol. 52 No. (12) (Dec 2005), pp. 3813-3818.

James, E. A.;Moustakas, A. K.;Bui, J., et al. (2010). HLA-DR1001 presents "altered-self" peptides derived from joint-associated proteins by accepting citrulline in three of its binding pockets. *Arthritis Rheum,*Vol. 62 No. (10) (Oct 2010), pp. 2909-2918.

Jaraquemada, D.;Ollier, W.;Awad, J., et al. (1986). HLA and rheumatoid arthritis: a combined analysis of 440 British patients. *Ann Rheum Dis,*Vol. 45 No. (8) (Aug 1986), pp. 627-636.

Kastbom, A.;Strandberg, G.;Lindroos, A., et al. (2004). Anti-CCP antibody test predicts the disease course during 3 years in early rheumatoid arthritis (the Swedish TIRA project). *Ann Rheum Dis,*Vol. 63 No. (9) (Sep 2004), pp. 1085-1089.

Klareskog, L.;Ronnelid, J.;Lundberg, K., et al. (2008). Immunity to citrullinated proteins in rheumatoid arthritis. *Annu Rev Immunol,*Vol. 26 No. 2008), pp. 651-675.

Klareskog, L.;Stolt, P.;Lundberg, K., et al. (2006). A new model for an etiology of rheumatoid arthritis: smoking may trigger HLA-DR (shared epitope)-restricted immune reactions to autoantigens modified by citrullination. *Arthritis Rheum,*Vol. 54 No. (1) (Jan 2006), pp. 38-46.

Kroot, E. J.;de Jong, B. A.;van Leeuwen, M. A., et al. (2000). The prognostic value of anti-cyclic citrullinated peptide antibody in patients with recent-onset rheumatoid arthritis. *Arthritis Rheum,*Vol. 43 No. (8) (Aug 2000), pp. 1831-1835.

Kubilus, J.;Waitkus, R. W.& Baden, H. P. (1979). The presence of citrulline in epidermal proteins. *Biochim Biophys Acta,*Vol. 581 No. (1) (Nov 23 1979), pp. 114-121.

Kurki, P.;Aho, K.;Palosuo, T., et al. (1992). Immunopathology of rheumatoid arthritis. Antikeratin antibodies precede the clinical disease. *Arthritis Rheum,*Vol. 35 No. (8) (Aug 1992), pp. 914-917.

Lacki, J. K.;Wassmuth, R.;Korczowska, I., et al. (2000). Does the presence of HLA-DR B1 shared motif affect progression of the disease in rheumatoid arthritis patients? *Int J Immunopathol Pharmacol,*Vol. 13 No. (2) (May-Aug 2000), pp. 83-89.

Ling, S.;Li, Z.;Borschukova, O., et al. (2007). The rheumatoid arthritis shared epitope increases cellular susceptibility to oxidative stress by antagonizing an adenosine-mediated anti-oxidative pathway. *Arthritis Res Ther,*Vol. 9 No. (1) 2007), pp. R5.

Makrygiannakis, D.;af Klint, E.;Lundberg, I. E., et al. (2006). Citrullination is an inflammation-dependent process. *Ann Rheum Dis,*Vol. 65 No. (9) (Sep 2006), pp. 1219-1222.

Makrygiannakis, D.;Hermansson, M.;Ulfgren, A. K., et al. (2008). Smoking increases peptidylarginine deiminase 2 enzyme expression in human lungs and increases citrullination in BAL cells. *Ann Rheum Dis,*Vol. 67 No. (10) (Oct 2008), pp. 1488-1492.

Masson-Bessiere, C.;Sebbag, M.;Girbal-Neuhauser, E., et al. (2001). The major synovial targets of the rheumatoid arthritis-specific antifilaggrin autoantibodies are deiminated forms of the alpha- and beta-chains of fibrin. *J Immunol*,Vol. 166 No. (6) (Mar 15 2001), pp. 4177-4184.

Migliorini, P.;Pratesi, F.;Tommasi, C., et al. (2005). The immune response to citrullinated antigens in autoimmune diseases. *Autoimmun Rev*,Vol. 4 No. (8) (Nov 2005), pp. 561-564.

Mody, G. M.& Hammond, M. G. (1994). Differences in HLA-DR association with rheumatoid arthritis among migrant Indian communities in South Africa. *Br J Rheumatol*,Vol. 33 No. (5) (May 1994), pp. 425-427.

Muntasell, A.;Carrascal, M.;Alvarez, I., et al. (2004). Dissection of the HLA-DR4 peptide repertoire in endocrine epithelial cells: strong influence of invariant chain and HLA-DM expression on the nature of ligands. *J Immunol*,Vol. 173 No. (2) (Jul 15 2004), pp. 1085-1093.

Mydel, P.;Wang, Z.;Brisslert, M., et al. (2010). Carbamylation-dependent activation of T cells: a novel mechanism in the pathogenesis of autoimmune arthritis. *J Immunol*,Vol. 184 No. (12) (Jun 15 2010), pp. 6882-6890.

Nemazee, D. A. (1985). Immune complexes can trigger specific, T cell-dependent, autoanti-IgG antibody production in mice. *J Exp Med*,Vol. 161 No. (1) (Jan 1 1985), pp. 242-256.

Neogi, T.;Aletaha, D.;Silman, A. J., et al. (2010). The 2010 American College of Rheumatology/European League Against Rheumatism classification criteria for rheumatoid arthritis: Phase 2 methodological report. *Arthritis Rheum*,Vol. 62 No. (9) (Sep 2010), pp. 2582-2591.

Nicholas, A. P.& Whitaker, J. N. (2002). Preparation of a monoclonal antibody to citrullinated epitopes: its characterization and some applications to immunohistochemistry in human brain. *Glia*,Vol. 37 No. (4) (Mar 15 2002), pp. 328-336.

Nicholas, A. P.;King, J. L.;Sambandam, T., et al. (2003). Immunohistochemical localization of citrullinated proteins in adult rat brain. *J Comp Neurol*,Vol. 459 No. (3) (May 5 2003), pp. 251-266.

Nielen, M. M.;van Schaardenburg, D.;Reesink, H. W., et al. (2004). Specific autoantibodies precede the symptoms of rheumatoid arthritis: a study of serial measurements in blood donors. *Arthritis Rheum*,Vol. 50 No. (2) (Feb 2004), pp. 380-386.

Nijenhuis, S.;Zendman, A. J.;Vossenaar, E. R., et al. (2004). Autoantibodies to citrullinated proteins in rheumatoid arthritis: clinical performance and biochemical aspects of an RA-specific marker. *Clin Chim Acta*,Vol. 350 No. (1-2) (Dec 2004), pp. 17-34.

Nishimura, K.;Sugiyama, D.;Kogata, Y., et al. (2007). Meta-analysis: diagnostic accuracy of anti-cyclic citrullinated peptide antibody and rheumatoid factor for rheumatoid arthritis. *Ann Intern Med*,Vol. 146 No. (11) (Jun 5 2007), pp. 797-808.

Okada, Y.;Yamada, R.;Suzuki, A., et al. (2009). Contribution of a haplotype in the HLA region to anti-cyclic citrullinated peptide antibody positivity in rheumatoid arthritis, independently of HLA-DRB1. *Arthritis Rheum*,Vol. 60 No. (12) (Dec 2009), pp. 3582-3590.

Poor, G.;Nagy, Z. B.;Schmidt, Z., et al. (2007). Genetic background of anticyclic citrullinated peptide autoantibody production in Hungarian patients with rheumatoid arthritis. *Ann N Y Acad Sci*,Vol. 1110 No. (Sep 2007), pp. 23-32.

Pritzker, L. B.;Joshi, S.;Gowan, J. J., et al. (2000). Deimination of myelin basic protein. 1. Effect of deimination of arginyl residues of myelin basic protein on its structure and susceptibility to digestion by cathepsin D. *Biochemistry,*Vol. 39 No. (18) (May 9 2000), pp. 5374-5381.

Proost, P.;Loos, T.;Mortier, A., et al. (2008). Citrullination of CXCL8 by peptidylarginine deiminase alters receptor usage, prevents proteolysis, and dampens tissue inflammation. *J Exp Med,*Vol. 205 No. (9) (Sep 1 2008), pp. 2085-2097.

Rantapaa-Dahlqvist, S.;de Jong, B. A.;Berglin, E., et al. (2003). Antibodies against cyclic citrullinated peptide and IgA rheumatoid factor predict the development of rheumatoid arthritis. *Arthritis Rheum,*Vol. 48 No. (10) (Oct 2003), pp. 2741-2749.

Ronnelid, J.;Wick, M. C.;Lampa, J., et al. (2005). Longitudinal analysis of citrullinated protein/peptide antibodies (anti-CP) during 5 year follow up in early rheumatoid arthritis: anti-CP status predicts worse disease activity and greater radiological progression. *Ann Rheum Dis,*Vol. 64 No. (12) (Dec 2005), pp. 1744-1749.

Rosloniec, E. F.;Ivey, R. A., 3rd;Whittington, K. B., et al. (2006). Crystallographic structure of a rheumatoid arthritis MHC susceptibility allele, HLA-DR1 (DRB1*0101), complexed with the immunodominant determinant of human type II collagen. *J Immunol,*Vol. 177 No. (6) (Sep 15 2006), pp. 3884-3892.

Salvarani, C.;Boiardi, L.;Mantovani, V., et al. (1999). HLA-DRB1 alleles associated with polymyalgia rheumatica in northern Italy: correlation with disease severity. *Ann Rheum Dis,*Vol. 58 No. (5) (May 1999), pp. 303-308.

Salvat, S.;Auger, I.;Rochelle, L., et al. (1994). Tolerance to a self-peptide from the third hypervariable region of HLA DRB1*0401 in rheumatoid arthritis patients and normal subjects. *J Immunol,*Vol. 153 No. (11) (Dec 1 1994), pp. 5321-5329.

Sanchez, B.;Moreno, I.;Magarino, R., et al. (1990). HLA-DRw10 confers the highest susceptibility to rheumatoid arthritis in a Spanish population. *Tissue Antigens,*Vol. 36 No. (4) (Oct 1990), pp. 174-176.

Schellekens, G. A.;de Jong, B. A.;van den Hoogen, F. H., et al. (1998). Citrulline is an essential constituent of antigenic determinants recognized by rheumatoid arthritis-specific autoantibodies. *J Clin Invest,*Vol. 101 No. (1) (Jan 1 1998), pp. 273-281.

Schellekens, G. A.;Visser, H.;de Jong, B. A., et al. (2000). The diagnostic properties of rheumatoid arthritis antibodies recognizing a cyclic citrullinated peptide. *Arthritis Rheum,*Vol. 43 No. (1) (Jan 2000), pp. 155-163.

Sebbag, M.;Simon, M.;Vincent, C., et al. (1995). The antiperinuclear factor and the so-called antikeratin antibodies are the same rheumatoid arthritis-specific autoantibodies. *J Clin Invest,*Vol. 95 No. (6) (Jun 1995), pp. 2672-2679.

Senshu, T.;Sato, T.;Inoue, T., et al. (1992). Detection of citrulline residues in deiminated proteins on polyvinylidene difluoride membrane. *Anal Biochem,*Vol. 203 No. (1) (May 15 1992), pp. 94-100.

Senshu, T.;Kan, S.;Ogawa, H., et al. (1996). Preferential deimination of keratin K1 and filaggrin during the terminal differentiation of human epidermis. *Biochem Biophys Res Commun,*Vol. 225 No. (3) (Aug 23 1996), pp. 712-719.

Simon, M.;Girbal, E.;Sebbag, M., et al. (1993). The cytokeratin filament-aggregating protein filaggrin is the target of the so-called "antikeratin antibodies," autoantibodies specific for rheumatoid arthritis. *J Clin Invest,*Vol. 92 No. (3) (Sep 1993), pp. 1387-1393.

Stastny, P. (1978). Association of the B-cell alloantigen DRw4 with rheumatoid arthritis. *N Engl J Med,*Vol. 298 No. (16) (Apr 20 1978), pp. 869-871.

Stensland, M.;Holm, A.;Kiehne, A., et al. (2009). Targeted analysis of protein citrullination using chemical modification and tandem mass spectrometry. *Rapid Commun Mass Spectrom,*Vol. 23 No. (17) (Sep 2009), pp. 2754-2762.

Stern, L. J.;Brown, J. H.;Jardetzky, T. S., et al. (1994). Crystal structure of the human class II MHC protein HLA-DR1 complexed with an influenza virus peptide. *Nature,*Vol. 368 No. (6468) (Mar 17 1994), pp. 215-221.

Suzuki, A.;Yamada, R.;Chang, X., et al. (2003). Functional haplotypes of PADI4, encoding citrullinating enzyme peptidylarginine deiminase 4, are associated with rheumatoid arthritis. *Nat Genet,*Vol. 34 No. (4) (Aug 2003), pp. 395-402.

Tarcsa, E.;Marekov, L. N.;Mei, G., et al. (1996). Protein unfolding by peptidylarginine deiminase. Substrate specificity and structural relationships of the natural substrates trichohyalin and filaggrin. *J Biol Chem,*Vol. 271 No. (48) (Nov 29 1996), pp. 30709-30716.

Tarkowski, A.;Czerkinsky, C.& Nilsson, L. A. (1985). Simultaneous induction of rheumatoid factor- and antigen-specific antibody-secreting cells during the secondary immune response in man. *Clin Exp Immunol,*Vol. 61 No. (2) (Aug 1985), pp. 379-387.

Tutturen, A. E.;Holm, A.;Jorgensen, M., et al. (2010). A technique for the specific enrichment of citrulline-containing peptides. *Anal Biochem,*Vol. 403 No. (1-2) (Aug 2010), pp. 43-51.

van der Helm-van Mil, A. H.;Huizinga, T. W.;Schreuder, G. M., et al. (2005). An independent role of protective HLA class II alleles in rheumatoid arthritis severity and susceptibility. *Arthritis Rheum,*Vol. 52 No. (9) (Sep 2005), pp. 2637-2644.

van der Helm-van Mil, A. H.;Verpoort, K. N.;Breedveld, F. C., et al. (2006). The HLA-DRB1 shared epitope alleles are primarily a risk factor for anti-cyclic citrullinated peptide antibodies and are not an independent risk factor for development of rheumatoid arthritis. *Arthritis Rheum,*Vol. 54 No. (4) (Apr 2006), pp. 1117-1121.

van Gaalen, F. A.;Linn-Rasker, S. P.;van Venrooij, W. J., et al. (2004). Autoantibodies to cyclic citrullinated peptides predict progression to rheumatoid arthritis in patients with undifferentiated arthritis: a prospective cohort study. *Arthritis Rheum,*Vol. 50 No. (3) (Mar 2004), pp. 709-715.

van Venrooij, W. J.& Pruijn, G. J. (2000). Citrullination: a small change for a protein with great consequences for rheumatoid arthritis. *Arthritis Res,*Vol. 2 No. (4) 2000), pp. 249-251.

Verpoort, K. N.;Cheung, K.;Ioan-Facsinay, A., et al. (2007). Fine specificity of the anti-citrullinated protein antibody response is influenced by the shared epitope alleles. *Arthritis Rheum,*Vol. 56 No. (12) (Dec 2007), pp. 3949-3952.

Verreck, F. A.;van de Poel, A.;Drijfhout, J. W., et al. (1996). Natural peptides isolated from Gly86/Val86-containing variants of HLA-DR1, -DR11, -DR13, and -DR52. *Immunogenetics,*Vol. 43 No. (6) 1996), pp. 392-397.

Vincent, C.;Nogueira, L.;Sebbag, M., et al. (2002). Detection of antibodies to deiminated recombinant rat filaggrin by enzyme-linked immunosorbent assay: a highly effective test for the diagnosis of rheumatoid arthritis. *Arthritis Rheum,*Vol. 46 No. (8) (Aug 2002), pp. 2051-2058.

von Delwig, A.;Locke, J.;Robinson, J. H., et al. (2010). Response of Th17 cells to a citrullinated arthritogenic aggrecan peptide in patients with rheumatoid arthritis. *Arthritis Rheum,*Vol. 62 No. (1) (Jan 2010), pp. 143-149.

Vossenaar, E. R.;Zendman, A. J.;van Venrooij, W. J., et al. (2003). PAD, a growing family of citrullinating enzymes: genes, features and involvement in disease. *Bioessays,*Vol. 25 No. (11) (Nov 2003), pp. 1106-1118.

Vossenaar, E. R.;Smeets, T. J.;Kraan, M. C., et al. (2004a). The presence of citrullinated proteins is not specific for rheumatoid synovial tissue. *Arthritis Rheum,*Vol. 50 No. (11) (Nov 2004a), pp. 3485-3494.

Vossenaar, E. R.;Despres, N.;Lapointe, E., et al. (2004b). Rheumatoid arthritis specific anti-Sa antibodies target citrullinated vimentin. *Arthritis Res Ther,*Vol. 6 No. (2) 2004b), pp. R142-150.

Vossenaar, E. R.;Radstake, T. R.;van der Heijden, A., et al. (2004c). Expression and activity of citrullinating peptidylarginine deiminase enzymes in monocytes and macrophages. *Ann Rheum Dis,*Vol. 63 No. (4) (Apr 2004c), pp. 373-381.

Wysocka, J.;Allis, C. D.& Coonrod, S. (2006). Histone arginine methylation and its dynamic regulation. *Front Biosci,*Vol. 11 No. 2006), pp. 344-355.

Yelamos, J.;Garcia-Lozano, J. R.;Moreno, I., et al. (1993). Association of HLA-DR4-Dw15 (DRB1*0405) and DR10 with rheumatoid arthritis in a Spanish population. *Arthritis Rheum,*Vol. 36 No. (6) (Jun 1993), pp. 811-814.

Yue, D.;Brintnell, W.;Mannik, L. A., et al. CTLA-4Ig blocks the development and progression of citrullinated fibrinogen-induced arthritis in DR4-transgenic mice. *Arthritis Rheum,*Vol. 62 No. (10) (Oct pp. 2941-2952.

5

Cell Surface Glycans at SLE – Changes During Cells Death, Utilization for Disease Detection and Molecular Mechanism Underlying Their Modification

Bilyy Rostyslav[1,2], Tomin Andriy[1], Yaroslav Tolstyak[2], Havrylyuk Anna[2], Chopyak Valentina[2], Kit Yuriy[1] and Stoika Rostyslav[1]

[1]*Institute of Cell Biology, National Academy of Sciences of Ukraine, Lviv,*
[2]*Danylo Halytsky Lviv National Medical University, Lviv,*
Ukraine

1. Introduction

Autoimmune diseases develop when the immune system starts producing antibodies and T cells that are targeting components of the body. Such state occurs when the ability to recognition of self is disturbed and the immune cells attack healthy cells. The autoimmune diseases are frequently accompanied by self-destruction which is realized via apoptosis. There are two signaling pathways how the immune cells induce apoptosis in the target cells: 1) receptor-mediated; 2) receptor-independent. In the first mechanism, so called "death receptors" that are located on plasma membrane of the target cell are involved, while their "death ligands" are either located on the surface of the immune cell, or released by these cells and acting in free form. The corresponding ligand-receptor interactions cause activation of "death receptors" which use special "death domains" for contacting with specific intracellular signaling proteins and formation of death-inducing signaling complex (DISC). It is considered that this complex is capable of interacting with procaspase 8 and activating this initiator caspase. It is also probable that from this moment (activation of caspase 8), cascade of the apoptotic events gains irreversible character (Ashkenazi & Dixit, 1998). The receptor-independent mechanisms of apoptosis induction in which the immune cells take part, differ significantly (Vermijlen et al., 2001). These mechanisms are based on the ability of cytotoxic T cells to induce formation of special pores in plasma membrane of the target cells. Through these pores, calcium cations and protein granzyme B penetrates the target cells where they directly activate apoptotic enzymes - the caspases.

Fas-receptor that belongs to a family of tumor necrosis factor (TNF) receptors (Orlinick & Chao, 1998) is a typical "death receptor". It is known that TNF is produced by activated macrophages and T cells as a host response to infection (Tartaglia & Goeddel, 1992). Its interaction with specific plasma membrane receptors induces production of transcription factors NF-kB and AP-1 which take part in the activation of specific genes whose products are involved in the inflammation and immunomodulation (Tartaglia & Goeddel, 1992).

After association with the adaptor protein TRADD, TNF receptor can interact with the procaspase 8, and this occurs during the TNF-induced apoptosis.
Apo2L or TRAIL is another TNF-like ligand that can induce apoptosis in various cell lines including tumor ones (Pradhan, Krahling, Williamson, & Schlegel, 1997). Since the population of mature T cells gains sensitivity to the TRAIL-induced apoptosis after their stimulation with the interleukin 2, it is considered that TRAIL takes part in elimination of the peripheral T lymphocytes.
The receptor-independent apoptosis is the main mechanism by which the cytotoxic lymphocytes destroy virus-infected cells, as well as tumor cells (Ploegh, 1998). This mechanism is based on exocytosis of special dense granules which interact with plasma membrane of the target cells. These granules contain cytolytic substances which can polymerize in the presence of calcium cations and form macromolecular channels in the plasma membrane of the target cells. These channels are used for penetration of the granzyme B - serine protease that is capable of activating various caspases, for example the procaspase 3 (Goping et al., 2003). An elevated expression of the antiapoptotic mitochondrial protein Bcl-2 blocks such activation of the caspase 3, while the granzyme B blocks functioning of the Bcl-2. Thus, granzyme B is critical agent in the induction of apoptosis caused by the cytotoxic T cells.

1.1 SLE

Systemic Lupus Erythematosus (SLE) is a chronic, usually life-long, potentially fatal autoimmune disease characterized by unpredictable exacerbations and remissions with variable clinical manifestations. In SLE patients, there is a high probability for clinical involvement of the joints, skin, kidney, brain, lung, heart, serosa and gastrointestinal tract. Women and minorities are disproportionately affected, and Lupus SLE is most common in women of child-bearing age. A recent study identified a prevalence in the Unites States of 500 per 100,000 (1:200) in women (Belmont, 2010). SLE is a multifactorial disease involving genetic, environmental and hormonal factors. Its precise pathogenesis is unclear. There is growing evidence in favor of clearance deficiency of apoptotic cells as a core mechanism in SLE pathogenesis.

1.2 Clearance and SLE

Defective clearance of apoptotic cells causes secondary necrosis with a release of intracellular content and inflammatory mediators. This occurrence is considered as an intrinsic defect that can cause permanent presence of cellular debris responsible for the initiation of systemic autoimmunity in such diseases as SLE (for details see the review (Munoz, Lauber, Schiller, Manfredi, & Herrmann, 2010)). Macrophages respond and present self-antigens to T and B cells. Pathogenic autoantibodies are the primary cause of tissue damage in patients with lupus. The production of these antibodies arises by means of complex mechanisms involving every key facet of the immune system. Thus, restoring organism's ability to remove dying cells and impaired macromolecules (improving clearance efficiency) can serve as a perspective approach to treatment of autoimmune disorders and achieving clinical remission.

1.3 Ways to improve clearance

The apoptotic markers located in plasma membrane of the cell are very important, since they allow detecting apoptosis without violation of cell integrity. At present, phosphatidyl serine externalization is the most widely used apoptotic marker on PM (Fadok et al., 1992). It is detected by the annexin V binding test (Reutelingsperger & Christiaan Peter, 1998). Recently, we found that apoptosis is accompanied by not only the loss of plasma membrane asymmetry caused by phosphatidyl serine externalization, but also by changes in cell surface glycoconjugates described by us (R. Bilyy & Stoika, 2007; R. O. Bilyy, Antonyuk, & Stoika, 2004; R. O. Bilyy & Stoika, 2003). Similar results were obtained by the group headed by Prof. Martin Herrmann (Heyder et al., 2003). Further findings of our (R. Bilyy et al., 2005; R. O. Bilyy et al., 2004) and other groups (Batisse et al., 2004; Franz et al., 2006; Franz et al., 2007) allowed us to consider that an increase in the exposure levels of α-D-mannose- and β-D-galactose-rich GPs of the PM is a characteristic feature of the apoptotic cells. Their expression is substantially increased after apoptosis induction. Two independent mechanisms can lead to the appearance of altered surface glycoepitopes. One mechanism is the activation of surface sialidases resulting in exposure of desialylated (galactose-rich) surface glycoepitopes.

These glyconeoepitopes have been proposed for both the detection of apoptotic cells (R. O. Bilyy et al., 2004) and their isolation from the mixed populations (Stoika, Bilyy, & Antoniuk, 2006). Moreover, these glycoepitops can be directly involved in clearance of the apoptotic cells by the macrophages, serving as an "eat-me" signals of the apoptotic cells, as we have shown in (Meesmann et al., 2010). Our finding explains the previously known fact of surface glycopattern contribution to the clearance of dying and aged cells (Savill, Fadok, Henson, & Haslett, 1993). We effectively used changed apoptotic cell glycopattern for detection of dying cells in blood samples at the autoimmune disorders (R. Bilyy et al., 2009). We have proved that artificial desialylation of apoptotic and viable cells enhances their clearance by macrophages. This was confirmed in both cell lines and isolated human PMN and monocytes differentiated to macrophages (Meesmann et al., 2010).

Detection of both annexin V (van den Eijnde et al., 1997) and fluorescent conjugates of lectins (Heyder et al., 2003) usually requires using complex equipment like flow cytometer and/or fluorescent microscope. Evaluation of phosphatidyl serine externalization should be conducted as soon as possible after blood isolation, and cannot be done after the majority of available fixation procedure, since it would result in false-positive results; while the GPs are not affected by cell fixation or staining procedure. We have focused at the development of a test aimed to detect cell surface glycoconjugate changes during apoptotic cell death. We utilized the multivalency of lectin molecules for inducing agglutination of apoptotic cells, resulting from their altered surface GP content, and developed a specific test for apoptosis measurement (R. Bilyy & Stoika, 2007; Stoika et al., 2006).

2. Lymphocyte desialylation at SLE

Previously, we (R. Bilyy et al., 2009) demonstrated a significant increase in apoptosis incidence in the perypheral blood lymphocytes of RA patients comparing with lymphocytes of clinically healthy donors. That increase was detected by both flow cytometry and lectin-induced agglutination testing of apoptosis. We concluded that apoptosis-related changes in glycoconjugates of plasma membrane of the peripheral blood lymphocytes in RA patients can be used as a reliable and simple tool for apoptosis measurement during this and, probably, other autoimmune disorders. Detection of glycoconjugates via specific lectin binding is compatible with other available fixation/staining procedures, and can be recommended as an additional indicator in the multi-parameter automated detection systems.

Here we estimated changes in cell surface GP expression, namely changes in ß-D-containing glycans, in the peripheral blood lymphocytes of SLE patients and clinically healthy donors, and compared these changes with the level of apoptotic cells detected by the alternative methods. Detection of ß-D-containing glycans was performed by using VAA lectin staining, since this lectin binds to the surface of both early and late apoptotic cells, as can be seen at the confocal image on Fig. 1.

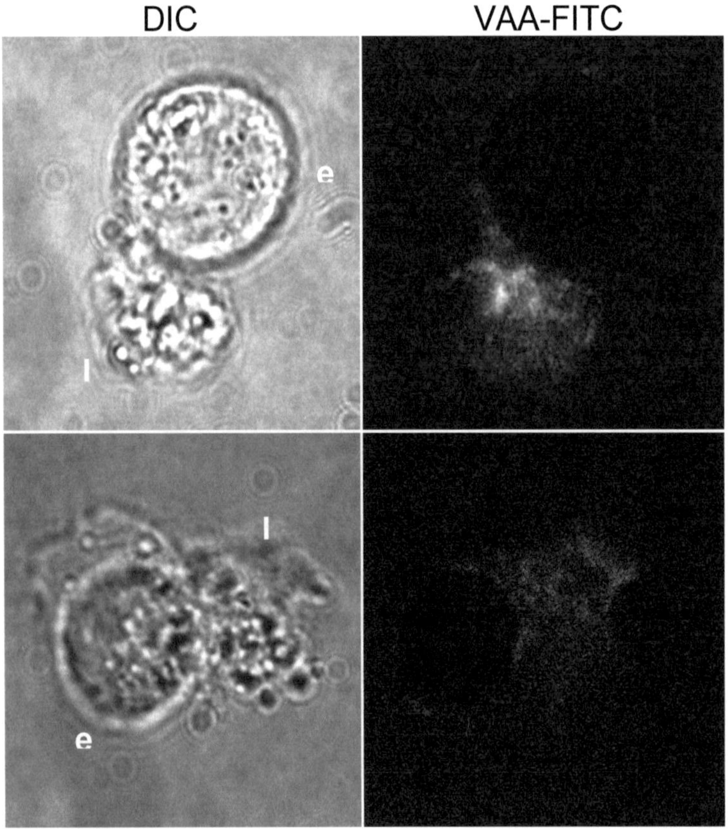

Fig. 1. Confocal microscopy of Jurkat T-cells at early (e) and late (l) stages of apoptosis progression, staining with VAA lectin. Lectin binds with cell surface, both cells are PI-negative.

Study of the peripheral blood lymphocytes of healthy donors revealed that their populations contained 0.707±0.121 % of cells with noticeable pre-G1 peak in cell cycle, with a range of 1.95% (minimal value - 0.14% and maximal value – 2.09), while the SLE patients were characterized by a markedly increased number of apoptotic cells (if judged by the appearance of G1 peak) – 4.47±0.50 %, with a wide range of 10.72% (minimal value – 0.86% and maximal value 11.62 %) (significance of the difference between two groups was $P<0.001$).

The lectin-induced agglutination test is based on the evaluation of minimal concentration of ß-D-galactose specific *Viscum album* lectin (VAA) used for cell agglutination. The principle of lectin-induced agglutination test is described in Fig. 2. Previously, it was proved that the level of these GPs was increased at apoptosis, and the concentration of lectin used for agglutination is in a reverse dependence upon the amount of cell surface GPs - the higher amount of the apoptotic like GPs is present on the cell surface - the less amount of lectin is needed for agglutination of these cells. Agglutination of lymphocytes of clinically healthy donors (0.32% and 0.12% of apoptotic cells), and of SLE patients (4.91% and 2.37% of apoptotic cells), as well as flow cytometry data on pre-G1 cell content are presented in Fig. 2.

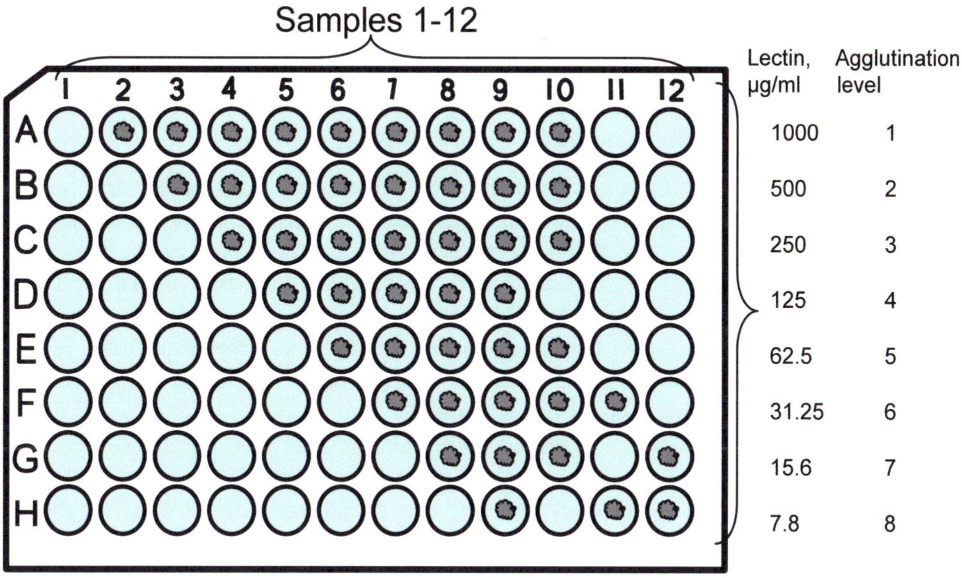

Interpretation:												
0	1	2	3	4	5	6	7	8	7[2]	-[3]	-[4]	Agglutination level
2000[1]	1000	500	250	125	62,5	31,3	15,6	7,8	15,6	-	-	Lectin concentration

Fig. 2. Principle of lectin-stimulated agglutination test. Agglutination level corresponds to minimal lectin concentration, needed for cell agglutination. Notes: 1 – our data indicate that lectin concentration, 2000 µg/ml agglutinates almost all intact cells. 2,3,4 – this conditions indicates possible errors in sample preparation and needs to be re-tested.

In the group of healthy donors, the mean lectin concentration needed to agglutinate lymphocytes was 1,500±121.27 µg/ml, while in the group of SLE patients, this indicator equaled 306.19±128.17 (significance of the difference between two groups was $P<0.001$) (Table 1). Thus, the ratio between the lectin concentrations in two studied groups constituted almost 4 times. This could be caused by two reasons: 1. increased basal (overall) lectin binding by cells in population; 2. increased number of cells that specifically bind the lectin. To clarify these mechanisms, smears of peripheral blood lymphocytes were subjected to lectin-cytochemical analysis based on using VAA lectin with subsequent microphotography and densitometric study. It revealed that basal staining in control group was 0.153±0.013 a.u., while in the SLE patients it was 0.144±0.01 a.u. There was no significant differences between two cell populations, while the number of cells that were intensively stained in both populations was significantly different (see Table 1). Thus, we suggested that difference in agglutination between lymphocytes of two groups is due to an increased percentage of cells exposing galactose-rich glycoconjugates on their surface.

	Healthy donors, n=18	SLE patients, n=23	p
% of apoptotic cells[1]	0.707 ± 0.121%	4.471 ±0.502 %	p<0.001
Agglutination[2]	1,500 ± 121.27 µg/ml	306.19±128.17 µg/ml	p<0.001
Basal VAA staining[3]	0.153 ± 0.013 a.u.	0.144 ± 0.010 a.u.	0.061
% of VAA stained cells	4.783 ± 0.936 %	8.27 ± 1.30 %	p<0.05

1 - judged by content of pre-G1 cells, measured by flow cytometry;
2 - measured by lectin-induced agglutination;
3 - measured by lectin-cytochemical analysis.

Table 1. Number of apoptotic cells and changes in plasma membrane glycoconjugates of lymphocytes in clinically healthy donors and SLE patients.

Correlation analysis of the amount of apoptotic cells detected by flow cytometry, and of minimal lectin concentration, needed for cell agglutination detected by lectin-stimulated agglutination, revealed a strong negative correlation between these two parameters (R=-0,764, P<0.001, see Fig.4). As previously established, the agglutinating lectin concentration is reversely proportional to the amount of apoptotic cells. Thus, the amount of apoptotic cells established by both methods - pre-G1 cell detection by flow cytometry and the lectin-induced agglutination - is well correlated. It should be noted that lectin-induced agglutination is much easier and cheaper in performing.

The correlation study between the amount of apoptotic cells detected by the Annexin V-FITC labeling and by testing based on using mannose-specific lectin from *Narcissus pseudonarcissus* (both detected by flow cytometry) was performed, and strong correlation between both parameters (R=0.725) was demonstrated (Heyder et al., 2003). Thus, specific changes in cell surface glycoconjugate pattern can be effectively used for detection of apoptotic cells at SLE and, probably, other at other autoimmune disorders.

The study of peripheral blood lymphocytes of 23 SLE patients and that of 18 clinically healthy donors revealed a significantly increased incidence of apoptosis in the SLE patients. That was detected by both flow cytometry and lectin-induced agglutination testing. High correlation between these results obtained by using two different methods suggests that apoptosis-related changes in plasma membrane glycoconjugates of the peripheral blood lymphocytes at SLE can be used as a reliable and easy tool for apoptosis measurement during autoimmune disorders. Detection of glycoconjugates via specific lectin binding is compatible with other available fixation/staining procedures. It can be recommended as an additional indicator in the multi-parameter automated detection systems.

Thus, the obtained data demonstrated that SLE was accompanied by an appearance of apoptotic cells possessing desialylated glycoepitopes (rich in terminal ß-D-containing glycans). Taking into account the above described clauses that desialylated glycans are important for cell clearance and that SLE potentially results from insufficient cell clearance, an intriguing question appears- are there any desialylating agents in blood of SLE patients.

3. Desialylating abzymes at SLE

Mammalian sialidases (related enzymes including bacterial and viral are also referred as neuraminidases) are glycosidases responsible for the removal of sialic acids from the glycoproteins and glycolipids. They have been implicated to participate in many biological processes, particularly in lysosomal catabolism (Miyagi, Wada, Yamaguchi, Hata, &

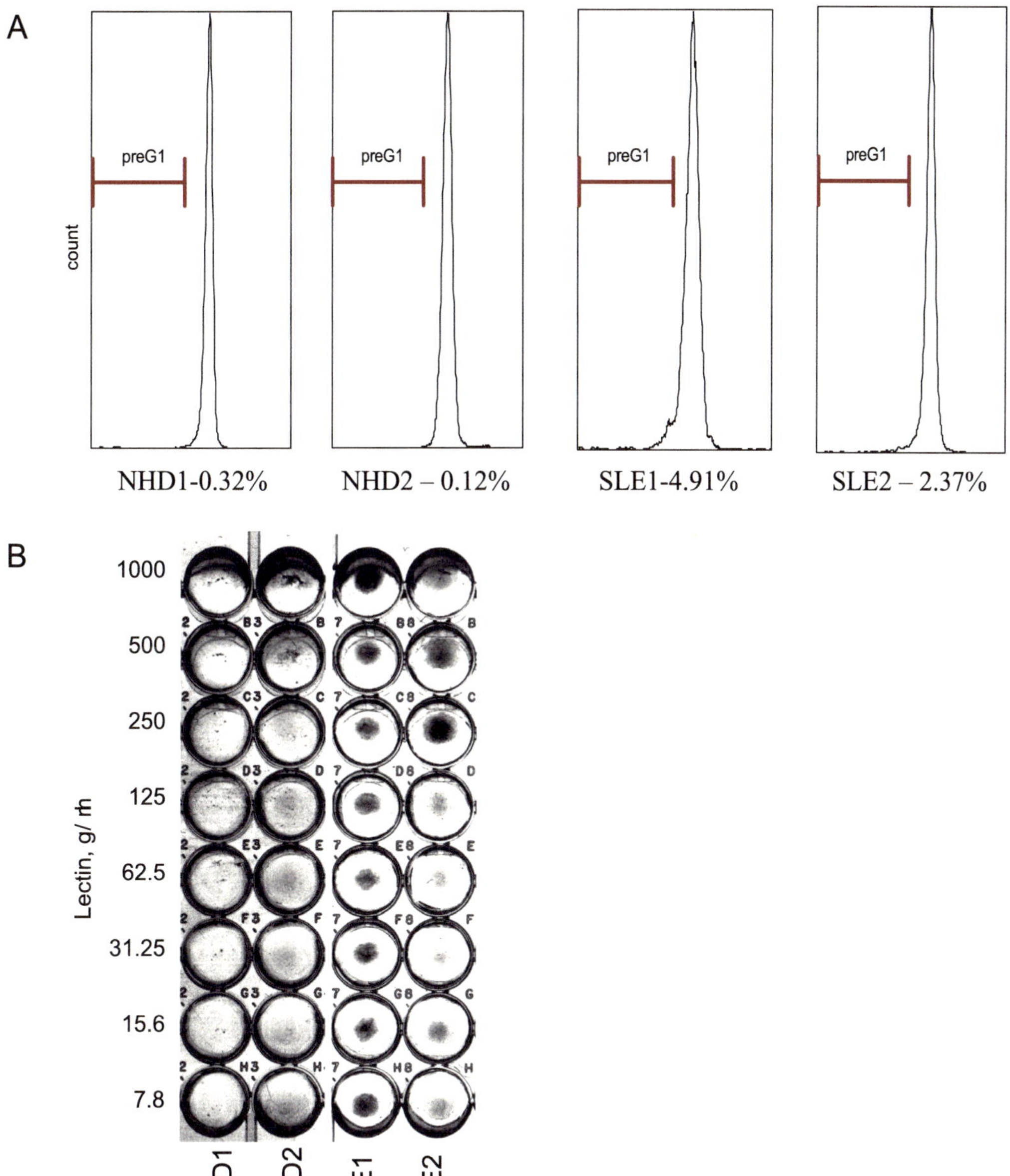

Fig. 3. Detection of apoptotic cells by measuring amount of pre-G1 cells using PI staining by flow cytometry (A) and minimal concentration needed for lectin-induced agglutination (B) of peripheral blood lymphocytes of two normal healthy donors and two SLE patients.

Shiozaki, 2008; Monti, Preti, Venerando, & Borsani, 2002). Altered sialylation of glycoproteins and glycolipids is observed as a ubiquitous phenotype in cancer. It leads to an appearance of tumor-associated antigens, aberrant adhesion and disturbance of transmembrane signalling (Miyagi, Wada, & Yamaguchi, 2008; Miyagi, Wada, Yamaguchi, & Hata, 2004). Aberrant sialylation is closely associated with the malignant phenotype of cancer cells, including metastatic potential and invasiveness (Miyagi, Wada, & Yamaguchi, 2008; Miyagi et al., 2004; Miyagi, Wada, Yamaguchi, Shiozaki, et al., 2008). However, its biological significance and molecular mechanisms have not been fully elucidated.

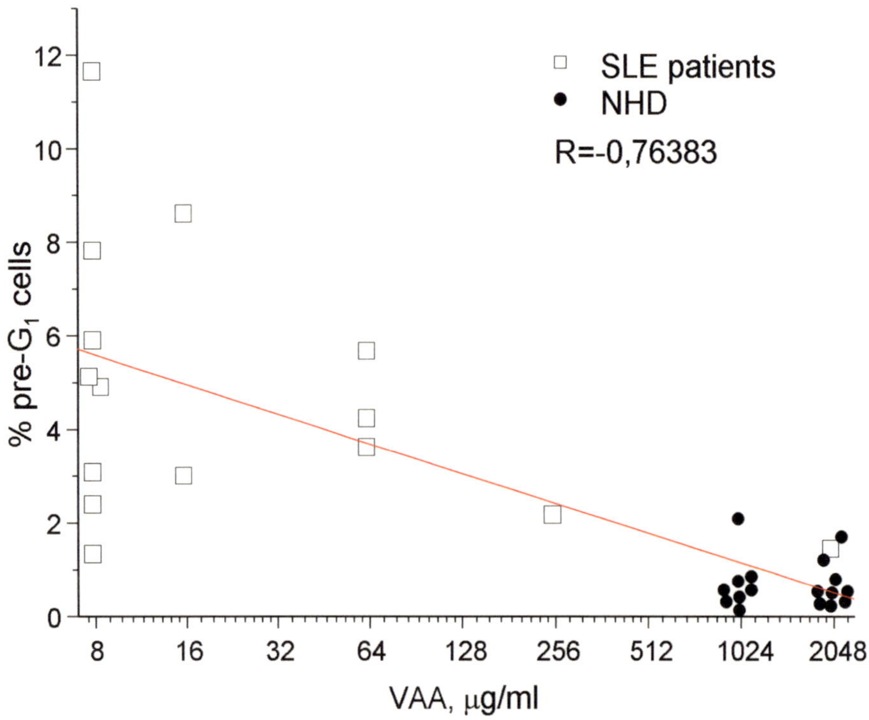

Fig. 4. Correlation analysis between specific lectin concentrations needed for lymphocyte agglutination and a percentage of the apoptotic cells. Lectin concentration needed for agglutination is reversely proportional to the amount of apoptotic cells.

Neuraminidases are abundant in prokaryotes and viruses, while only 4 sialidases are known in human (Miyagi, Wada, Yamaguchi, Shiozaki, et al., 2008). The last described one, Neu4, was reported only in 2003 (Comelli, Amado, Lustig, & Paulson, 2003). Neu 1 is a lysosomal sialidase, and Neu2 is localized in lysosomes and involved in digestion of N-glycans, and Neu3, known as ganglioside sialidase, is localized in plasma membrane and involved in ganglioside metabolism (Monti et al., 2000). Neu4 is localized in lysosomes (Seyrantepe et al., 2004) and can be translocated to mitochondria (Yamaguchi et al., 2005) and endoplasmic reticulum (Bigi et al.). However, none of known sialidases is active in the body fluids (blood or lymph). There is no evidence that plasma membrane sialidase Neu3 (or any other sialidase) can be shed from cell surface into the blood flow (Miyagi, Wada, Yamaguchi, Shiozaki, et al., 2008). While detecting increased neuraminidase activity on the surface of apoptotic cells (R. Bilyy, Tomin, & Stoika, 2010), we failed to detect any sialidase activity in culture media that could result from enzyme secretion/release during cell death.

We have focused our attention at the catalytic antibodies. These antibodies, now named as "abzymes", were first obtained in 1986 (Pollack, Jacobs, & Schultz, 1986; Tramontano, Janda, & Lerner, 1986), the first example of natural abzymes was IgG found in bronchial asthma patients, cleaving intestinal vasoactive peptide (Paul et al., 1989). Abzyme's properties were discussed in more detail in recent reviews (Belogurov, Kozyr, Ponomarenko, & Gabibov, 2009; Georgy A. Nevinsky & Buneva, 2005; Planque et al., 2008; Taguchi et al., 2008). Abzymes were detected in human organism at a variety of autoimmune and non-autoimmune pathologies (Gabibov, Ponomarenko, Tretyak, Paltsev, & Suchkov, 2006; G. A. Nevinsky & Buneva, 2003), and various peptides, proteins, nucleic acids and oligosaccharides can serve as substrates for the catalytically active antibodies in human and other mammalians (Hanson, Nishiyama, & Paul, 2005; Lacroix-Desmazes et al., 2006). The involvement of abzymes in pathogenesis of autoimmune disorders has been documented (Gabibov et al., 2006; Hanson et al., 2005; Lacroix-Desmazes et al., 2006; G. A. Nevinsky & Buneva, 2003). Catalytically active antibodies are typically found in patients with autoimmune disorders, however, they have also been detected in cancer patients. DNA-hydrolyzing activity of IgG auto-Ab from blood serum of patients with various types of lymphoproliferative diseases was described (Kozyr et al., 1998; Kozyr et al., 1996). Testing of the abzymes in patients with hematological tumors and SLE revealed a linkage of anti-DNA

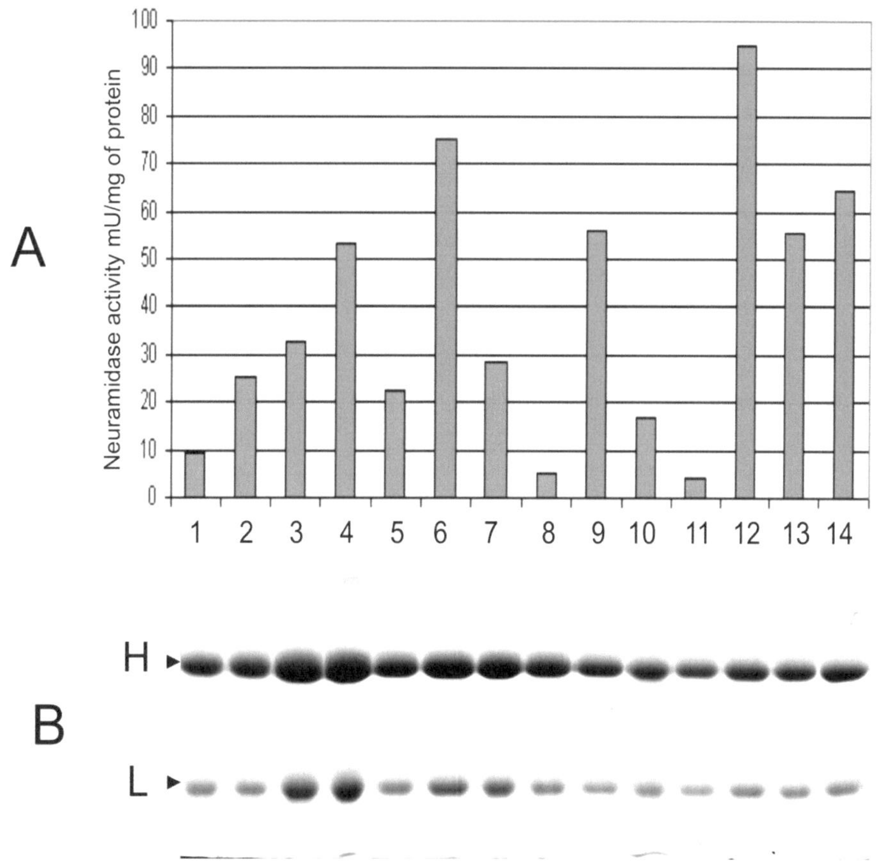

Fig. 5. Comparative analysis of sialidase activity of IgGs obtained by chromatography on Protein G - Sepharose from blood serum of SLE patients (A) and SDS-PAG electrophoresis of IgG-preparations (B), n = 14. The position on the gel of heavy (H) and light (L) chains of IgGs molecules is indicated.

Ab catalysis with mature B-cell tumors, and an increased probability of DNA-abzymes formation at the autoimmune conditions (Gabibov et al., 2006). These data suggest a similarity between the mechanisms of abzyme formation at SLE and B-cell lymphomas. Peptide-hydrolyzing and DNA-hydrolyzing activities of Bence Jones proteins isolated from blood serum of myeloma patients are well studied (Paul et al., 1995; Sun, Gao, Kirnarskiy, Rees, & Paul, 1997). There are numerous data demonstrating that the catalytic activity of anti-DNA IgGs and Bence Jones proteins are associated with their cytotoxic activity and correlate with the disease pathogenesis (Gabibov, Kozyr, & Kolesnikov, 2000; Kozyr et al., 2002; Matsuura, Ohara, Munakata, Hifumi, & Uda, 2006; Sashchenko et al., 2001; Sinohara & Matsuura, 2000). Recently, we demonstrated that anti-histone H1 IgGs isolated from blood serum of multiple sclerosis patients, were capable of hydrolyzing histone H1 (Kit, Starykovych, Richter, & Stoika, 2008). IgGs with similar proteolytic activity were also found in blood serum of patients with SLE (Magorivska et al., 2010) and multiple myeloma (Magorivska et al., 2009). Recently, we have shown that in the blood serum of some multiple myeloma patients there are immunoglobulins IgG possessing sialidase activity (R. Bilyy, Tomin, Mahorivska, et al., 2010). These data suggest an important role of abzymes at the autoimmune and oncological diseases. However, further studies are needed for better understanding of humoral immunity functions under normal and pathological conditions.

Here we demonstrated for the first time that blood serum of SLE patients contains catalytically active IgGs possessing sialidase activity. Biological consequences of such phenomenon are discussed.

The reason for studying neuraminidase activity of Ab in SLE patients is based on data showing that Ig preparations obtained by precipitation with 50% saturated ammonium sulphate from blood serum of 14 SLE patients possessed a significant capability of hydrolyzing neuramidase substrate 4-MUNA (Fig. 5), while Ig preparations of 12 healthy

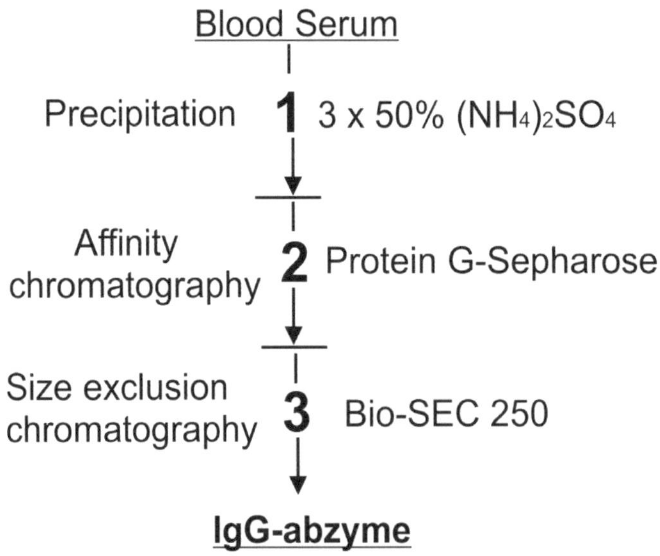

Fig. 6. Purification of IgG-abzymes from blood serum of SLE patients. Step 1 - Three-fold Ab precipitation with ammonium sulfate. Step 2 - IgG isolation by affinity chromatography on protein G-Sepharose column. Step 3 - HPLC size exclusion chromatography at pH 2.6, favoring dissociation of the immune complexes on Bio-Sec 250 column.

donors, obtained in the similar manner, were devoid of significant level of sialidase activity. Thus, we suggested that at least a part of this catalytic activity could be linked to abzymes present in the Ig preparations. To verify this suggestion, the catalytically active Ig preparations obtained with ammonium sulphate precipitation were further purified by the chromatography on protein G-sepharose column (Fig. 6) and additionally purified by HPLC SEC at neutral and acidic conditions (Fig.7). Besides, we obtained $(Fab)_2$-fragments of this

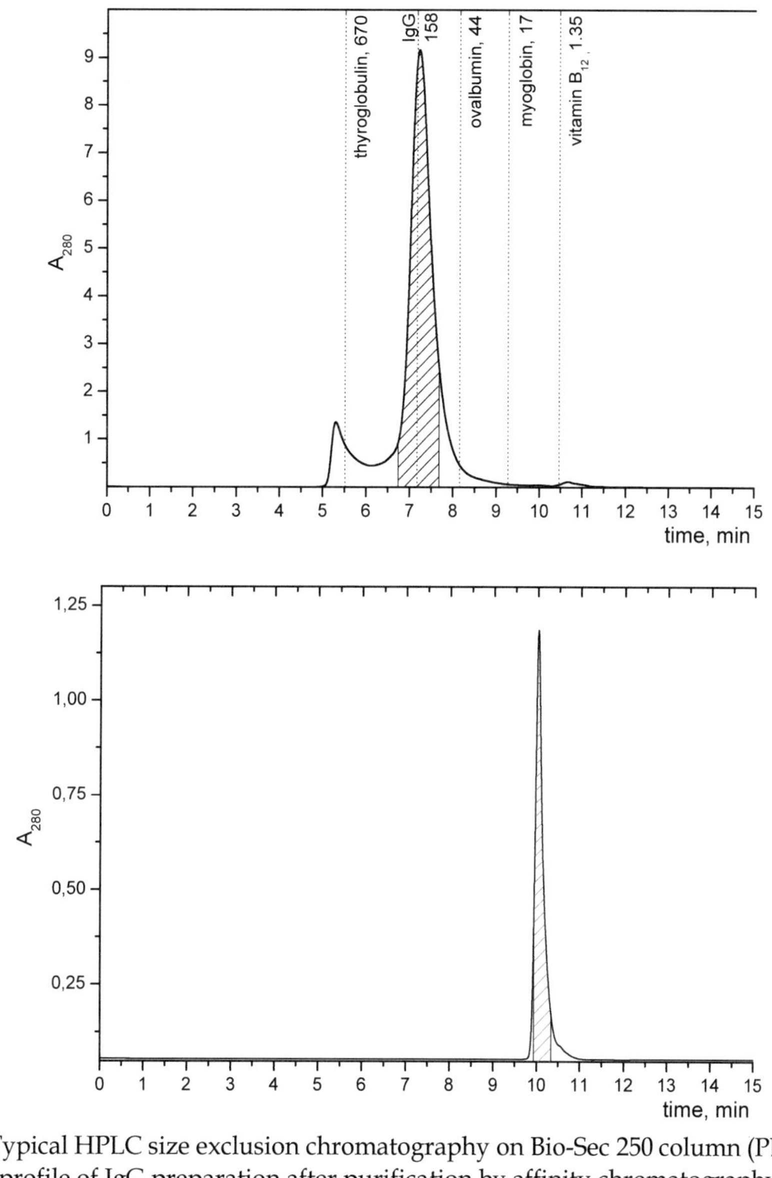

Fig. 7. Typical HPLC size exclusion chromatography on Bio-Sec 250 column (PBS, pH 6.8) elution profile of IgG preparation after purification by affinity chromatography on protein G-Sepharose (top) and additional size exclusion chromatography of this IgG sample at pH 2.6 (glycine*HCl), favoring dissociation of the immune complexes on Bio-Sec 250 column (bottom). Peaks indicated by shading were collected and used for further analysis.

IgG, and studied their sialidase activity. It was found that both IgG preparation and its $(Fab)_2$ fragments possessed sialidase activity towards 4-MUNA, but not galactosidase activity towards 4-MU-Gal (Fig. 8). Sialidase activity towards 4-MUNA was not inhibited in the presence of 10 mM 4-MU ($p<0.05$).

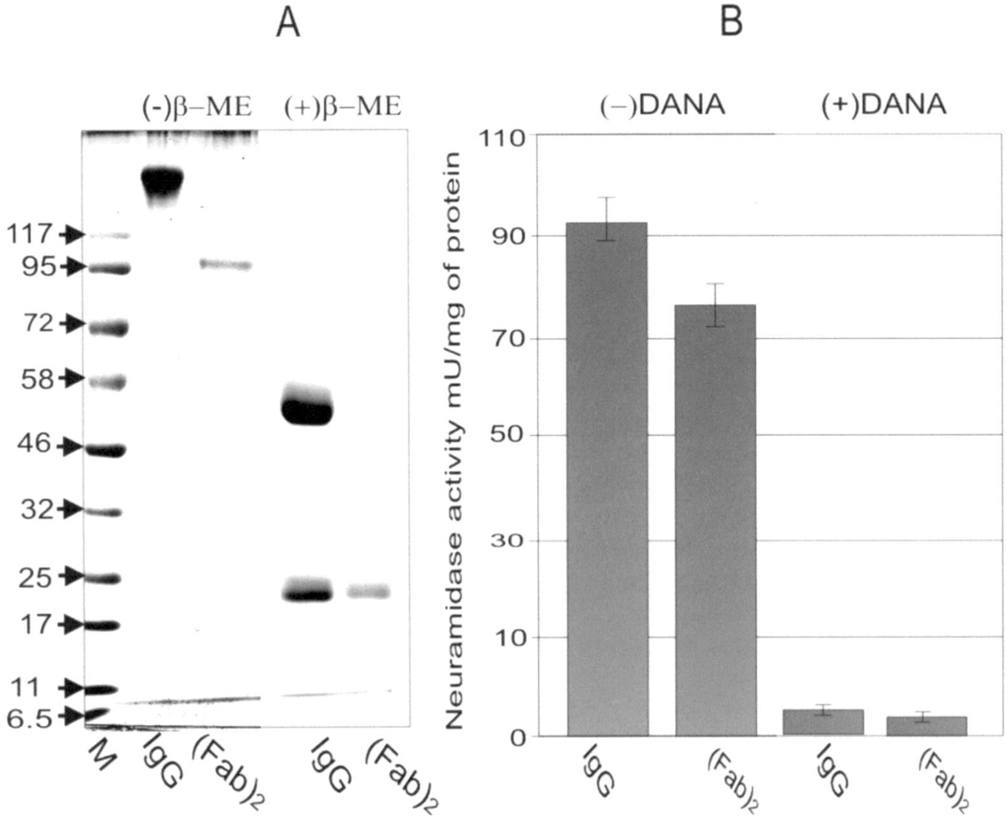

A - Homogeneity determination of IgGs and their (Fab)2 by SDS electrophoresis in gradient PAGE (5–16%) in the absence (-) or presence (+) of beta-mercaptoethanol (in non-reducing and reducing conditions, respectively). M: protein molecular mass markers (kDa).
B - Sialidase activity of IgGs and their (Fab)2 in the absence (-) or presence (+) of specific sialidase inhibitor DANA.

Fig. 8. Evidences that sialidase activity of IgG preparations purified by the affinity chromatography on protein G-sepharose from blood serum of SLE patient is an intrinsic properties of antibodies.

To prove that sialidase activity of IgG fractions isolated from the SLE patients is an intrinsic property of the abzymes and is not caused by the co-purified enzymes/impurities, we applied the same criteria to the purity of catalytic Ab which have been proposed earlier (G. A. Nevinsky & Buneva, 2003; Paul et al., 1989). To rule out possible enzymatic contamination tightly bound to IgG molecule, we performed HPLC-SEC chromatography at the acidic conditions (pH 2.6), that are known to guarantee dissociation of antibody-antigen complexes (Hanson et al., 2005; G. A. Nevinsky & Buneva, 2003) (Fig. 7). It was confirmed by the SDS-PAGE electrophoresis and Western-blot analysis using anti(human)-IgG Ab that the main chromatographic peak is an electrophoretically homogeneous IgG. Its sialidase activity was tested and shown to be attributable to IgG fraction. HPLC purification resulted in the retention of ~50% of original sialidase activity of protein-G purified IgG sample. Sialidase activity was significantly decreased when the reaction was performed in the presence of pan-neuraminidase inhibitor DANA that excludes a possibility of non-specific hydrolysis reaction. The mechanism of DANA action is connected with its resemblance of the unhydrolyzable transition-state analogue formed during sialic acid cleavage which is irreversibly bound by active centers of most neuraminidases (Chavas et al., 2005).

It is known, that the pH optimum of different sialidases is in range of pH 4–6.5. We have shown that isolated IgG is active under the physiological pH of blood serum. By using buffer systems in the pH range 3-9, we found that studied IgG samples revealed maximum speed reaction at pH range of 4.5÷6.0, nevertheless at pH 7.4 all samples retained from 27 to 52% of their maximal activity, measured at NaCl concentration equal to that of blood serum. This suggests its potential enzymatic effectiveness in blood serum.

In order to determine the speed of catalytic reaction of both IgG and corresponding $(Fab)_2$-fragments, we have calculated kinetic parameters (K_m, V_{max}, k_{cat}) for sialidase reaction at 0.1–100 μM concentrations of the substrate. Computer analysis demonstrated that the observed reaction belongs to a single substrate type, described by classical Michaelis-Menten equation. The calculated data for different studies sialyl abzymes were: Km=44.4÷1600 μM and kcat=0.045÷23.1 min-1 (Fig. 9). The catalysis mediated by an artificial abzymes is usually characterized by relatively low reaction rates: k_{cat} values are 10^2–10^6-fold lower than for the canonical enzymes (Georgy A. Nevinsky & Buneva, 2005). The known kcat values for natural abzymes vary in the range of 0.001–40 min^{-1}. The kcat values detected for MUNA hydrolysis (0.045÷23.1 depending on sample) are comparable with the typical k_{cat} values established for others abzymes. To validate the kinetics assay, we have used *C. perfringens* neuraminidase as standard for kinetic parameters measurement. According to the obtained results, *C. perfringens* Km equals to 89.2 μM for 4-MUNA, which is in a good accordance with the literature data of 120 μM (Li et al., 1994)(Inoue & Kitajima, 2006), while V_{max} was detected to be 2856 μmol/min/mg. The obtained Km value of IgG were of similar range, while V_{max} of IgG was significantly lower (k_{cat} significantly higher) than that of *C. perfringens* neuraminidase.

Principal question concerning a role of the discovered abzymes possessing sialidase activity is whether they can use as potential desialylation substrates also glycoproteins and glycolipids that are present in human's blood plasma and cells. Earlier, we have shown that sialyl-abzymes from multiple myeloma patients act towards human RBC by desialylating them and promoting agglutination with PNA lectins (R. Bilyy, Tomin, Mahorivska, et al., 2010). It is known that the peanut agglutinin (PNA) agglutinates human RBC after their sialidase treatment resulting in the exposure of sub-terminal Gal-residues (Nakano, Fontes Piazza, & Avila-Campos, 2006). Here, by incubating IgG preparation form SLE sera with RBC of NHD (blood group A(0)) and using subsequent agglutination test with different PNA lectin concentrations, we demonstrated an ability of IgG-abzyme obtained from blood serum of SLEs patient desialylate human RBCs directly. Agglutination was observed at PNA concentration 7 μg/ml, while when the IgG preparation from NHD was used, agglutination was achieved at 250 μg/ml; PBS served here as a negative control (no agglutination at 1,000 μg/ml, and *Clostridium perfringens* neuraminidase (10 mU) served as a positive control, agglutination at 7μg/ml of PNA. Thus treatment with sialyl abzymes from

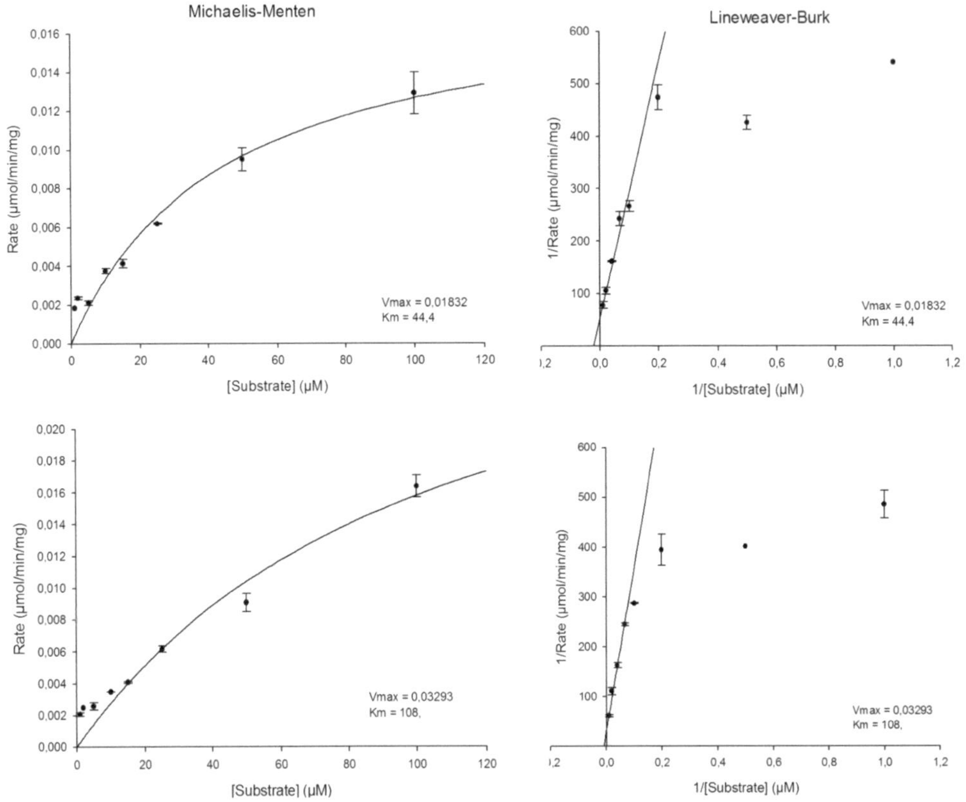

Fig. 9. Kinetic parameters (Michaelis-Menten and Lineweaver-Burk plots) of sialidase reaction catalyzed by the IgG (A) or its $(Fab)_2$-fragments (B). The incubation time for all samples was 180 min.

SLE patient have increased the amount of desialylated glycoepitopes for 250 µg /7 µg =35 times. We also used as substrates for sialyl abzymes: a) gangliodes of mouse brain and b) total surface glycans on eukaryotic (human T-leukemia Jurkat) cells. Ganglioside fraction was isolated from mouse brain and was incubated with sialil-abzyme and neuraminidase. Both sialil-abzyme and neuraminidase caused desialylation of GM3 and increase in the content of free sialic (neuraminic) acid (Fig.10). Treatment of human leukemia Jurkat cells with sialil-abzyme and neuraminidase caused a decrease in the level of a2,6-sialil-reach surface glycoconjugates (if judged by binding of FITC-labeled SNA lectin analyzed by flow cytometry) (Fig 11). Moreover, treatment of Jurkat cells with sialil-abzyme and neuraminidase also caused an increase in the level of desialylated glycoepitopes, if judged by binding of PNA lectin (biotynilated, treated with streptavidin-FITC and analyzed by flow cytometry) (Fig. 11).

Thus, isolated sialyl abzymes were desialylating both human RBC, gangliosides and total surface glycoepitopes of the eukaryotic cells and were active under pH and ion content values of human blood serum.

We have demonstrated previously unknown catalytic activity in the IgG antibodies of SLE patients - an intrinsic sialidase activity. Such activity was present in the IgG of blood serum

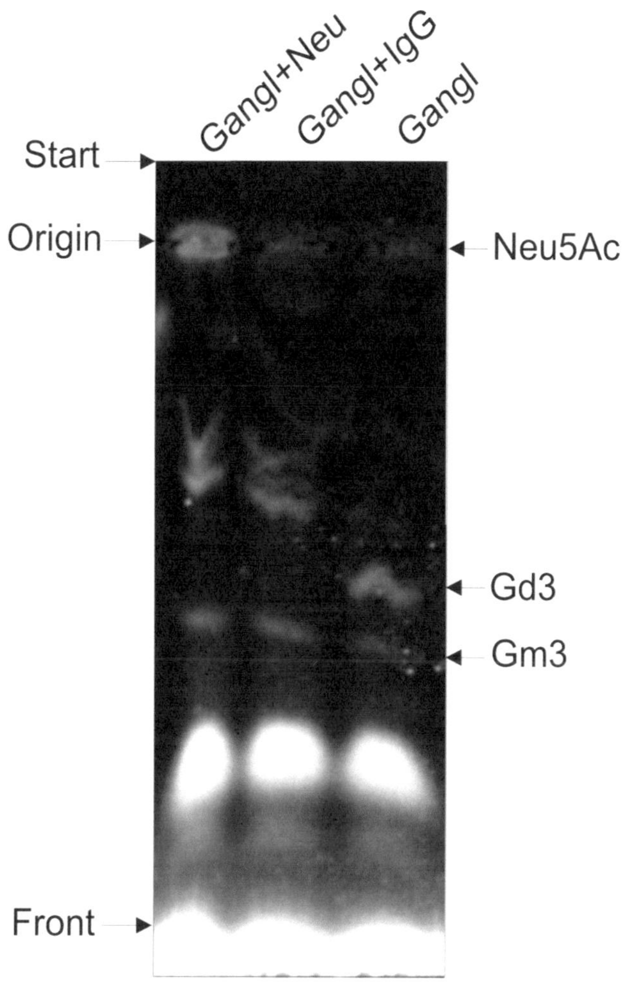

Fig. 10. Desialation of gangliosids by sialidase active IgGs obtained from blood serum of SLE patients possessing highest sialidase activity. Gangl+Neu - gangliosides incubated with neuramidase from *C. perphringers*; Gangl+IgG - gangliosides incubated with sialidase active IgGs; Gangl - gangliosides without incubation (control). The positions of free neuraninic acid (Neu5Ac), gangliosides GM3 and GD3 are shown by arrows on the right hand.

of SLE patients and absent in the IgG of NHD. Sialidase activity was detected under different conditions which exclude a possibility of contamination or artefacts. It was blocked by typical sialidase inhibitor (DANA), expressed under physiological pH, and corresponded to classical Michaelis-Menten kinetics. Since DANA is an unhydrolyzable transitional state analogue of hydrolysis reaction, one can assume that the mechanism of action of IgG with sialidase activity is similar to that of sialidase enzyme. Moreover, the described IgGs possessing sialidase activity were capable of direct desialylation of human RBCs, ganglyosides and T-lymphocytes. The reason for appearance of discovered sialidase activity is not fully understood. One of the possible suggestions is their anti-idiotypic antibody as the "internal image" of an active site of endo- or exogenic sialidases, as known for other abzymes (Friboulet, Izadyar, Avalle, Roseto, & Thomas, 1994).

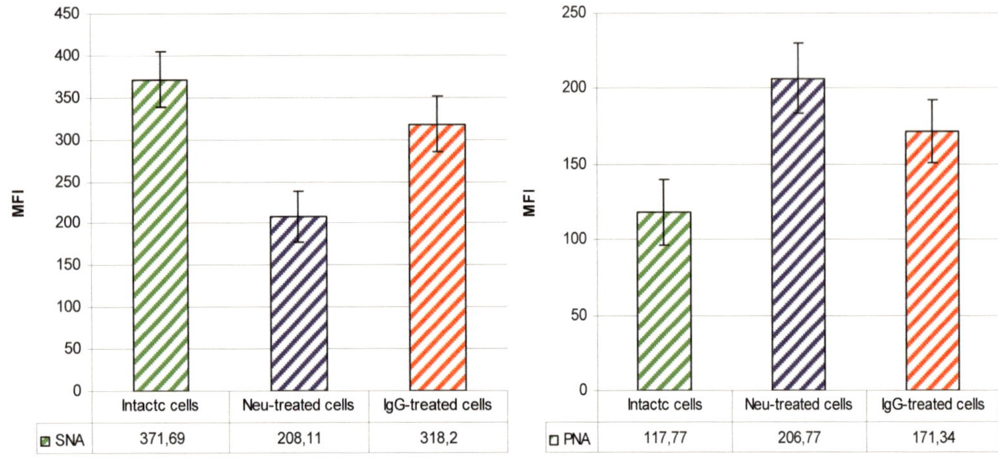

Jurkat cells were stained with FITC-labeled SNA (left), or biotinilated PNA lectin (right), stained with streptavidin-FITC. Cells were either treated with Neuraminidase, 10mU or sialil-abzyme, 10 uM for 3h at 37°C. Data represent normalized MFI of lectin binding. SNA lectin binds terminal a2,6-sialic acid residues, while PNA lectin binds desialylated glycoepitopes (Antonyuk, 2005).

Fig. 11. Analysis of lectin binding to human Jurkat T-cells.

The level of IgG molecule's sialylation was reported to be critical in defining their pro- or anti-inflamatory properties (Kaneko, Nimmerjahn, & Ravetch, 2006). Anti-inflamatory activity of immunoglobulins was tightly connected with the presence of α2,6-sialylated Asn^{297} in the IgG molecule (Anthony, Nimmerjahn, et al., 2008). Macrophages receptors responsible for binding sialylated IgG and modulating its anti-inflamatory action were also described (Anthony, Wermeling, Karlsson, & Ravetch, 2008). Agalactosylated and desialylated IgG antibodies' action *in vivo* depends on binding of cellular Fc receptors (Nimmerjahn, Anthony, & Ravetch, 2007). Specific glycoforms, if present in populations of immunoglobulin molecules, are connected with disease-associated alterations and can serve as diagnostic biomarkers at rheumatoid arthritis and other diseases (Arnold, Wormald, Sim, Rudd, & Dwek, 2007). Blood serum level of desialylylated form of IgG (IgG-G0) isolated from patients with rheumatoid arthritis, are more that 2 standard deviations above those levels in the age-matched healthy control (R. B. Parekh et al., 1985). They correlate with the disease activity and fall during remission periods (Rook et al., 1991). High levels of desialylylated IgG-G0 are also characteristic for other disorders: Crohn's disease, SLE complicated by Sjogren's syndrome, and tuberculosis (Bond et al., 1997; R. Parekh et al., 1989; R. B. Parekh et al., 1985). The enzyme EndoS from *Streptococcus pyogenes* that cleaves IgG glycan between two GlcNAc residues, was used for "making autoantibodies safe" (Scanlan, Burton, & Dwek, 2008). The action of EndoS truncated IgG glycans and IgG molecules lost the ability to initiate activating signals through C1q, FcγRs and MBL, while the ability to interact with inhibitory FcγRIIB was preserved (Collin, Shannon, & Bjorck, 2008).

4. Summary

In previous studies, we have shown that cell surface glycopattern is changed during apoptosis. This, in part, results from activation of surface sialidases, with desialylated glycoproteins being characteristic markers of apoptosis (R. Bilyy & Stoika, 2007). Such feature was successfully utilized for lymphocyte screening in the autoimmune patients (R. Bilyy et al., 2009). It is widely accepted that altered glycoepitopes (desialylaed) are important surface markers for clearance of apoptotic cells (R. Bilyy & Stoika, 2007). We have shown (Meesmann et al., 2010) that desialylation of cell surface epitopes in viable cells, caused by sialidase, acts as an "eat-me" signal for macrophages and is needed for elimination of late apoptotic cells along with phosphatydilserine exposure, needed for elimination of early apoptotic cells. Apoptotic cells possess an elevated neuraminidase activity on their surface, however, we failed to detect any sialidase activity in culture media that could result from enzyme secretion/release during cell death. As we have shown, SLE – a disease resulting from insufficient cell clearance (Munoz et al., 2010) - is accompanied by the appearance of desialylated lymphocytes in blood stream. At the same time, some of SLE patients possessed abzymes with sialydase activity in their blood. The exact role of sialyl abzymes at SLE is currently unclear, as well as their relation to apoptotic cell desialylation and clearance. The abzymes possessing sialidase activity can change surface sialylation level and, thus, alter the glycocalyx of SLE patients' cells and promote their clearance. They can also influence the immune response by acting towards blood serum IgG molecules.

5. Acknowledgements

The authors would like to acknowledge I. Kril' who greatly contributed to this work. The work was supported by the National Academy of Sciences of Ukraine, and grants awarded to R. Bilyy by the WUBMRC and the President of Ukraine.

6. Abbreviations

GP - glycoprotein, PI - propidium iodide, PM – plasma membrane, RA - rheumatoid arthritis, Ab – antibodies, DANA - 2,3-dehydro-2-deoxy-N-acetylneuraminic acid, SLE- multiple myeloma, 4-MUNA - 2'-(4-Methylumbelliferyl)-α-D-N-acetylneuralminic acid, 4-MU-Gal - 4-Methylumbelliferyl-β-D-galactopyranoside, NHD – normal healthy donors, RBC – red blood cells, SLE - systemic lupus erymatosus.

7. References

Anthony, R. M., Nimmerjahn, F., Ashline, D. J., Reinhold, V. N., Paulson, J. C. and Ravetch, J. V. (2008), Recapitulation of IVIG anti-inflammatory activity with a recombinant IgG Fc, *Science,* Vol. 320 No. 5874, pp. 373-376.

Anthony, R. M., Wermeling, F., Karlsson, M. C. and Ravetch, J. V. (2008), Identification of a receptor required for the anti-inflammatory activity of IVIG, *Proc Natl Acad Sci U S A,* Vol. 105 No. 50, pp. 19571-19578.

Antonyuk, V. O. (2005), *The lectins and their resources [in Ukrainian]*, Quart, Lviv. 554 p.

Arnold, J. N., Wormald, M. R., Sim, R. B., Rudd, P. M. and Dwek, R. A. (2007), The impact of glycosylation on the biological function and structure of human immunoglobulins, *Annu Rev Immunol,* Vol. 25, pp. 21-50.

Ashkenazi, A. and Dixit, V. M. (1998), Death Receptors: Signaling and Modulation, *Science,* Vol. 281 No. 5381, pp. 1305-1308.

Batisse, C., Marquet, J., Greffard, A., Fleury-Feith, J., Jaurand, M. C. and Pilatte, Y. (2004), Lectin-based three-color flow cytometric approach for studying cell surface glycosylation changes that occur during apoptosis, *Cytometry A,* Vol. 62 No. 2, pp. 81-88.

Belmont, M. (2010), Lupus Clinical Overview, http://cerebel.com/lupus/

Belogurov, A., Jr., Kozyr, A., Ponomarenko, N. and Gabibov, A. (2009), Catalytic antibodies: balancing between Dr. Jekyll and Mr. Hyde, *BioEssays,* Vol. 31 No. 11, pp. 1161-1171.

Bigi, A., Morosi, L., Pozzi, C., Forcella, M., Tettamanti, G., Venerando, B., Monti, E. and Fusi, P. (2010), Human sialidase NEU4 long and short are extrinsic proteins bound to outer mitochondrial membrane and the endoplasmic reticulum, respectively, *Glycobiology,* Vol. 20 No. 2, pp. 148-157.

Bilyy, R., Kit, Y., Hellman, U., Tryndyak, V., Kaminskyy, V. and Stoika, R. (2005), In vivo expression and characteristics of novel alpha-D-mannose-rich glycoprotein markers of apoptotic cells, *Cell Biol Int,* Vol. 29 No. 11, pp. 920-928.

Bilyy, R., Nemesh, L., Antonyuk, V., Kit, Y., Valchuk, I., Havryluk, A., Chopyak, V. and Stoika, R. (2009), Apoptosis-related changes in plasma membrane glycoconjugates of peripheral blood lymphocytes in rheumatoid arthritis, *Autoimmunity,* Vol. 42 No. 4, pp. 334 - 336.

Bilyy, R. and Stoika, R. (2007), Search for novel cell surface markers of apoptotic cells, *Autoimmunity,* Vol. 40 No. 4, pp. 249-253.

Bilyy, R., Tomin, A., Mahorivska, I., Shalay, O., Lohinskyy, V., Stoika, R. and Kit, Y. (2010), Antibody-Mediated Sialidase Activity in Blood Serum of Patients With Multiple Myeloma, *Journal of Molecular Recognition,* Vol. 23 No. 6, pp. DOI:10.1002/jmr.1071.

Bilyy, R., Tomin, A. and Stoika, R. (2010), Method of neuraminidase activity detection in cells and cellular compartments, in a201003168, U. (Ed.), *Bul.13, 12.07.2010,* UA.

Bilyy, R. O., Antonyuk, V. O. and Stoika, R. S. (2004), Cytochemical study of role of alpha-d-mannose- and beta-d-galactose-containing glycoproteins in apoptosis, *J Mol Histol,* Vol. 35 No. 8-9, pp. 829-838.

Bilyy, R. O. and Stoika, R. S. (2003), Lectinocytochemical detection of apoptotic murine leukemia L1210 cells, *Cytometry A,* Vol. 56 No. 2, pp. 89-95.

Bond, A., Alavi, A., Axford, J. S., Bourke, B. E., Bruckner, F. E., Kerr, M. A., Maxwell, J. D., Tweed, K. J., Weldon, M. J., Youinou, P. and Hay, F. C. (1997), A detailed lectin analysis of IgG glycosylation, demonstrating disease specific changes in terminal galactose and N-acetylglucosamine, *J Autoimmun,* Vol. 10 No. 1, pp. 77-85.

Chavas, L. M., Tringali, C., Fusi, P., Venerando, B., Tettamanti, G., Kato, R., Monti, E. and Wakatsuki, S. (2005), Crystal structure of the human cytosolic sialidase Neu2. Evidence for the dynamic nature of substrate recognition, *J Biol Chem,* Vol. 280 No. 1, pp. 469-475.

Collin, M., Shannon, O. and Bjorck, L. (2008), IgG glycan hydrolysis by a bacterial enzyme as a therapy against autoimmune conditions, *Proc Natl Acad Sci U S A,* Vol. 105 No. 11, pp. 4265-4270.

Comelli, E. M., Amado, M., Lustig, S. R. and Paulson, J. C. (2003), Identification and expression of Neu4, a novel murine sialidase, *Gene,* Vol. 321, pp. 155-161.

Fadok, V. A., Voelker, D. R., Campbell, P. A., Cohen, J. J., Bratton, D. L. and Henson, P. M. (1992), Exposure of phosphatidylserine on the surface of apoptotic lymphocytes triggers specific recognition and removal by macrophages, *J Immunol.,* Vol. 148 No. 7, pp. 2207-2216.

Franz, S., Frey, B., Sheriff, A., Gaipl, U. S., Beer, A., Voll, R. E., Kalden, J. R. and Herrmann, M. (2006), Lectins detect changes of the glycosylation status of plasma membrane constituents during late apoptosis, *Cytometry A,* Vol. 69 No. 4, pp. 230-239.

Franz, S., Herrmann, K., Fuhrnrohr, B., Sheriff, A., Frey, B., Gaipl, U. S., Voll, R. E., Kalden, J. R., Jack, H. M. and Herrmann, M. (2007), After shrinkage apoptotic cells expose internal membrane-derived epitopes on their plasma membranes, *Cell Death.Differ.,* Vol. 14 No. 4, pp. 733-742.

Friboulet, A., Izadyar, L., Avalle, B., Roseto, A. and Thomas, D. (1994), Abzyme generation using an anti-idiotypic antibody as the "internal image" of an enzyme active site, *Appl Biochem Biotechnol,* Vol. 47 No. 2-3, pp. 229-237; discussion 237-229.

Gabibov, A. G., Kozyr, A. V. and Kolesnikov, A. V. (2000), Disease association and cytotoxic effects of DNA-hydrolyzing autoantibodies, *Chem Immunol,* Vol. 77, pp. 130-156.

Gabibov, A. G., Ponomarenko, N. A., Tretyak, E. B., Paltsev, M. A. and Suchkov, S. V. (2006), Catalytic autoantibodies in clinical autoimmunity and modern medicine, *Autoimmun Rev,* Vol. 5 No. 5, pp. 324-330.

Goping, I. S., Barry, M., Liston, P., Sawchuk, T., Constantinescu, G., Michalak, K. M., Shostak, I., Roberts, D. L., Hunter, A. M., Korneluk, R. and Bleackley, R. C. (2003), Granzyme B-Induced Apoptosis Requires Both Direct Caspase Activation and Relief of Caspase Inhibition, *Immunity,* Vol. 18 No. 3, pp. 355-365.

Hanson, C. V., Nishiyama, Y. and Paul, S. (2005), Catalytic antibodies and their applications, *Curr Opin Biotechnol,* Vol. 16 No. 6, pp. 631-636.

Heyder, P., Gaipl, U. S., Beyer, T. D., Voll, R. E., Kern, P. M., Stach, C., Kalden, J. R. and Herrmann, M. (2003), Early detection of apoptosis by staining of acid-treated apoptotic cells with FITC-labeled lectin from Narcissus pseudonarcissus, *Cytometry,* Vol. 55A No. 2, pp. 86-93.

Inoue, S. and Kitajima, K. (2006), KDN (deaminated neuraminic acid): dreamful past and exciting future of the newest member of the sialic acid family, *Glycoconj J,* Vol. 23 No. 5-6, pp. 277-290.

Kaneko, Y., Nimmerjahn, F. and Ravetch, J. V. (2006), Anti-inflammatory activity of immunoglobulin G resulting from Fc sialylation, *Science,* Vol. 313 No. 5787, pp. 670-673.

Kit, Y. Y., Starykovych, M. A., Richter, V. A. and Stoika, R. S. (2008), Detection and characterization of IgG- and sIgA-Abzymes capable of hydrolyzing histone H1, *Biochemistry (Mosc),* Vol. 73 No. 8, pp. 950-956.

Kozyr, A. V., Kolesnikov, A. V., Aleksandrova, E. S., Sashchenko, L. P., Gnuchev, N. V., Favorov, P. V., Kotelnikov, M. A., Iakhnina, E. I., Astsaturov, I. A., Prokaeva, T. B., Alekberova, Z. S., Suchkov, S. V. and Gabibov, A. G. (1998), Novel functional activities of anti-DNA autoantibodies from sera of patients with lymphoproliferative and autoimmune diseases, *Appl Biochem Biotechnol,* Vol. 75 No. 1, pp. 45-61.

Kozyr, A. V., Kolesnikov, A. V., Iakhnina, E. I., Astsaturov, I. A., Varlamova, E., Kirillov, E. V. and Gabibov, A. G. (1996), [DNA-hydrolyzing antibodies in lymphoproliferative disorders], *Biull Eksp Biol Med,* Vol. 121 No. 2, pp. 204-206.

Kozyr, A. V., Sashchenko, L. P., Kolesnikov, A. V., Zelenova, N. A., Khaidukov, S. V., Ignatova, A. N., Bobik, T. V., Gabibov, A. G., Alekberova, Z. S., Suchkov, S. V. and

Gnuchev, N. V. (2002), Anti-DNA autoantibodies reveal toxicity to tumor cell lines, *Immunol Lett,* Vol. 80 No. 1, pp. 41-47.

Lacroix-Desmazes, S., Wootla, B., Delignat, S., Dasgupta, S., Nagaraja, V., Kazatchkine, M. D. and Kaveri, S. V. (2006), Pathophysiology of catalytic antibodies, *Immunol Lett,* Vol. 103 No. 1, pp. 3-7.

Li, Y. T., Yuziuk, J. A., Li, S. C., Nematalla, A., Hasegawa, A., Kimura, M. and Nakagawa, H. (1994), A novel sialidase capable of cleaving 3-deoxy-D-glycero-D-galacto-2-nonulosonic acid (KDN), *Arch Biochem Biophys,* Vol. 310 No. 1, pp. 243-246.

Magorivska, I., Bilyy, R., Havryluk, A., Chop'yak, V., Stoika, R. and Kit, Y. (2010), Anti-histone H1 IgGs from blood serum of systemic lupus erythematosus patients are capable of hydrolyzing histone H1 and myelin basic protein, *Journal of Molecular Recognition,* Vol. 23, pp. DOI:10.1002/jmr.1033.

Magorivska, I., Bilyy, R., Shalay, O., Loginsky, V., Kit, Y. and Stoika, R. (2009), Blood serum immunoglobulins of patients with multiple myeloma are capable of hydrolysing histone H1, *Exp Oncol,* Vol. 31 No. 2, pp. 97-101.

Matsuura, K., Ohara, K., Munakata, H., Hifumi, E. and Uda, T. (2006), Pathogenicity of catalytic antibodies: catalytic activity of Bence Jones proteins from myeloma patients with renal impairment can elicit cytotoxic effects, *Biol Chem,* Vol. 387 No. 5, pp. 543-548.

Meesmann, H. M., Fehr, E.-M., Kierschke, S., Herrmann, M., Bilyy, R., Heyder, P., Blank, N., Krienke, S., Lorenz, H.-M. and Schiller, M. (2010), Decrease of sialic acid residues as an eat-me signal on the surface of apoptotic lymphocytes, *J Cell Sci,* Vol. 123 No. 19, pp. 3347-3356.

Miyagi, T., Wada, T. and Yamaguchi, K. (2008), Roles of plasma membrane-associated sialidase NEU3 in human cancers, *Biochim Biophys Acta,* Vol. 1780 No. 3, pp. 532-537.

Miyagi, T., Wada, T., Yamaguchi, K. and Hata, K. (2004), Sialidase and malignancy: a minireview, *Glycoconj J,* Vol. 20 No. 3, pp. 189-198.

Miyagi, T., Wada, T., Yamaguchi, K., Hata, K. and Shiozaki, K. (2008), Plasma membrane-associated sialidase as a crucial regulator of transmembrane signalling, *J Biochem,* Vol. 144 No. 3, pp. 279-285.

Miyagi, T., Wada, T., Yamaguchi, K., Shiozaki, K., Sato, I., Kakugawa, Y., Yamanami, H. and Fujiya, T. (2008), Human sialidase as a cancer marker, *Proteomics,* Vol. 8 No. 16, pp. 3303-3311.

Monti, E., Bassi, M. T., Papini, N., Riboni, M., Manzoni, M., Venerando, B., Croci, G., Preti, A., Ballabio, A., Tettamanti, G. and Borsani, G. (2000), Identification and expression of NEU3, a novel human sialidase associated to the plasma membrane, *Biochem J,* Vol. 349 No. Pt 1, pp. 343-351.

Monti, E., Preti, A., Venerando, B. and Borsani, G. (2002), Recent development in mammalian sialidase molecular biology, *Neurochem Res,* Vol. 27 No. 7-8, pp. 649-663.

Munoz, L. E., Lauber, K., Schiller, M., Manfredi, A. A. and Herrmann, M. (2010), The role of defective clearance of apoptotic cells in systemic autoimmunity, *Nat Rev Rheumatol,* Vol. 6 No. 5, pp. 280-289.

Nakano, V., Fontes Piazza, R. M. and Avila-Campos, M. J. (2006), A rapid assay of the sialidase activity in species of the Bacteroides fragilis group by using peanut lectin hemagglutination, *Anaerobe,* Vol. 12 No. 5-6, pp. 238-241.

Nevinsky, G. A. and Buneva, V. N. (2003), Catalytic antibodies in healthy humans and patients with autoimmune and viral diseases, *J Cell Mol Med,* Vol. 7 No. 3, pp. 265-276.

Nevinsky, G. A. and Buneva, V. N. (2005), Natural Catalytic Antibodies - Abzymes, in Prof. Dr. Ehud, K. (Ed.), *Catalytic Antibodies,* pp. 505-569.

Nimmerjahn, F., Anthony, R. M. and Ravetch, J. V. (2007), Agalactosylated IgG antibodies depend on cellular Fc receptors for in vivo activity, *Proc Natl Acad Sci U S A,* Vol. 104 No. 20, pp. 8433-8437.

Orlinick, J. R. and Chao, M. V. (1998), TNF-Related Ligands and Their Receptors, *Cellular Signalling,* Vol. 10 No. 8, pp. 543-551.

Parekh, R., Isenberg, D., Rook, G., Roitt, I., Dwek, R. and Rademacher, T. (1989), A comparative analysis of disease-associated changes in the galactosylation of serum IgG, *J Autoimmun,* Vol. 2 No. 2, pp. 101-114.

Parekh, R. B., Dwek, R. A., Sutton, B. J., Fernandes, D. L., Leung, A., Stanworth, D., Rademacher, T. W., Mizuochi, T., Taniguchi, T., Matsuta, K. and et al. (1985), Association of rheumatoid arthritis and primary osteoarthritis with changes in the glycosylation pattern of total serum IgG, *Nature,* Vol. 316 No. 6027, pp. 452-457.

Paul, S., Li, L., Kalaga, R., Wilkins-Stevens, P., Stevens, F. J. and Solomon, A. (1995), Natural catalytic antibodies: peptide-hydrolyzing activities of Bence Jones proteins and VL fragment, *J Biol Chem,* Vol. 270 No. 25, pp. 15257-15261.

Paul, S., Volle, D. J., Beach, C. M., Johnson, D. R., Powell, M. J. and Massey, R. J. (1989), Catalytic hydrolysis of vasoactive intestinal peptide by human autoantibody, *Science,* Vol. 244 No. 4909, pp. 1158-1162.

Planque, S., Nishiyama, Y., Taguchi, H., Salas, M., Hanson, C. and Paul, S. (2008), Catalytic antibodies to HIV: physiological role and potential clinical utility, *Autoimmun Rev,* Vol. 7 No. 6, pp. 473-479.

Ploegh, H. L. (1998), Viral Strategies of Immune Evasion, *Science,* Vol. 280 No. 5361, pp. 248-253.

Pollack, S. J., Jacobs, J. W. and Schultz, P. G. (1986), Selective chemical catalysis by an antibody, *Science,* Vol. 234 No. 4783, pp. 1570-1573.

Pradhan, D., Krahling, S., Williamson, P. and Schlegel, R. (1997), Multiple systems for recognition of apoptotic lymphocytes by macrophages, *Mol. Biol. Cell,* Vol. 8 No. 5, pp. 767-778.

Reutelingsperger, C. P. and Christiaan Peter, M. (1998), Method for detecting and/or optionally quantifying and/or separating apoptotic cells in or from a sample, in, United States, pp. 1-9.

Rook, G. A., Steele, J., Brealey, R., Whyte, A., Isenberg, D., Sumar, N., Nelson, J. L., Bodman, K. B., Young, A., Roitt, I. M. and et al. (1991), Changes in IgG glycoform levels are associated with remission of arthritis during pregnancy, *J Autoimmun,* Vol. 4 No. 5, pp. 779-794.

Sashchenko, L. P., Khaidukov, S. V., Kozyr, A. V., Luk'yanova, T. I., Gabibov, A. G., Suchkov, S. V., Bobik, T. V., Alekberova, Z. S. and Gnuchev, N. V. (2001), Caspase-dependent cytotoxicity of anti-DNA autoantibodies, *Dokl Biochem Biophys,* Vol. 380, pp. 313-315.

Savill, J., Fadok, V., Henson, P. and Haslett, C. (1993), Phagocyte recognition of cells undergoing apoptosis, *Immunol.Today,* Vol. 14 No. 3, pp. 131-136.

Scanlan, C. N., Burton, D. R. and Dwek, R. A. (2008), Making autoantibodies safe, *Proc Natl Acad Sci U S A,* Vol. 105 No. 11, pp. 4081-4082.

Seyrantepe, V., Landry, K., Trudel, S., Hassan, J. A., Morales, C. R. and Pshezhetsky, A. V. (2004), Neu4, a novel human lysosomal lumen sialidase, confers normal phenotype to sialidosis and galactosialidosis cells, *J Biol Chem,* Vol. 279 No. 35, pp. 37021-37029.

Sinohara, H. and Matsuura, K. (2000), Does catalytic activity of Bence-Jones proteins contribute to the pathogenesis of multiple myeloma?, *Appl Biochem Biotechnol,* Vol. 83 No. 1-3, pp. 85-92; discussion 93-84, 145-153.

Stoika, R. S., Bilyy, R. O. and Antoniuk, V. O. (2006), Agglutination-based method for fast detection, isolation and quantification of apoptotic cells, in *WO/2007/053654* USA, UA, pp. 1-85.

Sun, M., Gao, Q. S., Kirnarskiy, L., Rees, A. and Paul, S. (1997), Cleavage specificity of a proteolytic antibody light chain and effects of the heavy chain variable domain, *J Mol Biol,* Vol. 271 No. 3, pp. 374-385.

Taguchi, H., Planque, S., Nishiyama, Y., Szabo, P., Weksler, M. E., Friedland, R. P. and Paul, S. (2008), Catalytic antibodies to amyloid beta peptide in defense against Alzheimer disease, *Autoimmun Rev,* Vol. 7 No. 5, pp. 391-397.

Tartaglia, L. A. and Goeddel, D. V. (1992), Two TNF receptors, *Immunology Today,* Vol. 13 No. 5, pp. 151-153.

Tramontano, A., Janda, K. D. and Lerner, R. A. (1986), Catalytic antibodies, *Science,* Vol. 234 No. 4783, pp. 1566-1570.

van den Eijnde, S. M., Luijsterburg, A. J., Boshart, L., De Zeeuw, C. I., van Dierendonck, J. H., Reutelingsperger, C. P. and Vermeij-Keers, C. (1997), In situ detection of apoptosis during embryogenesis with annexin V: from whole mount to ultrastructure, *Cytometry,* Vol. 29 No. 4, pp. 313-320.

Vermijlen, D., Froelich, C. J., Luo, D., Suarez-Huerta, N., Robaye, B. and Wisse, E. (2001), Perforin and granzyme B induce apoptosis in FasL-resistant colon carcinoma cells, *Cancer Immunology, Immunotherapy,* Vol. 50 No. 4, pp. 212-217.

Yamaguchi, K., Hata, K., Koseki, K., Shiozaki, K., Akita, H., Wada, T., Moriya, S. and Miyagi, T. (2005), Evidence for mitochondrial localization of a novel human sialidase (NEU4), *Biochem J,* Vol. 390 No. Pt 1, pp. 85-93.

6

Regulatory T Cell Deficiency in Systemic Autoimmune Disorders – Causal Relationship and Underlying Immunological Mechanisms

Fang-Ping Huang and Susanne Sattler
Division of Immunology and Inflammation, Department of Medicine,
Imperial College London,
Great Britain

1. Introduction

Systemic lupus erythematosus (SLE), formerly named 'disseminated lupus erythematosus', is an organ-non-specific autoimmune disease that has a largely unknown aetiology. Multiple susceptibility genes as well as environmental factors are found to be involved in the lupus pathogenesis (multi-factorial) [1, 2]. Also known as the prototype of autoimmune diseases, lupus is very intriguing both clinically and immunologically for its systemic nature and complexity in pathogenesis. The disease is characterized by multi-organ involvement and presence of autoantibodies to a variety of self antigens, particularly of the nuclear components [3]. Deposition of the immune complexes may trigger complement activation causing tissue damages. The broad auto-reactivities and hyperactivity of B cells are known to be predominately T cell-dependent [4], but the cellular and molecular mechanisms underlying such a systemic loss of B and T cell tolerance are yet to be fully understood. In contrast to B cell hyperactivity [5], reduced Interleukin 2 (IL-2) production and aberrant responsiveness of T cells are characteristic of SLE [6, 7]. Moreover, impaired cellular immunity, complement deficiency, defects in the clearance of dying cells by macrophages [8-10], roles of DC and the disrupted mechanisms of tolerance induction [11-14] are among many immunological characteristics of, or potential mechanisms proposed for, the disease.

2. Regulatory T cells

Regulatory T cells (Treg) belong to a specialized group or subsets of $CD4^+$ T cells with immunoregulatory capacity, which have been shown to play many important roles in maintaining peripheral tolerance [15, 16]. Treg can actively suppress self–reactive lymphocytes that escape central tolerance. The so-called naturally occurring Treg cells (nTreg), which constitutively express high levels of surface IL-2 receptor α chain (IL-2Rα, CD25) [17, 18], are originated from the thymus. Mice deficient in the $CD4^+CD25^{hi}$ Treg cells developed a multi-systemic autoimmune disease, including gastritis, oophoritis, arthritis, and thyroiditis. Co-transfer of Treg cells with self-reactive cells could prevent the development of experimentally-induced autoimmune diseases [17, 19]. Another relatively more specific marker of Treg cells is the intracellular molecule *Foxp3* (forkhead box P3). The *Foxp3* gene is crucial in the development and function of Treg cells in both humans [20, 21] and mice [22-24], and defective *Foxp3* expression generates strong activation of the immune system resulting in multi-organ autoimmune diseases [25, 26]. *Foxp3* transduction has been shown to convert naive $CD4^{+}CD25^{-}$ T cells into $CD25^{+}$ regulatory cells with suppressive activity [22]. Expression of *Foxp3* can also be induced in $CD4^{+}CD25^{-}$ T cells upon activation [27] or in the presence of TGF-ß [28, 29]. These findings suggest that the microenvironment could influence the expression of *Foxp3* during an immune response, inducing and promoting the expansion of peripheral Treg, also known as the inducible or adaptive Treg cells [27].

Treg may exert their immunosuppressive effects through cell-cell contacts and by the release of immunosuppressive cytokines such as IL-10 and TGF-β [30]. More recently, IL-35 has been identified to be the very cytokine not only directly associated with Treg functions but also their peripheral expansion [31, 32] [33, 34], including the induction of a unique human Treg subset (iT_R35) which could exert its immunosuppressive functions in an IL-35-dependent, but IL-10, TGF-β and Foxp3-independent, mechanism. Thus, although the induction and activation of Treg may be individually and cumulatively antigen-driven [35], these cells can suppress T effector cell (Teff) activation in an antigen non-specific manner [36, 37], e.g. by the release of immunosuppressive cytokines and via their inhibitory effects on antigen presenting cells (APC), DC in particular [38]. Indeed, the lack of Treg has been associated with many organ-specific autoimmune diseases [15, 17, 39] and, more recently, systemic autoimmune disorders including SLE [40-90].

3. Aberrant Treg frequencies and functions associated with lupus disorders

In recent years, Treg aberrations have been widely demonstrated in both SLE patients [40, 41, 43-48, 51-67, 71-80, 82-86, 88] and lupus mouse models [42, 49, 50, 68-70, 81, 87, 89-98]. These studies provided thus a plausible explanation for the systemic nature of the disease. A lack of Treg-mediated immune regulation in lupus is now a general consensus, although there have been differences in the findings as to whether a reduced Treg frequency [40-46, 49-53, 58-61, 68, 71-75, 82-84, 88, 90], defective Treg functions [44, 48, 53, 57, 59, 60, 66, 70, 76, 80, 89, 90] or both, or alternatively an insensitivity of the Treg target cells [66, 67, 70, 89, 99], are truly accountable.

By using CD25 as the marker, an early study by Crispin and colleagues first showed that, in lupus patients with active disease, the frequencies of Treg ($CD4+CD25^{+/bright}$) were significantly decreased, while T cells with an activated T helper (Th) effector phenotype ($CD4^{+}CD69^{+}$) increased [40]. An imbalance of Treg versus Teff was therefore proposed as a potential mechanism of disease development, and similar findings from many subsequent clinical studies mentioned above also confirmed this notion. Since IL-2 receptor (IL-2R) can be up-regulated on activated effector T and B lymphocytes too, the use of CD25 (alpha chain of IL-2R) as a Treg marker has understandably its limitation. Nevertheless, the identification of Foxp3, a relatively more specific if not exclusive marker of Treg, later allowed further verifications for the proposed link between Treg aberrations and systemic autoimmunity [49-51, 53, 57, 61, 68, 71, 73, 74, 76, 83, 88, 100].

However, there have also been controversial findings from other studies showing that the frequency of Treg cells, either defined as $CD4^{+}CD25^{bright}$ or $CD4^{+}Foxp3^{+}$, could be normal

[48, 66, 67, 70, 85, 86] or even increased [47, 54-56, 58, 62-65, 69, 74, 76-79, 81] in lupus disease. Instead, some of these studies suggested that Treg were functionally defective and less capable of suppressing those potentially auto-reactive lymphocytes in lupus patients [44, 48, 53, 57, 59, 60, 66, 76, 80], and the mouse models [70, 89, 90]. Again, alternative findings demonstrating lupus Treg being functionally normal [49, 50, 62, 67, 85], or at least normal in majority of patients tested [48, 64], or even enhanced in some way [68, 80, 87] added further confusion as well as interest to the matter.

Upon a closer examination, these seemingly discrepant findings can in fact be logically explained. Two most critical issues to be addressed are about the true causal relationship between the Treg changes and disease kinetics, and the complex underlying immunological mechanisms involved as discussed below.

4. Treg deficiency in systemic autoimmunity – the mutually causative relationship

In terms of disease kinetics, for example, low Treg frequencies are often found to be associated with SLE patients having active, but less so inactive, disease [40, 45, 83], or in patients on certain anti-inflammatory drugs undergoing clinical remission [47, 55, 56, 86]. Considering the multi-factorial nature, variability in disease onset and genetic heterogeneity of human lupus, however, it is also not surprising to note that such clinical association has not been always an obvious case [43, 48, 54, 62, 64].

Nevertheless, findings from studies using animal models especially inbred strains of mice which develop spontaneously a lupus like disease have offered some useful insights in this regard. The MRL/MpJ-*lpr/lpr* (MRL/*lpr*) mice develop spontaneously an age-dependent lupus-like disease and have been widely used as an animal model of human lupus. We have previously shown how the characteristic age-dependent biphasic changes of Treg frequency in the mice could reflect vividly a desperate, though eventually failed, attempt of the immune system trying to control auto-aggression [68]. After an early increase, Treg frequency (ratio) within the total CD4 T cell population in the peripheral lymphoid organs rapidly declined with age (**Fig. 1A-1B**), followed immediately by the onset and exacerbation of clinical disease [68], yet the total Treg number were in general higher compared to those in the control MRL/+ mouse strain (**Fig. 1C**).

Interestingly, in a similar study, it was demonstrated that peripheral Treg frequency in the NZB/W F1 strain of mice, another spontaneous lupus mouse model, was rather reduced at young age. In contrast, in the aged and diseased mice, a higher Treg frequency was detected in the renal draining lymph nodes, though also decreased in the spleen, as compared to normal BALB/c mice [50]. This may again reflect the differences in severity and kinetics of disease progression, in relation to the age-dependent Treg cell changes, between the MRL/*lpr* and NZB/W F1 strains. As shown in **Fig. 1C**, the total Treg numbers were constantly higher in the MRL/lpr strain too. This suggests that it is the Treg:Teff balance, rather than absolute Treg number, which is more relevant and critical to the disease kinetics. Such balance appears to have been maintained in the young MRL/*lpr* mice at least until 2-3 months of age, a stage prior to the development of overt clinical disease [2]. Compared to the MRL/*lpr* strain, NZB/W F1 mice develop a relatively milder clinical disease and at a much later stage [2]. The increased Treg frequency in the NZB/W F1 diseased mice could also reflect similarly the ongoing feedback regulatory mechanism yet relatively more sustainable in this mouse strain.

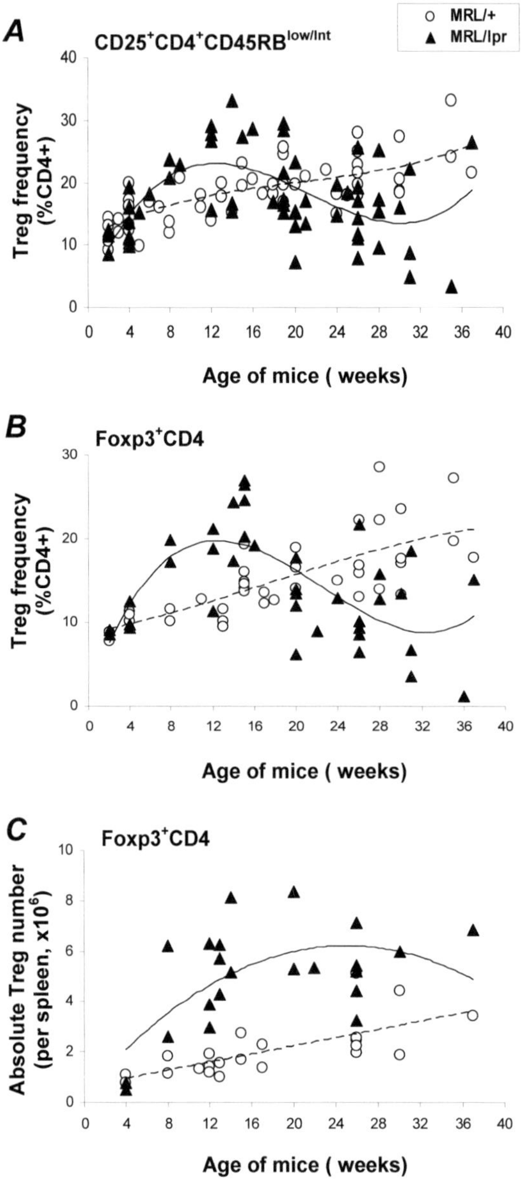

(Data from EJI 2008. **38**:1664-76 with permission)

Fig. 1. **Age-dependent bi-phasic changes of splenic Treg frequency in MRL/lpr mice.** Freshly isolated splenocytes were stained for CD4, CD25, CD45RB and Foxp3 in different combinations, and analyzed by multicolor flow cytometry. Treg cells were identified by means of **(A)** $CD4^+CD25^{hi}CD45RB^{low/Int}$ and (**B**, and **C**) $CD4^+Foxp3^+$, and shown as the percentage of total $CD4^+$ cell population (**A**, and **B**) and absolute Treg number per spleen (**C**) for each mouse. Data shown are Treg frequencies calculated from individual mice of different age (female), of the MRL/+ (open circles, n=58) and MRL/**lpr** (filled triangles, n=60) strains respectively, where each symbol represents one individual animal.

In other words, although the original defect(s) leading to the initiation of lupus may differ in SLE patients and these different lupus mouse models, changes in Treg versus Teff can be a true reflection of the capacity, or limitation, of the immune system trying to control the pathogenic autoimmune responses.

5. Defective Treg-mediated suppression in systemic autoimmunity – the underlying immunological mechanisms

The next important question concerns the complex immunological mechanisms underlying Treg deficiency in lupus disorders. Defects in the Teff cells and DC in particular have been found to contribute either directly or indirectly to the aberrant Treg-mediated suppression. These include abnormal Teff and DC functional status, and their expression of, or responsiveness to, certain cytokines critically involved in Treg and/or Teff functions.

5.1 Teff resistance

It was demonstrated that Teff cells isolated from lupus patients were less susceptible to Treg-mediated suppression [66, 67], and the level of resistance inversely correlated with patients' clinical disease activities [67]. Similar findings have also been shown in several lupus-prone mouse strains [70, 89, 99]. Based on their findings, the authors concluded that it was the enhanced resistance of responder cells (i.e. Teff), rather than defects in Treg themselves, that was to be blamed for the defective Treg-mediated suppression. A lack of Fas-mediated Teff activation induced cell death (AICD) and low surface expression of T cell inhibitory molecules (e.g. CTLA-4), or their ligands (CD80, CD86) on APC, are among the possible mechanisms proposed.

Moreover, it was also shown that the aberrant resistance of Teff could be associated with the activation state or lineage-commitment of Teff cells. While Treg isolated from the autoimmune BALB/c-lpr/lpr and gld/gld Fas/FasL-deficient mice could block naïve T cell activation and differentiation into the Th1 phenotype, they were unable to suppress those pre-existing lineage-committed IFN-γ-producing effector Th1 cells [99].

5.2 Lack of Teff-derived soluble factors essential for Treg functions & expansion

However, soluble factors produced by Teff cells are also known to be crucial for normal Treg functions. IL-2 produced by activated Teff, for example, is an essential growth factor for Treg cell differentiation and proliferation, and a potent inducer of Treg IL-10 expression [101]. We have previously demonstrated that, in two unrelated lupus mouse models, IL-2 deficiency is responsible for an early and progressive defect in T cell proliferation, which could be restored by exogenous IL-2 [7]. The cytokine was indeed later found to be able to restore Treg expansion and functions, both in vitro and *in vivo*, in the lupus mice [68, 87]. In other words, under normal physiological conditions, the Treg-mediated suppressive action has to be 'endorsed' by their 'target cells' too. When such a 'mutual agreement' is no longer in order, i.e. the lack of 'informed consent' from their target cells, Treg cells are left functionally powerless allowing subsequently the rapid expansion of autoreactive T and B cells.

5.3 Imbalanced peripheral Treg versus Teff expansion

The imbalance between Treg and Teff, including Th1 [99], expansion has provided a good basis and some mechanistic explanations for the systemic nature of lupus disorders [14, 68].

Th17 is another subset of specialized T helper cells, which produce the signature cytokine IL-17, or IL-17A. IL-17 mediates various inflammatory responses such as recruitment of monocytes and neutrophils [102], T cell infiltration and activation [103], induction of further proinflammatory cytokine expression [104] and, Th17 as a new pathogenic cell type, has been implicated in many autoimmune inflammatory diseases (reviewed in [105]). IL-17 producing Th17 cells also contribute to the pathogenesis and development of SLE. Several groups have shown that the numbers of Th17 cells and notably the ratio between Th17 and Treg were altered in SLE patients [75, 82, 106-108]. The number of Th17 cells in the blood of SLE patients was elevated [82] and accordingly serum IL-17 levels were increased [82, 109, 110]. However, the changes in the number of Th17 cells itself did not seem to correlate with lupus disease development, whereas the ratio between Treg and Th17 cells had a very clear inverse correlation with disease activity, especially in those patients with acute nephritis [107]. Moreover, the low Treg:Th17 ratios were also found to be restorable following clinical treatment that controlled disease activity [108].

5.4 Cytokines differentially involved in driving Treg & Teff differentiation

Naive $CD4^+$ T helper cells can be induced to differentiate into Th1, Th2, Th17 and Treg phenotypes depending to the local cytokine milieu. The presence of IL-12 signalling through STAT-4 (signal transduction and activator of transcription-4) drives towards Th1, whereas IL-4 (signalling through STAT-6) skews towards Th2 [111]. Interestingly, the differentiation of pro-inflammatory Th17 and anti-inflammatory Treg cells, two seemingly mutually exclusive cell types, follows a very similar pattern. Differentiation into both of these T cell subsets requires TGF-β, a cytokine capable of inducing expression of Foxp3 and RORγt, which are essential transcription factors for the development of Treg and Th17 cells, respectively [28, 112]. Under homeostatic non-inflammatory conditions, TGF-β induces only Treg, as Treg expressed Foxp3 itself is capable of suppressing Th17 development by binding to RORγt and thereby inhibiting its activity as a transcriptional activator [113]. Only in the presence of certain potent pro-inflammatory cytokines including IL-6, IL-21 and IL-23, the Foxp3 mediated inhibition of RORγt can be abrogated and differentiation into Th17 cells initiated [113, 114].

5.5 Roles of DC

Aberrant DC functions play evidently crucial roles in lupus disease induction, e.g. by driving the pathogenic Th1 type of responses [14] or skewing Teff versus Treg expansion [68]. **Fig. 2A** shows clearly that the DC generated from MRL/lpr mice are functionally defective in driving Treg, but not Teff, cell expansion. The importance of Treg:Th17 ratio for lupus disease activity has also been highlighted by work performed by Kang et al on the role of tolerogenic DC. The authors showed that injection of lupus-prone mice with a nucleosomal histone peptide epitope ($H4_{71\text{-}94}$) induced TGF-β producing Treg while suppressing inflammatory Th17 cells, with a general increase in survival. This was attributed to the induction of tolerogenic DC which produced enhanced levels of TGF-β, but decreased IL-6 expression [115]. Another study by Wan et al also pointed to the role of IL-6 produced by DC in blocking Treg function, and its genetic linkage (sle1) in mice originated from the NZM2410 lupus mouse strain [90]. In addition, aberrant expression of Type 1 interferon (IFN-α) by APC has also been shown to block Treg functions contributing to the Treg versus Teff imbalance in lupus disease [65, 81, 116].

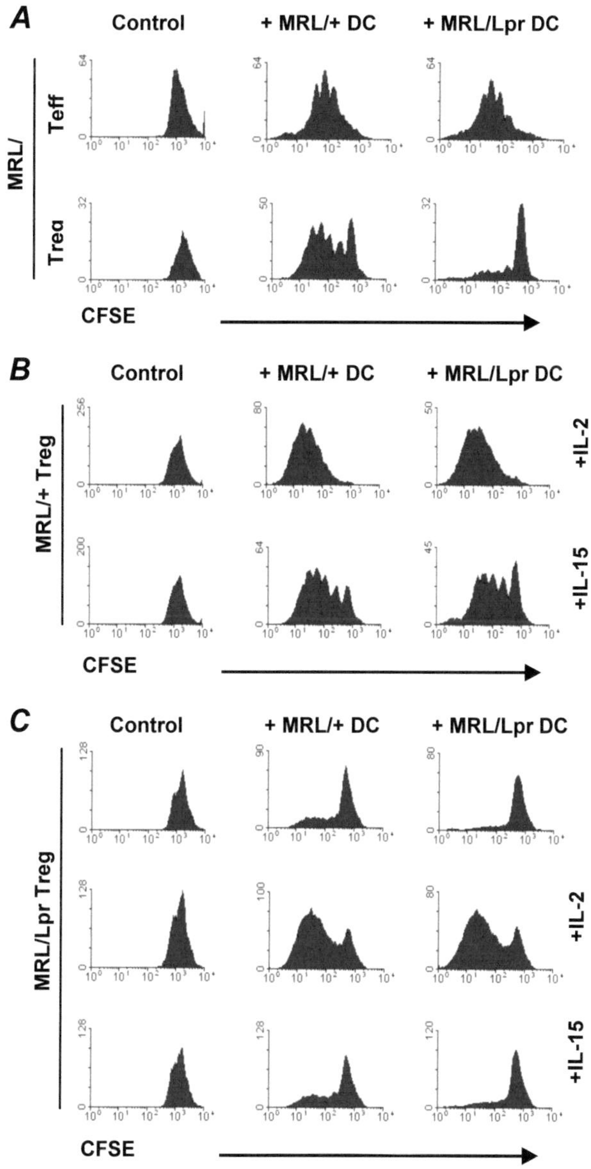

(Data from EJI 2008. 38:1664-76 with permission)

Fig. 2. **Defects in DCs and Treg cells of MRL/lpr mice.** *A. MRL/lpr DCs are defective in promoting Treg but not Teff cell proliferation.* Treg and Teff cells were purified from spleens of MRL/+ mice (3-month, female), and DCs were generated from bone marrow precursor cells of age-sex-matched MRL/+ or MRL/**lpr** mice (3-month, female). After labeling with CFSE, the Treg or Teff cells were stimulated with anti-CD3 mAb for 5 days, in the presence or absence of live MRL/**lpr** or MRL/+ DCs (as indicated in the graphs). *B. Restoration of Treg promoting capacity of MRL/lpr DCs by exogenous IL-2 and IL-15.* The CSFE-labeled splenic Treg cells purified from MRL/+ mice (as described in A) were stimulated with anti-CD3 mAb for

5 days, in the presence or absence of live MRL/**lpr** or MRL/+ DCs, and with or without addition of recombinant mouse IL-2 (10 ng/ml) or IL-15 (40 ng/ml), as indicated in the respective graphs. *C. Restoration of a defect in MRL/lpr Treg proliferation by IL-2, but not IL-15.* CSFE-labeled splenic Treg cells purified from MRL/**lpr** mice were stimulated with anti-CD3 mAb for 5 days, in the presence or absence of live MRL/**lpr** or MRL/+ DCs, and with or without addition of recombinant mouse IL-2 (10 ng/ml) or IL-15 (40 ng/ml). Cell division (CFSE dilution) was determined by flow cytometry. Controls were cells stimulated in the same way but in the absence of DCs. CM: culture medium control. Data shown were representative FACS profiles of more than 3 repeated experiments.

5.6 Possible Treg intrinsic defects

Furthermore, certain intrinsic defects associated with Treg themselves might also be involved [68]. IL-15 is a pleiotropic cytokine akin to IL-2 [117, 118], which is produced by monocytic cells including DC [119, 120] rather than T cells. IL-15 mediates its functions through the β- and γ-chains of the IL-2 receptor together with an unique IL-15 α-chain, and is known to be involved in the regulation of normal differentiation and expansion of T cells including Treg [121]. While the defect of MRL/lpr DC in driving expansion of the wild type (MRL/+) control Treg mentioned above (**Fig. 2A**) could be restored by adding exogenous IL-2 or IL-15 (**Fig. 2B**), the MRL/lpr Treg though also restorable by IL-2 failed completely to respond to IL-15 (**Fig. 2C**). These findings suggest that the MRL/lpr Treg possibly have an intrinsic defect as well in their responsiveness to the IL-2-like non-T cell-derived cytokine. It would also be very interesting to know how these cells may respond to other factors, such as IL-35 known to be closely associated with Treg functions [32].

6. Therapeutic implications of Treg in systemic autoimmune disorders

As discussed above, though also a result of overt autoimmune response itself, the lack of Treg mediated immune regulation contributes evidently to the early onset and kinetics of lupus disease development. Normalization of Treg frequencies and functions by restoring the Treg:Teff balance, may therefore prove to be clinically beneficial, hence a reasonable treatment strategy for the human disease. This concept has recently been tested in animal models by direct adoptive transfer of *ex vivo* derived, or *in vitro* expanded, Treg with encouraging results [68, 96, 122]. The treated mice had significantly delayed clinical disease as evident by delayed onset of glomerulonephritis, reduced proteinuria and skin lesions, and prolonged mouse survival [68, 96, 122].

Besides reconstitution of the Treg population by adoptive transfer, potential treatment methods to achieve an *in vivo* expansion of endogenous Treg and a normalization of the ratio between Treg and Teff, might be as diverse as the initial reasons for the deficiency in the Treg population. Accordingly, it has been shown that administration of rIL-2 promotes the proliferation of endogenous Treg and delays the progression of established disease, most likely by re-establishing the homeostatic balance of Treg and effector T cells [87]. Supporting evidence from earlier studies also indicates that tolerance induction by injecting various tolerogenic peptides [91, 115, 123], anti-thymocyte globulin agents [95], or oral administration of anti-CD3 antibodies [97], are all associated with *in vivo* Treg expansion.

It needs to be clearly pointed out that, while transfer of Treg may be beneficial against autoimmune syndromes [68], severe side effects such as infections following excessive (high dose) Treg treatment especially in non-adult mice can also occur (Yang et al, unpublished observations). Therefore, similar to the use of any immunosuppressive drug, caution should be taken about potential side effects of the treatment, for patients of young ages in particular.

7. Concluding remarks

In summary, immune regulation by Treg is an important mechanism against systemic autoimmunity, and a general lack of Treg-mediated suppression is evident in lupus disorder. Different findings from studies of lupus patients and various animal disease models about the aberrant changes in Treg frequency and functionality reflect vividly the disease kinetics, severity, and often the on-going desperate attempts of the immune system to control auto-aggression. Clarification of their true causal relationship is undoubtedly very important not only for our understanding of the complex disease mechanisms, but also for rational design of therapeutic strategies for our patients.

8. Acknowledgements

We wish to thank Dr Cui-Hong Yang and Dr Lina Tian for some of their important findings mentioned in this book chapter. We would also like to acknowledge the funding support which we have received for our research projects. SS is supported by the Arthritis Research UK (ARUK18523). FPH is currently supported by the Higher Education Funding Council UK (HEFC UK), and has received research funding support from the Arthritis Research UK (ARUK18523), the Hong Kong Research Grant Committee (RGC HKU 7246/01M, 7291/02M, 7410/03M, 7397/04M, 7580/06M), the MacFeat Bequest Fund (Glasgow) and the Li Ka Sheng Academic Foundation (Shantou). All correspondence should be addressed to FPH (fp.huang@imperial.ac.uk, or fphuang@hkucc.hku.hk)

9. References

[1] Vyse, T.J. and B.L. Kotzin, *GENETIC SUSCEPTIBILITY TO SYSTEMIC LUPUS ERYTHEMATOSUS.* Annu. Rev. Immunol., 1998. 16(1): p. 261-292.
[2] Theofilopoulos, A.N. and F.J. Dixon, *Murine models of systemic lupus erythematosus.* Adv Immunol, 1985. 37: p. 269-390.
[3] Mills, J.A., *Systemic lupus erythematosus.* N Engl J Med, 1994. 330(26): p. 1871-9.
[4] Rahman, A. and D.A. Isenberg, *Systemic lupus erythematosus.* N Engl J Med, 2008. 358(9): p. 929-39.
[5] Lipsky, P.E., *Systemic lupus erythematosus: an autoimmune disease of B cell hyperactivity.* Nat Immunol, 2001. 2(9): p. 764-6.
[6] Altman, A., et al., *Analysis of T cell function in autoimmune murine strains. Defects in production and responsiveness to interleukin 2.* J Exp Med, 1981. 154(3): p. 791-808.
[7] Huang, F.P. and D.I. Stott, *Restoration of an early, progressive defect in responsiveness to T-cell activation in lupus mice by exogenous IL-2.* Autoimmunity, 1993. 15(1): p. 19-29.
[8] Manderson, A.P., M. Botto, and M.J. Walport, *The role of complement in the development of systemic lupus erythematosus.* Annu Rev Immunol, 2004. 22: p. 431-56.
[9] Cook, H.T. and M. Botto, *Mechanisms of Disease: the complement system and the pathogenesis of systemic lupus erythematosus.* Nat Clin Pract Rheumatol, 2006. 2(6): p. 330-7.

[10] Pickering, M.C., et al., *Prevention of C5 activation ameliorates spontaneous and experimental glomerulonephritis in factor H-deficient mice.* Proc Natl Acad Sci U S A, 2006. 103(25): p. 9649-54.
[11] Matsumoto, K., et al., *Defect in negative selection in lpr donor-derived T cells differentiating in non-lpr host thymus.* J Exp Med, 1991. 173(1): p. 127-36.
[12] Mok, C.C. and C.S. Lau, *Pathogenesis of systemic lupus erythematosus.* J Clin Pathol, 2003. 56(7): p. 481-90.
[13] Watanabe-Fukunaga, R., et al., *Lymphoproliferation disorder in mice explained by defects in Fas antigen that mediates apoptosis.* Nature (London), 1992. 356(6367): p. 314-7.
[14] Ma, L., et al., *Systemic autoimmune disease induced by dendritic cells that have captured necrotic but not apoptotic cells in susceptible mouse strains.* Eur J Immunol, 2005. 35(11): p. 3364-75.
[15] Sakaguchi, S., *Naturally arising CD4+ regulatory t cells for immunologic self-tolerance and negative control of immune responses.* Annu Rev Immunol, 2004. 22: p. 531-62.
[16] Wing, K. and S. Sakaguchi, *Regulatory T cells exert checks and balances on self tolerance and autoimmunity.* Nat Immunol, 2010. 11(1): p. 7-13.
[17] Sakaguchi, S., et al., *Immunologic self-tolerance maintained by activated T cells expressing IL-2 receptor alpha-chains (CD25). Breakdown of a single mechanism of self-tolerance causes various autoimmune diseases.* J Immunol, 1995. 155(3): p. 1151-64.
[18] Saoudi, A., et al., *The thymus contains a high frequency of cells that prevent autoimmune diabetes on transfer into prediabetic recipients.* J Exp Med, 1996. 184(6): p. 2393-8.
[19] Asano, M., et al., *Autoimmune disease as a consequence of developmental abnormality of a T cell subpopulation.* J Exp Med, 1996. 184(2): p. 387-96.
[20] Yagi, H., et al., *Crucial role of FOXP3 in the development and function of human CD25+CD4+ regulatory T cells.* Int Immunol, 2004. 16(11): p. 1643-56.
[21] Bacchetta, R., et al., *Defective regulatory and effector T cell functions in patients with FOXP3 mutations.* J Clin Invest, 2006. 116(6): p. 1713-22.
[22] Hori, S., T. Nomura, and S. Sakaguchi, *Control of regulatory T cell development by the transcription factor Foxp3.* Science, 2003. 299(5609): p. 1057-61.
[23] Fontenot, J.D., M.A. Gavin, and A.Y. Rudensky, *Foxp3 programs the development and function of CD4+CD25+ regulatory T cells.* Nat Immunol, 2003. 4(4): p. 330-6.
[24] Khattri, R., et al., *An essential role for Scurfin in CD4+CD25+ T regulatory cells.* Nat Immunol, 2003. 4(4): p. 337-42.
[25] Brunkow, M.E., et al., *Disruption of a new forkhead/winged-helix protein, scurfin, results in the fatal lymphoproliferative disorder of the scurfy mouse.* Nat Genet, 2001. 27(1): p. 68-73.
[26] Gambineri, E., T.R. Torgerson, and H.D. Ochs, *Immune dysregulation, polyendocrinopathy, enteropathy, and X-linked inheritance (IPEX), a syndrome of systemic autoimmunity caused by mutations of FOXP3, a critical regulator of T-cell homeostasis.* Curr Opin Rheumatol, 2003. 15(4): p. 430-5.
[27] Curotto de Lafaille, M.A., et al., *CD25- T cells generate CD25+Foxp3+ regulatory T cells by peripheral expansion.* J Immunol, 2004. 173(12): p. 7259-68.
[28] Chen, W., et al., *Conversion of peripheral CD4+CD25- naive T cells to CD4+CD25+ regulatory T cells by TGF-beta induction of transcription factor Foxp3.* J Exp Med, 2003. 198(12): p. 1875-86.

[29] Fantini, M.C., et al., *Cutting edge: TGF-beta induces a regulatory phenotype in CD4+CD25- T cells through Foxp3 induction and down-regulation of Smad7.* J Immunol, 2004. 172(9): p. 5149-53.

[30] Kitani, A., et al., *Transforming growth factor (TGF)-beta1-producing regulatory T cells induce Smad-mediated interleukin 10 secretion that facilitates coordinated immunoregulatory activity and amelioration of TGF-beta1-mediated fibrosis.* J Exp Med, 2003. 198(8): p. 1179-88.

[31] Niedbala, W., et al., *IL-35 is a novel cytokine with therapeutic effects against collagen-induced arthritis through the expansion of regulatory T cells and suppression of Th17 cells.* Eur J Immunol, 2007. 37(11): p. 3021-9.

[32] Collison, L.W., et al., *The inhibitory cytokine IL-35 contributes to regulatory T-cell function.* Nature, 2007. 450(7169): p. 566-9.

[33] Seyerl, M., et al., *Human rhinoviruses induce IL-35-producing Treg via induction of B7-H1 (CD274) and sialoadhesin (CD169) on DC.* Eur J Immunol, 2009.

[34] Collison, L.W., et al., *IL-35-mediated induction of a potent regulatory T cell population.* Nat Immunol, 2010. 11(12): p. 1093-101.

[35] Tarbell, K.V., S. Yamazaki, and R.M. Steinman, *The interactions of dendritic cells with antigen-specific, regulatory T cells that suppress autoimmunity.* Semin Immunol, 2006. 18(2): p. 93-102.

[36] Thornton, A.M. and E.M. Shevach, *CD4+CD25+ immunoregulatory T cells suppress polyclonal T cell activation in vitro by inhibiting interleukin 2 production.* J Exp Med, 1998. 188(2): p. 287-96.

[37] Yu, P., et al., *Specific T regulatory cells display broad suppressive functions against experimental allergic encephalomyelitis upon activation with cognate antigen.* J Immunol, 2005. 174(11): p. 6772-80.

[38] Yamazaki, S., et al., *Dendritic cells expand antigen-specific Foxp3+ CD25+ CD4+ regulatory T cells including suppressors of alloreactivity.* Immunol Rev, 2006. 212: p. 314-29.

[39] Saoudi, A., et al., *The physiological role of regulatory T cells in the prevention of autoimmunity: the function of the thymus in the generation of the regulatory T cell subset.* Immunol Rev, 1996. 149: p. 195-216.

[40] Crispin, J.C., A. Martinez, and J. Alcocer-Varela, *Quantification of regulatory T cells in patients with systemic lupus erythematosus.* J Autoimmun, 2003. 21(3): p. 273-6.

[41] Liu, M.F., et al., *Decreased CD4+CD25+ T cells in peripheral blood of patients with systemic lupus erythematosus.* Scand J Immunol, 2004. 59(2): p. 198-202.

[42] Wu, H.Y. and N.A. Staines, *A deficiency of CD4+CD25+ T cells permits the development of spontaneous lupus-like disease in mice, and can be reversed by induction of mucosal tolerance to histone peptide autoantigen.* Lupus, 2004. 13(3): p. 192-200.

[43] Fathy, A., et al., *Diminished CD4+CD25+ T-lymphocytes in peripheral blood of patients with systemic lupus erythematosus.* Egypt J Immunol, 2005. 12(1): p. 25-31.

[44] Miyara, M., et al., *Global natural regulatory T cell depletion in active systemic lupus erythematosus.* J Immunol, 2005. 175(12): p. 8392-400.

[45] Lee, J.H., et al., *Inverse correlation between CD4+ regulatory T-cell population and autoantibody levels in paediatric patients with systemic lupus erythematosus.* Immunology, 2006. 117(2): p. 280-6.

[46] Mellor-Pita, S., et al., *Decrease of regulatory T cells in patients with systemic lupus erythematosus.* Ann Rheum Dis, 2006. 65(4): p. 553-4.

[47] Suarez, A., et al., *Enrichment of CD4+ CD25high T cell population in patients with systemic lupus erythematosus treated with glucocorticoids.* Ann Rheum Dis, 2006. 65(11): p. 1512-7.

[48] Alvarado-Sanchez, B., et al., *Regulatory T cells in patients with systemic lupus erythematosus.* J Autoimmun, 2006. 27(2): p. 110-8.

[49] Hsu, W.T., J.L. Suen, and B.L. Chiang, *The role of CD4CD25 T cells in autoantibody production in murine lupus.* Clin Exp Immunol, 2006. 145(3): p. 513-9.

[50] Scalapino, K.J., et al., *Suppression of disease in New Zealand Black/New Zealand White lupus-prone mice by adoptive transfer of ex vivo expanded regulatory T cells.* J Immunol, 2006. 177(3): p. 1451-9.

[51] Barath, S., et al., *The severity of systemic lupus erythematosus negatively correlates with the increasing number of CD4+CD25(high)FoxP3+ regulatory T cells during repeated plasmapheresis treatments of patients.* Autoimmunity, 2007. 40(7): p. 521-8.

[52] Barath, S., et al., *Measurement of natural (CD4+CD25high) and inducible (CD4+IL-10+) regulatory T cells in patients with systemic lupus erythematosus.* Lupus, 2007. 16(7): p. 489-96.

[53] Lyssuk, E.Y., et al., *Reduced number and function of CD4+CD25highFoxP3+ regulatory T cells in patients with systemic lupus erythematosus.* Adv Exp Med Biol, 2007. 601: p. 113-9.

[54] Lin, S.C., et al., *The quantitative analysis of peripheral blood FOXP3-expressing T cells in systemic lupus erythematosus and rheumatoid arthritis patients.* Eur J Clin Invest, 2007. 37(12): p. 987-96.

[55] Sfikakis, P.P., et al., *Increased expression of the FoxP3 functional marker of regulatory T cells following B cell depletion with rituximab in patients with lupus nephritis.* Clin Immunol, 2007. 123(1): p. 66-73.

[56] Vallerskog, T., et al., *Treatment with rituximab affects both the cellular and the humoral arm of the immune system in patients with SLE.* Clin Immunol, 2007. 122(1): p. 62-74.

[57] Valencia, X., et al., *Deficient CD4+CD25high T regulatory cell function in patients with active systemic lupus erythematosus.* J Immunol, 2007. 178(4): p. 2579-88.

[58] Bonelli, M., et al., *Foxp3 expression in CD4+ T cells of patients with systemic lupus erythematosus: a comparative phenotypic analysis.* Ann Rheum Dis, 2008. 67(5): p. 664-71.

[59] Bonelli, M., et al., *Quantitative and qualitative deficiencies of regulatory T cells in patients with systemic lupus erythematosus (SLE).* Int Immunol, 2008. 20(7): p. 861-8.

[60] Lee, H.Y., et al., *Altered frequency and migration capacity of CD4+CD25+ regulatory T cells in systemic lupus erythematosus.* Rheumatology (Oxford), 2008. 47(6): p. 789-94.

[61] Zhang, B., et al., *Reduction of forkhead box P3 levels in CD4+CD25high T cells in patients with new-onset systemic lupus erythematosus.* Clin Exp Immunol, 2008. 153(2): p. 182-7.

[62] Zhang, B., et al., *Clinical significance of increased CD4+CD25-Foxp3+ T cells in patients with new-onset systemic lupus erythematosus.* Ann Rheum Dis, 2008. 67(7): p. 1037-40.

[63] Azab, N.A., et al., *CD4+CD25+ regulatory T cells (TREG) in systemic lupus erythematosus (SLE) patients: the possible influence of treatment with corticosteroids.* Clin Immunol, 2008. 127(2): p. 151-7.

[64] Yates, J., et al., *Natural regulatory T cells: number and function are normal in the majority of patients with lupus nephritis.* Clin Exp Immunol, 2008. 153(1): p. 44-55.

[65] Yan, B., et al., *Dysfunctional CD4+,CD25+ regulatory T cells in untreated active systemic lupus erythematosus secondary to interferon-alpha-producing antigen-presenting cells.* Arthritis Rheum, 2008. 58(3): p. 801-12.
[66] Vargas-Rojas, M.I., et al., *Quantitative and qualitative normal regulatory T cells are not capable of inducing suppression in SLE patients due to T-cell resistance.* Lupus, 2008. 17(4): p. 289-94.
[67] Venigalla, R.K., et al., *Reduced CD4+,CD25- T cell sensitivity to the suppressive function of CD4+,CD25high,CD127 -/low regulatory T cells in patients with active systemic lupus erythematosus.* Arthritis Rheum, 2008. 58(7): p. 2120-30.
[68] Yang, C.H., et al., *Immunological mechanisms and clinical implications of regulatory T cell deficiency in a systemic autoimmune disorder: Roles of IL-2 versus IL-15.* Eur J Immunol, 2008. 38: p. 1664-1676.
[69] Abe, J., et al., *Increased Foxp3(+) CD4(+) regulatory T cells with intact suppressive activity but altered cellular localization in murine lupus.* Am J Pathol, 2008. 173(6): p. 1682-92.
[70] Parietti, V., et al., *Function of CD4+,CD25+ Treg cells in MRL/lpr mice is compromised by intrinsic defects in antigen-presenting cells and effector T cells.* Arthritis Rheum, 2008. 58(6): p. 1751-61.
[71] Atfy, M., et al., *Impact of CD4+CD25high regulatory T-cells and FoxP3 expression in the peripheral blood of patients with systemic lupus erythematosus.* Egypt J Immunol, 2009. 16(1): p. 117-26.
[72] Banica, L., et al., *Quantification and molecular characterization of regulatory T cells in connective tissue diseases.* Autoimmunity, 2009. 42(1): p. 41-9.
[73] Barreto, M., et al., *Low frequency of CD4+CD25+ Treg in SLE patients: a heritable trait associated with CTLA4 and TGFbeta gene variants.* BMC Immunol, 2009. 10: p. 5.
[74] Suen, J.L., et al., *Altered homeostasis of CD4(+) FoxP3(+) regulatory T-cell subpopulations in systemic lupus erythematosus.* Immunology, 2009. 127(2): p. 196-205.
[75] Yang, J., et al., *Th17 and natural Treg cell population dynamics in systemic lupus erythematosus.* Arthritis Rheum, 2009. 60(5): p. 1472-83.
[76] Bonelli, M., et al., *Phenotypic and functional analysis of CD4+ CD25- Foxp3+ T cells in patients with systemic lupus erythematosus.* J Immunol, 2009. 182(3): p. 1689-95.
[77] Dai, Z., et al., *Normally occurring NKG2D+CD4+ T cells are immunosuppressive and inversely correlated with disease activity in juvenile-onset lupus.* J Exp Med, 2009. 206(4): p. 793-805.
[78] Yang, H.X., et al., *Are CD4+CD25-Foxp3+ cells in untreated new-onset lupus patients regulatory T cells?* Arthritis Res Ther, 2009. 11(5): p. R153.
[79] Yan, B. and Y. Liu, *The Nature of Increased Circulating CD4CD25Foxp3 T Cells in Patients with Systemic Lupus Erythematosus: A Novel Hypothesis.* Open Rheumatol J, 2009. 3: p. 22-4.
[80] Gomez, J., et al., *Conserved anti-proliferative effect and poor inhibition of TNFalpha secretion by regulatory CD4+CD25+ T cells in patients with systemic lupus erythematosus.* Clin Immunol, 2009. 132(3): p. 385-92.
[81] Scaglione, B.J., et al., *Regulatory T cells as central regulators of both autoimmunity and B cell malignancy in New Zealand Black mice.* J Autoimmun, 2009. 32(1): p. 14-23.
[82] Henriques, A., et al., *Frequency and functional activity of Th17, Tc17 and other T-cell subsets in Systemic Lupus Erythematosus.* Cell Immunol, 2010. 264(1): p. 97-103.

[83] Habibagahi, M., et al., *Quantification of regulatory T cells in peripheral blood of patients with systemic lupus erythematosus.* Rheumatol Int, 2010.

[84] Chen, D.Y., et al., *The associations of circulating CD4(+)CD25(high) regulatory T cells and TGF-beta with disease activity and clinical course in patients with adult-onset Still's disease.* Connect Tissue Res, 2010. 51(5): p. 370-7.

[85] Mesquita, D., et al., *Systemic lupus erythematosus exhibits a dynamic and continuum spectrum of effector/regulatory T cells.* Scand J Rheumatol, 2011. 40(1): p. 41-50.

[86] Ma, J., et al., *The imbalance between regulatory and IL-17-secreting CD4+ T cells in lupus patients.* Clin Rheumatol, 2010. 29(11): p. 1251-8.

[87] Humrich, J.Y., et al., *Homeostatic imbalance of regulatory and effector T cells due to IL-2 deprivation amplifies murine lupus.* Proc Natl Acad Sci U S A, 2010. 107(1): p. 204-9.

[88] Xing, Q., et al., *Elevated Th17 cells are accompanied by FoxP3+ Treg cells decrease in patients with lupus nephritis.* Rheumatol Int, 2011.

[89] Monk, C.R., et al., *MRL/Mp CD4+,CD25- T cells show reduced sensitivity to suppression by CD4+,CD25+ regulatory T cells in vitro: a novel defect of T cell regulation in systemic lupus erythematosus.* Arthritis Rheum, 2005. 52(4): p. 1180-4.

[90] Wan, S., C. Xia, and L. Morel, *IL-6 produced by dendritic cells from lupus-prone mice inhibits CD4+CD25+ T cell regulatory functions.* J Immunol, 2007. 178(1): p. 271-9.

[91] Kang, H.K., et al., *Very low-dose tolerance with nucleosomal peptides controls lupus and induces potent regulatory T cell subsets.* J Immunol, 2005. 174(6): p. 3247-55.

[92] Reilly, C.M., et al., *The histone deacetylase inhibitor trichostatin A upregulates regulatory T cells and modulates autoimmunity in NZB/W F1 mice.* J Autoimmun, 2008. 31(2): p. 123-30.

[93] Tago, F., et al., *Repeated 0.5-Gy gamma irradiation attenuates autoimmune disease in MRL-lpr/lpr mice with suppression of CD3+CD4-CD8-B220+ T-cell proliferation and with up-regulation of CD4+CD25+Foxp3+ regulatory T cells.* Radiat Res, 2008. 169(1): p. 59-66.

[94] Sharabi, A. and E. Mozes, *The suppression of murine lupus by a tolerogenic peptide involves foxp3-expressing CD8 cells that are required for the optimal induction and function of foxp3-expressing CD4 cells.* J Immunol, 2008. 181(5): p. 3243-51.

[95] Kaplan, J., et al., *Therapeutic benefit of treatment with anti-thymocyte globulin and latent TGF-beta1 in the MRL/lpr lupus mouse model.* Lupus, 2008. 17(9): p. 822-31.

[96] Scalapino, K.J. and D.I. Daikh, *Suppression of glomerulonephritis in NZB/NZW lupus prone mice by adoptive transfer of ex vivo expanded regulatory T cells.* PLoS One, 2009. 4(6): p. e6031.

[97] Wu, H.Y., et al., *Suppression of murine SLE by oral anti-CD3: inducible CD4+CD25-LAP+ regulatory T cells control the expansion of IL-17+ follicular helper T cells.* Lupus, 2009. 18(7): p. 586-96.

[98] Zhang, J.L., et al., *CD3 mAb treatment ameliorated the severity of the cGVHD-induced lupus nephritis in mice by up-regulation of Foxp3+ regulatory T cells in the target tissue: kidney.* Transpl Immunol, 2010. 24(1): p. 17-25.

[99] Hondowicz, B.D., et al., *Autoantibody production in lpr/lpr gld/gld mice reflects accumulation of CD4+ effector cells that are resistant to regulatory T cell activity.* J Autoimmun, 2008. 31(2): p. 98-109.

[100] Cuda, C.M., et al., *Murine lupus susceptibility locus Sle1a controls regulatory T cell number and function through multiple mechanisms.* J Immunol, 2007. 179(11): p. 7439-47.

[101] Scheffold, A., J. Huhn, and T. Hofer, *Regulation of CD4+CD25+ regulatory T cell activity: it takes (IL-)two to tango.* Eur J Immunol, 2005. 35(5): p. 1336-41.

[102] Witowski, J., et al., *IL-17 stimulates intraperitoneal neutrophil infiltration through the release of GRO alpha chemokine from mesothelial cells.* J Immunol, 2000. 165(10): p. 5814-21.
[103] Albanesi, C., A. Cavani, and G. Girolomoni, *IL-17 is produced by nickel-specific T lymphocytes and regulates ICAM-1 expression and chemokine production in human keratinocytes: synergistic or antagonist effects with IFN-gamma and TNF-alpha.* J Immunol, 1999. 162(1): p. 494-502.
[104] Schwarzenberger, P., et al., *Requirement of endogenous stem cell factor and granulocyte-colony-stimulating factor for IL-17-mediated granulopoiesis.* J Immunol, 2000. 164(9): p. 4783-9.
[105] Xu, S. and X. Cao, *Interleukin-17 and its expanding biological functions.* Cell Mol Immunol. 2010 May, 7(3): p. 164-74.
[106] Wong, C.K., et al., *Hyperproduction of IL-23 and IL-17 in patients with systemic lupus erythematosus: implications for Th17-mediated inflammation in auto-immunity.* Clin Immunol, 2008. 127(3): p. 385-93.
[107] Xing, Q., et al., *Elevated Th17 cells are accompanied by FoxP3+ Treg cells decrease in patients with lupus nephritis.* Rheumatol Int. 2011 Jan 18. [Epub ahead of print]
[108] Ma, J., et al., *The imbalance between regulatory and IL-17-secreting CD4+ T cells in lupus patients.* Clin Rheumatol. 2010 Nov; 29(11): p. 1251-8.
[109] Mok, M.Y., et al., *The relation of interleukin 17 (IL-17) and IL-23 to Th1/Th2 cytokines and disease activity in systemic lupus erythematosus.* J Rheumatol. 2010 Oct; 37(10): p. 2046-52.
[110] Chen, X.Q., et al., *Plasma IL-17A is increased in new-onset SLE patients and associated with disease activity.* J Clin Immunol. 2010 Mar; 30(2): p. 221-5.
[111] Nelms, K., et al., *The IL-4 receptor: signaling mechanisms and biologic functions.* Annu Rev Immunol, 1999. 17: p. 701-38.
[112] Mangan, P.R., et al., *Transforming growth factor-beta induces development of the T(H)17 lineage.* Nature, 2006. 441(7090): p. 231-4.
[113] Zhou, L., et al., *TGF-beta-induced Foxp3 inhibits T(H)17 cell differentiation by antagonizing RORgammat function.* Nature, 2008. 453(7192): p. 236-40.
[114] Bettelli, E., et al., *IL-10 is critical in the regulation of autoimmune encephalomyelitis as demonstrated by studies of IL-10- and IL-4-deficient and transgenic mice.* J Immunol, 1998. 161(7): p. 3299-306.
[115] Kang, H.K., M. Liu, and S.K. Datta, *Low-dose peptide tolerance therapy of lupus generates plasmacytoid dendritic cells that cause expansion of autoantigen-specific regulatory T cells and contraction of inflammatory Th17 cells.* J Immunol, 2007. 178(12): p. 7849-58.
[116] Golding, A., et al., *Interferon-alpha regulates the dynamic balance between human activated regulatory and effector T cells: implications for antiviral and autoimmune responses.* Immunology, 2010. 131(1): p. 107-17.
[117] Grabstein, K.H., et al., *Cloning of a T cell growth factor that interacts with the beta chain of the interleukin-2 receptor.* Science, 1994. 264(5161): p. 965-8.
[118] McInnes, I.B., et al., *The role of interleukin-15 in T-cell migration and activation in rheumatoid arthritis [see comments].* Nat Med, 1996. 2(2): p. 175-82.
[119] Ruckert, R., et al., *Dendritic cell-derived IL-15 controls the induction of CD8 T cell immune responses.* Eur J Immunol, 2003. 33(12): p. 3493-503.
[120] Ohteki, T., et al., *Essential roles of DC-derived IL-15 as a mediator of inflammatory responses in vivo.* J Exp Med, 2006. 203(10): p. 2329-38.

[121] Koenen, H.J., E. Fasse, and I. Joosten, *IL-15 and cognate antigen successfully expand de novo-induced human antigen-specific regulatory CD4+ T cells that require antigen-specific activation for suppression.* J Immunol, 2003. 171(12): p. 6431-41.

[122] Su, H., et al., *Transforming growth factor-beta1-induced CD4+CD25+ regulatory T cells in vitro reverse and prevent a murine lupus-like syndrome of chronic graft-versus-host disease.* Br J Dermatol, 2008. 158(6): p. 1197-209.

[123] Sharabi, A., et al., *A peptide based on the complementarity-determining region 1 of an autoantibody ameliorates lupus by up-regulating CD4+CD25+ cells and TGF-beta.* Proc Natl Acad Sci U S A, 2006. 103(23): p. 8810-5.

7

Postinfectious Autoimmune Syndrome as a Key Factor in Chronization of the Infectious Disease

Natalia Cherepahina, Murat Agirov, Jamilyia Tabaksoeva,
Kusum Ahmedilova and Sergey Suchkov
First Moscow State Medical University
Russian State Medical University
Russia

1. Introduction

Disturbances in immune tolerance provoke autoimmune aggression, i.e., a specific immune response to auto-Ags with subsequent development of an autoimmune syndrome or an autoimmune disease (Suchkov et al., 2007).

A crucial role in formation of autoimmune syndromes and progression of autoimmune diseases is played by inborn (in the first place, HLA-associated) predisposition coupled with impaired immune responsiveness of the invaded organism. Noteworthy, initiation and progression of autoaggressive reactions cannot be triggered without preliminary activation of signaling reaction cascades, which include:

i. polyclonal activation of autoreactive cytotoxic T lymphocytes (CTL) by super-Ag (multimolecular protein complexes composed of microbial Ags, Ags and/or haptens of the carrier or intermediary drug-related metabolites) demonstrating broad spectrum of epitopes;
ii. release of sequestered or intramolecular (cryptic) autoepitopes after the tissue damage or organ injures during the inflammatory process;
iii. anti-idiotypic Ab formation that can damage own tissue and promote autoagression;
iv. effect of mimicking epitopes (microbial Ags cross-reacting with autoepitopes of human tissues and organs).

Of particular interest in this respect is so-called *molecular mimicry*. Its biological mechanism is based on cross-reactivity, i.e., ability of the infected organism to cross-react, by virtue of structural homology between its auto-Ags and microbial Ags, with the microbial antigen thereby triggering miscellaneous immune reactions. Under these conditions, the role of autoaggressors is played simultaneously by two different groups of Ags, namely, mimicking Ags of the microbial pathogen and patient's own autoAgs. Their interactions form the clinical picture of the postinfectious autoimmune syndrome (PIFA), one of main clinical variants of syndromeal immune pathology (Paltsev et al., 2009a).

Today, the key role of the immune system in the pathogenesis of chronically relapsing infectious diseases (CRID) leaves no doubt. Their clinical course is controlled by an immense variety of factors and their combinations among which the immunologic syndrome (IS) reflecting the origin and severity of disturbances in immune homeostasis occupies a special niche. The concept of IS is not new in principle and is widely met in the current literature.

However, the term "*clinico-immunological syndrome*" (CIS) is far less explicit and needs to be supplemented with a pathogenetically rationalized, clinically significant formulaic definition encompassing the tremendous body of evidence accumulated thus far in the modern literature (Paltsev et al., 2009b) (Fig. 1).

CLINICAL CRITERIA

- Causal factor
- Lingering or chronic course of inflammatory processes (irrespective of localization) associated with frequent relapses
- Activation of conditionally pathogenic microflora, mixed infections; changes in the infectious pathogen during progression of the disease; involvement of other internal organs in autoimmune process
- Resistance to antibacterial therapy

CRITERIA OF STRUCTURAL IMMUNODEFICIENCY

- Clinical picture
- Deterioration of parameters reflecting populational magnitude and functional activity of lymphocytes, their subpopulations and non-specific protective factors to levels below the physiological level
- Diagnostically significant deterioration of 2–3 parameters in one component of the immune system or associated disturbances

CRITERIA OF FUNCTIONAL IMMUNODEFICIENCY

- Clinical picture
- Laboratory findings (content and functional activity of T and B lymphocytes, monocytes/macrophages and their subpopulations and other significant nonspecific protective factors)

Fig. 1. Clinical and immunological criteria of PIFSI

PIFSI – postinfectious secondary immunodeficiency syndrome.

In this section, we shall consider one of the most important clinical aspects of CIS, viz., *postinfectious CIS (PICIS)* whose role for practitioners in clinical medicine can hardly be overestimated. PICIS being a form of secondary (*syndromal*) immune pathology associated with the underlying (infectious) disease is provoked by a variety of factors including infectious pathogens of various etiology, clinical progression and complication of the disease proper, or inadequately applied antimicrobial therapy. The most common forms of this syndrome are as follows:

i. postinfectious secondary immunodeficiency syndrome (PIFSI);
ii. (ii) postinfectious autoimmune syndrome (PIFA);
iii. autoimmune syndrome coupled with postinfectious secondary immunodeficiency (PIFASID) (Suchkov et al., 2004).

Predisposition to one or another form of syndromeal immune pathology depends on a great number of genetically determined factors, which play a key role in the formation of patient's own immune resources. Its functional activity is controlled by coordinated functioning of *innate* and *adaptive* immune mechanisms; however, their role in the development and chronization of infectious processes is still open to question, which strongly impedes the construction of state-of-art immunopathogenetic models (Fig. 2).

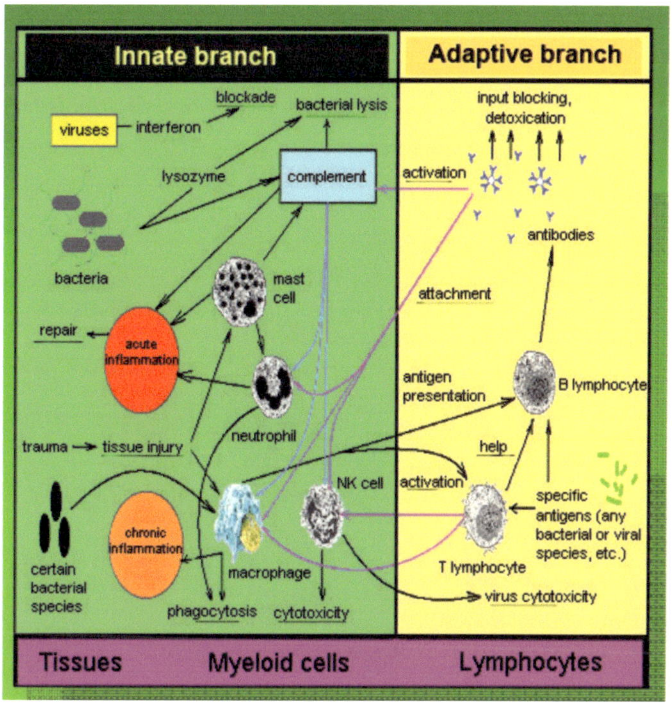

Fig. 2. The innate and adaptive branches of immunity.

In this context, analysis of major immunopathologic manifestations in patients with PICIS-related chronically relapsing infectious diseases and construction of basic algorithms for state-of-art immunogenetic diagnostic protocols becomes a prime target for clinical medicine.

Human immune system is a complex physiological mechanism whereby the human organism protects itself from exogenous etiopathogenic attacks. Its functional activity is provided by two types of protective immune mechanisms, one of which is *specific* and the other one is *nonspecific*. The main outcome of the immune response to etiopathogenic attacks is formation of two populations of regulatory T helper cells (Th cells). The Th population is further subdivided into Th1 cells responsible for activation of effector links of cell-mediated immunity (macrophages and cytotoxic T lymphocytes/CTL) and Th2 cells exerting control over antibody (AB) production (McGuirk & Mills, 2002) (Fig. 3).

However, the key factor in determining a particular type of the immune response and, correspondingly, a particular form of CIS, is localization (*extracellular* or *intracellular*) of the etiopathogen (Fig. 4).

The latter circumstance is of particular importance from both pathogenetic and clinical points of view, since the majority of currently known pathogenic microorganisms can escape from immune control and, in doing so, change the scenario of genetically programmed immune responsiveness thereby provoking unpredictable complications for the patient and hindering physician's attempts to implement adequate treatment strategies (Azikury, 1985; Aitpaev & Seisembekov, 1987).

Two major disturbances in immune responsiveness are presently recognized as causal factors in chronization of infectious diseases and formation of PICIS:

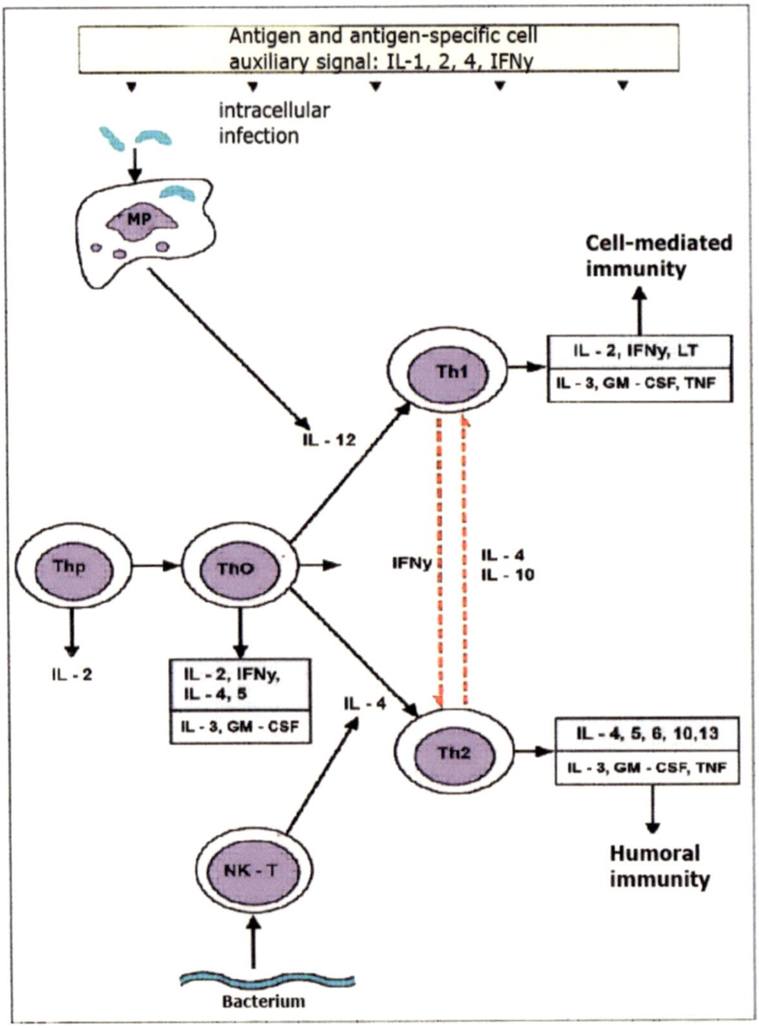

Note: In the presence of IL-4, precursor Th0 cells are transformed into Th2 cells whose main function consists in activation of humoral immunity and production of definite classes of cytokins, viz., IL-3, IL-4, IL-5, IL-6, IL-10, IL-13, TNF, etc. Under the action of IL-12, Th0 precursors are transformed into Th2 cells stimulating the production of other cytokin populations, e.g., IL-2, IL-3, IFN -γ, TNF-α, TNF-β, etc., able to activate cell-mediated immune responses. Other Th1/Th2 classes are represented by natural killer cells (NK cells), helper T cells (Th cells), granulocytic macrophageal colony-stimulating factors (GM-CSF), interferon (IFN), interleukin (IL), macrophages (MØ) and tumor necrosis factor (TNF).

Fig. 3. The pathways of formation of Th1/Th2 lymphocytes.

i. deficiency of effector links of immunity with predominant involvement of the T link (as in the case of isolated forms of PIFSI);
ii. disbalance of intercellular immunoregulatory mechanisms responsible for the formation of associated forms of syndromeal immune pathologies, e.g., PIFA and PIFASID).

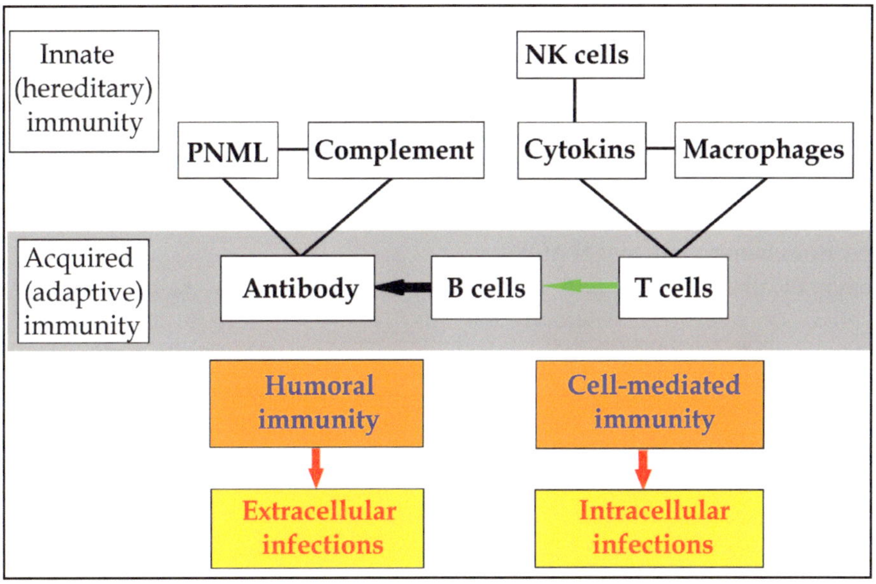

Note: PMNL and NK are polymorphonuclear leukocytes and natural killer cells, respectively.

Fig. 4. The contribution of the innate and adaptive branches of immunity to control over intra- and extracellular infections.

2. Clinical manifestations of PICIS in the framework of clinical models of CRID

As targets for our investigation, we chose three classical models of CRID, namely, intracranial infectious inflammatory pathologies (ICIIP), chronic pyelonephrites (CPN) and myocardites (M). All these pathologies have one common feature (i.e., association with a concrete organ or a tissue), but differ from one another both topically and pathogenetically. Although the panel of immunologic disturbances varies substantially depending on the clinical form of PICIS, immune statuses of patients and clinical manifestations of the diseases are very similar (Antonov & Tsinzerling, 2001; Borisov, 2000; Kukhtevich et al., 1997; Morozov, 2001; Paukov, 1996).

2.1 Immunopathological factors as biomarkers and biopredictors of chronization of infectious diseases

2.1.1 Inflammation mediators as PICIS-related factors

Emergence and accumulation, in patient's blood, of inflammation markers whose concentration reaches the highest level in patients with PIFA and degresses in the direction from PIFASID to PIFSI are the most common markers of chronization of infectious diseases and formation of syndromeal immune pathologies (Mazo et al., 2007; Litvinov et al., 2008; Zhmurov et al., 2000; Rumyantsev & Goncharova, 2000).

2.1.2 Abnormalities in the innate branch of immunity as a PICIS-related factor

Miscellaneous shifts in the innate branch of immunity play a no less important role in chronization of infectious diseases. Thus, pronounced suppression of innate immune mechanisms is a salient feature of PIFSI, while PIFA and PIFASID are distinguished for disproportions in individual links of innate immunity and/or disbalance in the functional activity of its specific mechanisms (Bauer et al., 2001; Bingen-Bidois et al., 2002; Blackwell et al., 1987; Carballido et al., 2003; Dantzer & Wollman, 2003).

Complement deficiency. In patients with PIFA and PIFASID, outbursts of activity in the C5 and C5a components of the complement are usually observed against the background of stable operation of the majority of other links of the immune system (PIFA) or pronounced disproportions between them (PIFASID).

Deficiency of phagocytosis and cytotoxicity mechanisms. To factors responsible for chronization of infectious diseases, one may relate oppositely directed changes in phagocytosis and cytotoxicity parameters. In PIFSI, both mechanisms are strongly suppressed, while in PIFA and PIFASID relative stability of certain components of both systems is concomitant with disproportions in other components.

Deficiency of dendritic cells. Dendritic cells (DCs) are among the most essential regulatory factors in the innate branch of immunity. In patients with PIFSI, the specific contribution of these cells is rather small, while in case of PIFASID and PIFA DCs play a prominent role and show a tendency for activation (Sanaev et al., 2008; Cherepakhina et al., 2009).

2.1.3 Abnormalities in the adaptive branch of immunity as a PICIS-related factor

Deficiency of T cell-mediated immunity. Among other disturbances in the adaptive branch of immunity, special attention should be given to differently directed changes in T cell-mediated immunity. PIFSI, for example, is characterized by enhanced suppression of T cell functions resulting from disproportions in immunoregulatory components and massive apoptosis of T cells. In contrast, activation of T cell-mediated immunity is critical for PIFA and PIFASID, being more pronounced for the former and less pronounced for the latter.

Deficiency of humoral immunity. Suppression of humoral immunity is a characteristic feature of PIFSI, while PIFA and PIFASID are associated with its activation. The activating effect of quantitative and qualitative (functional) mechanisms of humoral immunity is especially apparent in PIFA, while in patients with PIFASID this effect is far less expressed.

Disproportions in the cytokin spectrum of the blood. PIFSI is associated with significant reduction of the population of antiinflammatory cytokins, while in PIFA this population is predominant. PIFASID is characterized by general disproportions in the cytokin spectrum at large (Cherepakhina et al., 2010a).

3. PICIS and its main clinical forms

3.1 PIFSI

The main clinical manifestations of PIFSI are related to disturbances in antimicrobial protective mechanisms due to deficiency of the innate branch of immunity and development of secondary immune pathologies in the adaptive branch of immunity. The latter manifest themselves as chronically relapsing infectious diseases of bacterial or mixed origin (Shogenov et al., 2006).

3.2 PIFA

During induction and progression of CRID, some autoreactive CTL cross-reacting with microbial antigens (Ags) in the paradigm of the infectious process undergo activation by hazardous factors including *molecular mimicry* (Khitrov et al., 2007a; Fujinami et al., 2006; Rose & Mackay, 2000; Benoist & Mathis, 2001). Its consequences are especially apparent during recognition of determinant autoAgs by T cells and subsequent formation of the PIFA syndrome (Fig. 5). The latter attack any target organ or tissue of the infected organism by a rocket mechanism. The risk of PIFA development increases dramatically with increasing incidence of infectious diseases and the panel of infecting pathogens (*mixed* infections).

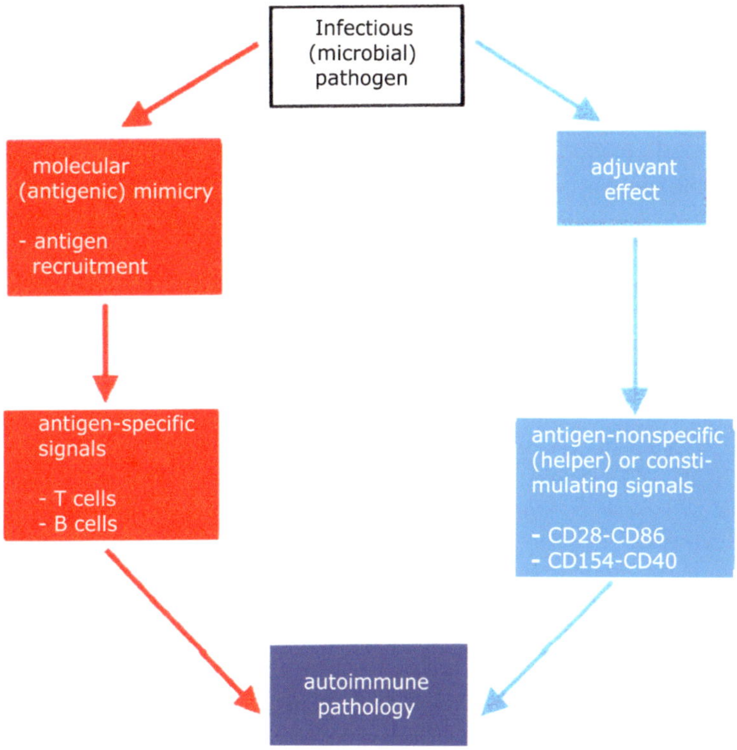

Note: The primary infectious (microbial) pathogen triggers a postinfectious autoimmune syndrome (PIFA) through activation of two different mechanisms: (i) depletion of intrinsic (antigenic) molecular mimicry pools of cross-reacting (mimicking) antigenic determinants of the infecting pathogen (red arrows); (b) generation, by the infectious pathogen, of antigen-nonspecific signals (blue arrows) able to induce inflammation and thus enhance immune responsiveness (so-called adjuvant effect).

Fig. 5. A schematic representation of the postinfectious autoimmune syndrome (PIFA).

There exist at least three different interpretations for the relatedness of the infectious process to the risk of PIFA in response to activation of autoreactive clones of T and B lymphocytes, namely: (i) stimulation by microbial *superAgs*; (ii) secretion of *cryptic* (intramolecular) autoAg determinants in response to cell damage induced by persisting infections and (iii) molecular mimicry. These pathogenetic mechanisms are not mutually exclusive and play a crucial role in definite (as a rule, early) steps of PIFA-related CRID. The main triggering factors in the PIFA initiation step are: (i) antigenic activity of the microbial pathogen and (ii) tropism of the microbial pathogen towards definite cell populations, organs and tissues as targets for its cytopathic effect (Vturin et al., 1994; Manges et al., 2004).

Contrary to PIFSI, all classes of antimicrobial ABs (antibacterial, antiviral, antiparasitic, etc.) are morbid in PIFA. Although in the majority of patients the incidence and titers of antibacterial and antiviral ABs are more or less identical, in certain forms of CRID (e.g., CPN or M) antiparasitic ABs are detected in highest titers, while in patients with other pathologies (e.g., ICIIP) they are absent. These findings can be attributed to clinical manifestations of the underlying diseases rather than to inadequate functioning of triggering mechanisms of PIFA) (Cherepakhina et al., 2010b).

Indeed, autoaggression provoked by insufficient coordination between two branches of immunity and hyperfunction of its adaptive branch is a dominant feature of PIFA. Its unique feature is a vast repertoire of antiorganic and antitissue autoABs responsible for *multiseropositivity* and specific autoimmune inflammation markers, e.g., anti-B7-HI autoABs) (Khitrov et al., 2007).

By illustration, antimyelin and antineuronal autoABs are usually associated with ICIIP. Patients with CPN contain predominantly anti-THG autoABs as highly specific markers of autoimmune inflammation in renal tissue, while the presence of anti-KM autoABs indicates AIM (Miller et al., 1970).

To the most informative models of PIFA one may relate autoimmune myocarditis (AIM), autoimmune encephalomyelitis (AEM), ICIIP, rheumatoid arthritis (PA), autoimmune hepatitis (AIHe), autoimmune colienteritis (AICE), autoimmune pancreatitis (AIPCT), autoimmune gastritis (AIGa), autoimmune (streptococcal) glomerulonephritis (AGN), CPN, etc.

Autoimmune myocarditis (AIM) usually develops in genetically predisposed individuals infected with the Coxsackievirus-3 virus (CVB3) and is one of the most typical manifestations of *molecular mimicry*. The presence, in circulating blood, of cardiomyosin-autoreactive cytotoxic T lymphocytes (KM-autoreactive CTL) and anti-KM autoABs is prerequisite to AIM development. Their interactions in patients with *PIFA* or *PIFASID* initiate myocardial lesions in response to enhanced secretion of sequestered autoAgs (Shogenov et al., 2010) (Fig. 6).

In type I diabetes mellitus (DM I), *insulitis* develops in genetically predisposed individuals at the earliest (preclinical) stages of the disease (as a rule, against the background of infection with the Coxsackie-4 virus (CVB4)), and is further transformed into PIFA. This pathological process is mediated by autoreactive CTL and autoABs against islet autoAgs. Their coordinated functioning initiates the destruction (direct or indirect) of beta cells, e.g., through secretion of cytokins, generation of free radicals or apoptosis of beta cells, eventually resulting in *PIFA* or *PIFASID*.

The main causal factors in initiation of chronically relapsing autoimmune colienteritis (AICE) are mimicking AGs of microbial or dietary origin. These AGs are localized in the intestinal lumen where they activate immune cells of intestinal mucosa. Having penetrated into these cells, AGs begin to interact with tissue immunocytes (most frequently, with lymphocytes and DCs) thereby triggering adaptive immune responses. Innate immune resources also become activated under the stimulating effect of microbial products due to activation of specific surface receptors of intestinal epithelium. This reaction cascade stimulates the secretion of numerous cytokins and chemokins able to activate immunocytes of intestinal mucosa. Activation of antigen-presenting cells (APC) (e.g., DCs) initiate enhanced production of Th1 cells (Crohn's disease) or atypical Th2 cells (ulcerative colitis). In addition to major cytokins stimulating the activity of Th1 cells (IL-12, IL-18, etc.), activated macrophages give rise to a great diversity of antiinflammatory cytokins (IL-1, IL-6,

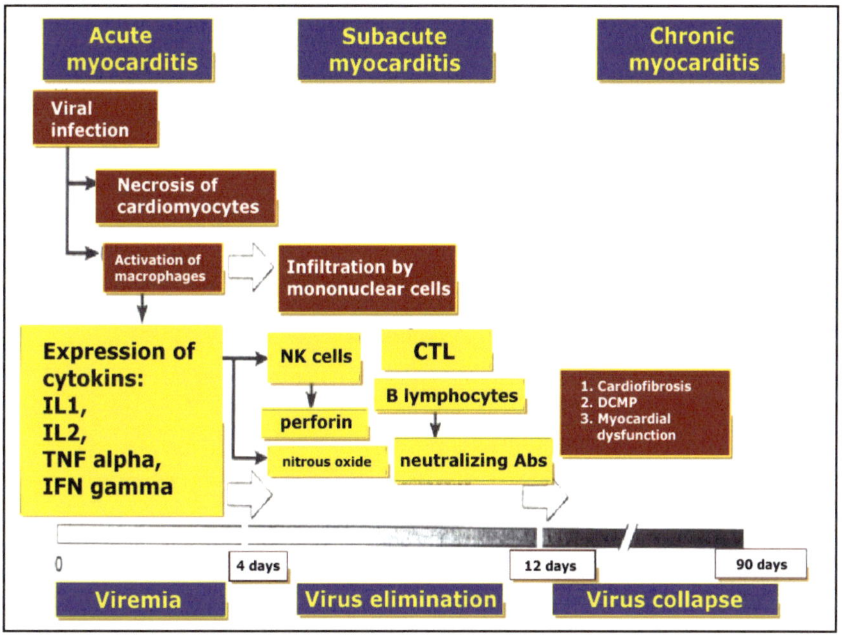

Note: AB - antibody; CTL - cytotoxic T lymphocyte; IFN - interferon; IL - interleukin; NK - natural killer cell; DCMП - dilated cardiomyopathy.

Fig. 6. Initiation and progression of myocarditis

TNF alpha, etc.) endowed with an ability to stimulate the activity of different cell populations (including endothelial cells) in inflammation foci by promoting enhanced migration of lymphocytes, fibroblasts and epithelial cells from the vascular network to inflammation niduses, which significantly deteriorates the clinical picture of autoimmune nidal inflammation (Khaitov & Pinegin, 2000; Bach, 2005).

3.3 PIFASID

A salient feature of this syndrome is equal contribution of associated abnormalities to both branches of immunity. Its clinical picture is distinguished for mixed-type immunopathology, viz., autoimmune syndrome coupled with immunodeficiency and concurrent deterioration of antiinfectious protection.

4. Associative correlation between clinical manifestations of PICIS and CRID

The associativity between microbial infection and various immunopathological states with PICIS can be correlative or causal. In patients with CRID, syndromal forms of immune pathologies depend critically on the stage of the inflammatory process occurring in target organs or tissues and general chronization of the disease (Sanaev et al., 2007).

For example, early stages of CRID are concomitant with PIFSI (› 50%), whereas the contribution of PIFA and PIFASID does not exceed 20%. At the subsequent stages, the clinical picture is different, viz., the contribution of the autoimmune syndrome increases dramatically (to 50% at the intermediate stages (PIFA) and to 60% at the final stage (PIFASID).

The correlation between the stage of CRID and the form of PICIS is also characterized by the involvement of an additional (third) component, viz., clinical form or variant of CRID. Here are several analytical examples related to:

1. *clinical form of CRID*. In patients with primary pyelonephritis (PPNP) and infectious myocarditis (IM), PIFSI is detected in 75% of cases, whereas in patients with secondary pyelonephrites (SPNP) and AIM the contribution of PIFSI is notably decreased (to 25%) giving way to autoaggression (the contribution of PIFA and PIFASID increases to 60% and 85%, respectively);
2. *stage of CRID*. At early stages (< 3 months for CPN and < 1 month for myocarditis (M)), PIFSI is detected in 40% of cases; however, at later stages of CRID its share decreases appreciably, while that of autoimmune syndromes increases in contrast;
3. *rate of progression and chronization of CRID*. In patients with relapsing or rapidly progressing CRID (e.g., ICIIP or AIM), the contribution of PIFSI does not exceed 32-36%, while the share of autoimmune syndromes reaches 80-100%. In such patients, persistent forms of meningoencephalitis (e.g., ICIIP) or AIM associated with myocardial dystrophies are predominant.

These findings suggest that PIFSI is not only the outcome of the infectious process, but also represents a factor responsible for its lingering and chronically relapsing course. Further progression and *chronization* of CRID are controlled by postinfectious autoaggression factors, such as PIFA and PIFASID.

5. Clinico-immunological criteria of PICIS and state-of-art immunogenetic diagnostic algorithms

So far, there is no unique set of criteria for adequate assessment of immune statuses of patients with different forms of PICIS, most probably, due to immense diversity of clinical manifestations of syndromal immunopathologies and factors responsible for their emergence. Moreover, existing laboratory protocols for assessing immune statuses are nonspecific and do not include specific analyses of microbial pathogens (Vinnitskij, 2002; Kolesnikov et al., 2001; Cherepakhina et al., 2010c).

With this in mind and in order to procure adequate evaluation of many syndromal immune pathologies, we developed a series of clinical and immunologic tests and criteria for more precise diagnosis of PICIS. The criteria for constructing immunogram charts include:

i. *screening of abnormalities in the innate branch of immunity* (selective markers of phagocytosis, natural cytotoxicity (NCT), basic functional parameters of DC- and Ag-presenting cells (APC) and complement components (if necessary);
ii. *screening of abnormalities in the adaptive branch of immunity* (selective markers of effector or regulatory links of the immune system, serotyping of blood elements for anti-organic and anti-tissue autoABs concurrently with identification of Abs against mimicking Ag determinants of infecting pathogens).

The main criteria in the etiotropic diagnosis step (design of microbial landscape maps) include:

i. identification and localization of microbial gene pools;
ii. serological profiles of antimicrobial ABs.

The novel diagnostic ideology is based on a combination of two categories of investigations:

i. pathogenetically oriented diagnosis of PICIS and (ii) etiotropic diagnosis of microbial pathogens as the main causal factors of PICIS.

The most efficient technological strategies will be based on:
i. at the *immunodiagnostics* stage (cytofluorimetric analysis of processing and presentation of AGs on the surface of APC, monitoring of antiorganic and antitissue autoAB pools, analysis of metabolic profiles of individual cells, etc.);
ii. *etiotropic diagnostics* (combination of conventional techniques for culturing microbial cells with advanced molecular diagnostics strategies based on sequencing of microbial genomes, screening of biological fluids and tissues for antimicrobial ABs, etc.).

6. Conclusion

Morbidity from infectious pathologies (e.g., CRID), in the first place, those provoked by viruses, conditionally pathogenic ("opportunistic") microflora and/or pathogens endowed with atypical properties including muiltiple resistance to antibacterial drugs, is steadily increasing. Among other things, CRID-affected individuals are characterized by lowering general immune responsiveness concurrent with unusual forms of immune responses to the clinical course of the infectious pathology. Studies in this field including our own investigations established that PICIS is one of the most important clinical manifestations of CRID, since it determines, in many features, the progression and chronization of underlying pathologies and their possible complications. The *monosyndromal* dominant form of PICIS in patients with CRID is PIFSI. However, more than 30% of CRID patients suffer from more specific forms of PICIS concomitant with autoimmune aggression (PIFA) or from combined immunopathological forms (e.g., PIFASID).

Clinical forms of PICIS and, correspondingly, immunologic disturbances in patients with CRID correlate associatively with the clinical picture of the disease. It is not excluded that chronization of infectious inflammatory processes involves a general sequence of pathogenetically important factors, which differ in inner architechtonics of each of PICIS variants and thus demonstrate their high criterial significance.

Future progress in clinical immunology and immune biotechnology may open up fresh opportunities for introduction into routine clinical practice of advanced protocols for immunogenetic diagnostics of PICIS-related infectious diseases and design of state-of-art treatment-and-rehabilitation protocols based on the use of the most advanced immunogenetic tools and strategies.

7. References

Suchkov S.V.; Shogenov Z.S. & Khitrov A.N. (2007). Postinfectious autoimmune syndrome: features of pathogenesis and modern protocols of clinical immunogenodiagnostics. *Therapeutic Archives*. Vol.79, No.4, (April 2007), pp. 71-76, ISSN 0040-3660

Paltsev M.A.; Cherepakhina N.E. & Suchkov S.V. (2009). Postinfectious clinical immunologic syndrome: foundations of etiopathogenesis and strategy of immunogenodiagnostics. *Bulletin of the Russian Academy of Medical Sciences*. Vol.10, (October, 2009), pp. 25-31, ISSN 0869-6047

Paltsev M.A. Clinical and immune-mediated syndrome (CAIMS) in clinical practice: features and strategies in immune and molecular diagnostics. (2009). *New Horizons in Allergy, Asthma & Immunology*, pp. 177-181, ISBN 978-88-7587-505-3, Dubai, UAE, April 24-27, 2009

Suchkov S.V.; Blagoveschenskij S.V. & Vinnitskij L.I. (2004). Modern aspects of immunopathogenesis and immunocorrection in patients with intracranial infectious inflammatory diseases. *Allergology and Immunology*. Vol.5, No.2, (2004), pp. 323-330, ISSN 1562-3637

McGuirk P. & Mills K.H. Pathogen-specific regulatory T cells provoke a shift in the Th1/Th2 paradigm in immunity to infectious diseases. (2002). *Trends in Immunology*. Vol.23, No.9, (September 2002), pp. 450-455, ISSN 1471-4906

Azikury O.I. Cellular and humoral immunity at pyelonephritis. (1985). *Urology and Nephrology*. Vol.2, (March 1985), pp. 10-11, ISSN 0042-1154

Aitpaev B. K. & Seisembekov T.Z. (1987). Cellular and humoral factors of nonspecific resistance and immunologic reactivity at chronic pyelonephritis. *Therapeutic Archives*. Vol.8, (August 1987), pp. 59-63, ISSN 0040-3660

Antonov V.P. & Tsinzerling V.A. Contemporary status of the problem of chronic and slow neuroinfections. (2001). *Archieves of Pathology*. Vol.63(1), (January 2001), pp. 47-51, ISSN 0004-1955

Borisov I.A. Pyelonephritis. (2000). In: *Nephrology*, Tareeva I.E. (Ed.), pp. 383-399, Medicine, ISBN 5-225-04195-7, Moscow, Russia

Kukhtevich A.V.; Gordovskaya N.B. & Kozlovskaya N.L. Pyelonephritis. *Russian Medical Journal*. Vol.5, No.23, (December 1997), pp. 54-62, ISSN 0869-7760

Morozov A.V. Chronic infection of urinary tract (pathogenesis, diagnostic and treatment principles). *Russian Medical Journal*. Vol.9, No.23, (December 2001), pp. 1074-1077, ISSN 0869-7760

Paukov V.S. Immunology and morphology of chronic inflammation. *Achieves of Pathology*. Vol.58(1), (January 1996), pp. 28-33, ISSN 0869-7760

Mazo E.B.; Vinnitskij L.I. & Litvinov V.A. (2007). Chronic pyelonephritis: features of immunopathogenesis and its' clinical and diagnostical values. *Therapeutic Archives*. Vol.79(1), (January 2007), pp. 85-89, ISSN 0040-3660

Litvinov V.A.; Cherepakhina N.E. & Suchkov S.V. (2008). Chronic pyelonephritis: features of immunopathogenesis and principles of clinical immunogenetic diagnostics. *Physician*. Vol.1, (January 2008), pp. 12-17, ISSN 0236-3054

Zhmurov V.A.; Oskolkov V.A. & Malishevskij M.V. (2000). Correlation between immunogenetic markers and metabolic processes at chronic pyelonephritis. *Urology*. Vol.3, (2000), pp. 9-13, ISSN 0042-1154

Rumyantsev A.S. & Goncharova I.S. Etiology and pathogenesis of pyelonephritis. *Nephrology*. Vol.4, No.3, (2000), pp. 40-52, ISSN 1561-6274

Bauer J.; Rauschka H. & Lassmann H. Inflammation in the nervous system: the human perspective. *Glia*, Vol.36, No.2, (November 2001), pp. 235-243, ISSN 1098-1136

Bingen-Bidois M.; Clermont O. & Bonacorsi S. Phylogenetic analysis and prevalence of urosepsis strains of Escherichia coli bearing pathogenicity island-like domains. *Infect Immun*. Vol. 70, No.6, (June 2002), pp. 3216-3226, ISSN 1098-5522

Blackwell C.C.; May S.J. & Brettle R.P. Secretor state and immunoglobulin levels among women with recurrent urinary tract infections. *J Clin Lab Immunol*. Vol.22, No.3, (1987), pp. 133-137, ISSN 0141-2760

Carballido J.A.; Alvarez-Mon M. & Olivier C. Inflammatory pathology in urology. Standardization. *Actas Urol Esp*. Vol.27, No.3, (March 2003), pp. 173-179, ISSN 0210-4806

Dantzer R. & Wollman E.E. Relationships between the brain and the immune system. *J Soc Biol.* Vol.197, No.2, (2003), pp. 81-88, ISSN 0037-766X

Sanaev A.O.; Kachkov I.A. & Vinnitskij L.I. (2008). Immunomonitoring and immunorehabilitation in case of intracranial infectious inflammatory diseases. *Russian Journal of Immunology.* Vol.2(11), No.1, (2008), pp. 78-82, ISSN 1028-7221

Cherepakhina N.E.; Shogenov Z.S. & Elbeik T. (2009). Postinfectious clinical-and-immunologic syndrome and its place in clinical practice. *Therapeutic Archives.* Vol.81(1), No.12, (December 2009), pp. 71-78, ISSN 0040-3660

Cherepakhina N.E.; Tabaksoeva D.A. & Suchkov S.V. (2010). Associative relation of microbial factor and postinfectious clinical-and-immunologic syndrome in case of chronic relapsing diseases. *Clinical Microbiology and Antimicrobial Chemotherapy.* Vol.12, No.2, suppl.1, (2010), p. 54, ISSN 1684-4386

Shogenov Z.S.; Cherepakhina N.E. & Suchkov S.V. (2006). Immunogenetic diagnostics and postinfectious immunodeficiency syndrome in physicians' practice. *Clinical Laboratory Diagnostics.* Vol.11, (November 2006), pp. 36-43, ISSN 0869-2084

Khitrov A.N.; Shogenov Z.S. & Suchkov S.V. (2007). Molecular mimicry phenomenon and its place in postinfectious autoimmune syndrome (PIFA) pathogenesis. *Molecular Medicine.* Vol.4, (2007), pp. 24-32, ISSN 1728-2918

Fujinami R.S.; von Herrath M.G. & Christen U. Molecular mimicry, bystander activation, or viral persistence: infections and autoimmune disease. *Clin. Microbiol. Rev.* Vol.19, No.1, (January 2006), pp. 80-94, ISSN 0893-8512

Rose N.R. & Mackay I.R. Molecular mimicry: a critical look at exemplary instances in human diseases . *Cell Mol. Life Sci.* Vol.57, No.4 (April 2000), pp. 542-551, ISSN 1420-682X

Benoist C. & Mathis D. Autoimmunity provoked by infection: how good is the case for T cell epitope mimicry? *Nat. Immunol.* Vol.2, No.9, (September 2001), pp. 797-801, ISSN 1529-2908

Vturin B.V.; Delektorskij V.V. & Kovalchuk V.K. Pathogenic mechanisms of bacteria at different infections. (1994). *Archives of pathology.* Vol.56, No.5, (September 1994), pp. 10-15, ISSN 0004-1955

Manges A.R.; Dietrich P.S. & Riley L.W. Multidrug-resistant Escherichia coli clonal groups causing community-acquired pyelonephritis. *Clin Infect Dis.* Vol.38, No.3, (February 2004), pp. 329-334, ISSN 0934-9723

Cherepakhina N.E.; Maksimenko D.M. & Suchkov S.V. (2010). Microbial landscape and its value for the modern model of immunopathogenesis of chronic relapsing infectious diseases. *Proceedings of the III World asthma & COPD forum and World forum of pediatrics*, pp. 99-102, ISBN 978-88-7587-558-9, Dubai, UAE, April 24-27, 2010

Khitrov A.N.; Shogenov Z.S. & Tretyak E.B. (2007). Postinfectious immunodeficiency and autoimmunity: pathogenic and clinical values and implications. *Expert Review of Clinical Immunology.* Vol.3, No.3, (May 2007), pp. 323-331, ISSN 1744-666X

Miller T.E.; Smith J.W. & Lehmann J.W. Autoimmunity in chronic experimental pyelonephritis. *J Infect Dis.* Vol.122, No.3, (September 1970), pp. 191-195, ISSN 1344-6304

Shogenov Z.S.; Akhmedilova K.A. & Tabaksoeva D.A. Features of immunopathogenesis and chronization of myocarditis as the basis of immunogenetic diagnostic and immunogenetic monitoring protocols development. *Russian cardiology journal.* Vol.6(86), (November 2010), pp. 76-87, ISSN 1560-4071

Khaitov R.M. & Pinegin B.V. Contemporary conceptions of safeguard of host organism against infection. *Immunology.* Vol.1, (January 2000), pp. 61-64, ISSN 0206-4952

Bach J.F. Infections and autoimmunity. *Rev. Med. Interne.* Vol.1, (October 2005), pp. 32-34, ISSN 0248-8663

Sanaev A.O.; Kachkov I.A. & Vinnitskij L.I. (2007). Modern aspects of immunotherapy at intracranial infectious inflammatory diseases therapy by example of brain abscesses. *Allergology and Immunology.* Vol.8, No.4, (2007), pp. 384-387, ISSN 1562-3637

Vinnitskij L.I. Diagnostic facilities of contemporary immune technologies in surgical clinic. (2002) *Allergology and Immunology.* Vol.3, No.1, (2002), pp. 198-203, ISSN 1562-3637

Kolesnikov A.P.; Khabarov A.S. & Kozlov V.A. (2001). Diagnostics and differentiated treatment of secondary immunodeficiencies. *Therapeutic Archives.* Vol.73(4), (April 2001), pp. 55-59, ISSN 0040-3660

Cherepakhina N.E.; Maksimenko D.M. & Suchkov S.V. (2010). Strategy of immunotherapy and immunorehabilitation of chronic relapsing infectious. *International Journal on Immunorehabilitation.* Vol.12, No.2, (May 2010), p. 139, ISSN 1562-3629

8

Contribution of Peroxynitrite, a Reactive Nitrogen Species, in the Pathogenesis of Autoimmunity

Rizwan Ahmad[1] and Haseeb Ahsan[2]
[1]*Department of Biochemistry, Oman Medical College, Sohar,*
[2]*Department of Biochemistry, Faculty of Dentistry, Jamia Millia Islamia, New Delhi,*
[1]*Sultanate of Oman*
[2]*India*

1. Introduction

Peroxynitrite is a member of reactive nitrogen species that also includes nitric oxide (·NO) and nitrogen dioxide radical ($NO_2^{\cdot}$). Peroxynitrite is a reactive nitrogen species and an anion with the formula ($ONOO^-$). It is an unstable 'valence isomer' of nitrate (NO_3^-), making it an oxidant and nitrating agent. Because of its oxidizing properties, peroxynitrite can damage a wide range of molecules in cells, including DNA and proteins (1). It is produced by the body in response to a variety of environmental toxins, stress, ultraviolet light and many other stimuli. It is also produced in the body due to ischemia/ reperfusion injury and inflammation (2, 3). *In vivo,* peroxynitrite is formed in the macrophages, endothelial cells, platelets, leukocytes, neurons, etc by the reaction between $O_2^{\cdot -}$ and ·NO (4, 5). Tissue inflammation and chronic infection lead to the overproduction of ·NO and $O_2^{\cdot -}$, which rapidly combine to yield peroxynitrite: $O_2^{\cdot -} + {\cdot}NO \rightarrow ONO_2^-$. Endothelial ·NO synthase (eNOS) is responsible for most of the vascular ·NO produced. The eNOS oxidizes its substrate L-arginine to L-citrulline and ·NO. A functional eNOS requires dimerization of the enzyme, the substrate L-arginine, and an essential cofactor, BH4 (5,6,7,8-tetrahydro-L-biopterin). The $O_2^{\cdot -}$ produced can react with vascular ·NO to form peroxynitrite. Diminished levels of BH4 promote $O_2^{\cdot -}$ production by eNOS. The transformation of eNOS from a vasoprotective enzyme to a contributor to oxidative stress has been observed in several *in vitro* systems, animal models of cardiovascular diseases and in patients with cardiovascular risk factors (6). In inflammation or septic shock, ·NO is also synthesized by the inducible ·NO synthase (iNOS), an isoform that is expressed in many cell types including vascular endothelial cells, vascular smooth muscle and inflammatory cells in response to pro-inflammatory cytokines. Peroxynitrite, can be formed intravascularly in various disease conditions when there is overproduction of either ·NO or $O_2^{\cdot -}$ (7). The intravascular formation of peroxynitrite can result in oxidative modifications of plasma and vessel wall proteins including the formation of protein-3-nitrotyrosine. Protein tyrosine nitration in plasma or vessel wall proteins may be indicative of peroxynitrite formation, and constitutes a good biomarker of ·NO-derived oxidant production in the vascular space. Detection of 3-nitrotyrosine *in vivo* has attracted considerable interest not only as a biomarker of peroxynitrite formation but also as a predictor of vascular risk (8).

Peroxynitrite is a potent oxidant and nitrating species formed by rapid reaction of two free radicals - nitric oxide and superoxide anion (9). It can modify variety of biomolecules but possesses high affinity for tyrosine residues in proteins, and 3-nitrotyrosine is a relatively specific marker of peroxynitrite mediated damage to proteins (10). Other markers of peroxynitrite-induced protein modifications are; cysteine oxidation, oxidation/nitration of tryptophan and tyrosine, protein carbonyls, dityrosine and fragmentation. In view of numerous reports on detection of significant amount of 3-nitrotyrosine in various pathological conditions, the significance of non-enzymatic tyrosine nitration in health and disease has become a subject of great interest. Protein nitration has been observed in atherosclerosis, hypertension, Parkinson's, Huntington's and Alzheimer's disease (11-13), multiple sclerosis (14), autoimmune myocarditis (15), systemic lupus erythematosus (SLE) (16) and rheumatoid arthritis (17). Furthermore, self proteins become immunologically active if their structure is altered. Accumulations of a variety of chemically modified proteins have been reported in inflamed tissues or apoptotic cells (18).

Histones are highly conserved proteins but poorly immunogenic. These positively charged proteins were found to be immunogenic after acetylation or complexation with RNA. Autoantibodies against histones are present as often as anti-DNA antibodies in SLE. It has been demonstrated that anti-native DNA autoantibodies are commonly co-present with anti-histone autoantibodies and may react with each of the five chromatin-associated histones and also with H3-H4 and H2A-H2B complex (19). However, importance of anti-histone antibodies in SLE is confounded by discrepancies in their reported prevalence, isotype, specificity and correlation with symptoms. Over expression of inducible nitric oxide synthase enzyme has been seen in numerous tissues of active SLE patients, *vis-à-vis* higher level of serum nitrotyrosine. Nitrotyrosine serves as a long-term indicator of peroxynitrite-mediated protein modification and it is not affected by endogenous source of NOx or serum thiol (20). The *in vivo* nitration of histones (as shown in cultured cells exposed to nitric oxide donors and mutatect tumour tissues) appears to be a potentially useful marker for demonstrating extended exposure of cells/tissues to NO derived reactive nitrogen species. The generation of peroxynitrite by activated macrophages, neutrophils and endothelial cells and presence of nitrotyrosine in human tissues, fluids and in animal models of various diseases needs further investigation on protein-peroxynitrite interactions (21).

2. Cellular biochemistry and pathology

Peroxynitrite is a relatively long-lived oxidant that may serve as an important cytotoxic agent. Its biological effects are due to its reactivity toward a large number of molecules including lipids, amino acids, and nucleic acids. It is involved in tissue damage in a number of pathophysiological conditions such as neurodegenerative diseases, cardiovascular disorders, etc. (1-3). Evidence suggests that most of the cytotoxicity attributed to nitric oxide is due to peroxynitrite, produced from the reaction between the free radical species, $^{\cdot}NO$ and $O_2^{\cdot -}$. Peroxynitrite interacts with lipids, DNA and proteins causing oxidative damage and other free radical induced chain reactions. These reactions trigger cellular responses such as cell signaling, oxidative injury, committing cells to necrosis or apoptosis. *In vivo*, peroxynitrite generation represents a crucial pathological mechanism in conditions such as stroke, myocardial infarction, chronic heart failure, diabetes, inflammation, neurodegenerative disorders and cancer. Even though nucleic acid antigens are by themselves poorly immunogenic, their antigenicity can be enhanced by modification through different free radicals (8).

Peroxynitrite exhibits unique chemical reactivities such as protein nitration, DNA strand breakage, base modification, etc., which may have cytotoxic effects and also lead to mutagenesis. It is thought to be involved in both cell death and an increased cancer risk (8-22,23). The reaction of peroxynitrite with lipids leads to peroxidation (malondialdehyde and conjugated diene formation) and formation of nitrito-, nitro-, nitrosoperoxo-, and nitrated lipid oxidation derivatives (24-26). Peroxynitrite is a particularly effective oxidant of aromatic molecules, thioethers and organosulfur compounds that include free amino acids and polypeptide residues.

The reaction of various amino acids with peroxynitrite leads to the following products: 1) cysteine and glutathione are converted to disulfides; 2) methionine is converted to sulfoxide or is fragmented to ethylene and dimethyl disulfides. Dimethyl sulfoxide is oxidized to formaldehyde; and 3) tyrosine and tryptophan undergo one electron oxidation to radical cations, which are hydroxylated, nitrated and dimerized (27-29). Exposure of amino acids, peptides and proteins to ionizing radiation such as gamma radiation and peroxynitrite in the presence of O_2, give rise to hydroperoxides. These hydroperoxides decompose to oxygen and carbon centered radicals on exposure to copper (Cu^+) and other transition metal ions. Hydroperoxide formation on nuclear proteins results in oxidative damage to associated DNA. These hydroperoxide-derived radicals react readily with pyrimidine DNA bases and nucleosides to form adduct species, for example 8-oxo-dG. This adduct is highly mutagenic and induces G:C to T:A transversions in human DNA after replication (30).

A change in the structure of DNA could either be due to radiation or due to interaction with different free radicals (31). Since there are many polybasic compounds in the vicinity of DNA, there exists a possibility of their interaction with DNA on exposure to radiation or free radicals. Lysine and arginine-rich histones in nucleosomes on modification by environmental agents form histone-DNA adducts, making it immunogenic. It appears that the pathogenic anti-DNA autoantibodies are generated through some modified epitopes on nucleic acids (32-34). Prominent DNA modifications induced by exposure to peroxynitrite include the formation of 8-nitro-guanine and 8-oxyguanine, as well as the induction of single-strand breaks (35). Peroxynitrite reacts significantly only with guanine, which upon oxidation and nitration leads to mutagenicity and strand breaks, respectively. Peroxynitrite also damages DNA by covalent bond formation and removal of DNA bases (36).

Purine nucleotides are vulnerable to oxidation and to adduct formation (37,38). Peroxynitrite is a mutagenic agent with a potential to produce nitration, nitrosation and deamination of DNA bases. Methylation of cytosine in DNA is important for the regulation of gene expression and normal methylation patterns are altered by the carcinogenic effect of peroxynitrite (39). Prominent DNA modifications induced by peroxynitrite include the formation of 8-nitro-guanine and 8-oxyguanine, as well as the induction of single strand breaks (40). DNA single strand breaks generated by peroxynitrite leads to activation of the nuclear enzyme, poly (ADP-ribose) synthetase (PARS), which can trigger cellular suicidal pathway. Single strand breaks generated by peroxynitrite can arise from two processes: 1) sugar damage, which involves abstraction of hydrogen leading to the formation of sugar radical or 2) base damage, which rapidly depurinates to generate abasic sites, finally resulting in single strand breaks (41). Peroxynitrite is mutagenic in the *supF* gene inducing G to T transversions and deletions clustered at the 5′ end of the gene. The mutagenicity of peroxynitrite is believed to result from chemical modifications at guanine leading to miscoding (42). Carcinogenesis is induced by altered DNA or tissue damage, mutations and chromosomal aberrations (43,44). Peroxynitrite is a mutagenic agent with the potential to produce nitration, nitrosation and deamination reactions on DNA bases. It reacts significantly only with guanine, which upon oxidation and nitration leads to mutagenicity and strand breaks, respectively (45,46). Peroxynitrite levels are elevated in inflammation and infection and play an important role in autoimmunity and carcinogenesis (Figure 1). It damages tumor suppressor genes and leads to the expression of proto-oncogenes. Peroxynitrite induced DNA damage leading to mutations has been strongly implicated in carcinogenesis (47) (Figure 1).

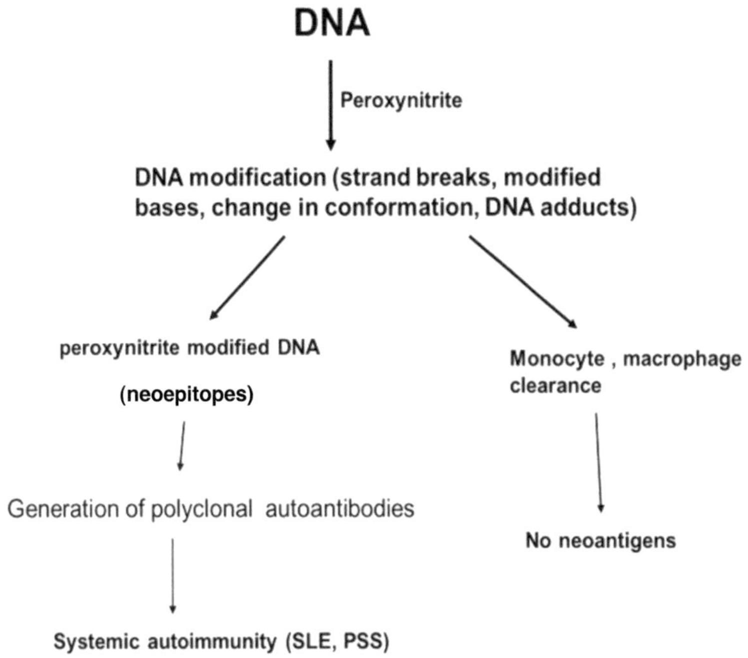

Fig. 1. The role of peroxynitrite, a reactive nitrogen species, in the etiopathogenesis of autoimmune disorders, such as systemic lupus erythematosus (SLE) and progressive systemic sclerosis (PSS).

Proteins are targets of reactive nitrogen species such as peroxynitrite and NO_2. Among the various amino acids in proteins, tryptophan residues are especially susceptible to attack by reactive nitrogen species (48). Peroxynitrite is capable of oxidizing protein and non-protein sulfhydryl (-SH) groups including lipid peroxidation and reactivity with aromatic amino acid side chain in proteins to form nitroadducts (49). Peroxynitrite induced tyrosine nitration may lead to dysfunction of nitrated proteins, SOD, cytoskeletal proteins, neuronal tyrosine hydroxylase, cytochrome P450 and prostacyclin synthase (50-53). Oxidation of critical -SH groups is responsible for the inhibition of mitochondrial and cytosolic aconitase and other critical enzymes in the mitochondrial respiratory chain (54). Peroxynitrite mediated nitration of myofibrillar creatine kinase activity may lead to contractile dysfunction of the heart (55). Peroxynitrite-modified cellular proteins are subject to accelerated degradation via the proteosome (56).

Adducts arise from the chemical modification of bases in DNA or amino acids in proteins by toxic chemicals and high energy UV radiation. Many chemicals known to be carcinogenic in humans have been shown to form adducts. Ultraviolet radiation is regarded as one of the major environmental factors responsible for the photoconjugation of DNA with amino acid residues. Lysine is an amino acid of particular interest as a potential participant in DNA-protein photo-cross-linking. Nearly 60% of thymine and cytosine bases in DNA are modified due to lysine photoaddition and approximately every helical turn of DNA contains one lysine molecule in the photobound state (57). It appears to enhance the antigenicity of the DNA-lysine adduct, suggesting possible roles of peroxynitrite-induced neoepitopes in damaged DNA in the production of autoantibodies in cancer patients (58).

Ahmad et al have characterised the peroxynitrite treated human-DNA lysine photoadduct (59). We have investigated the photochemical addition of lysine to native DNA in view of its potential importance in the photo-cross-linking of histones to DNA in chromatin. The C-2 carbon atom of thymine in DNA undergoes a covalent photoaddition reaction with the ε-amino group of lysine on UV irradiation to form a DNA-lysine photoconjugate or photoadduct (57). The UV spectroscopic analysis of the DNA-lysine photoadduct showed hyperchromism, indicating either the formation of single-stranded breaks in DNA or "breathing" of a double-stranded polymer at the site of lysine conjugation. Peroxynitrite caused substantial damage to the DNA-lysine adduct as evident from the hyperchromicity of the spectral curve, which could be attributed to the generation of strand breaks (Figure 2A). On peroxynitrite modification, the hypochromicity increased, which may be due to the shielding effect of lysine, limiting the sites for peroxynitrite action. Hypochromicity may also be attributed to the extensive cross-linking between peroxynitrite and the DNA-lysine adduct (31).

As shown in Figure 2B, the fluorescence emission intensity (FI) was highest for native DNA (curve 1) and least for the DNA-lysine photoadduct (curve 3). However, on peroxynitrite modification there was a change in the emission intensity, as seen in the figure (curve 2). A decrease in FI of 45.2% for the DNA-lysine photoadduct in comparison to the peroxynitrite-modified DNA-lysine adduct was observed from fluorescence spectroscopy measurements. Loss of FI of 21.3% in the peroxynitrite-modified adduct with respect to native DNA is indicative of the loss of structural integrity in DNA and generation of single-strand regions (59). The UV absorption and fluorescence characteristics of native and modified lysine photoadduct have been summarized in Table 1.

Properties	Native DNA	Native adduct	Modified adduct
A260/280 ratio	1.74	1.20	1.01
Melting temperature (°C)	75	70	85
Hyperchromicity (%)	–	52	84
Loss of FI (%)	–	76.1	21.3

Table 1. Absorption and fluorescence characteristics of native DNA, DNA-lysine photoadduct (native adduct) and peroxynitrite-modified photoadduct (modified adduct)

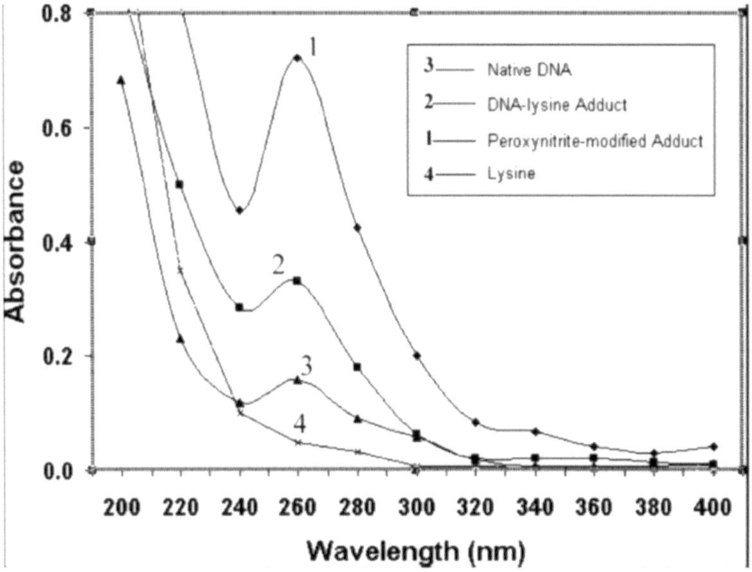

(a)

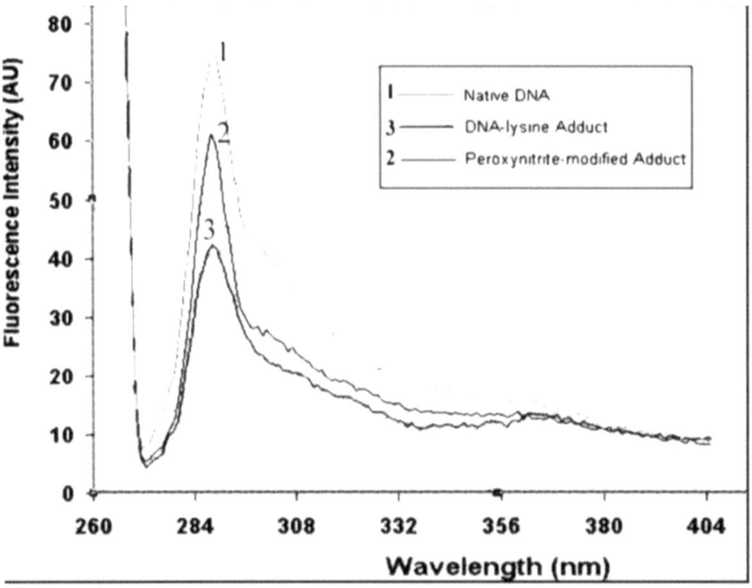

(b)

Fig. 2. UV absorption spectra of native DNA (curve 3), DNA-lysine photoadduct (curve 2) and peroxynitrite-modified adduct (curve 1). **2B:** Fluorescence spectra of native DNA (curve 1), DNA-lysine photoadduct (curve 3), and peroxynitrite-modified adduct (curve 2).

The melting profile of the DNA-lysine photoadduct reveals that the ultraviolet radiation induced covalent incorporation of lysine into the native DNA. The photoaddition of lysine to DNA might have obliterated the favorable A = T and G = C pairing interaction of double helical native DNA (57), thus decreasing the duplex melting temperature (Tm) by 5ºC relative to the fully paired parent native DNA. In the study, on peroxynitrite treatment, the Tm of the DNA-lysine adduct increased by 15°C with respect to the native DNA-lysine photoadduct (Figure 3). This may be due to shielding of the available sites for peroxynitrite action by lysine. Hence, more energy would be needed to break the covalent bonding between lysine and the DNA bases in order to denature the double helix (59).

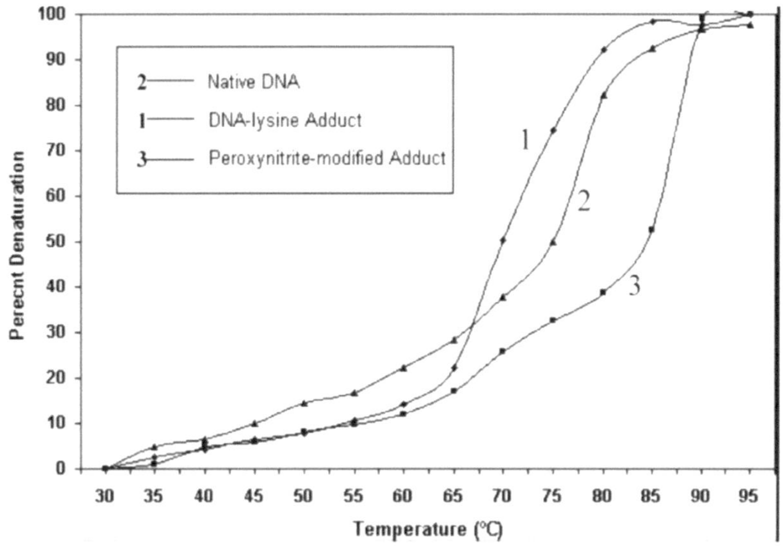

Fig. 3. Thermal melting profile of native DNA (curve 2), DNA-lysine photoadduct (curve 1), and peroxynitrite-modified photoadduct (curve 3).

Biological significance of tyrosine nitration has generated much interest among biomedical scientists because abnormal generation of 3-nitrotyrosine *in vivo* in diverse pathological conditions have been proved without doubt. Peroxynitrite is a strong oxidant that can oxidize a variety of biomolecules including proteins and non-protein thiol, protein sulphides, lipids and deoxyribose. The markers of oxidative damage to proteins include mainly carbonyls of lysine, arginine, threonine and proline, oxidized tryptophan, tyrosine and cysteine residues and fragmented protein. One persistent footprint left by peroxynitrite is nitration of phenolic ring of tyrosine residues in protein. The resultant 3-nitrotyrosine is a relatively specific marker of nitrosative stress. A recent study on repair of protein nitration in rat tissues by 3-nitrotyrosine denitrase activity suggests that a tyrosine nitration–denitration pathway participates in nitric oxide/peroxynitrite dependent signal transduction, a phenomenon similar to phosphorylation–dephosphorylation system. The reports suggest that 3-nitrotyrosine has importance not only as biomarker of nitrogen mediated tissue injury but also as a means to gain insight into molecular mechanisms of nitric oxide related physiological and pathophysiological phenomena. Furthermore, hypernitrotyrosinemia has also been reported in various inflammatory diseases including SLE, Sjogren's syndrome, vasculitis and rheumatoid arthritis (60).

Alteration of DNA or proteins resulting from photomodification or peroxynitrite could lead to the development of antibodies or mutations to modified DNA. Therefore, the DNA-lysine photoadduct and modified photoadduct could have important implications in various pathophysiological conditions such as toxicology, carcinogenesis, and autoimmune phenomena (57).

3. Autoimmune phenomenon

Manifestations of autoimmunity are often complex and heterogenous. It has been postulated that the immune response against host antigens could be due to genetic predisposition, exaggerated B cell activity, cross-reactivity between foreign and host antigens, etc. The foreign antigens arise as a consequence of infection, inflammation, drug administration, environmental factors, free radicals, etc (57,61). It has been established that not only oxygen but nitrogen free radicals play an important role in the pathogenesis of several human diseases. Reactive nitrogen species is produced by the reaction of nitric oxide with superoxide. Nitric oxide radical participate in some pathological conditions such as arthritis, vasculitis, asthma, hypertension, etc. It is also an unstable molecule like oxygen free radical but less reactive and can react with proteins (31).

Two diseases that are considered as a prototype for systemic autoimmunity are systemic lupus erythematosus (SLE) and rheumatoid arthritis (RA). SLE is a multi-systemic disorder characterized by a variety of autoantibodies and abnormal lymphocyte function that are responsible for many of the clinical manifestations important in diagnosis. A hallmark of SLE is the presence of antinuclear antibodies (ANA). ANA are prototype autoantibodies that mark the course of rheumatic diseases (62). Because of the close association between ANA and clinical diagnosis, these antibodies have become a key component in the evaluation of patients. These antibodies target a diverse range of macromolecules including DNA, RNA, proteins and protein-nucleic acid (PNA) complexes. Antibodies to DNA have been particularly associated with SLE which is considered to be a prototype autoimmune disease. Native DNA is no longer regarded as the antigen initiating the disease mainly immunization with nDNA does not produce SLE like symptoms. A few of the possible candidates could be polynucleotides, denatured DNA, RNA or modified DNA. While antibodies to single stranded DNA are formed in several inflammatory complexes including RA; antibodies to double stranded DNA serve as an immunochemical marker in the diagnosis of SLE (63). Serum obtained form SLE individuals have been shown to possess anti-DNA antibodies of diverse antigenic specificity. These anti-DNA autoantibodies have been used to evaluate therapeutic effect and clinical features of SLE patients (64,65).

The origin of autoantibody remains an enigma and the production of anti-DNA antibodies is even more complicated. Even though nucleic acid antigens are themselves poorly immunogenic, their antigenicity can be enhanced by modification with agents such as free radicals. Autoantibodies produced against such modified macromolecule are the hallmark of systemic human disease, SLE. B cell hyperactivity and the production of pathogenic autoantibodies is the main immunonological event in the pathogenesis of this disease. One approach to study the pathogenesis of SLE and determine how the autoantibody response is initiated and sustained is to analyse variable genes expressed by antibodies. Quantification of this repertoire has revealed the presence of a specific expansion of IgG clonotypes that impart reactivity with disease related autoantigens. The amino acid and nucleotide sequence of autoantibodies derived from human lupus present in immune complexes and renal eluates of subjects with active disease show features of diversification with a high rate of replacement or silent mutations and the clustering of mutations in the hypervariable region. This distinctive feature implies that a pure polyclonal activation cannot be the only mechanism responsible for autoantibody production. An antigen-driven process is more likely to play a role in their generation. It has been suggested that the antibodies may be stimulated by nucleic acid antigens or pathogens. B cells whose paratopes have complementary determining regions (CDR) which are formed by amino acids that can promote DNA binding may be selectively stimulated by nucleic acid related structures (31). A number of studies support the role of free radicals in the initiation and progression of autoimmune response. Therefore, in chronic inflammatory diseases, peroxynitrite generated by phagocytic cells may cause damage to DNA and proteins, generating neoepitopes that lead to the production of antibodies cross-reacting with nDNA or histone proteins. Modification of native DNA or proteins by peroxynitrite might also lead to the generation of neoepitopes on the molecule, and may be one of the factors for the induction of the immune responses as seen in an autoimmune disease like systemic lupus erythematosus (SLE) (58). The peroxynitrite modified human DNA was found to be highly immunogenic in rabbits inducing high titre immunogen specific antibodies (Figure 4). The data demonstrate that the antibodies, though cross-reactive with various nucleic acids and polynucleotides, preferentially bind peroxynitrite-modified epitopes on DNA (58).

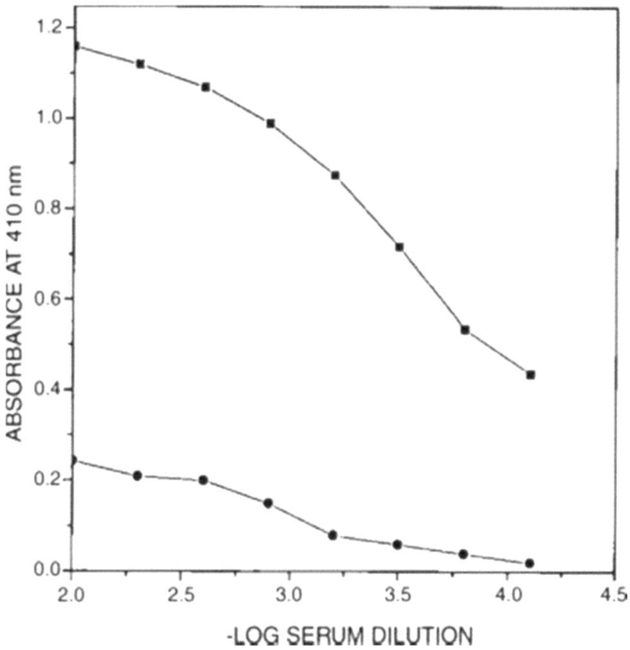

Fig. 4. Antigenicity of peroxynitrite modified human DNA. Direct binding ELISA of anti-peroxynitrite-human DNA antisera (○) and pre-immune sera (●). The microtitre plates were coated with peroxynitrite modified-human DNA (2.5 µg/ml).

DNA is a non-immunogenic entity, but any significant unrepaired alteration in its basic structure could render it "foreign," leading to the activation of immune pathways. A change in the structure of DNA could either be due to radiation or interaction with different free radicals. NO and its derivatives are among the radicals known to interact with DNA and are primarily involved in deamination of DNA bases. Peroxynitrite, on the other hand, leads to more extensive damage than that caused by an equivalent dose of ·NO. Formation occurs both intracellularly inside macrophages and extracellularly, and causes DNA strand breaks and modification of guanine (66). The two main products identified from the reaction of deoxyguanosine with peroxynitrite are 8-oxodeoxyguanine and 8-nitroguanine. The former has long been regarded as a reliable biomarker for monitoring DNA damage in studies with various oxidizing agents. The peroxynitrite-modified DNA has been shown to acquire immunogenicity and was suspected to be one of the causes for generation of autoantibodies in cancer and autoimmune disorders (12,67). The peroxynitrite modified DNA is a potent immunizing stimulus, inducing high-titer immunogen-specific antibodies in rabbits. Peroxynitrite modification might have generated potential neoepitopes against which antibodies are raised. The analysis of cross-reactivity indicates that anti-peroxynitrite-DNA IgG is immunogen-specific, showing various extents of cross-reactivity attributable to sharing of common antigenic determinants. The common antigenic determinants between peroxynitrite-DNA and nDNA could possibly be the sugar-phosphate backbone, since peroxynitrite attacks DNA and causes single strand breaks through sugar fragmentation. Induced antibodies also recognized synthetic polynucleotides, representing A/B conformations, with a preference for the B-form (12). Elevated levels of ·NO in systemic lupus erythematosus (SLE) patients suggest a role for ·NO in the pathogenesis of the disease. Murine models of SLE demonstrate abnormally high levels of ·NO compared with normal mice, whereas systemic blockade of ·NO production reduces disease activity. Elevated serum nitrate levels correlate with indices of disease activity and, along with serum titers of anti-(ds DNA) antibodies, serve as indicators of SLE (68-69). Auto-antibody production in SLE has been attributed to either selective stimulation of autoreactive B-cells by self-antigens or antigens crossreactive with self. The persistence of anti-DNA antibodies in SLE patients, despite systems to suppress self-recognition, suggests that the response is driven by an antigen resembling nDNA. The DNA damage by peroxynitrite is far more lethal than that caused by ·NO alone, leading to the perturbations in nDNA that render it immunogenic. This modified DNA might therefore play a role in the induction of circulating anti-DNA autoantibodies in various autoimmune disorders including SLE (12,59)

Histones are small, highly conserved cationic proteins which bind DNA. They are weak immunogen because of their conserved nature. Histones are major constituent of cells' chromatin and remain confined to nucleus. However, after apoptosis they may appear in circulation as nucleosomes. Incidence of autoantibodies against histone H1, H2A, H2B, H3 and H4 are 60%, 53%, 48%, 36% and 29.5% respectively in the sera of SLE patients (70). Histones also act as autoantigens in humorally-mediated paraneoplastic diseases (71). Furthermore, anti-histone antibodies have also been reported in polymyositis / dermatomyositis (72).

As peroxynitrite reaction involves free radical intermediates, it may favor cross-linking and aggregation during nitration. The extent of cross-linking depends on type of reagent used, protein concentration, type of protein and solvent conditions including pH. The exact chemical nature of the cross-linking is disputed but linkage of side chains of tyrosine residue is the common answer. Formation of tyrosyl radical by peroxynitrite and its reaction with another tyrosyl radical (on same or different histone molecule) may generate O,O'-dityrosine covalent cross-links. Peroxynitrite induces an array of modifications in H2A structure namely-tyrosine nitration, formation of protein carbonyl, dityrosine and cross-linking. Such gross structural changes might favor polymerization of native epitopes of H2A histone into potent immunogenic neo-epitopes. The histone proteins are conserved proteins and act as weak immunogens. However, they show strong immunogenicity after acetylation and alterations in amino acid structure or sequence can generate neo-epitopes on self proteins causing and immune attack. The oxidative and nitrative action of peroxynitrite confers additional immunogenicity on H2A histone and probably there is a direct correlation between nitration and immunogenicity. In another words, peroxynityrite-modified H2A still has some old epitopes which are scattered among neo-epitopes. Hence, immunization with peroxynityrite-modified H2A may produce polyspecific antibodies which can recognize both old and neo-epitopes or altogether there are two types of antibodies, one recognizing nitrated neo-epitopes and other binding exclusively with old epitopes (73).

The mechanism of autoantibody production in diseases such as SLE has not yet been clearly identified. If antigen selection is an important aspect of differentiation, the nature of the stimulating antigen also remains to be determined. The origin of antibodies remains obscure, although modified DNA appears to be a causative factor in RA and SLE. It is possible that the production of autoantibodies may be the result of free radical attack on DNA or histone proteins causing changes at the macromolecule level. It is therefore postulated that in chronic inflammatory diseases, free radicals generated by phagocytic cells may cause damage to DNA and proteins and antibodies to self-antigen are produced. Also, a defect in the control of apoptosis and delayed clearance of apoptotic debris provide sustained interaction between free radicals and macromolecules, generating neoepitopes which subsequently result in autoimmunity and generating polyspecific autoantibodies (73).

Sera of animals immunized with native and peroxynitrite-modified histones were tested on polysorp wells coated with respective immunogens (Figure 5). Modification by 100 µm peroxynitrite conferred more high immunogenicity on H2A histone (73).

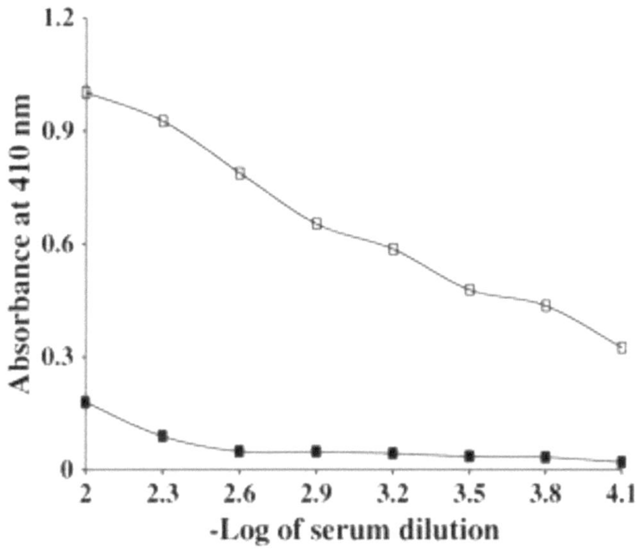

Fig. 5. Antigenicity of peroxynitrite modified proteins. Direct binding ELISA of experimentally induced antibodies against peroxynitrite-modified H2A (□) and native histone H2A (■).

Accumulation of a variety of post-translationally modified self-proteins during inflammation may lead to generation or unmasking of new antigenic epitopes that in turn activate B-and/or T-cells, thereby impairing or bypassing immunological tolerance. Peroxynitrite-modified H2A

histone could act as an autoantigen leading to generation of anti-H2A histone antibodies. It is envisaged that anti-histone antibodies seen in a sub-group of SLE patients might originate from immunological activity of peroxynitrite-modified histones due to their protection from digestion by normal proteolytic machinery (61). In the context of anti-histone antibodies in drug induced lupus erythematosus, it is quite possible that the drug itself might mimic reaction(s) pathway(s) leading to abnormal synthesis of peroxynitrite. The peroxynitrite may then modify the structure of histone making it immunogenic (76).
Hence, alteration of DNA or proteins resulting from photomodification or peroxynitrite could lead to the development of antibodies or mutations to modified DNA. Therefore, the DNA-lysine photoadduct and modified photoadducts could have important implications in toxicology, carcinogenesis, and autoimmune phenomena. Hence, understanding the pathophysiology of peroxynitrite could lead to important therapeutic interventions against this increasingly important and physiologically relevant reactive nitrogen species.

4. References

[1] Szabo C. Multiple pathways of peroxynitrite cytotoxicity. Toxicol Lett. (2003) 140–141: 105–112.
[2] Pacher P, Beckman JS, Liaudet L. Nitric oxide and peroxynitrite in health and disease. Physiol Rev. (2007) 87(1): 315–424.
[3] Szabo C, Ischiropoulos H, Radi R. Peroxynitrite: biochemistry, pathophysiology and development of therapeutics. Nat Rev Drug Discov. (2007) 6(8): 662–80.
[4] Squadrito GL, Pryor WA . Oxidative chemistry of nitric oxide: the roles of superoxide, peroxynitrite, and carbon dioxide. Free Rad Biol Med (1998), 25(4-5):392-403.
[5] Radi R, Peluffo G, Alvarez MN, Naviliat M, Cayota A. Unraveling peroxynitrite formation in biological systems. Free Radic Biol Med. (2001) 30(5): 463–88.
[6] Forstermann U, Munzel T. Endothelial nitric oxide synthase in vascular disease: from marvel to menace. Circulation. (2006) 113(13): 1708–14.
[7] Romero N, Denicola A, Radi R. Red blood cells in the metabolism of nitric oxide-derived peroxynitrite. IUBMB Life. (2006) 58(10): 572–80.
[8] Ahmad R, Rasheed Z Ahsan H. Biochemical and cellular toxicology of peroxynitrite: implications in cell death and autoimmune phenomenon. Immunopharmacology and Immunotoxicology (2009) 18(7): 388–396.
[9] Pryor W A, Squandrito G I. Chemistry of peroxynitrite: aproduct from the reaction of nitrite oxide with superoxide. Am J Physiol. (1995),268, L699-22.
[10] Oshima H,Frisen M, Bruer I, Bartsch H. Nitrotyrosine as a marker for endogenous nitrosation and nitration of proteins. Food Chem Toxicol (1990), 28: 647-52.
[11] Good P F, Hsu A, Werner P, Perl DP, Olanow C W. Protein nitration in Parkinson's disease. J Neuropathol Exp Neurol (1998), 57:338-42.
[12] Browne S E, Ferrante R J , Beal M F. Oxidative stress in Huntington's disease, Brain Pathol. (1999): 147-63
[13] Smith M A, Richey harris P L, Sayre L M, Beckman J S, Perry G. Widespread peroxynitrite-mediated damage in Alzheimer's disease. J Neurosci (1997), 17:2653-7
[14] Bagasra O, Michaelis FH, Zheng YM et al. Activation of the inducible form of nitric oxide synthase in the brains of patients with multiple sclerosis. Proc Natl Acad Sci (USA) (1995), 92: 12041-5

[15] Bachmaier K, Nikolaus N, Pommerer C et al. iNOS expression and nitrotyrosine formation in the myocardium in response to inflammation is controlled by the interferon transcription factor 1. Circulation (1997), 96:585-91

[16] Oates J C, Christensen E F, Reilly C M, Self S E, Gilkeson G S. Prospective measure of serum 3-nitrotyrosine levels in systemic lupus erythmatosus:correlation with disease activity. Proc Assoc Am Physicians (1995), 111:611-21

[17] Kaur H,Halliwell B. Evidence for nitric oxide mediated oxidative damage in chronic inflammation. Nitrotyrosine in serum and synovial fluid from rheumatoid patients. FEBS Lett (1994),350:9-12

[18] Anderson S M. Post translational modification of self antigens: implications for autoimmunity.Curr Opin Immunol (2004), 16:753-8

[19] Olins A L, Olins D E. Stereo electron microscopy of the 25-nm chromatin fibres in isolated nuclei.J Cell Biol (1979), 81:260-5

[20] Monesteir M, Kortzin B L. Antibodies to histones in systemic lupus erythmatosus and drug-induced lupus syndromes. Rheum Dis Clin North Am (1992), 18: 415-536

[21] Haqqani A S, Kelly J F, Birnboin H C. Selective nitration of histone tyrosine residues *in vivo* mutatect tumors. J Biol Chem (2002), 277:3614-21

[22] Maeda H, Akaike T. Nitric oxide and oxygen radicals in infection, inflammation, and cancer. Biochemistry (Mosc). (1998) 63(7): 854–865.

[23] Ohshima H, Bartsch H. Chronic infections and inflammatory processes as cancer risk factors: possible role of nitric oxide in carcinogenesis. Mutat Res. (1994) 305(2): 253–264.

[24] Rubbo H. Nitric oxide and peroxynitrite in lipid peroxidation. Medicina (B Aires). (1998) 58(4), 361–366.

[25] Rubbo H, Freeman BA. Nitric oxide regulation of lipid oxidation reactions: formation and analysis of nitrogen-containing oxidized lipid derivatives. Methods Enzymol. (1996) 269: 385–394.

[26] Rubbo H, Radi R, Trujillo M, Telleri R, Kalyanaraman B, Barnes S, Kirk M, Freeman B A. Nitric oxide regulation of superoxide and peroxynitrite-dependent lipid peroxidation. Formation of novel nitrogen-containing oxidized lipid derivatives. J Biol Chem (1994) 269(42): 26066–26075.

[27] Ramezanian MS, Padmaja S, Koppenol WH. Nitration and hydroxylation of phenolic compounds by Peroxynitrite. Chem Res Toxicol. (1996) 9(1): 232–240.

[28] Ramezanian MS, Padmaja S, Koppenol WH Nitration and hydroxylation of phenolic compounds by Peroxynitrite. Methods Enzymol. (1996) 269: 195–201.

[29] Alvarez B, Radi R. Peroxynitrite reactivity with amino acids and proteins. Amino Acids. (2003) 25(3–4): 295–311.

[30] Luxford C, Morin B, Dean RT, Davies MJ Histone H1 and other protein- and amino acid-hydroperoxides can give rise to free radicals which oxidize DNA. Biochem J. (1999); 344(1), 125–134.

[31] Ahsan H, Ali A, Ali R (2003). Oxygen free radicals and systemic autoimmunity. Clin. Exp. Immunol. 131(3):398–404.

[32] Ahsan H, Abdi S, Ali A (2002) Recognition of DNA-arginine photoadduct by anti-DNA auto-antibodies in systemic lupus erythematosus. Ind. J. Med. Res. 115:201–211.

[33] Dixit K, Ahsan H, Ali A (2003) Polydeoxyribonucleotide C photoconjugated with lysine or arginine present unique epitopes for human anti-DNA autoantibodies. Hum. Immunol. 64(9): 880–886.
[34] Habib S, Moinuddin, Ali R (2006) Peroxynitrite modified DNA: a better antigen for systemic lupus erythematosus anti-DNA autoantibodies. Biotechnol. Appl. Biochem. 43(2): 65–70.
[35] Szabo C, Ohshima H (1997) DNA damage induced by peroxynitrite: subsequent biological effects. Nitric Oxide 1(7):373–385.
[36] Yermilov V, Rubio J, Becchi M, Friesen MD, Pignatelli B, Ohshima H (1995) Formation of 8-nitroguanine by the reaction of guanine with peroxynitrite *in vitro.* Carcinogenesis 16(9): 2045–2050.
[37] Douki T, Cadet J. Peroxynitrite mediated oxidation of purine bases of nucleosides and isolated DNA. Free Rad Res. (1996) 24(5): 369–380.
[38] Douki T, Cadet J, Ames BN. An adduct between peroxynitrite and 2′-deoxyguanosine: 4,5-dihydro-5-hydroxy-4-(nitrosooxy)-2′-deoxyguanosine. Chem Res Toxicol. (1996) 9(1): 3–7.
[39] Wiseman H, Halliwell B. Damage to DNA by reactive oxygen and nitrogen species: role in inflammatory disease and progression to cancer. Biochem J. (1996) 313(1): 17–29.
[40] Ohshima H, Virág L, Souza J, Yermilov V, Pignatelli B, Masuda M, Szabo C. Detection of certain peroxynitrite-induced DNA modifications. Methods Mol Biol. (2002) 186: 77–88.
[41] Ohshima H, Virág L, Souza J, Yermilov V, Pignatelli B, Masuda M, Szabo C. Detection of certain peroxynitrite-induced DNA modifications. Methods Mol Biol. (2002) 186: 77–88.
[42] Tretyakova NY, Burney S, Pamir B, Wishnok JS, Dedon PC, Wogan GN, Tannenbaum, SR. Peroxynitrite-induced DNA damage in the sup F gene: correlation with the mutational spectrum. Mutat Res (2000) 447(2): 287–303.
[43] Ames BN, Shigenaga MK, Gold LS. DNA lesions, inducible DNA repair, and cell division: three key factors in mutagenesis and carcinogenesis. Environ Health Perspect. (1993) 101(suppl 5): 35–44.
[44] Ames BN, Shigenaga MK, Hagen TM Oxidants, antioxidants, and the degenerative diseases of aging. Proc Natl Acad Sci (USA) (1993) 90(17): 7915–7922.
[45] Sawa T, Ohshima H. Nitrative DNA damage in inflammation and its possible role in carcinogenesis. Nitric Oxide. (2006) 14(2): 91–100.
[46] Yermilov V, Rubio J, Becchi M, Friesen MD, Pignatelli B, Ohshima H. Formation of 8-nitroguanine by the reaction of guanine with peroxynitrite *in vitro*. Carcinogenesis. (1995) 16(9): 2045–2050.
[47] Ohshima H. Genetic and epigenetic damage induced by reactive nitrogen species: implications in carcinogenesis. Toxicol Lett (2003) 140–141: 99–104.
[48] Suzuki T, Mower HF, Friesen MD, Gilibert I, Sawa T, Ohshima, H. Nitration and nitrosation of N-acetyl-L-tryptophan and tryptophan residues in proteins by various reactive nitrogen species. Free Rad Biol Med. (2004) 37(5): 671–681.
[49] Beckman JS, Koppenol WH. Nitric oxide, superoxide, and peroxynitrite: the good, the bad, and ugly. Am J Physiol. (1996) 271(5 Pt 1): C1424–1437.

[50] Beckman JS. Oxidative damage and tyrosine nitration from Peroxynitrite. Chem Res Toxicol. (1996) 9(5): 836–844.
[51] Beckman JS. Protein tyrosine nitration and peroxynitrite. FASEB J. (2002) 16(9): 1144.
[52] Greenacre SA, Ischiropoulos H. Tyrosine nitration: localisation, quantification, consequences for protein function and signal transduction. Free Rad Res. (2001) 34(6): 541–581.
[53] Ischiropoulos H, Zhu L, Chen J, Tsai M, Martin JC, Smith CD, Beckman JS. Peroxynitrite-mediated tyrosine nitration catalyzed by superoxide dismutase. Arch Biochem Biophy. (1992) 298(2): 431–437.
[54] Hausladen A, Fridovich I. Superoxide and peroxynitrite inactivate aconitases, but nitric oxide does not. J Biol Chem. (1994) 269(47): 29405–29408.
[55] Mihm MJ, Yu F, Carnes CA, Reiser PJ, McCarthy PM, Van Wagoner DR, Bauer JA Impaired myofibrillar energetics and oxidative injury during human atrial fibrillation. Circulation. (2001) 104(2): 174–180.
[56] Grune T, Blasig IE, Sitte N, Roloff B, Haseloff R, Davies KJ. Peroxynitrite increases the degradation of aconitase and other cellular proteins by proteasome. J Biol Chem. (1998) 273(18): 10857-10862.
[57] Islam N, Ali R. (1998) Immunological studies on DNA-lysine photoadduct. Biochem. Mol. Biol. Int. 45(3):453–464.
[58] Dixit K, Moinuddin, Ali A (2005) Immunological studies on peroxynitrite modified DNA. Life Sci. 77(21):2626–2642.
[59] Ahmad R, Rasheed Z, Kaushal E, Singh D, Ahsan H. Biochemical evaluation of human DNA-lysine photoadduct treated with peroxynitrite. Toxicol Mech Meth. (2008) 18(7): 589–595.
[60] Gong C X, Liu F, Grundke-Iqbal I, Iqbal K.Dysregulation of protein phosphorylation/dephosphorylation in Alzheimer's disease: atherapeutic target.J Biomed Biotechnol (2006), 2006:31825.
[61] Ahmad R, Alam K, Ali R. Antigen binding characteristics of antibodies against hydroxyl radical modified thymidine monophosphate. Immunol Lett (2000),71:111-115
[62] Pisetsky DS. Antinuclear antibodies. Diagn Lab Immunol (1994),14:371-85
[63] Isenberg D, Shenfeld Y.The origin and significance of anti-DNA antibodies.Immunol Today (1997),8:279-81
[64] Tan EM. Autoantibody to nuclear antigens (ANA):their immunobiology and medicine. Adv Immunol (1982),33:167-208
[65] Pollard KM, Jones JE, TanEM, Theofilopoulos AN, Dixon FJ, Rubin RL. Polynucleotide specificity of murine monoclonal anti-DNA antibodies. Clin Immunol Immunopathol (1986), 40:197-208.
[66] Burney S, Caulfield JL, Niles JC, Wishnok JS, Tannenbaum SR. The chemistry of DNA damage from nitric oxide and peroxynitrite. Mutat Res (1999),424 (1-2):37-49.
[67] Habib S, Moinuddin, Ali R. Acquired antigenicity of DNA after modification with peroxynitrite. Int J Biol macromol (2005),35(3-4):221-225.
[68] Wanchu A, Khullar M, Deodhar SD bambery P, Sud A. Nitric oxide synthesis is increased in patients with systemic lupus erythmatosus. Rheumatol Int. (1998),18(2):41-43.

[69] Oates JC, Ruiz P, Alexander A, Pippen AM, Gilkeson GS. Effect of late modulation of nitric oxide production on murine lupus. Clin Immunol Immunopathol. (1997), 83(1):86-92.
[70] Gheidira I, Andolsi H, Mankai A, Fabien N, Jeddi M. Anti-histone antibodies in systemic lupus erythmatosus, comparison of three assays:ELISA, dot blot and immunoblot. Pathol Biol (2006), 54: 148-54
[71] Marc M, Thomas M, Lothar B, Frank SL. Anti-histone antibodies in subacute sensory neuropathy. J Neurooncol (1991),11:71-75.
[72] Masahidi K, Hironobu I, Norhito Y, Shinichi S, Kanako K, Kunihiko T. Prevelance and antigen specificity of anti-histone antibodies in patients with polymyositis/ dermatomyositis. J Invest Dermatol (1999), 112:1523-747.
[73] Khan MA, Dixit K, Jabeen S, Moinuddin, Alam K. Impact of peroxynitrite modification on structure and immunogenicity of H2A histone. Scan J Immunol (2008), 69:99-109.

9

Immunological Effects of Silica and Related Dysregulation of Autoimmunity

Naoko Kumagai[1], Hiroaki Hayashi[2], Megumi Maeda[1], Yoshie Miura[3], Hidenori Matsuzaki[1], Suni Lee[1], Yasumitsu Nishimura[1], Wataru Fujimoto[2] and Takemi Otsuki[1]

[1]Department of Hygiene,
[2]Department of Dermatology,
[1,2]Kawasaki Medical School, Kurashiki,
[3]Division of Molecular and Clinical Genetics, Department of Molecular Genetics, Medical Institute of Bioregulation, Kyushu University, Higashi-ku, Fukuoka, Japan

1. Introduction

Silicosis is known as environmental and occupational pulmonary fibrosis and the most typical form of pneumoconiosis results from long-term exposure (ten years or more) to relatively low concentrations of silica dust and usually appears ten to thirty years after the first exposure (Hoffman & Wanderer, 2010; Madl, 2008; Rimal, 2005). Patients with this type of silicosis, especially in the early stages, may not have obvious signs or symptoms of disease, but abnormalities may be detected by x-ray. Chronic cough and exertional dyspnea are common clinical findings. Radiographically, chronic simple silicosis reveals a profusion of small (less than 10 mm in diameter) opacities, typically rounded, and predominating in the upper lung zones. Patients with silicosis are particularly susceptible to tuberculosis infection—known as silicotuberculosis (Brown, 2009). It is thought that silica damages pulmonary macrophages, inhibiting their ability to kill mycobacteria. Pulmonary complications of silicosis also include chronic bronchitis and airflow limitation, non-tuberculous *Mycobacterium* infection, fungal lung infection, compensatory emphysema, and pneumothorax (Cohe & Velho, 2002; Rees & Murray, 2007). Lung cancer is also considered to be associated with silicosis and the International Agency for Research on Cancer (IARC) categorized crystalline silica as a causative of lung cancer (Cocco, 2007; IARC, 1997; Pelucchi, 2006). In addition, it is well known that silicosis patients (SILs) often experience complications due to autoimmune diseases (Shanklin & Smalley, 1998; Steenland & Goldsmith, 1995; Uber & McReynolds, 1982) such as rheumatoid arthritis (known as Caplan syndrome) (Caplan, 1959, 1962), systemic lupus erythematosus (SLE) (Bartsch, 1980; Yamazaki 2007), systemic scleroderma (SSc) (Barnadas, 1986; Cowie, 1987 Haustein, 1990; Haustein & Anderegg, 1998; Sluis-Cremer, 1985) and anti-neutrophil cytoplasmic autoantibody (ANCA)-related vasculitis/nephritis (Bartůnková, 2006; Mulloy, 2003; Tervaert, 1998).

Silica-induced dysregulation of autoimmunity has been thought to be caused by the adjuvant effect of silica (Cooper, 2008; Davis, 2001, Parks, 1999). Although this represents one mechanism by which silica might be involved in the development of autoimmune diseases, silica can influence circulating immunocompeting cells and dysregulate the T responder (Tresp) survival and activation status, since several different autoimmune diseases may be associated with silica dust exposure as mentioned above. In addition, silica may affect the regulatory T cell (Treg, CD4+25+FoxP3+), since Treg has been considered the most important subpopulation of T cells for the control of Tresp activation by the recognition of foreign and/or auto-antigens (Baecher-Allan, 2004; Bluestone & Tang, 2005; Schwartz, 2005). If the function or number of Treg is reduced, continuous stimulation of Tresp is thought to be maintained.

Furthermore, recent findings regarding the NOD-like receptor family, pryin domain containing 3 (NLRP3, Nalp3)-inflammasome, have contributed substantially to our understanding of the sequential cellular events occurring when silica is inhaled into the pulmonary region and alveolar macrophages try to treat silica particles as a foreign substance (Cassel, 2008; Dostert, 2008; Hormung, 2008).

At first, initial recognition of silica occurs by cell membrane receptors such as the macrophage receptor with collagenous structure (MARCO), scavenger receptor (SR)-AI and SR-AII (Brown, 2007; Hamilton, 2006; Thakur, 2009). The next stage involves capture of silica by macrophages and entrapment within lysosomes and their activation of the nucleotide-binding domain and leucine-rich repeat containing proteins, the NLRP3 inflammasome, to cleave pro-caspase 1 to an active form (Cassel, 2008; Dostert, 2008; Hormung, 2008). Thereafter, cleavage of pro-interleukin (IL)-1β occurs to an active form for release to form fibrotic nodules and production of reactive oxygen species (ROS) and reactive nitrogen species (RNS) in the macrophages yielded (37-40). As a consequence, the induction of cellular and tissue damages occur due to the production of ROS and RNS and the apoptosis of alveolar macrophages. Various cytokines/chemokines such as IL-1β, tumor necrosis factor (TNF)-α, macrophage inflammatory protein (MIP)-1/2, monocyte-chemoattractant protein-1 (MCP-1) and IL-8 are produced that cause chronic inflammation and proliferation of collagenic fibers (Barrett, 1999; Hamilton, 2008; Hubbard, 2001; Porter, 2002). Silica particles are released from alveolar macrophages and the similar cellular reactions described above by newly-recognizing nearby macrophages will be repeated. Finally, silica particles are transferred to regional lymph nodes. As these cellular and molecular reactions are continuously repeated, pulmonary fibrosis will gradually and progressively appear.

Even though details of these initial biological sequential reactions are recognized, it is still unclear how silica causes dysregulation of autoimmunity. From this viewpoint, we have been investigating the following perspectives:

1. Alteration of Fas and related molecules to affect long-term survival of lymphocytes.
2. Chronic activation of Tresp exposed to silica particles.
3. Alteration of Treg function and/or numbers exposed to silica particles.

In this chapter, we describe and summarize our experimental findings regarding the above three viewpoints, and insights concerning silica-induced dysregulation of autoimmunity will be discussed. Investigation using patient materials such as serum and lymphocytes were approved by the Institutional Ethics Committee of Kawasaki Medical School, Kusaka Hospital or Hinase-Urakami Iin. The specimens were only obtained from patients who gave documented informed consent. All of the patients were Japanese brickyard workers in Bizen City (Okayama prefecture, Japan), and were monitored at either Kusaka Hospital or the Hinase-Urakami Clinic. The silica in materials handled by these workers (e.g., dirt, sand, mud, concrete), and thus presenting the potential risk of being inhaled by these individuals in their work environment, was estimated to reach levels as high as 40–60% (by mass). The subjects were diagnosed with pneumoconiosis according to the ILO 2000 Guideline (ILO, 2004). These patients displayed neither clinical symptoms related to autoimmune diseases (e.g., sclerotic skin, Raynaud's phenomenon, facial erythema, or arthralgia) nor any cancers.

2. Alteration of Fas/CD95 and its related molecules in SILs

The discovery of Fas has led to a remarkable improvement in our understanding of apoptosis and its signal transduction (Matiba, 1997; Nagata, 1996; Nagata & Golstein, 1995). Abnormal regulation of apoptosis, particularly in relation to the Fas/Fas ligand (FasL) pathway, has been thought to play a role in the pathogenesis of autoimmune diseases (Eguchi, 2001; Rudin, 1996; Yonehara, 2002). Mutations of the *fas* gene and the *fas ligand* gene which lead to defects in apoptosis have been found in autoimmune strains of mice (*lpr* mice and *gld* mice, respectively) and human autoimmune lymphoproliferative syndrome (ALPS) in childhood (Nagata, 1998; Nagata & Suda, 1995, Mountz & Edwards, 1992; Steinberg, 1994). Fas/CD95, which is mainly expressed on the cell membrane of lymphocytes, usually exists as membrane-type Fas and forms a Fas-trimer after binding with FasL (Matiba, 1997; Nagata, 1996; Nagata & Golstein, 1995). The signal-transducing death domain located in the intracellular domain of Fas then recruits Fas-associated protein with Death Domain (FADD) and pro-caspase 8 to form the active death-inducing signaling complex (DISC) (Curtin & Cotter, 2003; Yu & Shi, 2008). Thereafter, activated caspase-8 triggers a caspase-cascade involving the activation of CAD/CPAN/DFF40 by removing its inhibitor, ICAD/DFF45, DNA fragmentation, and finally apoptotic cell death (Sabol, 1998; Sakahira, 1998).

The most typical alternatively spliced variant of the wild-type *fas* gene transcript is known as soluble Fas (sFas). Since this variant transcript lacks 63 bp of the transmembrane domain, its product (sFas) can be secreted from cells to suppress membrane Fas-mediated apoptosis by blocking the binding between membrane Fas and the FasL in the extracellular region (Matiba, 1997; Nagata, 1996; Nagata & Golstein, 1995). If there is a high level of sFas in the extracellular regions, lymphocytes in these regions may avoid apoptosis and survive longer. Actually, there have been several studies showing elevated serum levels of sFas in patients with autoimmune diseases (Cheng, 1994; Knipping, 1995; Tokano, 1996).

The following findings were obtained from our series of analyses of specimens from SILs. The detection of autoantibody to Fas and caspase-8, as well as topoisomerase I and desmoglein (Takata-Tomokuni, 2005; A. Ueki, 2001a, 2002; H. Ueki, 2001). Anti-Fas autoantibody detected in SILs was functionally active and caused Fas-mediated apoptosis (takata-Tomokuni, 2005). The level of serum sFas was higher in SILs than healthy volunteers (HVs), although the level of serum soluble FasL did not differ between SILs and HVs (Tomokuni, 1997, 1999). The mean fluorescent intensity (MFI) of membrane Fas was lower with lymphocytes from SILs than those from HVs, although total numbers of Fas-positive lymphocytes (membrane Fas expression) did not differ between the two populations (Otsuki, 2005). The weaker membrane Fas expressers (among lymphocytes) were identified to be weaker *fas* message expressers (Otsuki, 2005). The gene expression levels of extracellular inhibitor competing membrane Fas-FasL binding such as sFas, decoy receptor 3 (DCR3), and other alternatively spliced variants of the *fas* gene were higher in peripheral blood mononuclear cells (PBMC) from SILs than HVs (Otsuki, 2000a, 2000b). The intracellular apoptosis-inhibitory genes including *i-flice*, *sentrin*, *survivine* and *icad* showed a lower expression in PBMC from SILs than HDs (Guo, 2001; Otsuki, 2000c).

Although significant mutations of *fas* and *fas ligand* genes were not detected, these results indicated that two populations of lymphocytes may exist in the peripheral blood of SILs. As shown on the right side of Fig. 1, one population is a weaker membrane Fas expresser and these cells may have developed out of an excessive transcription of the alternatively spliced *fas* gene and other variant messages. Therefore, these cells may be resistant to the functional anti-fas autoantibody, secrete higher levels of sFas, DCR3 and spliced variants, and are resistant to Fas-mediated apoptosis (Murakami, 2007, Otsuki, 2005, 2007). As reported previously (Otsuki, 2005), patients with a weaker MFI of membrane Fas often have a higher titer of anti-nuclear antibodies (ANA), and self-recognizing clones in silicosis may be included in the fraction because these clones may survive longer and show resistance to apoptosis.

The other population, shown on the left side of Fig. 1, represents stronger membrane Fas expressers that may be sensitive to Fas-mediated apoptosis including cell death caused by anti-Fas autoantibody, show a reduced expression of intracellular inhibitor genes of Fas-mediated apoptosis, and undergo apoptosis. These cells may be recruited from bone marrow after reaching the final stage of cell death. This recruited fraction would not have encountered silica and would be sensitive to Fas-mediated apoptosis. As a result, cells in this fraction would be continuously undergoing renewal and then apoptosis (Murakami, 2007, Otsuki, 2005, 2007).

The overall findings support the supposition that the long-term surviving subpopulation of T cells may include self-recognizing clones. However, these results provide no evidence that the lymphocytes in SILs are activated continuously. Thus, an investigation that incorporates experimental and patient-oriented studies is required to observe the chronic activation of Tresp by silica.

3. Chronic activation of Tresp by exposure to silica

To investigate the hypothesis that silica chronically activates Tresp, we first examined the *in vitro* activation of Tresp by exposure to silica (Wu, 2005). Freshly isolated PBMCs from HVs were cultured with or without phytohaemagglutinin (PHA), Min-U-silica (25 or 50 μg/ml) or chrysotile A (an asbestos, 50 μg/ml) for ten days. The expression of CD69 was used as the marker for early activation of T cells. Results showed that only silica can upregulate CD69 expression in T cells slowly and gradually in a dose-dependent manner in regard to cell surface expression (as shown in Fig. 2-A) and the message level (Wu, 2005). Although the data is not shown here, it was evident that PHA can stimulate T cells and that CD69 expression was observed at day 1 as the peak and then gradually reduced until day 5 (Wu, 2005). Additionally, chrysotile A was not able to induce CD69 expression (Wu, 2005). In this study, the necessity of the existence of phagocytosed cells in contact with lymphocytes was also found, and soluble factors secreted from phagocytosed cells contributed to approximately half of the induced CD69 expression in T cells (Wu, 2005). These results indicated the importance of the NLRP3 inflammasome in these experimental situations. Moreover, if Tresp in SILs encounter silica at the pulmonary circulation and also regional lymph nodes where silica is accumulated after it is handled by alveolar macrophages, they can be exposed to silica chronically and recurrently. In view of this consideration, the activation of Tresp in circulating peripheral blood Tresp and collateral evidence of Tresp activation were then investigated.

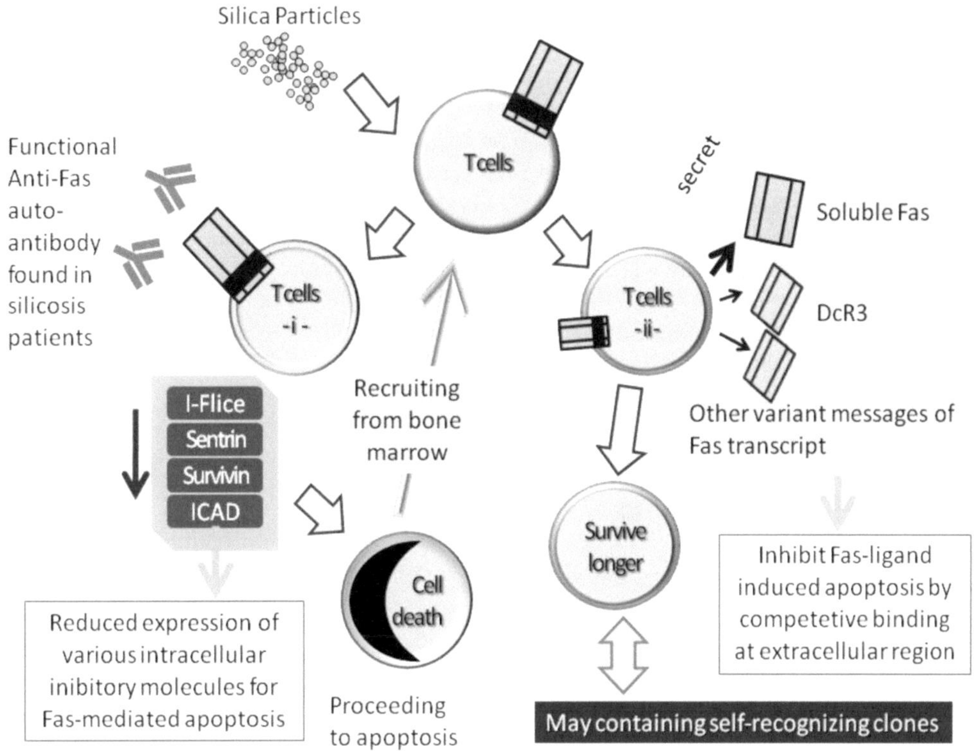

Fig. 1. Schematic model of the dysregulation of Fas and Fas-related molecules found in patients with silicosis. Two groups (temporarily designated T cell - i – and - ii -) may exist among lymphocytes from these patients: a population repeatedly undergoing apoptosis caused by silica and recruited from bone marrow, and another population surviving in the long term by avoiding apoptosis due to self-producing inhibitory molecules such as soluble Fas that may include self-recognizing clones.

With the recent recognition of Treg, most of the peripheral CD4+25+ T cells, particularly the higher expresser of CD25, are considered as Treg (Baecher-Allan, 2004; Bluestone & Tang, 2005; Schwartz, 2005). However, activated Tresp also express CD25 on their surface. Although Treg is defined in regard to the nuclear forkhead box P3 (FoxP3) gene as the master gene of Treg to manifest Treg function in order to inhibit the Tresp activation response against auto, foreign, cancerous and transplanted antigens (Baecher-Allan, 2004; Bluestone & Tang, 2005; Schwartz, 2005), observation of FoxP3 expression by flow cytometry requires the permeabilization of cell surface and nuclear membranes. This procedure is not suitable for subsequent biological examinations using sorted cells. Thus, in the following experiments, CD4+25+ cells were sorted to examine gene expression and the inhibitory function of the fraction.

As the marker for activation, we again used CD69 as an early activation marker and programmed cell death-1 (PD-1) genes (Saresella, 2008; Wang, 2009). Peripheral blood CD4+25- and CD4+25+ cells derived from HVs or SILs were collected by flow cytometry and relative gene expressions of CD69 and PD-1 were analyzed by real-time RT-PCR in comparison to glyceraldehyde-3-phosphate dehydrogenase (GAPDH) expression (Hayashi, 2010). As shown in Fig. 2-B, the CD4+25- fraction from both HVs and SILs revealed a higher expression of CD69 than CD25+ cells. In addition, CD69 expression in the CD25- fraction of SILs was significantly higher than that of HVs. Furthermore, as shown in Fig. 2-C, the expression of PD-1 was higher in the CD25- and CD25+ fractions of SILs than HVs. These findings supported the view that Tresp in SILs were chronically and recurrently activated and possessed long-term survival. Since CD69 expression was limited in the early stage of T cell activation, it is significant that the CD25+ fraction from both populations showed lower expression. However, both the CD25- and CD25+ fractions showed a higher expression of

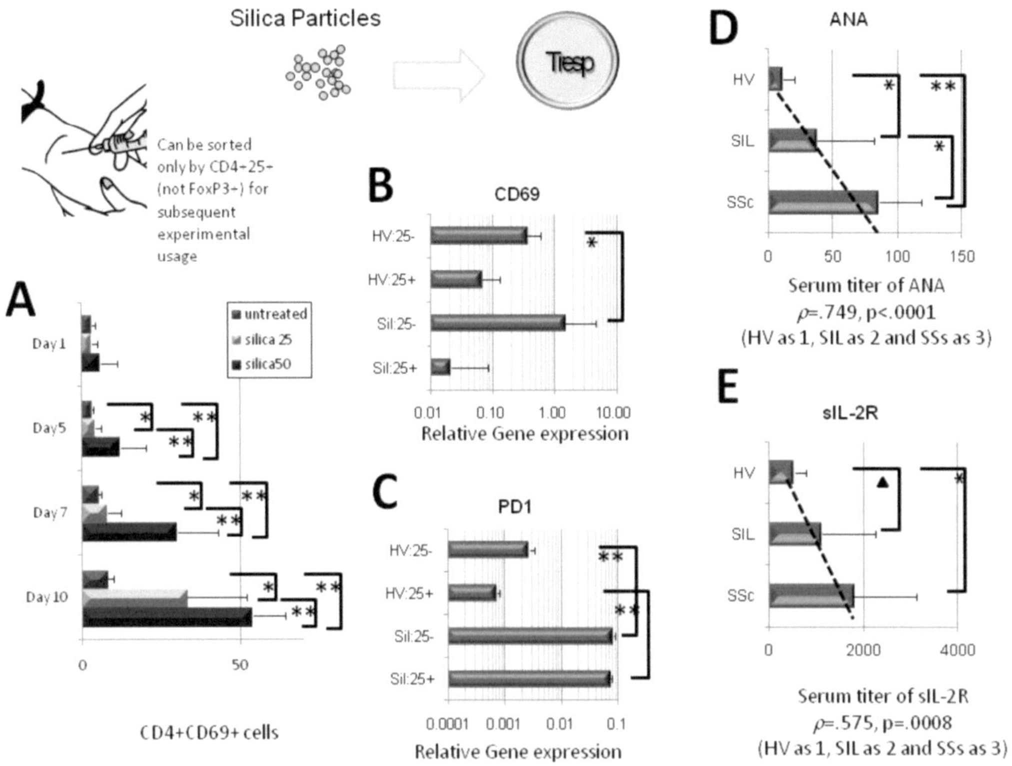

Fig. 2. Various examinations to recognize the effects of silica exposure on responder T cells (Tresp). ＊ : $p<0.05$, ＊＊<0.01 and ▲ : $0.05<p<0.1$. [A] Peripheral blood mononuclear cells from healthy volunteers (HVs) were incubated with or without silica particles (25 or 50 μg/ml) for ten days. CD69 expression in CD4+ cells was analyzed by flow cytometry. [B] and [C] Peripheral blood CD4+25- and CD4+25+ cell fractions derived from HVs and silicosis patients (SILs) were sorted by flow cytometry, extracted total RNAs from individual fractions, and synthesized cDNA. Real-time RT-PCR analyses were employed to compare the gene expression of CD69 and PD-1, respectively. [D] and [E] Serum levels of the ANA titer and soluble IL-2 receptor (sIL-2R), respectively, were measured by ELISA methods and compared among HVs, SILs and patients with systemic sclerosis (SSc). In addition, after a numbered disease status set to 1 for HVs, 2 for SILs and 3 for SSc, correlations between disease status number and titers of ANA or sIL-2R were analyzed.

PD-1 (Hayashi, 2010). This may suggest that silica can activate both Tresp and Treg, and that the CD25+ fraction in SILs may include chronically activated Tresp in which surface CD25 expression occurred continuously due to recurrent stimulation by silica (Hayashi, 2010).
To investigate another marker of Tresp activation, we measured the serum soluble IL-2 receptor (sIL-2R) in SILs and compared results with those obtained from HVs and patients with SSc, since sIL-2R is known to arise in the serum of apparently healthy individuals who subclinically possess neoplastic (i.e., certain lymphoid malignancies such as T cell leukemia and early cell leukemia), autoimmune or inflammatory diseases (Carlson, 1992; Nelson & Willerford, 1998; Pizzolo, 1991; Rubin & Nelson, 1990; Zerler, 1991). The high-affinity IL-2R is a multichain receptor which possesses at least three IL-2 binding chains: IL-2Rα/CD25 (55 kDa), IL-2Rβ/CD122 (75 kDa) and IL-2Rγ/CD132 (64 kDa). sIL-2R is the naturally occurring soluble form of IL-2Rα. For this analysis, the serum titer of anti-nuclear antigens (ANA) was measured in HVs, SILs and SSc using the Enzyme-Linked ImmunoSorbent Assay (ELISA)-based MESACUP ANA TEST (MBL Co. Ltd., Nagoya, Japan), which includes several recombinant proteins such as RNP, SS-A/Ro, SS-B/La, Scl-70, Jo-1 and Ribosomal P *in vitro* transcribed U1 RA and CENP-B protein, and purified antigen (Sm, SS-A/Ro, Scl-70m Histone and DNA) (Hayashi, 2009). As shown in Fig. 2-D, the ANA titer in SSc was the highest among the three groups, and significantly higher than that of HVs or SILs, whereas the ANA titer in SILs was also significantly higher than that of HVs. In addition, if disease status was numbered and set to 1 for HV, 2 for SIL and 3 for SSc, a significant positive correlation was obtained between the serum titer of ANA and disease status. Even our patients did not manifest any clinical symptoms for autoimmune diseases, and SILs subclinically tended to present a dysregulation of autoimmunity. Following these findings, serum sIL-2R was also analyzed in a manner similar to that used for the serum ANA titer. As shown in Fig. 2-E, SSc patients showed significantly higher serum sIL-2R than HVs or SILs, and the level shown by SILs tended to be higher than that shown by HVs. In addition, a significant positive correlation was detected between serum sIL-2R and disease status. These results suggest that sIL-2R may be used to detect immunological alteration in SILs, and that Tresp in SILs is activated chronically to an unknown higher level of sIL-2R (Hayashi, 2009).

4. Chronic activation of Treg by exposure to silica

As we have investigated Tresp activation in SILs as described above, the next point of interest was the function and activation of Treg. It has been revealed that CD4+25+ Treg contribute to maintaining self-tolerance by down-regulating the immune response to self and non-self antigens in an antigen-non-specific manner, presumably at the T cell activation stage (Baecher-Allan, 2004; Bluestone & Tang, 2005; Schwartz, 2005). Elimination and/or reduction of CD4+25+ T cells relieves this general suppression, thereby enhancing immune responses to non-self Ags and eliciting autoimmune responses to certain self-antigens. Recent studies have shown that CD4+25+ Treg specifically express transcription factor Foxp3 (Baecher-Allan, 2004; Bluestone & Tang, 2005; Schwartz, 2005). Genetic anomalies in Foxp3 cause autoimmune and inflammatory diseases in rodents and humans by affecting the development and function of CD4+CD25+ Treg (Baecher-Allan, 2004; Bluestone & Tang, 2005; Schwartz, 2005). Clinically, a deficiency in Treg function or decrease in the proportion of Treg has been shown to influence the pathogenesis of collagen or autoimmune diseases such as multiple sclerosis (O'Connor & Anderton, 2008), rheumatoid arthritis (Toh &

Miossec, 2007), systemic lupus erythematosus (Mudd, 2006), and pemphigus vulgaris (Yokoyama & Amagai, 2010). These findings at the cellular and molecular levels provide firm evidence that CD4+25+Foxp3+ Treg cells are an indispensable cellular constituent of the normal immune system, and that these cells play crucial roles in establishing and maintaining immunologic self-tolerance and immune homeostasis.

As mentioned above, CD25 molecules are also expressed on non-Treg subsets such as antigen-activated responder/effector T cells. Therefore, Foxp3 has been utilized as a useful marker to identify CD25+ regulatory T cells from CD25+ activated Tresp, although several distinguishable markers such as CD127 and PD-1 have been utilized to distinguish Treg from activated CD4+CD25+ Tresp (Liu, 2006; Hartigan-O'Connor, 2007; Saresella, 2008; Wang, 2009).

As described above, since the peripheral blood CD4+25+ fraction showed higher PD-1 expression (Fig. 2-C) and several findings demonstrate the chronic and recurrent activation of Tresp in SILs, the peripheral CD4+25+ fraction in SILs may be contaminated by these activated Tresp expressing CD25 on the base of Treg (Hayashi, 2010).

Thus, we first analyzed the function of the Treg fraction (actually, the peripheral CD4+25+ fraction sorted by flow cytometry in which Treg is mainly included and there is no availability of FoxP3-sorted cells for biological use as mentioned above) (Wu, 2006). As shown in Fig. 3-A, the inhibitory function of the CD4+25+ sorted fraction from SILs was lower than that of HVs when this fraction was added to the mixed lymphocyte culture (MLR) (Tresp was stimulated by irradiated allo-PBMCs) with the ratio $1{:}^1/_4$ or $1{:}^1/_2$, and tended to be lower when added with the ratio $1{:}^1/_8$ or 1:1. There may be a reduced number of true Treg in the CD4+25+ fraction from SILs or an impaired function of true Treg (wu, 2006). Taken together with the results of chronic and recurrent activation of Tresp in SILs (Hayashi, 2010; Wu, 2005), these findings support the possibility that the CD4+25+ fraction in SILs may include activated Tresp due to silica exposure. To examine this possibility, Treg-specific gene expression such as FoxP3 and cytotoxic T-lymphocyte antigen 4 (CTLA-4) was analyzed in CD4+25- and CD4+25+ fractions derived from HVs and SILs. As shown in Fig. 3-B and 3-C, the CD4+25+ fraction from SILs lost the dominant expression levels of both genes. These results suggested the CD4+25+ fraction in SILs was contaminated with chronically activated Tresp by exposure to silica (Hayashi, 2010; Wu, 2006). As expected and shown in Fig. 3-D, the percentage of the CD4+25+ fraction in peripheral lymphocytes was significantly smaller in HVs than SILs. Although the CD4+FoxP3+ fraction did not differ between HVs and SILs, the CD25+FoxP3- population was higher in SILs than HVs (Hayashi, 2010; Wu, 2006). These analyses indicated that the CD4+25+ fractions in SILs were contaminated by chronically activated Tresp due to exposure to silica (Hayashi, 2010; Wu, 2006). Although this may explain the results of reduced inhibitory function of the CD4+25+ fraction from SILs, there may be another possibility regarding the number of true Treg in SILs. Even the percentage of the CD4+FoxP3+ fraction did not differ between SILs and HVs, and a certain loss of Treg may occur, otherwise the reduced inhibitory function may not be fully explained.

We again take an interest with the Fas/CD95 molecule. As Tresp upregulated its CD25 expression due to chronic exposure to silica, Treg may have excess expression of Fas/CD95 because it has been shown that Treg expresses Fas/CD95 and is more sensitive to Fas-mediated apoptosis than Tresp (Fritzsching, 2005, 2006). To investigate this possibility, peripheral blood mononuclear cells from HVs and SILs were stained with CD4, CD25,

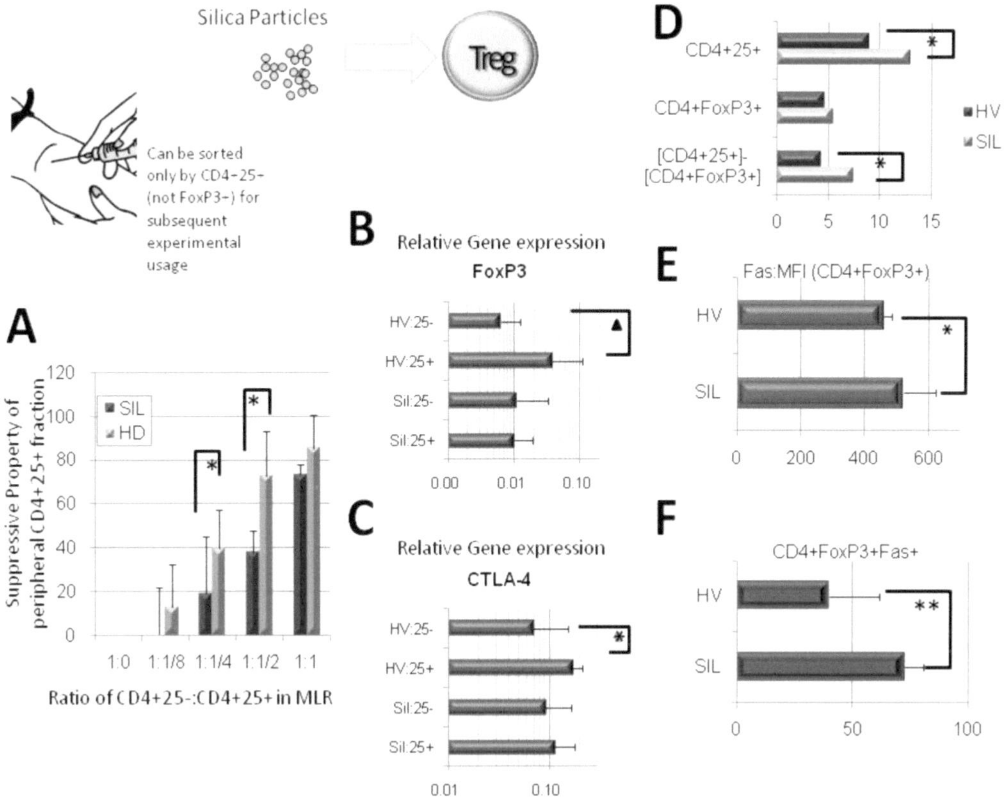

Fig. 3. Various examinations to recognize the effects of silica exposure on regulatory T cells (Treg). ＊ : $p<0.05$, ＊＊<0.01 and ▲ : $0.05<p<0.1$. [A] The CD4+25- and CD4+25+ fractions from healthy volunteers (HVs) and silicosis patients (SILs) were collected by flow cytometry. CD4+25- cells with or without various ratios of CD4+25+ cells, such as 1:0, 1:$^1/_8$, 1:$^1/_4$, 1:$^1/_2$ and 1:1, were applied to a mixed lymphocyte reaction (MLR). Allogenic irradiated peripheral blood mononuclear cells were used as a stimulator. Graphs express suppressive properties of added CD4+25+ fractions. The degree to which the added CD4+25+ fraction reduced Cd4+25- DNA synthesis was measured by the ^{3}H-thymidine incorporation assay. [B] and [C] Peripheral blood CD4+25- and CD4+25+ cell fractions derived from HVs and SILs were sorted by flow cytometry, extracted total RNAs from individual fractions, and synthesized cDNA. Real-time RT-PCR analyses were employed to compare the gene expression of FoxP3 and CTLA-4, respectively. [D] Peripheral blood CD4+25+ and CD4+FoxP2+ populations were compared between HVs and SILs. [E] and [F] Peripheral blood CD4+FoxP3+ cells derived from HVs and SILs were compared in regard to CD95/Fas expression by means of fluorescent intensity and positive cell percentage, respectively.

CD95/Fas and FoxP3, and CD95/Fas expression (MFI) and positive cell frequency were analyzed in the CD4+FoxP3+ cell fraction. As shown in Fig. 3-E (MFI) and 3-F (positive cell frequency), Treg from SILs showed significantly higher expression levels of CD95/Fas than those from HVs. In addition, CD4+25+ cells from SILs were significantly more sensitive against Fas-mediated apoptosis inducing monoclonal antibody (CH-11) than those from HVs (data not shown), and proceeded faster to apoptosis as previously reported (Hayashi,

2010). All of these findings indicate that Treg may lose its true Treg ability due to chronic activation of Treg by recurrent exposure to silica mediated by excess expression of Fas/CD95 on the Treg cell surface.

5. Silica-induced dysfunction of the Treg fraction in SILs

Our results and those of our previous findings suggest that silica can reconstitute the peripheral CD4+CD25+ fraction to facilitate a decline in the number and function of Treg by the activation of both Tresp and Treg cells (Hayashi, 2010; Maeda, 2010), as outlined in Fig. 4.

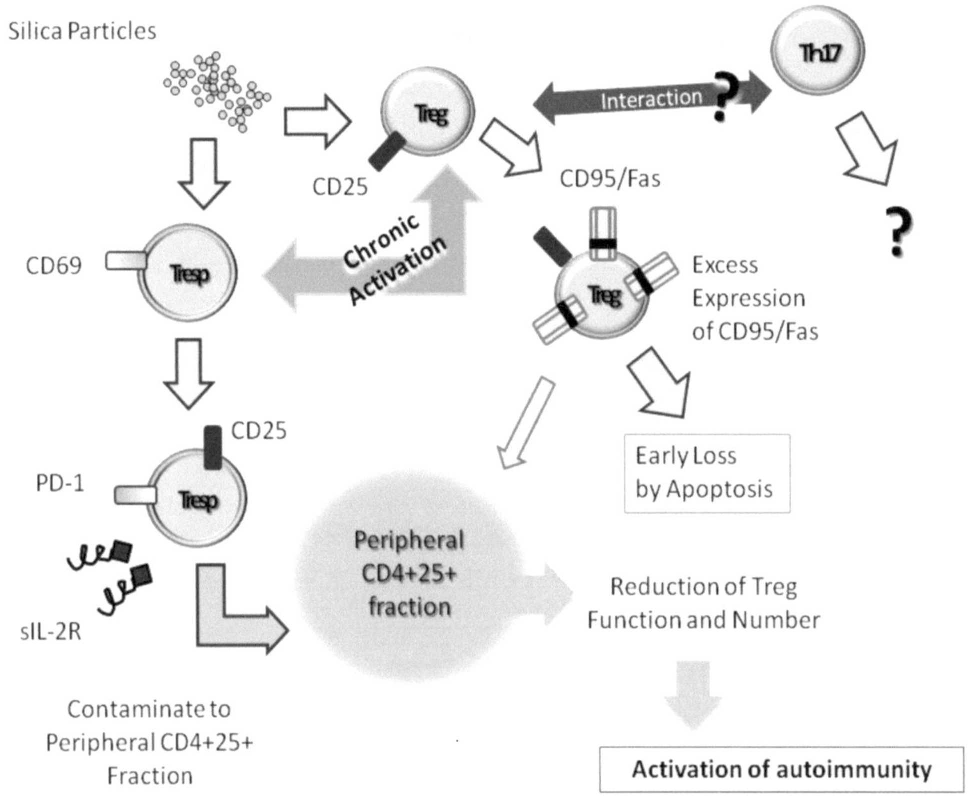

Fig. 4. Schematic representation of the immunological effects of silica exposure on alteration of autoimmunity. Silica chronically activates CD4+FoxP3 T cells (Treg), resulting in the induction of higher Fas expression. This up-regulated Fas marks Treg for Fas-mediated apoptosis. However, silica induces the change of CD4+FoxP3- T cells (Tresp) to CD4+25+FoxP3- activated Tresp. This population contaminates the peripheral CD4+25+ fraction in which Treg should be located. This imbalance between a decreased Treg and increased activated Tresp results in a dysfunction of the so-called CD4+25+ Treg fraction, which may trigger the occurrence of autoimmune diseases such as SSc. However, the roles and alterations of Th17 in silica-exposed patients are unknown and should be clarified through further research in order to obtain a better understanding of the immunological effects of silica on the human immune system.

Many issues remain to be resolved, such as delineating the complications of SSc in SILs (Barnadas, 1986; Cowie, 1987 Haustein, 1990; Haustein & Anderegg, 1998; Sluis-Cremer, 1985), or those complications associated with malignant tumors such as mesothelioma and lung cancer in patients exposed to the mineral silicate asbestos (Greillier, 2008; Toyokuni, 2009; Miura, 2008). Regarding the relationship between tumor immunity and Treg function, it may be that Treg enhances cell numbers or function to reduce tumor immunity (Chattopadhyay, 2005; Danese & Rutella, 2007; Kretschmer, 2006). If this is the case, future investigations will need to determine whether silica and asbestos possess opposite effects on Treg. Furthermore, specific parameters will need to be examined such as the degree of silica exposure, the progression of respiratory diseases (Otsuki, 1999), and identification of a possible individual factor such as the HLA type (A. Ueki, 2001b) that leads to the development of autoimmune complications in SILs.

In addition, the recent discovery of T helper type 17 cells (Th17) has contributed to the recognition of the occurrence of autoimmunity (Afzali, 2007; Awasthi & Kuchroo, 2009; Harrington, 2006; Jin, 2008; Louten, 2009; Stockinger, 2007). Research on the biology of Th17 cells suggests a critical role for Th17 in the development of inflammatory and autoimmune diseases. Furthermore, Th17 has been shown to interact with Treg cells (Afzali, 2007; Awasthi & Kuchroo, 2009; Harrington, 2006; Jin, 2008; Louten, 2009; Stockinger, 2007). TGF-β not only regulates the generation of Foxp3+ Treg cells, but together with IL-6 initiates Th17 differentiation. A reciprocal relationship between Th17 and Treg development has been proposed, since the generation of Foxp3+ Treg cells and Th17 cells both require TGF-β signaling. If the frequencies of Th17 and Treg were regulated by each other, silica-induced early loss of Treg may have an inverse effect by increasing the Th17 population, and represents another way to induce dysregulation of autoimmunity in SILs. Although we have just begun to investigate the status of Th17 in SILs, this is another important and critical issue to be resolved for a better understanding of environmental disturbance of autoimmunity such as that involving silica-induced autoimmune diseases (Shanklin & Smalley, 1998; Steenland & Goldsmith, 1995; Uber & McReynolds, 1982).

In the future, a comprehensive understanding of the immunological effects of silica may lead to the discovery of preventive and therapeutic molecular targets for autoimmune diseases, and will help to clarify the pathophysiological mechanisms involved in the development of dysregulation of autoimmunity.

6. Acknowledgments

The authors specially thank Dr. Masayasu Kusaka (Kusaka Hospital, 1122 Nishikatagami, Bizen, 705-0121, Japan) and Dr. Kozo Urakami (Hinase Urakami Iin, 243-4 Hinase, Hinase-cho, Bizen, 701-3204, Japan) for their particular contribution to the organization of patients. We also thank Ms. Tamayo Hatayama, Yoshiko Yamashita, Minako Kato, Tomoko Sueishi, Keiko Kimura, Misao Kuroki, Naomi Miyahara and Shoko Yamamoto for their technical help. This study was supported in part by Special Coordination Funds for Promoting Science and Technology (H18-1-3-3-1, Comprehensive approach on asbestos-related diseases), KAKENHI grants (18390186, 19659153 and 20390178), Kawasaki Medical School Project Grants (18-601, 19-603T, 20-410I, 20-603, 21-606 and 22-A7), a Sumitomo Foundation Grant (053027), a Yasuda Memorial Foundation Grant (H18), funding from the Takeda Science Foundation (I-2008) and Young Investigator Activating Grant in Japanese Society of Hygiene (H189).

7. References

Afzali, B., Lombardi, G., Lechler, R.I. and Lord, G.M. (2007) The role of T helper 17 (Th17) and regulatory T cells (Treg) in human organ transplantation and autoimmune disease. *Clin Exp Immunol.* 148, 32-46, ISSN:0009-9104

Awasthi, A. and Kuchroo, V.K. (2009) Th17 cells: from precursors to players in inflammation and infection. *Int Immunol.* 21, 489-498, ISSN:0953-8178

Baecher-Allan, C., Viglietta, V. and Hafler, D.A. (2004) Human CD4+CD25+ regulatory T cells. *Semin Immunol.* 16, 89-98, ISSN:1044-5323

Barnadas, M.A., Tuneu, A., Rajmil, H.O., Abud, O. and de Moragas, J.M. (1986) Impotence in silicosis-associated scleroderma. *J Am Acad Dermatol.* 15, 1294-1296, ISSN:0190-9622

Barrett, E.G., Johnston, C., Oberdörster, G. and Finkelstein, J.N. (1999) Silica-induced chemokine expression in alveolar type II cells is mediated by TNF-alpha-induced oxidant stress. *Am J Physiol Lung Cell Mol Physiol.* 276, L979-988, ISSN:1040-0605

Bartsch, P., Salmon, J. and Mahieu, P. (1980) Asbestosis and systemic lupus erythematosus. *Int Arch Allergy Appl Immunol.* 61, 28-31, ISSN:0020-5915

Bartůnková, J., Pelclová, D., Fenclová, Z., Sedivá, A., Lebedová, J., Tesar, V., Hladíková, M. and Klusácková, P. (2006) Exposure to silica and risk of ANCA-associated vasculitis. *Am J Ind Med.* 49, 569-576, ISSN:0271-3586

Bluestone, J.A. and Tang, Q. (2005) How do CD4+CD25+ regulatory T cells control autoimmunity? *Curr Opin Immunol.* 17, 638-642, ISSN:0952-7915

Brown, J.M., Swindle, E.J., Kushnir-Sukhov, N.M., Holian, A. and Metcalfe. D.D. (2007) Silica-directed mast cell activation is enhanced by scavenger receptors. Am J Respir *Cell Mol Biol.* 36, 43-52, ISSN:0145-5680

Brown, T. (2009) Silica exposure, smoking, silicosis and lung cancer--complex interactions. *Occup Med (Lond).* 59, 89-95, ISSN:0962-7480

Caplan, A. (1959) Rheumatoid disease and pneumoconiosis (Caplan's syndrome). *Proc R Soc Med.* 52, 1111-1113, ISSN:0035-9157

Caplan, A., Payne, R.B. and Withey, J.L. (1962) A broader concept of Caplan's syndrome related to rheumatoid factors. *Thorax.* 17, 205-212, ISSN:0040-6376

Carlson, I.H. (1992) New markers in serum for lymphocyte activation for predicting allograft rejection. Neopterin and soluble interleukin-2 receptor. *Clin Lab Med.* 12, 99-111, ISSN:0272-2712

Cassel, S.L., Eisenbarth, S.C., Iyer, S.S., Sadler, J.J., Colegio, O.R., Tephly, L.A., Carter, A.B., Rothman, P.B., Flavell, R.A. and Sutterwala, F.S. (2008) The Nalp3 inflammasome is essential for the development of silicosis. *Proc Natl Acad Sci U S A.* 105, 9035-9040, ISSN:0027-8424

Chattopadhyay, S., Chakraborty, N.G. and Mukherji, B. (2005) Regulatory T cells and tumor immunity. *Cancer Immunol Immunother.* 54, 1153-1161, ISSN:0340-7004

Cheng, J., Zhou, T., Liu, C., Shapiro, J.P., Brauer, M.J., Kiefer, M.C., Barr, P.J. and Mountz, J.D. (1994) Protection from Fas-mediated apoptosis by a soluble form of the Fas molecule. *Science.* 263, 1759-1762, ISSN:0036-8075

Cocco, P., Dosemeci, M. and Rice, C. (2007) Lung cancer among silica-exposed workers: the quest for truth between chance and necessity. *Med Lav.* 98, 3-17, ISSN:0025-7818

Cohen, R. and Velho, V. (20062 Update on respiratory disease from coal mine and silica dust. *Clin Chest Med.* 23, 811-826, ISSN:0272-5231

Cooper, G.S., Gilbert, K.M., Greidinger, E.L., James, J.A., Pfau, J.C., Reinlib, L., Richardson, B.C. and Rose, N.R. (2008) Recent advances and opportunities in research on lupus: environmental influences and mechanisms of disease. *Environ Health Perspect.* 116, 695-702, ISSN:0091-6765

Cowie, R.L. (1987) Silica-dust-exposed mine workers with scleroderma (systemic sclerosis). *Chest.* 92, 260-262, ISSN:0012-3692

Curtin, J.F. and Cotter, T.G. (2003) Live and let die: regulatory mechanisms in Fas-mediated apoptosis. *Cell Signal.* 15, 983-992, ISSN:0898-6568

Danese, S. and Rutella, S. (2007) The Janus face of CD4+CD25+ regulatory T cells in cancer and autoimmunity. *Curr Med Chem.* 14, 649-666, ISSN:0929-8673

Davis, G.S., Holmes, C.E., Pfeiffer, L.M. and Hemenway, D.R. (2001) Lymphocytes, lymphokines, and silicosis. *J Environ Pathol Toxicol Oncol.* 20S1, 53-65, ISSN:0731-8898

Dostert, C., Pétrilli, V., Van Bruggen, R., Steele, C., Mossman, B.T. and Tschopp, J. (2008) Innate immune activation through Nalp3 inflammasome sensing of asbestos and silica. *Science.* 320, 674-677, ISSN:0036-8075

Eguchi, K. (2001) Apoptosis in autoimmune diseases. *Intern Med.* 40, 275-284, ISSN:0918-2918

Fritzsching, B., Oberle, N., Eberhardt, N., Quick, S., Haas, J., Wildemann, B., Krammer, P.H. and Suri-Payer, E. (2005) In contrast to effector T cells, CD4+CD25+FoxP3+ regulatory T cells are highly susceptible to CD95 ligand- but not to TCR-mediated cell death. *J Immunol.* 175, 32-36, ISSN:0022-1767

Fritzsching, B., Oberle, N., Pauly, E., Geffers, R., Buer, J., Poschl, J., Krammer, P., Linderkamp, O. and Suri-Payer, E. (2006) Naive regulatory T cells: a novel subpopulation defined by resistance toward CD95L-mediated cell death. *Blood.* 108, 3371-3378, ISSN:0006-4971

Greillier, L. and Astoul, P. (2008) Mesothelioma and asbestos-related pleural diseases. Respiration. 76, 1-15, ISSN:0025-7931

Guo, Z-Q., Otsuki, T., Shimizu, T., Tachiyama, S., Sakaguchi, H., Isozaki, Y., Tomokuni, T., Hyodoh, F., Kusaka, M. and Ueki, A. (2001) Reduced expression of survivin gene in PBMC from silicosis patients. *Kwasaki Med J.* 27, 75-81, ISSN:0386-5924

Hamilton, R.F. Jr., Thakur, S.A., Mayfair, J.K. and Holian, A. (2006) MARCO mediates silica uptake and toxicity in alveolar macrophages from C57BL/6 mice. *J Biol Chem.* 281, 34218-23426, ISSN:0021-9258

Hamilton, R.F. Jr., Thakur, S.A. and Holian, A. (2008) Silica binding and toxicity in alveolar macrophages. *Free Radic Biol Med.* 44, 1246-1258, ISSN:0891-5849

Hartigan-O'Connor, D.J., Poon, C., Sinclair, E. amd McCune, J.M. (20079 Human CD4+ regulatory T cells express lower levels of the IL-7 receptor alpha chain (CD127), allowing consistent identification and sorting of live cells. *J Immunol Methods.* 319, 41-52, ISSN:0022-1759

Harrington, L.E., Mangan, P.R. and Weaver, C.T. (2006) Expanding the effector CD4 T-cell repertoire: the Th17 lineage. *Curr Opin Immunol.* 18, 349-356, ISSN:0952-7915

Hayashi, H., Maeda, M., Murakami, S., Kumagai, N., Chen, Y., Hatayama, T., Katoh, M., Miyahara, N., Yamamoto, S., Yoshida, Y., Nishimura, Y., Kusaka, M., Fujimoto, W. and Otsuki, T. (2009) Soluble interleukin-2 receptor as an indicator of immunological disturbance found in silicosis patients. *Int J Immunopathol Pharmacol.* 22, 53-62, ISSN:0394-6320

Hayashi, H., Miura, Y., Maeda, M., Murakami, S., Kumagai, N., Nishimura, M., Kusaka, M., Uragami, K., Fujimoto, W. and Otsuki, T. (2010) Reductive alteration of the regulatory function of the CD4+CD25+ T cell fraction in silicosis patients. *Int J Immunopathol Pharmacol.* 23, 1099-1109, ISSN:0394-6320

Haustein, U.F., Ziegler, V., Herrmann, K., Mehlhorn, J. and Schmidt, C. (1990) Silica-induced scleroderma. *J Am Acad Dermatol.* 22, 444-448, ISSN:0190-9622

Haustein, U.F and Anderegg, U. (1998) Silica induced scleroderma--clinical and experimental aspects. *J Rheumatol.* 25, 1917-1926, ISSN:0315-162X

Hoffman, H.M. and Wanderer, A.A. (2010) Inflammasome and IL-1β-mediated disorders. *Curr Allergy Asthma Rep.* 10, 229-235, ISSN:1529-7322

Hornung, V., Bauernfeind, F., Halle, A., Samstad, E.O., Kono, H., Rock, K.L., Fitzgerald, K.A. and Latz, E. (2008) Silica crystals and aluminum salts activate the NALP3 inflammasome through phagosomal destabilization. *Nat Immunol.* 9, 847-856, ISSN:1529-2908

Hubbard, A.K., Thibodeau, M. and Giardina, C. (2001) Cellular and molecular mechanisms regulating silica-induced adhesion molecule expression in mice. *J Environ Pathol Toxicol Oncol.* 20S1, 45-51, ISSN:0731-8898

IARC, IARC (ed) (1997) *Silica, Some Silicates, Coal Dust and para-Aramid Fibrils. IARC Monograph on the Evaluation of Carcinogenic Risks to Humans, IARC Monographs, Vol 68,* IARC Publisher, ISBN-13/9789283212683, ISBN-10/9283212681, Geneva , Switzerland

ILO, ILO (ed) (2002) Guidelines for the Use of the ILO International Classification of Radiographs of Pneumoconioses: *Revised Edition 2000,* ILO publisher, ISBN : 9789221108320, Geneva, Switzerland

Jin, D., Zhang, L., Zheng, J. and Zhao, Y. (2008) The inflammatory Th 17 subset in immunity against self and non-self antigens. *Autoimmunity.* 41, 154-162, ISSN:0891-6934

Knipping, E., Krammer, P.H., Onel, K.B., Lehman, T.J., Mysler, E. and Elkon, K.B. (1995) Levels of soluble Fas/APO-1/CD95 in systemic lupus erythematosus and juvenile rheumatoid arthritis. *Arthritis Rheum.* 38, 1735-1737, ISSN:0004-3591

Kretschmer, K., Apostolou, I., Jaeckel, E., Khazaie, K. and von Boehmer, H. (20069 Making regulatory T cells with defined antigen specificity: role in autoimmunity and cancer. *Immunol Rev.* 212, 163-169, ISSN:0105-2896

Liu, W., Putnam, A.L., Xu-Yu, Z., Szot, G.L., Lee, M.R., Zhu, S., Gottlieb, P.A., Kapranov, P., Gingeras, T.R., Fazekas de St Groth, B., Clayberger, C., Soper, D.M., Ziegler, S.F. and Bluestone, J.A. (2006) CD127 expression inversely correlates with FoxP3 and suppressive function of human CD4+ T reg cells. *J Exp Med.* 203, 1701-1711, ISSN:0022-1007

Louten, J., Boniface, K. and de Waal Malefyt, R. (2009) Development and function of TH17 cells in health and disease. *J Allergy Clin Immunol.* 123, 1004-10011, ISSN:0091-6749

Madl, A.K., Donovan, E.P., Gaffney, S.H., McKinley, M.A., Moody, E.C., Henshaw, J.L. and Paustenbach, D.J. (2008) State-of-the-science review of the occupational health hazards of crystalline silica in abrasive blasting operations and related requirements for respiratory protection. *J Toxicol Environ Health B Crit Rev.* 11, 548-608, ISSN:1093-7404

Maeda, M., Nishimura, Y., Kumagai, N., Hayashi, H., Hatayama, T., Katoh, M., Miyahara, N., Yamamoto, S., Hirastuka, J. and Otsuki, T. (2010) Dysregulation of the immune system caused by silica and asbestos. *J Immunotoxicol.* 7, 268-278, ISSN:1547-691X

Matiba, B., Mariani, S.M. and Krammer, P.H. (1997) The CD95 system and the death of a lymphocyte. *Semin Immunol.* 9, 59-68, ISSN:1044-5323

Miura, Y., Nishimura, Y., Maeda, M., Murakami, S., Hayashi, H., Fukuoka, K., Kishimoto, T., Nakano, T. and Otsuki, T. (2008) Immunological alterations found in mesothelioma patients and their experimental evidences. *Environ Health Prev Med.* 13, 55-59, ISSN:1342-078X

Mountz, J.D. and Edwards, C.K. 3rd. (19929 Murine models of autoimmunity: T-cell and B-cell defects. Curr Opin Rheumatol. 4, 612-620, ISSN:1040-8711

Mudd, P.A., Teague, B.N. and Farris, A.D. (2006) Regulatory T cells and systemic lupus erythematosus. *Scand J Immunol.* 64, 211-218, ISSN:0300-9475

Mulloy, K.B. (2003) Silica exposure and systemic vasculitis. Environ Health Perspect. 111, 1933-1938, ISSN:0091-6765

Murakami, S., Nishimura, Y., Maeda, M., Kumagai, N., Hayashi, H., Chen, Y., Kusaka, K., Kishimoto, T. and Otsuki, T. (2009) Cytokine alteration and speculated immunological pathophysiology in silicosis and asbestos-related diseases. *Environ Health Prev Med.* 14, 216-222, ISSN:1342-078X

Nagata, S. and Golstein, P. (1995) The Fas death factor. Science. 267, 1449-1456, ISSN:0036-8075

Nagata, S. and Suda, T. (1995) Fas and Fas ligand: lpr and gld mutations. *Immunol Today.* 16, 39-43, ISSN:0167-5699

Nagata, S. (1996) Fas-mediated apoptosis. *Adv Exp Med Biol.* 406, 119-124, ISSN:0065-2598

Nagata, S. (1998) Human autoimmune lymphoproliferative syndrome, a defect in the apoptosis-inducing Fas receptor: a lesson from the mouse model. *J Hum Genet.* 43, 2-8, ISSN:1434-5161

Parks, C.G., Conrad, K. and Cooper, G.S. (1999) Occupational exposure to crystalline silica and autoimmune disease. Environ Health Perspect. 107S5, 793-802, ISSN:0091-6765

Nelson, B.H. and Willerford, D.M. (1998) Biology of the interleukin-2 receptor. *Adv Immunol.* 70, 1-81, ISSN:0065-2776

O'Connor, R.A. and Anderton, S.M. (2008) Foxp3+ regulatory T cells in the control of experimental CNS autoimmune disease. *J Neuroimmunol.* 193, 1-11, ISSN:0165-5728

Otsuki, T., Ichihara, K., Tomokuni, A., Sakaguchi, H., Aikoh, T., Matsuki, T., Isozaki, Y., Hyodoh, F., Kusaka, M., Kita, S. and Ueki, A. (1999) Evaluation of cases with silicosis using the parameters related to Fas-mediated apoptosis. *Int J Mol Med.* 4, 407-411, ISSN:1107-3756

Otsuki, T., Tomokuni, A., Sakaguchi, H., Aikoh, T., Matsuki, T., Isozaki, Y., Hyodoh, F., Ueki, H., Kusaka, M., Kita, S. and Ueki, A. (2000a) Over-expression of the decoy receptor 3 (DcR3) gene in peripheral blood mononuclear cells (PBMC) derived from silicosis patients. *Clin Exp Immunol.* 119, 323-327, ISSN:0009-9104

Otsuki, T., Sakaguchi, H., Tomokuni, A., Aikoh, T., Matsuki, T., Isozaki, Y., Hyodoh, F., Kawakami, Y., Kusaka, M., Kita, S. and Ueki, A. (2000b) Detection of alternatively spliced variant messages of Fas gene and mutational screening of Fas and Fas ligand coding regions in peripheral blood mononuclear cells derived from silicosis patients. *Immunol Lett.* 72, 137-143, ISSN:0165-2478

Otsuki, T., Tomokuni, A., Sakaguchi, H., Hyodoh, F., Kusaka, M. and Ueki, A. (2000c) Reduced expression of the inhibitory genes for Fas-mediated apoptosis in silicosis patients. *J Occup Health.*42, 163-168, ISSN:1341-9145

Otsuki, T., Miura, Y., Nishimura, Y., Hyodoh, F., Takata, A., Kusaka, M., Katsuyama, H., Tomita, M., Ueki, A. and Kishimoto, T. (2006) Alterations of Fas and Fas-related molecules in patients with silicosis. *Exp Biol Med (Maywood).* 231, 522-533, ISSN:1535-3702

Otsuki, T., Maeda, M., Murakami, S., Hayashi, H., Miura, Y., Kusaka, M., Nakano, T., Fukuoka, K., Kishimoto, T., Hyodoh, F., Ueki. A. and Nishimura, Y. (2007) Immunological effects of silica and asbestos. *Cell Mol Immunol.* 4, 261-268, ISSN:1672-7681

Pelucchi, C., Pira, E., Piolatto, G., Coggiola, M., Carta, P. and La Vecchia, C.(2006) Occupational silica exposure and lung cancer risk: a review of epidemiological studies 1996-2005. *Ann Oncol.* 17, 1039-1050, ISSN:0923-7534

Pizzolo, G. (1991) The soluble interleukin-2 receptor as a new biological marker in diseases. *Allergol Immunopathol (Madr).* 19, 176-180, ISSN:0301-0546

Porter, D.W., Millecchia, L., Robinson, V.A., Hubbs, A., Willard, P., Pack, D., Ramsey, D., McLaurin, J., Khan, A., Landsittel, D., Teass, A. and Castranova, V. (2002) Enhanced nitric oxide and reactive oxygen species production and damage after inhalation of silica. *Am J Physiol Lung Cell Mol Physiol.* 283, L485-493, ISSN:1040-0605

Rees, D. and Murray, J. (2007) Silica, silicosis and tuberculosis. *Int J Tuberc Lung Dis.* 11, 474-484, ISSN:1027-3719

Rimal, B., Greenberg, A.K. and Rom, W.N. (2005) Basic pathogenetic mechanisms in silicosis: current understanding. *Curr Opin Pulm Med.* 11, 169-173, ISSN:1070-5287

Rubin, L.A. and Nelson, D.L. (1990) The soluble interleukin-2 receptor: biology, function, and clinical application. *Ann Intern Med.* 113, 619-627, ISSN:0003-4819

Rudin, C.M., Van Dongen, J. and Thompson, C.B. (1996) Apoptotic signaling in lymphocytes. *Curr Opin Hematol.* 3, 35-40, ISSN:1065-6251

Sabol, S.L., Li, R., Lee, T.Y. and Abdul-Khalek, R. (1998) Inhibition of apoptosis-associated DNA fragmentation activity in nonapoptotic cells: the role of DNA fragmentation factor-45 (DFF45/ICAD). *Biochem Biophys Res Commun.* 253, 151-158, ISSN:0006-291X

Sakahira, H., Enari, M. and Nagata, S. (1998) Cleavage of CAD inhibitor in CAD activation and DNA degradation during apoptosis. *Nature.* 391, 96-99, ISSN:0028-0836

Saresella, M., Marventano, I., Longhi, R., Lissoni, F., Trabattoni, D., Mendozzi, L., Caputo, D., and Clerici, M. (2008) CD4+CD25+FoxP3+PD1- regulatory T cells in acute and stable relapsing-remitting multiple sclerosis and their modulation by therapy. *FASEB J.* 22, 3500-3508, ISSN:0892-6638

Schwartz, R.H. (2005) Natural regulatory T cells and self-tolerance. *Nat Immunol.* 6, 327-330, ISSN:1529-2908

Shanklin, D.R. and Smalley, D.L. (1998) The immunopathology of siliconosis. History, clinical presentation, and relation to silicosis and the chemistry of silicon and silicone. *Immunol Res.* 18, 125-173, ISSN:0257-277X

Sluis-Cremer, G.K., Hessel, P.A., Nizdo, E.H., Churchill, A.R. and Zeiss, E.A. (1985) Silica, silicosis, and progressive systemic sclerosis. *Br J Ind Med.* 42, 838-843, ISSN:0007-1072

Steenland, K. and Goldsmith, D.F. (1995) Silica exposure and autoimmune diseases. *Am J Ind Med.* 28, 603-608, ISSN:0271-3586

Steinberg, A.D. (1994) MRL-lpr/lpr disease: theories meet Fas. *Semin Immunol.* 6, 55-69, ISSN:1044-5323

Stockinger, B., Veldhoen, M. and Martin, B. (2007) Th17 T cells: linking innate and adaptive immunity. *Semin Immunol.* 19, 353-361, ISSN:1044-5323

Takata-Tomokuni, A., Ueki, A., Shiwa, M., Isozaki, Y., Hatayama, T., Katsuyama, H., Hyodoh, F., Fujimoto, W., Ueki, H., Kusaka, M., Arikuni, H. and Otsuki, T. (2005) Detection, epitope-mapping and function of anti-Fas autoantibody in patients with silicosis. *Immunology.* 116, 21-29, ISSN:0019-2805

Tervaert, J.W., Stegeman, C.A. and Kallenberg, C.G. (1998) Silicon exposure and vasculitis. *Curr Opin Rheumatol.* 10, 12-17, ISSN:1040-8711

Thakur, S.A., Beamer, C.A., Migliaccio, C.T. and Holian, A. (2009) Critical role of MARCO in crystalline silica-induced pulmonary inflammation. *Toxicol Sci.* 108, 462-471, ISSN:1096-6080

Tokano, Y., Miyake, S., Kayagaki, N., Nozawa, K., Morimoto, S., Azuma, M., Yagita, H., Takasaki, Y., Okumura, K. and Hashimoto, H. (1996) Soluble Fas molecule in the serum of patients with systemic lupus erythematosus. *J Clin Immunol.* 16, 261-265, ISSN:0271-9142

Toh, M.L. and Miossec, P. (2007) The role of T cells in rheumatoid arthritis: new subsets and new targets. *Curr Opin Rheumatol.* 19, 284-288, ISSN:1040-8711

Tomokuni, A., Aikoh, T., Matsuki, T., Isozaki, Y., Otsuki, T., Kita, S., Ueki, H., Kusaka, M., Kishimoto, T. and Ueki, A. (1997) Elevated soluble Fas/APO-1 (CD95) levels in silicosis patients without clinical symptoms of autoimmune diseases or malignant tumours. *Clin Exp Immunol.* 110, 303-309, ISSN:0009-9104

Tomokuni, A., Otsuki, T., Isozaki, Y., Kita, S., Ueki, H., Kusaka, M., Kishimoto, T. and Ueki, A. (1999) Serum levels of soluble Fas ligand in patients with silicosis. *Clin Exp Immunol.* 118, 441-444, ISSN:0009-9104

Toyokuni, S. (2009) Mechanisms of asbestos-induced carcinogenesis. *Nagoya J Med Sci.* 71, 1-10, ISSN:0027-7622

Uber, C.L. and McReynolds, R.A. (1982) Immunotoxicology of silica. *Crit Rev Toxicol.* 10, 303-319, ISSN:1040-8444

Ueki, A., Isozaki, Y., Tomokuni, A., Otsuki, T., Hydoh, F., Sakaguchi, H., Tanaka, S. and Kusaka, M. (2001) Is the anti-topoisomerase I autoantibody response associated with a distinct amino acid sequence in the HLA-DQbeta1 domain? *Arthritis Rheum.* 44, 491-492, ISSN:0004-3591

Ueki, A., Isozaki, Y., Tomokuni, A., Hatayama, T., Ueki, H., Kusaka, M., Shiwa, M., Arikuni, H., Takeshita, T. and Morimoto, K. (2002) Intramolecular epitope spreading among anti-caspase-8 autoantibodies in patients with silicosis, systemic sclerosis and systemic lupus erythematosus, as well as in healthy individuals. *Clin Exp Immunol.* 129, 556-561, ISSN:0009-9104

Ueki, A., Isozaki, Y., Tomokuni, A., Tanaka, S., Otsuki, T., Kishimoto, T., Kusaka, M., Aikoh, T., Sakaguchi, H. and Hydoh, F. (2001) Autoantibodies detectable in the sera of silicosis patients. The relationship between the anti-topoisomerase I antibody response and HLA-DQB1*0402 allele in Japanese silicosis patients. *Sci Total Environ.* 270, 141-148.

Ueki, H., Kohda, M., Nobutoh, T., Yamaguchi, M., Omori, K., Miyashita, Y., Hashimoto, T., Komai, A., Tomokuni, A. and Ueki, A. (2001) Antidesmoglein autoantibodies in silicosis patients with no bullous diseases. *Dermatology.* 202, 16-21, ISSN:0742-3217

Wang, W., Lau, R., Yu, D., Zhu, W., Korman, A, and Weber, J. (2009) PD1 blockade reverses the suppression of melanoma antigen-specific CTL by CD4+ CD25(Hi) regulatory T cells. *Int Immunol.* 21, 1065-1077, ISSN:0953-8178

Wu, P., Hyodoh, F., Hatayama, T., Sakaguchi, H., Hatada, S., Miura, Y., Takata-Tomokuni. A., Katsuyama, H. and Otsuki, T. (2005) Induction of CD69 antigen expression in peripheral blood mononuclear cells on exposure to silica, but not by asbestos/chrysotile-A. *Immunol Lett.* 98, 145-152, ISSN:0165-2478

Wu, P., Miura, Y., Hyodoh, F., Nishimura, Y., Hatayama, T., Hatada, S., Sakaguchi, H., Kusaka, M., Katsuyama, H., Tomita, M. and Otsuki, T. (2006) Reduced function of CD4+25+ regulatory T cell fraction in silicosis patients. *Int J Immunopathol Pharmacol.* 19, 357-368, ISSN:0394-6320

Yamazaki, S., Yoshiike, F., Hirai, K., Kakegawa, T., Ikeda, M., Nagata, A., Saito, G., Nishimura, H., Hosaka, N. and Ehara, T. (2007) Silica-associated systemic lupus erythematosus in an elderly man. *Intern Med.* 46, 1867-1871, ISSN:0918-2918

Yokoyama, T. and Amagai, M. (2010) Immune dysregulation of pemphigus in humans and mice. *J Dermatol.* 37, 205-213, ISSN:0385-2407

Yonehara, S. (2002) Death receptor Fas and autoimmune disease: from the original generation to therapeutic application of agonistic anti-Fas monoclonal antibody. *Cytokine Growth Factor Rev.* 13, 393-402, ISSN:1359-6101

Yu, J.W. and Shi, Y. (2008) FLIP and the death effector domain family. *Oncogene.* 27, 6216-6227, ISSN:0950-9232

Zerler, B. (1991) The soluble interleukin-2 receptor as a marker for human neoplasia and immune status. *Cancer Cells.* 3, 471-479, ISSN:1042-2196

Part 2

Pathogenetic Aspects of Organ Specific Autoimmune Diseases

10

Tolerance and Autoimmunity in Type 1 Diabetes

Valentina Di Caro[1,2], Nick Giannoukakis[1] and Massimo Trucco[1]
[1]Division of Immunogenetics, Department of Pediatrics, School of Medicine, University of Pittsburgh,
[2]Rimed Foundation,
[1]USA
[2]Italy

1. Introduction

A functional immune system is able to distinguish between foreign antigens expressed by pathogens and self-antigens expressed by the body. The absence of a pathological response to self-antigens (e.g. tolerance) is dependent on a number of events that occur both centrally and peripherally. Central tolerance is induced at sites of lymphocyte development such as thymus and bone marrow for T cell and B cell respectively. On the other hand, peripheral tolerance occurs at sites of antigen recognition and processing, and includes secondary lymphoid as well as non-lymphoid tissues. Failure of central and/or peripheral tolerance can lead to increased development and expansion of pathogenic effector T cells and subsequent initiation and progression of autoimmunity.

Type 1 Diabetes (T1D) is an autoimmune disease due to a chronic inflammation in the pancreas that leads to the destruction of insulin-producing β-cells. The β-cells are selectively destroyed via both direct and indirect mechanisms by different immune cell types. Studies in animal models and humans have demonstrated that T cells play a major role in β-cell death. However, other cell types are present in the pancreatic infiltrate and in the pancreatic lymph node, where the initial presentation of islet antigen by dendritic cells (DC) to islet antigen specific T cells occurs. Besides different DC subsets, B cells and natural killer (NK) cells also contribute, with different roles, to β-cell destruction. This suggests a strong crosstalk between the immune cells that are involved in pathogenesis and those involved in immune regulation.

Herein, we will describe the autoimmune processes that result in clinical manifestation of this disease and we will discuss the immunologic basis supporting possible new therapeutic interventions.

2. The breakdown of self-tolerance in Type 1 Diabetes

T1D is the most common autoimmune disorder in childhood but the disease may become manifest at any age, even in adults. In the past decade, the incidence of T1D has increased considerably among children under the age of 15 years in most developed countries and, if the present trend continues, the current incidence is predicted to double in European children younger than 5 years, by 2020 (Patterson et al., 2009).

Despite a plethora of data in rodent models of the disease, the etiology and pathogenesis of T1D in humans is largely unknown. The onset of the disease and clinical/diagnostic signs are preceded by a long non-clinical phase during which an aggressive autoimmune reaction is proposed to be taking place. Clinical T1D is the result of end-stage insulitis, and it has been estimated that at the time of diagnosis only 10–20% of the β-cells are still functioning.

Studies in the non-obese diabetic (NOD) mouse, a mouse model that spontaneously develops autoimmune diabetes, have highlighted the critical role of adaptive immune responses in the pathogenesis of the disease. Initial β-cell death occurs physiologically in NOD mice, at 2-3 weeks of age, during tissue remodeling and β-cell metabolic changes or it could occur by injury mediated, for example, by viral infections (Turley et al., 2003). Such β-cell death leads to activation of DC, priming and expansion of specific β-cell-autoreactive T cells, initially in the pancreatic draining lymph nodes and subsequently in the pancreas itself. Ultimately, this chronic process ends with enough β-cell mass destruction to need insulin therapy.

It is now well established that a specific genetic constitution is required to develop diabetes. The most important genes contributing to disease susceptibility in humans are located in the HLA class II locus on chromosome 6. Additionally ten other genes or genetic regions have been associated with T1D (Morel et al., 1988; Todd et al., 2007). Nevertheless a relatively small proportion, less than 10%, of individuals with HLA-conferred diabetes susceptibility progress to clinical disease. This implies that additional factors, very likely environmental, are needed to trigger and drive β-cell destruction in genetically predisposed individuals.

Several models illustrate hypotheses on the outcome of the interplay between genetic and environmental factors. The linear β-cell decline hypothesis originally postulated by Eisenbarth remains the most widely referenced benchmark model for T1D (Eisenbarth, 1986). According to this model, genetically susceptible individuals at some point in time encounter certain environmental agents that trigger islet autoimmunity leading to a linear decay in β-cell mass, development of autoantibodies, hyperglycemia, and eventually complete loss of C-peptide. While this view provides an explanation for the sequence of events observed during the course of T1D, it does not integrate factors contributing to the variability along the time axis during the prediabetic phase. Some authors argue that disease progression in T1D is not a linear process, but rather proceeds at variable steps in patients (Chatenoud & Bluestone, 2007). As mentioned before, there is an effect of specific genetic polymorphisms on disease susceptibility but, on the other hand, predisposing DNA sequence variations may by themselves never lead to T1D, or require some degree of environmental insult (viral infection) to culminate in hyperglycemia. Today a more detailed version of the nonlinear model depicting T1D as a "relapsing-remitting" disease has been proposed (Bonifacio et al., 1999; von Herrath et al., 2007; van Belle et al., 2011). Specifically, this model posits that a disequilibrium between autoreactive effector T cells and T regulatory cells could develop over time and eventually lead to a decline in β-cell mass. Whereas the net balance shifts to islet autoimmunity, this effect is temporarily counteracted by the β-cells' proliferative response, perhaps resulting in a late transient phase of reduced insulin requirement called the "honeymoon phase". In an attempt to fit the role of infectious agents into this temporal T1D model, Von Herrath and colleagues introduced the "fertile field" hypothesis (von Herrath et al., 2003). The fertile field is described as a time window that follows viral infection. It can vary depending on the type, anatomical location, and duration of the virus-induced inflammatory response. This fertile field would allow autoreactive T cells to expand and lead to full-blown autoimmunity and clinical T1D (Figure 1).

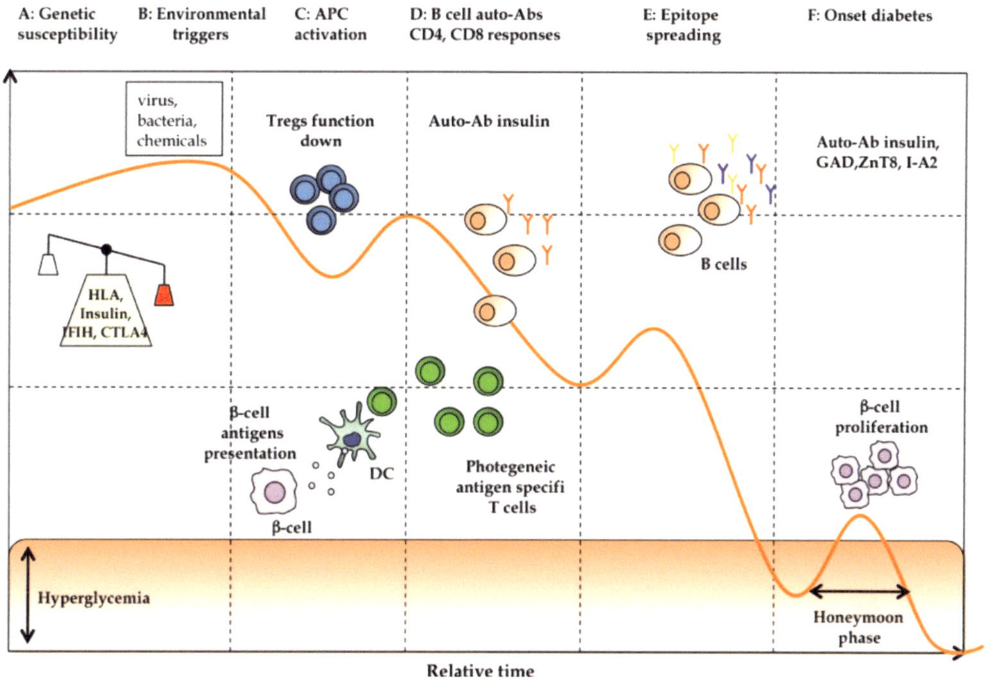

Fig. 1. How T1D might arise. The figure represents the β-cell mass or function (represented by the orange line) as well as the different immunological phases (columns with alphabetized tabs on top) that occur in the pancreas and peripherally. Once the orange line of β-cell function falls into the red zone, the individual is clinically diagnosed with T1D. Initially, a concurrence of genetic susceptibility and an environmental trigger sets an individual up for developing diabetes by causing β-cell death. In the pancreas, β-cell upregulate IFN and subsequently MHC class I. This exposes β-cell to attack by pathogenic antigen specific T cells. Consequently, the released β-cell antigens are picked up by resident APC and transferred to the pancreas-draining lymph nodes. Meanwhile in the periphery, a proinflammatory environment favors effector T cell responses over Treg function. β-cell antigens presented in this proinflammatory context and with CD4 help initiate conversion of B cells into plasma cells and the appearance of insulin autoantibodies . Also, autoreactive CD8 T cells are stimulated to proliferate and migrate into the pancreas. The stress induced by this second wave of β-cell killing causes some β-cell to stop insulin production. The killing also causes the release of new β-cell antigens that are picked up by APCs, including migrated B cells, which get shuttled to the pancreatic lymph node. This engages new antigen-specific clones of CD4 and CD8 T cells and B cells in a process called epitope spreading. Surprisingly, the autoimmune inflammation can also stimulate some β-cell proliferation so that the β-cell mass temporarily increases. The fluctuation between destructive autoreactive responses and β-cell proliferation may create a cyclical relapse-remitting profile of β-cell mass (orange line). Eventually, the autoreactive response wins though, and T1D is diagnosed when only 10 –30% of functional β-cell remains. The remission after clinically diagnosed diabetes is termed the honeymoon phase, a temporary state of relative self-sufficient insulin production.

3. Humoral β-cell autoimmunity

Human and murine T1D studies have shown that the appearance of autoantibodies is the first detectable pre-clinical sign of emerging β-cell autoimmunity. There are four disease-related autoantibodies that have been shown to predict clinical T1D (Knip et al., 2002). These include classical islet cell antibodies (ICA), insulin autoantibodies (IAA), and autoantibodies to the 65 kD isoform of glutamic acid decarboxylase (GADA) and the protein tyrosine phosphatase-related IA-2 molecule (IA-2A). Insulin is the first antigenic target detectable during the early progression of diabetes (Nakayama et al., 2005), although most autoantibodies are targeted against the β-cells themselves and other β-cell secreted proteins (Atkinson & Eisenbarth, 2001). Recently, ZnT8, a pancreatic β-cell specific zinc transporter, has been identified as a candidate autoantigen associated with T1D (Wenzlau et al., 2007). During the progression of T1D, a process of autoantigen epitope spreading occurs. Epitope spreading provides an explanation of how the immune system is capable of recognizing increasing numbers of autoantigens in correlation with increased T1D disease severity (von Herrath et al., 2007). Epitope spreading begins with the immune system recognizing and mounting an immune response against a single antigen, which is recognized via a single epitope. Over time, new antigens can be recognized, and previously recognized antigens can be differentially processed by antigen presenting cells to generate multiple epitopes for a single antigen (Morran et al., 2010).

The number and titer of detectable autoantibodies, rather than the specificity of the autoantibody, is unequivocally related to the risk of progression to overt T1D both in family studies and also in surveys based on general population cohorts. In family studies positivity for three to four autoantibodies is associated with a risk of developing clinical T1D in the range of 60–100% over the next 5–10 years (Barinas-Mitchell et al., 2004; Pietropaolo et al., 2005; Barker, 2006).

Islet specific autoantibodies are, however, considered more diagnostic than causative in T1D. It is generally accepted that the destruction of the β-cells is mediated by cellular immune responses. This is supported by the following facts: (a) T cells are present in insulitis; (b) disease progression is delayed by immunosuppressive drugs directed specifically against T cells; and (c) circulating autoreactive T cells can be detected in patients at clinical presentation of T1D (Roep, 2003).

4. Immune cell crosstalk in Type 1 Diabetes

4.1 T and B lymphocytes

Studies in NOD mice have shown that autoreactive T cells are released into the circulation because of faulty presentation of self-antigens by disease-susceptible MHC molecules that prevent negative selection in the thymus (Trucco, 1992; McDevitt, 2001). Central tolerance can be broken even in the presence of disease-resistant MHC molecules. Indeed, it has been demonstrated that disruption of thymic expression of a single tissue-specific gene self-molecule, as insulin for diabetes, is sufficient to trigger autoimmunity toward the specific tissue (Figure 2) (Fan et al., 2009).

In pre-diabetic mice, insulin specific T cells are the predominant component of islet-infiltrating T cells. Multiple $CD4^+$ and $CD8^+$ T cell clones, targeting different insulin epitopes, have been isolated (Wegmann et al., 1994) demonstrating that T1D development depends on both $CD4^+$ and $CD8^+$ T cells. Moreover, T1D can only be transferred to

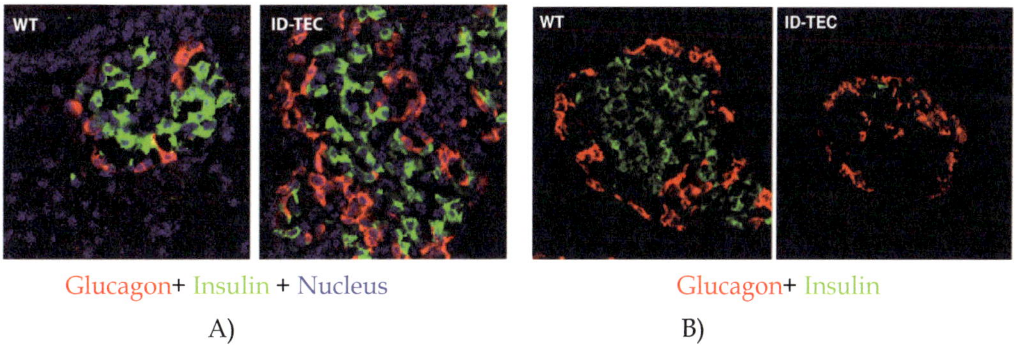

Fig. 2. Transgenic mice that do not express insulin in the thymus (ID-TEC) develop diabetes within 3 weeks. A) Normal islet development of transgenic mice at day 1 after birth; B) 4 week after birth only a small number of β-cells are still present in the islets. Pancreatic section stained using anti-insulin (green), and glucagon (red) antibodies (Fan et al., 2009).

immunocompromised syngeneic recipients by a combination of splenic $CD4^+$ and $CD8^+$ T cells from donor NOD mice but not by either T cell subset alone (Phillips et al., 2009).

There are several ways in which autoreactive T cells can mediate β-cell death. $CD8^+$ T cells may kill pancreatic β-cells through MHC class I mediated cytotoxicity, and both $CD4^+$ and $CD8^+$ T cells produce cytokines, such as interferon-γ (IFNγ), that induce expression of the death receptor Fas (CD95) and chemokine production by β-cells. Activation of Fas by Fas ligand (FasL)-expressing activated T cells can initiate β-cell apoptosis. Chemokine production by β-cells results in further recruitment of mononuclear cells to the site, thereby enhancing inflammation (Eizirik et al., 2009). In addition, IFNγ can activate macrophages and induce increased pro-inflammatory cytokine production, including interleukin-1β (IL-1β) and tumour necrosis factor (TNF). β-cells express high levels of IL-1 receptor and seem to be more sensitive to IL-1β-induced apoptosis than other endocrine cells in the islet. This crosstalk between T cells and macrophages undoubtedly exacerbates the immune-mediated stress on β-cells and contributes to their destruction. IFNγ, IL-1β and TNF also induce the expression of reactive oxygen species (ROS) including nitric oxide by β-cells, and ROS have the potential to mediate apoptosis.

Although T cells have a pathological role in T1D onset, there is also evidence supporting a role for a subset of T cells, the T regulatory cells (Tregs), able to prevent β-cell death.

Tregs play an indispensable role in maintaining homeostatic balance within the immune system. Tregs are involved in mediating normal immune responses against pathogens and terminating such responses when they are no longer required, as well as in preventing autoimmunity. Phenotypically, most Tregs express the surface marker CD25, the high affinity interleukin 2 (IL-2) receptor ligand-binding α chain, and Foxp3, an intracellular transcription factor (Fontenot et al., 2003). Because of that they are identified as $CD4^+CD25^+Foxp3^+$ cells. Both CD25 and Foxp3 coordinate Treg development and function. In the thymus, IL-2 is critical for the development of Tregs, while, in the periphery, it has been shown that interleukin 7 (IL-7) can complement potentially limiting amounts of IL-2 in promoting Treg survival and functional fitness (Di Caro et al., 2011).

Many studies in the NOD mouse strain have demonstrated the role of $CD4^+CD25^+Foxp3^+$ Tregs in the maintenance of self-tolerance. Indeed, depletion of CD25-expressing T cells results in a marked acceleration of T1D and $foxp3^{-/-}$ NOD mice display an increased incidence and earlier onset of the disease compared to wild type mice (Brunkow et al., 2001). In humans, patients with IPEX syndrome, who have a mutation in the *FOXP3* gene, develop endocrine autoimmune disease including T1D (Bennett et al., 2001). Tregs can control or limit the activation of $CD4^+$ and $CD8^+$ T cells at various stages such as differentiation and/or proliferation during priming in the draining lymph node, inhibition of IL-2 production or trafficking to the pancreas.

T cells are clearly of pivotal importance for T1D development, but there are also data suggesting an involvement of B-lymphocytes in initiation and progression of the disease. Recently, it was demonstrated that B cell depletion in NOD mice, either through gene targeting or antibody treatment, impaired the development of T1D (Hu et al., 2007) .

The investigation of the roles of B cells in autoimmune inflammatory diseases has focused mainly on the ability of B cells to secrete autoantibodies. More recently, B cells have been identified as important sources of pro- and anti-inflammatory cytokines, for example IL-6 and IL-10. B cells can either provide a quantitatively or functionally dominant source of cytokines. Moreover, they can have a role as antigen-presenting cells that maintain islet antigen-specific T cell activity (Hu et al., 2007; Pescovitz et al., 2009).

4.2 Innate immune cells

As islet antigen-specific T cells can differentiate into either pathogenic effector T cells or regulatory T cells, many studies have investigated the role of innate immune cells in T1D, as these cells usually determine a specific type of immune response. Innate cells producing pro- or anti-inflammatory cytokines define the milieu in which islet antigen specific T cells are activated and whether a deleterious or protective immune response occurs in the pancreas (Figure 3).

Macrophages are one of the two major antigen-presenting cells in islet infiltrates of NOD mice. It has been shown that inhibition of the macrophage influx into the pancreas, by blocking adhesion-promoting receptors on those cells, inhibited the development of T1D (Hutchings et al., 1990). *In vitro* and *in vivo* studies in mice and rats showed that the deleterious effect of macrophages on β-cells can be mediated through the production of TNF and IL-1β (Arnush et al., 1998; Dahlen et al., 1998). Interestingly, pro-inflammatory macrophages can be detected in pancreatic islets before T cell infiltration, as well as in NOD/*scid* (severe combined immunodeficient) mice, which lack functional B and T cells. Macrophages have been shown to produce IL-12 (Alleva et al., 2000) and to promote efficient differentiation of diabetogenic $CD8^+$ cytotoxic T lymphocytes (CTLs) leading to T1D onset (Jun et al., 1999). More recent data suggest that recruitment of macrophages to islets is mediated by the secretion of CC-chemokine ligand 1 (CCL1) and CCL2 by $CD4^+$ T cells and pancreatic β-cells, respectively (Cantor & Haskins, 2007; Martin et al., 2008). Macrophages recruited to the pancreas produce IL-1β, TNF and ROS that can cause β-cell death, revealing an additional role for macrophages in the destructive phase of T1D. Finally, TNF and IL-1β-producing macrophages have been observed in pancreatic islet infiltrates from patients with recent-onset T1D (Ueno et al., 2007). Together, these studies support a pathogenic role for macrophages in both the initiation and destruction phases of T1D at least in the mouse.

NK cells mediate early protection against viruses and are involved in the killing of infected cells and tumours. NK cells are both cytotoxic and producers of cytokines, particularly IFNγ. Thus, NK cells could contribute directly and indirectly to the destruction of β-cells.

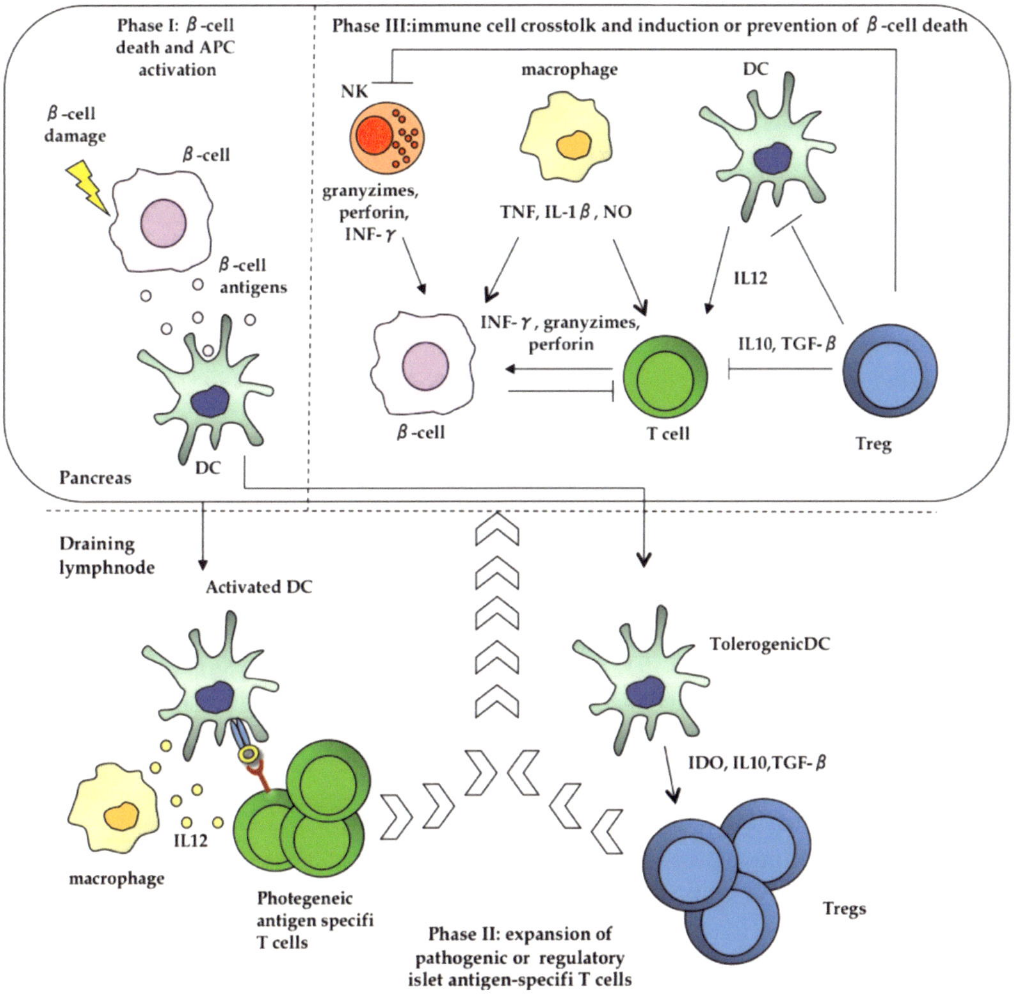

Fig. 3. Cellular and molecular mechanisms in the development or prevention of T1D. The initiation phase of T1D takes place in the pancreas, where DCs capture and process β-cell antigens. β-cell damage can occur by 'natural' apoptosis or after viral infections. Activated DCs prime pathogenic islet antigen-specific T cells after migration to the draining lymph nodes and macrophages promote this activation through IL-12 secretion. The activation of islet antigen-specific T cells can be inhibited by DCs through various mechanisms, such as expansion of Tregs through production of IDO, IL-10 and TGFβ. In the pancreas, β-cells can be killed by diabetogenic T cells and NK cells through the release of interferon-γ (IFNγ), granzymes and perforin, as well as by macrophages through the production of TNF, IL-1β and nitric oxide (NO). β-cell damage can be inhibited by Treg cells that inhibit diabetogenic T cells and innate immune cells through IL-10 and TGF-β. Tolerogenic DCs stimulated by NK cells could also control diabetogenic T cells through IDO production. Lastly, β-cells can inhibit diabetogenic T cells by expressing PDL1. This complex crosstalk between innate and adaptive immune cells results in the development or the prevention of T1D. (Figure adapted from Lehuen et al., 2010).

NK cells have been detected in the pancreas of patients with T1D and in T1D mouse models (Dotta et al., 2007; Alba et al., 2008; Brauner et al., 2010). Moreover, several reports have described a correlation between the frequency and/or activation of NK cells with the destructiveness of the pancreatic infiltrate (Poirot et al., 2004; Feuerer et al., 2009). NK cells isolated from the pancreas of diabetic mice have a more activated phenotype, proliferate more and spontaneously produce higher levels of IFNγ, which promote the effector function of diabetogenic $CD4^{+}$ T cell, and express CD107a on their cell surface, a marker of granule exocytosis, reflecting their cytotoxic function (Gur et al., 2010). Interestingly, NK cells were observed in the pancreas in NOD mice before T cell infiltration and in the pancreas of NOD-*Rag* mice, which lack mature B and T cells, suggesting that they could have a sentinel role in the pancreas.

Besides macrophages and NK cells, an important role in the pathogenesis of an autoimmune response is played by DCs. DCs are a heterogeneous population of antigen presenting cell that check tissue homeostasis, initiate T cell mediated immunity and control the maintenance of the immune tolerant state. It is known that patients with a congenital DC deficiency develop autoimmune diseases (Ohnmacht et al., 2009). This highlights their role in mediating peripheral tolerance. DCs, depending on their subset and function, can activate Tregs. It has been shown that they mediate peripheral tolerance by inducing T cell depletion or anergy and expansion of antigen specific Tregs (Ueno et al., 2007).

Studies aimed at elucidating the role of DCs in T1D have outlined beneficial as well as detrimental roles of this cell type in the autoimmune process. In the NOD/BDC2.5 transgenic mouse model, it was demonstrated that DCs prevent the inflammation process in the pancreas by producing indole 2,3-dioxygenase (IDO), a tryptophan catabolizing enzyme that arrests T cell proliferation (Saxena et al., 2007). However, in the same model, it was shown that IFN type 1 is more intimately involved in the initiation of the destructive autoimmunity and is correlated with the increased DC expression in the pancreatic lymph nodes (Li et al., 2008). Alternatively, these two opposite findings might point to a dual role of DC in the autoimmune process most probably depending on the stage of DC maturation and capacity to activate specific immunomodulatory cell types.

5. Immunotherapy to induce immunotolerance

Individuals with T1D develop hyperglycemia due to insufficient insulin production by β-cells in the pancreas. To prevent the rise of blood glucose to pathological levels, T1D patients have to receive a life long treatment with recombinant insulin. Despite insulin supplementation, rapid excursion of glucose levels, in these patients, increases the risk for severe complications such as cardiovascular diseases, nephropathy and neuropathy. Insulin replacement therapy cannot match the precision of endogenous insulin secretion, for this reason new treatments that, ideally, can cure the disease or at least delay/prevent the onset are needed.

The new emerging therapies for T1D, aimed at regulating the autoimmune response largely involve broad based immunoregulatory strategies, including the inhibition or deletion of lymphocytes subsets and/or the use of agents that induce or re-establish immune tolerance via activation of regulatory cells (Chatenoud, 2003; Luo et al., 2010).

5.1 Immunosuppressive drugs

Several randomized clinical trials (RCT), based on preclinical study in animal models, have been performed to test the effect of different immunosuppressive drugs on diabetes patients. Cyclosporin A (CSA) was employed in the first trials showing effects of immunosuppressive therapies on T1D. Continuous CSA treatment initiated soon after diagnosis eliminated the need for exogenous insulin (Bougneres et al., 1990; Carel et al., 1996). However, the lack of lasting effects and renal toxicity of the drug diminished enthusiasm for this approach. Indeed, in considering immunosuppressive therapies we have to remember that these drugs increase the risk of developing infections and malignancies and that some of them have been shown to inhibit β-cell regeneration (Nir et al., 2007). Within the multitude of immunosuppressive drugs, we are now focusing our overview on those drugs that are of particular interest because of their low levels of side effects and/or because they are able to induce Tregs or tolerogenic DCs.

5.1.1 Anti T-lymphocyte Globulin (ATG)

ATG is a very potent immunosuppressive drug. It depletes almost the entire T cell population in treated patients and is primarily used as inductive treatment after solid organ transplantation or in acute rejection settings in transplant patients. Since ATG is a polyclonal non-human protein mixture, common side effects include fever and serum sickness including arthralgia, rashes and lymphadenopathy. Administration over a longer period increases the risk for immunoproliferative disorders, which is why only short-term treatments are considered. A pilot trial involving new-onset T1D patients has shown a reduction of insulin requirement (Eisenbarth et al., 1985). In a more recent study, ATG (Fresenius) retarded the loss of C-peptide in new-onset patients without the need for continuous drug administration (Saudek et al., 2004) but additional studies are being performed to confirm these findings.

5.1.2 Anti-CD3

One of the most potent treatments at reversing new-onset diabetes in NOD mice is therapy with anti-CD3 mAb (Chatenoud et al., 1994). Chatenoud et al. showed that an intravenous treatment with anti-CD3 mAb resulted in a long-lasting restoration of normoglycemia in 80% of treated NOD mice. The treatment was given for only 5 days indicating that continuous administration might not be required to reach a beneficial effect through restoration of the immune balance in favor of endogens tolerance. These studies also showed that treatment was only effective if it was given shortly after the onset of hyperglycemia (Chatenoud, 2003). These results in NOD mice have led to trials in humans using humanized Fc-engineered monoclonal anti-CD3 antibodies. So far, two antibodies have been tested in diabetic patients, hOKT3 g1 Ala-Ala (Teplizumab) (Herold et al., 2005) and ChAglyCD3 (Otelixizumab) (Keymeulen et al., 2005), and both have shown positive results in patients with T1D in terms of C-peptide preservation and reduction of insulin requirements (Herold et al., 2002). Additionally, sustained C-peptide levels for approximately 2 years and in some cases up to 5 years were observed (Herold et al., 2005, Keymeulen et al., 2005). The side effects of anti-CD3 treatment were predominantly headaches, fever and arthralgia. Moreover gastrointestinal symptoms and most importantly transient EBV-viremia with symptoms of acute mononucleosis were observed. All patients however recovered spontaneously. The mechanism of action of this treatment has been extensively investigated. It can be demonstrated that anti-CD3 treatment modulates the T cell receptors in a way that renders T cells blind to antigens, induces T cell anergy, blocks the IL-2 signaling pathway, and induces apoptosis (Chatenoud & Blustone, 2007).

Interestingly, it has also been shown that Tregs are less susceptible to anti-CD3 induced apoptosis; at least when administered in low doses, thus leading to higher numbers of T regulatory cells under the generalized CD3+ T cell lymphopenia. Taken together, these data have made anti-CD3 antibody a possible candidate for future combination therapies. However, the anti CD3 based phase III clinical trial by Lilly didn't meet the target of the trial and the use of anti-CD3 is no longer being pursued by this commercial entity (http://www.fiercepharma.com/press_releases/macrogenics-and-lilly-announce-pivotal-clinical-trial-teplizumab-did-not-meet-primary).

5.1.3 Anti-CD20

B cells are implicated in the pathogenesis of diabetes. Hu et al., (2007) and Xiu et al., (2008) have shown that diabetes can be prevented in NOD mice by depleting B cells with anti-CD20 mAb before and at the time of onset of hyperglycemia (9–12-week-old mice) and can even reverse disease in about 30% of animals treated at the first appearance of hyperglycemia. Interestingly, cotransfer of B cells from the successfully treated mice diminished the rate of adoptive transfer of disease via T cells, suggesting a possible role for

Agent	Target mechanism	Phase/ ID	Details	Reference
Cyclosporin A	Immune suppression	Completed	Remission successful during treatment but severe side effects	Bougneres et al., 1990, Carel et al., 1996.
Teplizumab Anti CD3 (hOKT3) g1 Ala-Ala	T cell immunomodulation and treg generation by anti Cd3 mAb	Phase III	Primary end point not achieved	
Otelixizumab Anti CD3 (ChAgly CD3)	T cell immunomodulation and treg generation by anti Cd3 mAb	Phase II	6 day treatment: better maintenance of C-peptide levels, reduced insulin requirement out to 18 mo	Chatenoud et al., 1994; Keymeulen et al., 2005.
Rituximab (Anti-CD20 mAb)	B cell depletion	Phase II	Preservation of C-peptide levels for 3/6 months	Prescovitz et al., 2009; Hu et al., 2007.
ATG	T cell depletion generate Treg population	Phase II	Could cause cytokine release syndrome	Simon et al, 2008.

Table 1. Summary of immunotherapy approaches in T1D using antibodies.

activation of "regulatory" B cells. Others have shown that IL-10-producing B cells can be induced in mice depleted of $CD20^+$ B cells (Yanaba et al., 2008).
In a recent phase II clinical trial, depletion of B cells using an anti-CD20 mAb (Rituximab), has shown modest (23%) but significant improvement in β-cell function 3 months after diagnosis and overall at 1 year, in antibody-treated compared to placebo-treated subjects (Pescovitz et al., 2009). There were also significant improvements in clinical parameters including glycated hemoglobin A1c, C-peptide level and insulin use. Side effects that appear frequently are mostly related to the administration itself and decrease over the course of the therapy. However the patients eventually returned to hyperglycemia as B cells reappeared to a great extent (69%) by the end of the year and the C-peptide level started to decline.
This study could ultimately prove that there is a role for B cells in disease pathogenesis, which is scientifically of great interest. However, B cell depletion in this setting does not appear to mediate a significant deceleration of disease progression.

5.2 Anti-inflammatory treatments

5.2.1 Cytokine and cytokine receptor-directed therapies

Cytokine and cytokine receptor-directed therapies are also in development for treatment of T1D. Human insulitis shows a considerably greater infiltration of innate immune cells such as macrophages and NK compared to NOD insulitis (Itoh et al., 1993; Dotta et al., 2007). Moreover, innate mediators (TNF-α, IL-1, and type 1 interferons) were among the first molecules shown to have direct cytotoxic effects on β-cells and were postulated to be the direct cause of β-cell killing (Rabinovitch et al., 1990). Possibly because of its innate role in activating adaptive immune responses, it was not surprising that IL-1 receptor-deficient NOD mice had reduced development of diabetes (Thomas et al., 2004). Treatment with the IL-1 receptor antagonist (Anakinra) was shown to improve glucose control in patients with T2D (Donath & Mandrup-Poulsen, 2008). Interestingly, the drug mechanism appeared to involve a beneficial effect on β-cells, reflected by an increase in the insulin:proinsulin ratio. β-cells may be a source of IL-1, particularly in response to glucose, suggesting a destructive cycle in which hyperglycemia induces expression of the inflammatory mediator resulting in immune activation and further β-cell destruction. Initial preclinical data do not suggest that IL-1 blockade alone will prevent or reverse T1D, but this could be an important target of a combination strategy.
TNF-α is considered to play an active role in the pathogenesis of T1D. TNF-α is directly cytotoxic to β-cells, suggesting this cytokine as an additional possible target for immune therapy. In a small pilot trial in children and adolescents early after diagnosis (< 30 days on average), the use of a TNF antagonist (Etanercept) resulted in preservation of residual insulin secretion compared with placebo (Mastrandrea et al., 2009). C-peptide loss was reduced, as well as a decrease in insulin needs. However there are contrasting data about targeting the TNF-α pathways. Indeed, it has been shown, *in vitro*, that selective $CD8^+$ autoreactive Tcell death induction can be activated by TNF-α, suggesting the use of a TNF agonist instead of a TNF antagonist (Ban et al., 2008). The discrepancy could be due to the timing of TNF-α blockade/ TNF-α administration.

5.3 Antigen specific strategies

Establishment of a simple strategy that results in the emergence of antigen-specific regulatory T cells and the induction of tolerance to autoantigens is a desirable goal. It would ultimately stop the autoimmune process without inducing some of the major side effects that have been observed, for example, in chemical and antibody-based immunosuppressive treatments. Moreover, individuals at risk could be treated prior to significant destruction of β-cell mass and clinical onset of disease. However, the risk of boosting autoreactivity should never be underestimated. As outlined earlier, several autoantigens have been described in T1D; insulin and GAD65 are believed to be the major autoantigens that drive the autoreactivity. Consequently they have been studied most intensively in terms of inducing tolerance in humans.

5.3.1 Insulin

Several clinical trials target insulin because it is the initiating antigen in the NOD model and is also a major autoantigen in human T1D (Nakayama et al., 2005; Fan et al., 2009). There have been a number of human new-onset trials using insulin therapy. In the immunotherapy diabetes (IMDIAB) trial, a total of 82 patients with clinical T1D were randomized to receive oral insulin or placebo (Pozzilli et al., 2000). At a 1-year follow-up, there was no difference between the insulin-treated and the placebo-treated groups with respect to mean C-peptide secretion, requirement for insulin therapy, or IgG insulin antibodies. Furthermore, in patients younger than 15 years, a tendency for low C-peptide at 9 and 12 months was observed in the oral insulin group, suggesting acceleration in the decline of β-cell function. These results are consistent with those seen in murine models where oral insulin was shown not to reverse new-onset diabetes (Fousteri et al., 2007). Interestingly, if nasal insulin therapy is used in combination with anti-CD3 therapy, a significant benefit in reversing recent-onset diabetes is then achieved in two animal models of autoimmune diabetes (Bresson et al., 2006). Expansion of insulin-specific Treg cells producing IL-10, TGF-β, and IL-4, and possibly their modulation of antigen-presenting cells in local draining lymph nodes, were proposed as likely mechanisms. These findings should provide the basis for using combinatorial therapies in future trials for humans with recent-onset diabetes.

A recent phase I study using a single intramuscular injection of human insulin B chain in incomplete Freund's adjuvant in 12 subjects with recent-onset diabetes showed that this therapy led to the development of lasting (at a 2 year follow-up) insulin B chain-specific Tregs (Orban et al., 2009). This study provides the basis for testing this modality of insulin B chain therapy in a larger T1D trial to determine the effect on glycemic level. Another ongoing phase I–II clinical trial of subcutaneous BHT-3021, a plasmid encoding proinsulin, is testing the safety, dose, and preliminary efficacy of this therapeutic modality in recent-onset T1D patients

5.3.2 Glutamate decarboxylase 65

Immune therapies using GAD65 have also been tested in both animal models and human T1D. Interestingly, the initial antigenic region is confined to a few epitopes near the C terminus of the GAD protein but later spreads intramolecularly to other GAD determinants, followed by further intermolecular spreading to other β-cell antigens. Consequently, tolerance induction by intravenous or intrathymic injections of GAD in female NOD mice at 3 weeks of age eliminates the anti-GAD T cell responses, as well as subsequent spreading of the cascade of T cell responses to other β-cell antigens and the development of insulitis or clinical diabetes (Tisch et al., 1993). Intravenous injections of GAD during the later stages of disease still effectively blocked disease progression in prediabetic mice and protected syngeneic islet graft survival in diabetic NOD mice (Tian et al., 1996). The identification of Tregs in GAD-treated mice suggests a major role in the induction of tolerance by treatment with this autoantigen, which raises the question of whether GAD is targeted early in T1D (Tisch et al., 1998).

Agent	Target mechanism	Phase/ ID	Details	Reference
Anakinra (IL1 antagonist)	Anti-inflammatory and improve β-cell survival	Phase II/III	Recruiting	Pickersgill et al., 2009
Etanercept (TNF-α blockade)	Anti-inflammatory	Phase II/III	Low HbA1C and insulin need, increased C-peptide	Mastrandrea et al., 2009
Insulin in IFA	Tolerance vaccination to insulin B chain	Phase I/II	Ongoing	Orban et al., 2009.
BHT-3021	Tolerance vaccination to insulin	Phase I/II	Reduce insulin Ab titers, preserved C-peptide and reduce HbA1c	Gottlieb, 2009.
GAD-Alum	Tolerance to GAD65 skewing Th1 to Th2	Phase II Phase III	Preservation of residual insulin secretion, GAD specific humoral and cellular response, Ongoing in Europe and USA	Agardh et al., 2009; Ludvigsson et al., 2008
Diap277	Induction of Tregs via TLRs	Phase III	Phase I: preserved C-peptide Phase II: no effect in T1D adults and children Phase III: recruiting	Raz et al., 2001; Lazar et al., 2007; Schloot et al., 2007

Table 2. Summary of immunotherapy approach in T1D using autoantigens, cytokines or cytokine-specific antibodies.

Promising preclinical data in the NOD model prompted two clinical trials using alum-formulated human recombinant GAD65. A phase II safety and dose-finding trial conducted in patients with latent autoimmune diabetes in adults (LADA) (Agardh et al., 2005) showed the approach to be safe, and administration of two subcutaneous doses led to an increase of fasting and stimulated C-peptide at 24 weeks compared to baseline, a benefit that was associated with an increase in $CD4^{+}CD25^{+}$ Treg cells. In a second trial, in recent-onset T1D children between 10 and 18 years of age, a slower decline of fasting and stimulated C-peptide in the GAD-alum group was observed compared to the placebo (Ludvigsson et al., 2008). More importantly, the protective effect of GAD-alum was preferentially seen in those who received treatment within 6 months of diagnosis, suggesting that the autoimmune process is more susceptible to GAD-based modulatory therapy if initiated at an earlier stage.

5.3.3 Heat shock protein

Early controversies existed as to whether heat shock proteins (hsp) were true autoantigens implicated in the pathogenesis of T1D (Atkinson & Eisenbarth, 2001). However, extensive preclinical studies using the hsp60 peptide p277 demonstrated efficacy of peptide vaccination in halting disease progression in NOD mice (Elias et al., 1991; Elias & Cohen, 1995). p277 treatment appeared to promote Th2-type cell responses with upregulation of IL-10 and IL-13 and downregulation of IFN-γ (Elias et al., 1997; Jin et al., 2008). p277 also has inhibitory effects on the innate immune system via signaling through TLR-2, leading to inhibition of inflammatory lymphocyte chemotaxis (Nussbaum et al., 2006). The equivalent of human hsp60 p277 is a 24 amino acid synthetic peptide derived from the C terminus of the human hsp60, termed DiaPep277. Several phase I and II clinical trials in human T1D patients have been completed in Europe, and phase III trials are underway. A phase II trial was conducted in patients with established T1D but with residual β-cell function (Huurman et al., 2007) and used a range of doses of subcutaneously administered DiaPep277. Results showed a trend of dose-dependent preservation of stimulated C-peptide secretion. Three additional trials were conducted in new-onset T1D patients (Raz et al., 2001; Lazar et al., 2007; Schloot et al., 2007). Two of these trials enrolled adult TID patients, whereas the third enrolled pediatric T1D patients. The adult trials showed significantly better preservation of insulin synthesis as measured by C-peptide production in the treated groups compared with placebo, but this effect was not seen in the pediatric trial. Similar results were observed in one other trial performed in pediatric patients (Schloot et al., 2007), although in children with less aggressive disease progression based on genetic background, there appeared to be a trend to better preserved C-peptide at the end of the study period. In summary, phase II trials with DiaPep277 have shown some promise in preserving residual β-cell function, which appears to be less effective in patients with more aggressive disease. A phase III trial is underway with results expected in later 2011.

6. Cell therapy in type 1 diabetes

Cellular adoptive-transfer-based approaches have shown significant promise preclinically in the NOD model, both in prediabetic and postdiabetic stages. The idea is to compensate a presumed deficiency in tolerogenic cells or tolerogenic cell/molecular signaling pathways by transferring cell types with immunomodulatory capacity. Specifically, both *ex vivo* expanded Tregs or induced $CD4^{+}CD25^{+}Foxp3^{+}$ Tregs (iTreg) have been shown to control ongoing autoimmunity and either prevent progression to diabetes or protect syngeneic islet grafts and/or allow β-cell recovery, thus inducing diabetes remission in NOD mice (Tang & Bluestone, 2006; Weber et al., 2006; Luo et al., 2007; Godebu et al., 2008). It is unclear whether antigen specificity is critically important in this approach because both nonspecifically-expanded polyclonal or induced Tregs and islet antigen-specific Tregs have shown efficacy in controlling the disease. Additionally, it also appears that Tregs of one antigen specificity may be sufficient in controlling ongoing autoimmunity that is probably caused by autoaggressive T cells of multiple islet antigen specificities (Tarbell et al., 2004; Luo et al., 2007). Clearly delineating these characteristics of Treg adoptive-transfer therapy will have significant impact on the design of future clinical trials using this modality.

Another strategy for enhancing Treg numbers *in vivo* is by DC-based therapy. It has been shown that direct injection of either DC from pancreatic draining lymph nodes or β-cell antigen-pulsed immature DC protects prediabetic NOD mice from developing overt diabetes, possibly through the *in vivo* induction of Treg cells (Clare-Salzler et al., 1992; Lo et al., 2006). However, direct *ex vivo* DC therapy carries the potential risk of their acquiring an activated phenotype upon adoptive transfer, leading to immune activation to some antigen(s) rather than tolerance.

6.1 Diabetes-suppressive dendritic cells

Methods to stably maintain DC in an immature state, defined by low levels of surface costimulatory proteins that include CD80, CD86 and CD40, by downregulating these proteins or blocking their interaction with their ligands, are at the forefront of tolerogenic biologicals like the CTLA4-Ig protein. These strategies result in tolerance to allografts and prevention of autoimmune disease. We have considered two strategies to maintain DCs in a stably-immature state. The first involves *ex vivo* treatment with short double-stranded decoys of the NF-kappaB transcription factor and the second involves *ex vivo* treatment of DCs with antisense oligonucleotides (AS-ODN DC) targeting the primary transcripts of CD40, CD80 and CD86 concurrently. Both DC products are able to prevent and to reverse new onset T1D (Ma et al., 2003; Machen et al., 2004; Trucco & Giannoukakis, 2007; Giannoukakis et al., 2008). These preclinical studies have led to a recently completed phase I trial using autologous *ex vivo*-engineered DC from established diabetic patients (clinicaltrials.gov identifier NCT00445913), conducted at the University of Pittsburgh Medical Center (UPMC), to determine safety as a primary end-point (Figure 4).

Mechanistically, functionally immature DCs, with low to absent costimulatory molecule expression, mediate peripheral tolerance by inducing T cell anergy and the expansion of antigen specific $Foxp3^+$ $CD25^+$ $CD4^+$ Treg (Ueno et al., 2007).

In our approach, AS-ODN DCs promote Treg cell survival through IL-7 signaling in addition to impaired provision of CD40, CD80 and CD86 costimulation (Harnaha et al., 2006). AS-ODN DCs, but not control DC, produce IL-7, in response to a secondary action of the antisense oligonucleotides on Toll Like Receptor (TLR) signaling. It is known that CpG oligonucleotides, like the AS-ODN we use to make tolerogenic DCs, can activate TLR signaling and confer an immunoregulatory phenotype to DCs (Roberts et al., 2005; Jarnicki et al., 2008) and are thus useful for treatment of autoimmune conditions (Ho et al., 2005). It is possible that the oligonucleotides act in a sequence-nonspecific manner when interacting with TLRs, TLR9 in particular, based on conformation and higher order multistrand structures (Guiducci et al., 2008; Kindrachuk et al., 2008). For example, certain multimer formations or conformations would induce non-MyD88 signaling pathways, whereas others

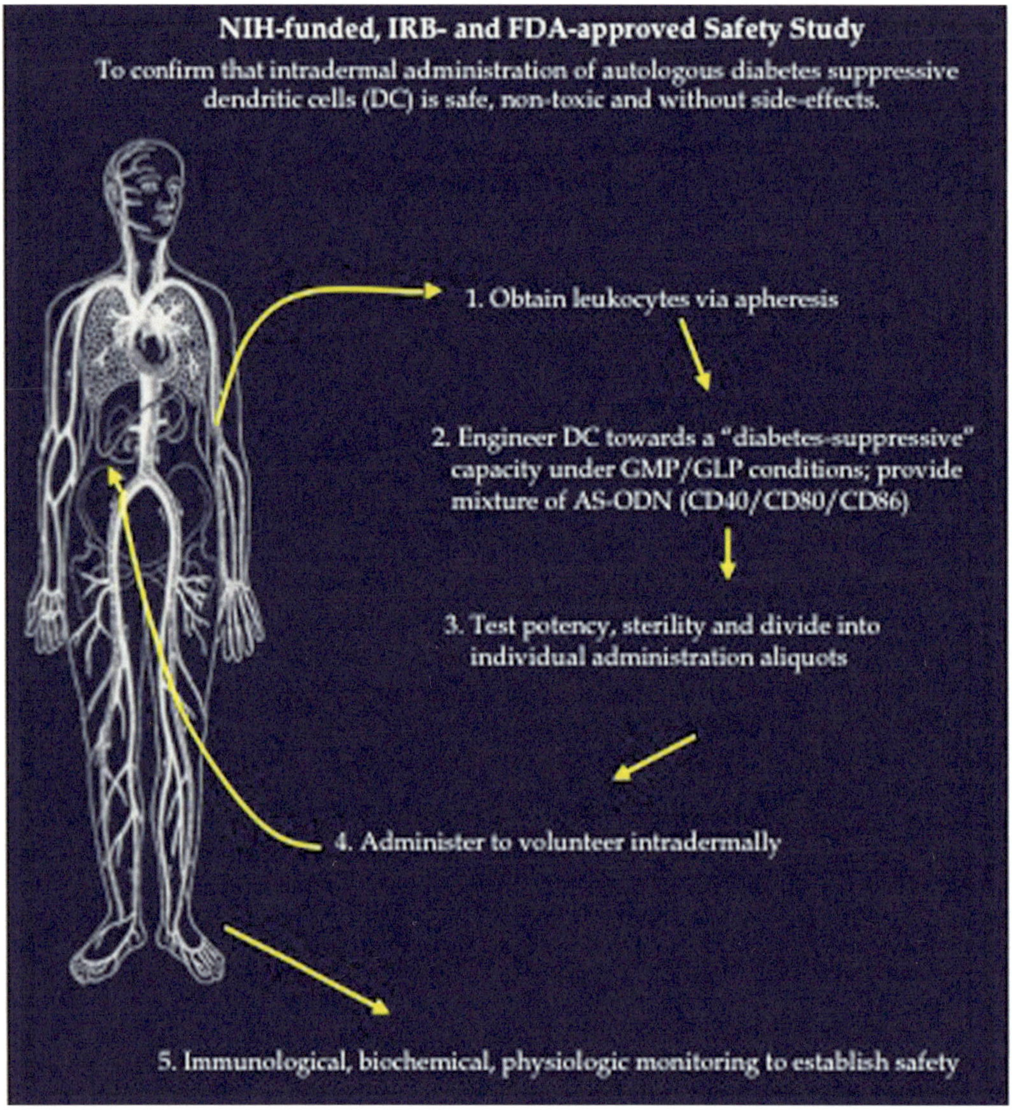

Fig. 4. DC-based clinical trial for T1D. Schematic of the procedures involved in the phase I clinical trial recently completed at the University of Pittsburgh to prove the safety of the DC-based vaccine. (Giannoukakis et al., 2008)

would recruit MyD88. We propose a model where AS-ODN treatment results in a coordinate downregulation of CD40, CD80 and CD86 and induction of IL-7 production via non-MyD88 TLR signals. At this time it is unclear which of the DNA-sensing TLRs transduces the AS-ODN effects. TLR3, TLR7, TLR8 and TLR9 are all equally possible, although the effect of chloroquine on IL- 7 production would suggest an endosomal TLR with TLR9 being the most likely candidate (Figure 5) (Di Caro & Giannoukakis, unpublished data). Indeed, the data indicating that CpG oligonucleotide-triggered TLR9 signaling confers immunosuppressive capacity to DC that can treat autoimmunity *in vivo* strengthens our hypothesis (Ho PP et al., 2005).

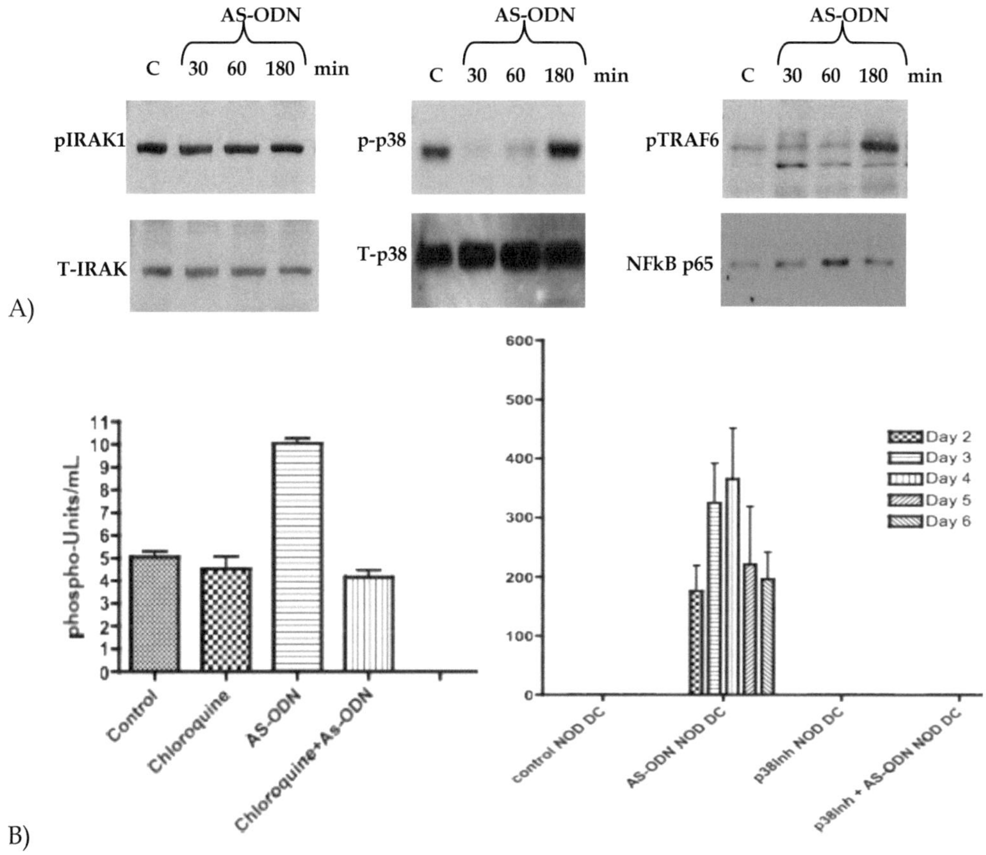

Fig. 5. AS-ODN treatment of DC *in vitro* activates TLRs signals leading to IL-7 production. A) Western blot analysis of protein extracts from DC treated with AS-ODN for CD40, CD80 and CD86 over time, using the indicated antibodies, shows activation of NFkB after 1 hour and activation of p38 MAP kinase and TRAF6 after 3 hours. B) p38 MAP kinase phosphorylation in AS-ODN DC in the presence of chloroquine, a specific inhibitor of endosomal TLR signaling (e.g. TLR9), is decreased, as demonstrated by LUMINEX-based nuclear transcription factor analysis. C) inhibition of p38 phosphorylation, using the p38 MAP Kinase inhibitor SB203580, shows a complete abrogation of IL-7 production for each of the 7 days of generation of the AS-ODN DC.

Recently, we identified a novel $CD127^+$ $CD25^+$ $Foxp3^+$ T cell subpopulation that expresses the IL-7 receptor (CD127) and has immunosuppressive activity (Figure 6). More interestingly, exposure of this novel T cell subpopulation to IL-7 *in vitro* results in the phenotypic maturation of $CD127^+$ $CD25^+$ $Foxp3^+$ T cells to the classical $CD25^{HIGH}$ $Foxp3^+$ Treg (Figure 7) (Di Caro et al., 2011).

IL-7 production by the AS-ODN DC could serve to mature the $CD127^+$ $Foxp3^+$ cells into powerfully suppressive $CD25^{HIGH}$ $Foxp3^+$ Tregs, and maintain their survival for a longer time period, especially when the IL-2 concentration in the lymphoid environment is expected to be limiting, given the competition among $CD25^+$ Tregs and $CD25^+$ effector T cells for this critical cytokine. Furthermore, the apparent biregulation of cell surface CD25

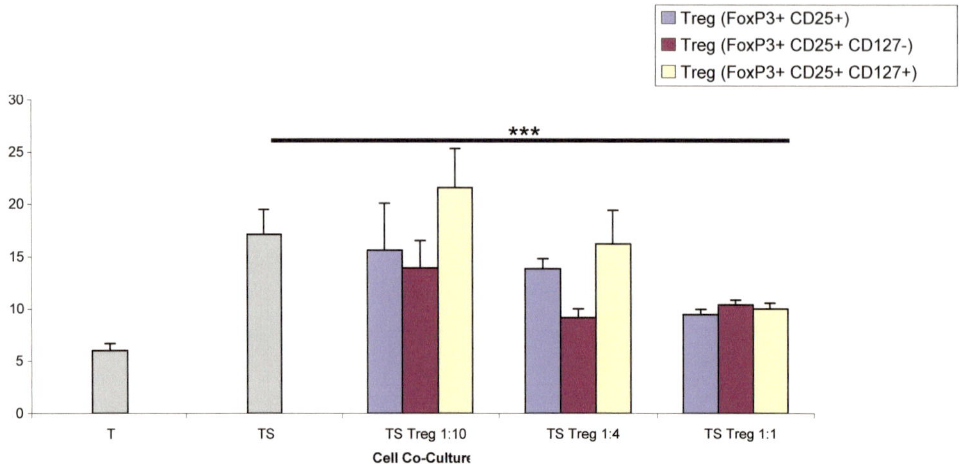

Fig. 6. CD127$^+$ CD25$^+$ Foxp3$^+$ T cell are functionally suppressive *in vitro*. Highly enriched, flow sorted CD4$^+$CD25$^+$CD127$^+$ splenic T cells, isolated form FoxP3 promoter-GFP transgenic mice, are suppressive when added to a co-culture of syngeneic T cells and allogeneic, irradiated, splenocytes (Di Caro et al., 2011).

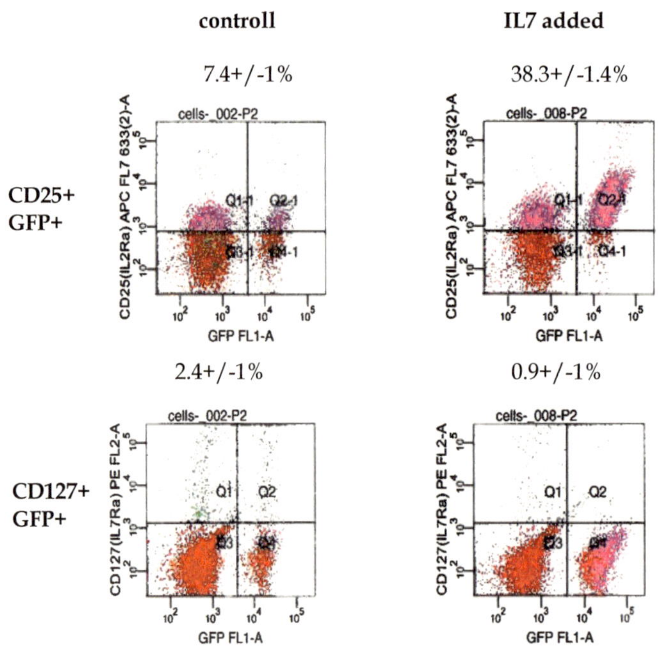

Fig. 7. IL-7 promotes an increase in prevalence of CD127$^-$CD25$^+$Foxp3$^+$ cells. Incubation of splenic CD4$^+$GFP$^+$ T cells from Foxp3 promoter-GFP transgenic mice with IL-7 overnight results in an increase in CD25$^+$GFP$^+$ T cells, whereas IL-7 downregulates the prevalence of CD127$^+$ GFP$^+$ cells (Di Caro et al., 2011).

and CD127 on Tregs in response to their respective ligand availability and signaling, in peripheral lymphoid organs, could have two functions; Treg maintenance and suppressive competency. IL-7 could best serve Tregs under homeostatic conditions in the periphery where IL-2 production would be low. This would maintain a pool of CD4+ $CD25^{HIGH}$ Tregs as some type of "memory" Treg population. In contrast, in an environment where IL- 2 would be acutely produced at high levels (i.e. vigorous proliferation of autoreactive T-cells), Tregs would compete as well as the effector T cells for IL-2 and therefore, IL-7 might not be as relevant.

Through these mechanisms and others yet unknown, tolerogenic DC could modulate and restore the balance of pro and anti-inflammatory components of the immune system. Our data and the work carried out by other groups highlights the relevance of using tolerogenic DC to treat autoimmune diabetes as well as other tissue specific autoimmune disorders.

7. Conclusion

T1D most likely results from a combination of genetic susceptibility and exposure to an environmental trigger. The main effector mechanism is clearly an autoimmune reaction, which is also evident at time of clinical diagnosis. A better knowledge of the causes that lead to T1D is critical for prevention as well as for developing new therapies. Early detection is also required to maximally preserve the remaining β-cell mass, because the ability to secrete even small amounts of insulin can make disease control easier and help minimize the complications due to chronic inadequate glycemic control.

Much of our current understanding of T1D comes from the NOD mouse model, this autoimmune diabetes model, so far, has been useful to discover and develop treatments even if some of them were not as successful in humans (e.g. the anti-CD3 therapy).

Today the landscape of possible treatment has been changed by the prospect that T1D progression may be blocked by the active stimulation of tolerance induced by autoantigen-specific Tregs or tolerogenic DCs. The ultimate goal of autoimmune therapy is to silence the immune attack against self without sacrificing the patient's protective immune response to pathogens. This will most likely be achieved by a therapy that combines a nonspecific immune suppressant and the induction of Tregs/ tolerogenic DCs. Regardless of the tolerogenic method employed for therapy, we think that early intervention in T1D patients is critical to prevent ongoing islet destruction and to establish an ideal microenvironment to allow the recovery of a normal β-cell mass from endogenous progenitor cells. The chances for disease prevention will be improved by the identification of biomarkers identifying patients at risk as early in the disease process as possible.

Major efforts on several fronts are still required to fully realize the benefits of the technological and scientific advances in autoimmune diabetes research even if substantial improvements in the cure of T1D patients were indeed promoted.

8. References

Agardh, C.D.; Cilio, C.M.; Lethagen, A.; Lynch, K.; Leslie, R.D.; Palmer, M.; Harris, R.A.; Robertson, J.A. & Lernmark, A. (2005). Clinical evidence for the safety of GAD65 immunomodulation in adult-onset autoimmune diabetes. *J Diabetes Complications*, Vol.19, (4), pp.238-246, ISSN 1056-8727

Alba, A.; Planas, R.; Clemente, X.; Carrillo, J.; Ampudia, R.; Puertas, M.C.; Pastor, X.; Tolosa, E.; Pujol-Borrell, R.; Verdaguer, J.&Vives-Pi, M. (2008). Natural killer cells are required for accelerated type 1 diabetes driven by interferon-beta. *Clin Exp Immunol*, Vol.151, (3), pp.467-475, ISSN 1365-2249

Alleva, D.G.; Pavlovich, R.P.; Grant, C.; Kaser, S.B. & Beller, D.I. (2000). Aberrant macrophage cytokine production is a conserved feature among autoimmune-prone mouse strains: elevated interleukin (IL)-12 and an imbalance in tumor necrosis factor-alpha and IL-10 define a unique cytokine profile in macrophages from young nonobese diabetic mice. *Diabetes*, Vol.49, (7), pp.1106-1115, ISSN 0012-1797

Arnush, M.; Scarim, A.L.; Heitmeier, M.R.; Kelly, C.B. & Corbett, J.A. (1998). Potential role of resident islet macrophage activation in the initiation of autoimmune diabetes. *J Immunol*, Vol.160, (6), pp.2684-2691, ISSN 0022-1767

Atkinson, M.A. & Eisenbarth, G.S. (2001). Type 1 diabetes: new perspectives on disease pathogenesis and treatment. *Lancet*, Vol.358, (9277), pp.221-229, ISSN 0140-6736

Ban, L.; Zhang, J.; Wang, L.; Kuhtreiber, W.; Burger, D. & Faustman, D.L. (2008). Selective death of autoreactive T cells in human diabetes by TNF or TNF receptor 2 agonism. *Proc Natl Acad Sci U S A*, Vol.105, (36), pp.13644-13649, ISSN 1091-6490

Barinas-Mitchell, E.; Pietropaolo, S.; Zhang, Y.J.; Henderson, T.; Trucco, M.; Kuller, L.H. & Pietropaolo. M. (2004). Islet cell autoimmunity in a triethnic adult population of the Third National Health and Nutrition Examination Surveys (NHANES) III. *Diabetes*, Vol.53, pp.1293- 1302, ISSN 0012-1797

Barker, J.M. (2006). Clinical review: Type 1 diabetes-associated autoimmunity: natural history, genetic associations, and screening. *J Clin Endocrinol Metab*, Vol.91, (4), pp.1210-1217, ISSN 0021-972X

Bennett, C.L.; Christie, J.; Ramsdell, F.; Brunkow, M.E.; Ferguson, P.J.; Whitesell, L.; Kelly, T.E.; Saulsbury, F.T.; Chance, P.F. & Ochs, H.D. (2001). The immune dysregulation, polyendocrinopathy, enteropathy, X-linked syndrome (IPEX) is caused by mutations of FOXP3. *Nat Genet*, Vol.27, (1), pp.20-21, ISSN 1061-4036

Bonifacio, E.; Scirpoli, M.; Kredel, K.; Fuchtenbusch, M. & Ziegler, A.G. (1999). Early autoantibody responses in prediabetes are IgG1 dominated and suggest antigen-specific regulation. *J Immunol*, Vol.163, (1), pp.525-532, ISSN 0022-1767

Bougneres, P.F.; Landais, P.; Boisson, C.; Carel, J.C.; Frament, N.; Boitard, C.; Chaussain, J.L. & Bach, J.F. (1990). Limited duration of remission of insulin dependency in children with recent overt type I diabetes treated with low-dose cyclosporin. *Diabetes*, Vol.39, (10), pp.1264-1272, ISSN 0012-1797

Brauner, H.; Elemans, M.; Lemos, S.; Broberger, C.; Holmberg, D.; Flodstrom-Tullberg, M.; Karre, K. & Hoglund, P. (2010). Distinct phenotype and function of NK cells in the pancreas of nonobese diabetic mice. *J Immunol*, Vol.184, (5), pp.2272-2280, ISSN 1550-6606

Bresson, D.; Togher, L.; Rodrigo, E.; Chen, Y.; Bluestone, J.A.; Herold, K.C. & von Herrath, M. (2006). Anti-CD3 and nasal proinsulin combination therapy enhances remission from recent-onset autoimmune diabetes by inducing Tregs. *J Clin Invest*, Vol.116, (5), pp.1371-1381, ISSN 0021-9738

Brunkow, M.E.; Jeffery, E.W.; Hjerrild, K.A.; Paeper, B.; Clark, L.B.; Yasayko, S.A.; Wilkinson, J.E.; Galas, D.; Ziegler, S.F. & Ramsdell, F. (2001). Disruption of a new forkhead/winged-helix protein, scurfin, results in the fatal lymphoproliferative disorder of the scurfy mouse. *Nat Genet*, Vol.27, (1), pp.68-73, ISSN 1061-4036

Cantor, J.& Haskins, K. (2007). Recruitment and activation of macrophages by pathogenic CD4 T cells in type 1 diabetes: evidence for involvement of CCR8 and CCL1. *J Immunol*, Vol.179, (9), pp.5760-5767, ISSN 0022-1767

Carel, J.C.; Boitard, C.; Eisenbarth, G.; Bach, J.F. & Bougneres, P.F. (1996). Cyclosporine delays but does not prevent clinical onset in glucose intolerant pre-type 1 diabetic children. *J Autoimmun*, Vol.9, (6), pp.739-745, ISSN 0896-8411

Chatenoud, L. (2003). CD3-specific antibody-induced active tolerance: from bench to bedside. *Nat Rev Immunol*, Vol.3, (2), pp.123-132, ISSN 1474-1733

Chatenoud, L. & Bluestone, J.A. (2007). CD3-specific antibodies: a portal to the treatment of autoimmunity. *Nat Rev Immunol*, Vol.7, (8), pp.622-632, ISSN 1474-1733

Chatenoud, L.; Thervet, E.; Primo, J. & Bach, J.F. (1994). Anti-CD3 antibody induces long-term remission of overt autoimmunity in nonobese diabetic mice. *Proc Natl Acad Sci U S A*, Vol.91, (1), pp.123-127, ISSN 0027-8424

Clare-Salzler, M.J.; Brooks, J.; Chai, A.; Van Herle, K. & Anderson, C. (1992). Prevention of diabetes in nonobese diabetic mice by dendritic cell transfer. *J Clin Invest*, Vol.90, (3), pp.741-748, ISSN 0021-9738

Dahlen, E.; Dawe, K.; Ohlsson, L. & Hedlund, G. (1998). Dendritic cells and macrophages are the first and major producers of TNF-alpha in pancreatic islets in the nonobese diabetic mouse. *J Immunol*, Vol.160, (7), pp.3585-3593, ISSN 0022-1767

Di Caro, V.; D'Anneo, A.; Phillips, B.; Engman, C.; Harnaha, J.; Lakomy, R.; Styche, A.; Trucco, M. & Giannoukakis, N. (2011). Interleukin-7 matures suppressive CD127(+) forkhead box P3 (FoxP3)(+) T cells into CD127(-) CD25(high) FoxP3(+) regulatory T cells. *Clin Exp Immunol*, ISSN 1365-2249

Donath, M.Y. & Mandrup-Poulsen, T. (2008). The use of interleukin-1-receptor antagonists in the treatment of diabetes mellitus. *Nat Clin Pract Endocrinol Metab*, Vol.4, (5), pp.240-241, ISSN 1745-8374

Dotta, F.; Censini, S.; van Halteren, A.G.; Marselli, L.; Masini, M.; Dionisi, S.; Mosca, F.; Boggi, U.; Muda, A.O.; Prato, S.D.; Elliott, J.F.; Covacci, A.; Rappuoli, R.; Roep, B.O. & Marchetti, P. (2007). Coxsackie B4 virus infection of beta cells and natural killer cell insulitis in recent-onset type 1 diabetic patients. *Proc Natl Acad Sci U S A*, Vol.104, (12), pp.5115-5120, ISSN 0027-8424

Eisenbarth, G.S. (1986). Type I diabetes mellitus. A chronic autoimmune disease. *N Engl J Med*, Vol.314, (21), pp.1360-1368, ISSN 0028-4793

Eisenbarth, G.S.; Srikanta, S.; Jackson, R.; Rabinowe, S.; Dolinar, R.; Aoki, T. & Morris, M.A. (1985). Anti-thymocyte globulin and prednisone immunotherapy of recent onset type 1 diabetes mellitus. *Diabetes Res*, Vol.2, (6), pp.271-276, ISSN 0265-5985

Eizirik, D.L.; Colli, M.L. & Ortis, F. (2009). The role of inflammation in insulitis and beta-cell loss in type 1 diabetes. *Nat Rev Endocrinol*, Vol.5, (4), pp.219-226, ISSN 1759-5037

Elias, D. & Cohen, I.R. (1995). Treatment of autoimmune diabetes and insulitis in NOD mice with heat shock protein 60 peptide p277. *Diabetes*, Vol.44, (9), pp.1132-1138, ISSN 0012-1797

Elias, D.; Meilin, A.; Ablamunits, V.; Birk, O.S.; Carmi, P.; Konen-Waisman, S. & Cohen, I.R. (1997). Hsp60 peptide therapy of NOD mouse diabetes induces a Th2 cytokine burst and downregulates autoimmunity to various beta-cell antigens. *Diabetes*, Vol.46, (5), pp.758-764, ISSN 0012-1797

Elias, D.; Reshef, T.; Birk, O.S.; van der Zee, R.; Walker, M.D. & Cohen, I.R. (1991). Vaccination against autoimmune mouse diabetes with a T-cell epitope of the human 65-kDa heat shock protein. *Proc Natl Acad Sci U S A*, Vol.88, (8), pp.3088-3091, ISSN 0027-8424

Fan, Y.; Rudert, W.A.; Grupillo, M.; He, J.; Sisino, G.&Trucco, M. (2009). Thymus-specific deletion of insulin induces autoimmune diabetes. *EMBO J*, Vol.28, (18), pp.2812-2824, ISSN 1460-2075

Feuerer, M.; Shen, Y.; Littman, D.R.; Benoist, C. & Mathis, D. (2009). How punctual ablation of regulatory T cells unleashes an autoimmune lesion within the pancreatic islets. *Immunity*, Vol.31, (4), pp.654-664, ISSN 1097-4180

Fontenot, A.P.; Gharavi, L.; Bennett, S.R.; Canavera, S.J.; Newman, L.S. & Kotzin, B.L. (2003). CD28 costimulation independence of target organ versus circulating memory antigen-specific CD4+ T cells. *J Clin Invest*, Vol.112, (5), pp.776-784, ISSN 0021-9738

Fousteri, G.; von Herrath, M. & Bresson, D. (2007). Mucosal exposure to antigen: cause or cure of type 1 diabetes? *Curr Diab Rep*, Vol.7, (2), pp.91-98, ISSN 1534-4827

Giannoukakis, N.; Phillips, B. & Trucco, M. (2008). Toward a cure for type 1 diabetes mellitus: diabetes-suppressive dendritic cells and beyond. *Pediatr Diabetes*, Vol.9, (3 Pt 2), pp.4-13, ISSN 1399-5448

Godebu, E.; Summers-Torres, D.; Lin, M.M.; Baaten, B.J. & Bradley, L.M. (2008). Polyclonal adaptive regulatory CD4 cells that can reverse type I diabetes become oligoclonal long-term protective memory cells. *J Immunol*, Vol.181, (3), pp.1798-1805, ISSN 1550-6606

Gottlieb, P.A. BHT-3021 DNA vaccine trial type 1 diabetes. *ADA conference*, June 2009, new Orlens LA.

Guiducci, C.; Ghirelli, C.; Marloie-Provost, M.A.; Matray, T.; Coffman, R.L.; Liu, Y.J.; Barrat, F.J. & Soumelis, V. (2008). PI3K is critical for the nuclear translocation of IRF-7 and type I IFN production by human plasmacytoid predendritic cells in response to TLR activation. *J Exp Med*, Vol.205, (2), pp.315-322, ISSN 1540-9538

Gur, C.; Porgador, A.; Elboim, M.; Gazit, R.; Mizrahi, S.; Stern-Ginossar, N.; Achdout, H.; Ghadially, H.; Dor, Y.; Nir, T.; Doviner, V.; Hershkovitz, O.; Mendelson, M.; Naparstek, Y. & Mandelboim, O. (2010). The activating receptor NKp46 is essential for the development of type 1 diabetes. *Nat Immunol*, Vol.11, (2), pp.121-128, ISSN 1529-2916

Harnaha, J.; Machen, J.; Wright, M.; Lakomy, R.; Styche, A.; Trucco, M.; Makaroun, S. & Giannoukakis, N. (2006). Interleukin-7 is a survival factor for CD4+ CD25+ T-cells and is expressed by diabetes-suppressive dendritic cells. *Diabetes*, Vol.55, (1), pp.158-170, ISSN 0012-1797

Herold, K.C.; Gitelman, S.E.; Masharani, U.; Hagopian, W.; Bisikirska, B.; Donaldson, D.; Rother, K.; Diamond, B.; Harlan, D.M. & Bluestone, J.A. (2005). A single course of anti-CD3 monoclonal antibody hOKT3gamma1(Ala-Ala) results in improvement in C-peptide responses and clinical parameters for at least 2 years after onset of type 1 diabetes. *Diabetes*, Vol.54, (6), pp.1763-1769, ISSN 0012-1797

Herold, K.C.; Hagopian, W.; Auger, J.A.; Poumian-Ruiz, E.; Taylor, L.; Donaldson, D.; Gitelman, S.E.; Harlan, D.M.; Xu, D.; Zivin, R.A. & Bluestone, J.A. (2002). Anti-CD3 monoclonal antibody in new-onset type 1 diabetes mellitus. *N Engl J Med*, Vol.346, (22), pp.1692-1698, ISSN 1533-4406

Ho, P.P.; Fontoura, P.; Platten, M.; Sobel, R.A.; DeVoss, J.J.; Lee, L.Y.; Kidd, B.A.; Tomooka, B.H.; Capers, J.; Agrawal, A.; Gupta, R.; Zernik, J.; Yee, M.K.; Lee, B.J.; Garren, H.; Robinson, W.H. & Steinman, L. (2005). A suppressive oligodeoxynucleotide enhances the efficacy of myelin cocktail/IL-4-tolerizing DNA vaccination and treats autoimmune disease. *J Immunol*, Vol.175, (9), pp.6226-6234, ISSN 0022-1767

Hu, C.Y.; Rodriguez-Pinto, D.; Du, W.; Ahuja, A.; Henegariu, O.; Wong, F.S.; Shlomchik, M.J. & Wen, L. (2007). Treatment with CD20-specific antibody prevents and reverses autoimmune diabetes in mice. *J Clin Invest*, Vol.117, (12), pp.3857-3867, ISSN 0021-9738

Hutchings, P.; Rosen, H.; O'Reilly, L.; Simpson, E.; Gordon, S. & Cooke, A. (1990). Transfer of diabetes in mice prevented by blockade of adhesion-promoting receptor on macrophages. *Nature*, Vol.348, (6302), pp.639-642, ISSN 0028-0836

Huurman, V.A.; Decochez, K.; Mathieu, C.; Cohen, I.R.&Roep, B.O. (2007). Therapy with the hsp60 peptide DiaPep277 in C-peptide positive type 1 diabetes patients. *Diabetes Metab Res Rev*, Vol.23, (4), pp.269-275, ISSN 1520-7552

Itoh, N.; Hanafusa, T.; Miyazaki, A.; Miyagawa, J.; Yamagata, K.; Yamamoto, K.; Waguri, M.; Imagawa, A.; Tamura, S.; Inada, M. & et al. (1993). Mononuclear cell infiltration and its relation to the expression of major histocompatibility complex antigens and adhesion molecules in pancreas biopsy specimens from newly diagnosed insulin-dependent diabetes mellitus patients. *J Clin Invest*, Vol.92, (5), pp.2313-2322, ISSN 0021-9738

Jarnicki, A.G.; Conroy, H.; Brereton, C.; Donnelly, G.; Toomey, D.; Walsh, K.; Sweeney, C.; Leavy, O.; Fletcher, J.; Lavelle, E.C.; Dunne, P. & Mills, K.H. (2008). Attenuating regulatory T cell induction by TLR agonists through inhibition of p38 MAPK signaling in dendritic cells enhances their efficacy as vaccine adjuvants and cancer immunotherapeutics. *J Immunol*, Vol.180, (6), pp.3797-3806, ISSN 0022-1767

Jin, L.; Zhu, A.; Wang, Y.; Chen, Q.; Xiong, Q.; Li, J.; Sun, Y.; Li, T.; Cao, R.; Wu, J. & Liu, J. (2008). A Th1-recognized peptide P277, when tandemly repeated, enhances a Th2 immune response toward effective vaccines against autoimmune diabetes in nonobese diabetic mice. *J Immunol*, Vol.180, (1), pp.58-63, ISSN 0022-1767

Jun, H.S.; Yoon, C.S.; Zbytnuik, L.; van Rooijen, N. & Yoon, J.W. (1999). The role of macrophages in T cell-mediated autoimmune diabetes in nonobese diabetic mice. *J Exp Med*, Vol.189, (2), pp.347-358, ISSN 0022-1007

Keymeulen, B.; Vandemeulebroucke, E.; Ziegler, A.G.; Mathieu, C.; Kaufman, L.; Hale, G.; Gorus, F.; Goldman, M.; Walter, M.; Candon, S.; Schandene, L.; Crenier, L.; De Block, C.; Seigneurin, J.M.; De Pauw, P.; Pierard, D.; Weets, I.; Rebello, P.; Bird, P.; Berrie, E.; Frewin, M.; Waldmann, H.; Bach, J.F.; Pipeleers, D. & Chatenoud, L. (2005). Insulin needs after CD3-antibody therapy in new-onset type 1 diabetes. *N Engl J Med*, Vol.352, (25), pp.2598-2608, ISSN 1533-4406

Kindrachuk, J.; Potter, J.; Wilson, H.L.; Griebel, P.; Babiuk, L.A. & Napper, S. (2008). Activation and regulation of toll-like receptor 9: CpGs and beyond. *Mini Rev Med Chem*, Vol.8, (6), pp.590-600, ISSN 1389-5575

Knip, M.; Kukko, M.; Kulmala, P.; Veijola, R.; Simell, O.; Akerblom, H.K. & Ilonen, J. (2002). Humoral beta-cell autoimmunity in relation to HLA-defined disease susceptibility in preclinical and clinical type 1 diabetes. *Am J Med Genet*, Vol.115, (1), pp.48-54, ISSN 0148-7299

Lazar, L.; Ofan, R.; Weintrob, N.; Avron, A.; Tamir, M.; Elias, D.; Phillip, M. & Josefsberg, Z. (2007). Heat-shock protein peptide DiaPep277 treatment in children with newly diagnosed type 1 diabetes: a randomised, double-blind phase II study. *Diabetes Metab Res Rev*, Vol.23, (4), pp.286-291, ISSN 1520-7552

Lehuen, A.; Diana, J.; Zaccone, P. & Cooke, A. (2010). Immune cell crosstalk in type 1 diabetes. *Nat Rev Immunol*, Vol.10, (7), pp.501-513, ISSN 1474-1741

Li, Q.; Xu, B.; Michie, S.A.; Rubins, K.H.; Schreriber, R.D. & McDevitt, H.O. (2008). Interferon-alpha initiates type 1 diabetes in nonobese diabetic mice. *Proc Natl Acad Sci U S A*, Vol.105, (34), pp.12439-12444, ISSN 1091-6490

Lo, J.; Peng, R.H.; Barker, T.; Xia, C.Q. & Clare-Salzler, M.J. (2006). Peptide-pulsed immature dendritic cells reduce response to beta cell target antigens and protect NOD recipients from type I diabetes. *Ann N Y Acad Sci*, Vol.1079, pp.153-156, ISSN 0077-8923

Ludvigsson, J.; Faresjo, M.; Hjorth, M.; Axelsson, S.; Cheramy, M.; Pihl, M.; Vaarala, O.; Forsander, G.; Ivarsson, S.; Johansson, C.; Lindh, A.; Nilsson, N.O.; Aman, J.; Ortqvist, E.; Zerhouni, P. & Casas, R. (2008). GAD treatment and insulin secretion in recent-onset type 1 diabetes. *N Engl J Med*, Vol.359, (18), pp.1909-1920, ISSN 1533-4406

Luo, X.; Herold, K.C. & Miller, S.D. (2010). Immunotherapy of type 1 diabetes: where are we and where should we be going? *Immunity*, Vol.32, (4), pp.488-499, ISSN 1097-4180

Luo, X.; Tarbell, K.V.; Yang, H.; Pothoven, K.; Bailey, S.L.; Ding, R.; Steinman, R.M. & Suthanthiran, M. (2007). Dendritic cells with TGF-beta1 differentiate naive CD4+CD25- T cells into islet-protective Foxp3+ regulatory T cells. *Proc Natl Acad Sci U S A*, Vol.104, (8), pp.2821-2826, ISSN 0027-8424

Ma, L.; Qian, S.; Liang, X.; Wang, L.; Woodward, J.E.; Giannoukakis, N.; Robbins, P.D.; Bertera, S.; Trucco, M.; Fung, J.J. & Lu, L. (2003). Prevention of diabetes in NOD mice by administration of dendritic cells deficient in nuclear transcription factor-kappaB activity. *Diabetes*, Vol.52, (8), pp.1976-1985, ISSN 0012-1797

Machen, J.; Bertera, S.; Chang, Y.; Bottino, R.; Balamurugan, A.N.; Robbins, P.D.; Trucco, M. & Giannoukakis, N. (2004). Prolongation of islet allograft survival following ex vivo transduction with adenovirus encoding a soluble type 1 TNF receptor-Ig fusion decoy. *Gene Ther*, Vol.11, (20), pp.1506-1514, ISSN 0969-7128

Martin, A.P.; Rankin, S.; Pitchford, S.; Charo, I.F.; Furtado, G.C. & Lira, S.A. (2008). Increased expression of CCL2 in insulin-producing cells of transgenic mice promotes mobilization of myeloid cells from the bone marrow, marked insulitis, and diabetes. *Diabetes*, Vol.57, (11), pp.3025-3033, ISSN 1939-327X

Mastrandrea, L.; Yu, J.; Behrens, T.; Buchlis, J.; Albini, C.; Fourtner, S. & Quattrin, T. (2009). Etanercept treatment in children with new-onset type 1 diabetes: pilot randomized, placebo-controlled, double-blind study. *Diabetes Care*, Vol.32, (7), pp.1244-1249, ISSN 1935-5548

McDevitt, H. (2001). Closing in on type 1 diabetes. *N Engl J Med*, Vol.345, (14), pp.1060-1061, ISSN 0028-4793

Morel, P.A.; Dorman, J.S.; Todd, J.A.; McDevitt, H.O. & Trucco, M. (1988). Aspartic acid at position 57 of the HLA-DQ beta chain protects against type I diabetes: a family study. *Proc Natl Acad Sci U S A*, Vol.85, (21), pp.8111-8115, ISSN 0027-8424

Morran, M.P.; Casu, A.; Arena, V.C.; Pietropaolo, S.; Zhang, Y.J.; Satin, L.S.; Trucco, M.; Becker, D.J. & Pietropaolo, M. (2010). Humoral autoimmunity against theextracellular domain of the neuroendocrine autoantigen IA-2 heightens the risk of type 1 diabetes. *Endocrinology*, Vol.151, pp.2528-2537, ISSN 1945-7170

Nakayama, M.; Abiru, N.; Moriyama, H.; Babaya, N.; Liu, E.; Miao, D.; Yu, L.; Wegmann, D.R.; Hutton, J.C.; Elliott, J.F. & Eisenbarth, G.S. (2005). Prime role for an insulin epitope in the development of type 1 diabetes in NOD mice. *Nature*, Vol.435, (7039), pp.220-223, ISSN 1476-4687

Nir, T.; Melton, D.A. & Dor, Y. (2007). Recovery from diabetes in mice by beta cell regeneration. *J Clin Invest*, Vol.117, (9), pp.2553-2561, ISSN 0021-9738

Nussbaum, G.; Zanin-Zhorov, A.; Quintana, F.; Lider, O. & Cohen, I.R. (2006). Peptide p277 of HSP60 signals T cells: inhibition of inflammatory chemotaxis. *Int Immunol*, Vol.18, (10), pp.1413-1419, ISSN 0953-8178

Ohnmacht, C.; Pullner, A.; King, S.B.; Drexler, I.; Meier, S.; Brocker, T. & Voehringer, D. (2009). Constitutive ablation of dendritic cells breaks self-tolerance of CD4 T cells and results in spontaneous fatal autoimmunity. *J Exp Med*, Vol.206, (3), pp.549-559, ISSN 1540-9538

Orban, T.; Sosenko, J.M.; Cuthbertson, D.; Krischer, J.P.; Skyler, J.S.; Jackson, R.; Yu, L.; Palmer, J.P.; Schatz, D. & Eisenbarth, G. (2009). Pancreatic islet autoantibodies as predictors of type 1 diabetes in the Diabetes Prevention Trial-Type 1. *Diabetes Care*, Vol.32, (12), pp.2269-2274, ISSN 1935-5548

Patterson, C.C.; Dahlquist, G.G.; Gyurus, E.; Green, A. & Soltesz, G. (2009). Incidence trends for childhood type 1 diabetes in Europe during 1989-2003 and predicted new cases 2005-20: a multicentre prospective registration study. *Lancet*, Vol.373, (9680), pp.2027-2033, ISSN 1474-547X

Pescovitz, M.D.; Greenbaum, C.J.; Krause-Steinrauf, H.; Becker, D.J.; Gitelman, S.E.; Goland, R.; Gottlieb, P.A.; Marks, J.B.; McGee, P.F.; Moran, A.M.; Raskin, P.; Rodriguez, H.; Schatz, D.A.; Wherrett, D.; Wilson, D.M.; Lachin, J.M. & Skyler, J.S. (2009). Rituximab, B-lymphocyte depletion, and preservation of beta-cell function. *N Engl J Med*, Vol.361, (22), pp.2143-2152, ISSN 1533-4406

Phillips, J.M.; Parish, N.M.; Bland, C.; Sawyer, Y.; De La Pena, H. & Cooke, A. (2009). Type 1 Diabetes Development Requires Both CD4+ and CD8+ T cells and Can Be Reversed by Non-Depleting Antibodies Targeting Both T Cell Populations. *Rev Diabet Stud*, Vol.6, (2), pp.97-103, ISSN 1614-0575

Pickersgill, L.M. & Mandrup-Poulsen, T.R. (2009). The anti-interleukin-1 in type 1 diabetes action trial–background and rationale. *Diabetes Metab Res Rev*, Vol.25, pp. 321–324, ISSN1520-7560

Pietropaolo, M.; Yu, S.; Libman, I.M.; Pietropaolo, S.L.; Riley, K.; LaPorte, R.E.; Drash, A.L.; Mazumdar, S.; Trucco, M. & Becker, D.J. (2005). Cytoplasmic islet cell antibodies remain valuable in defining risk of progression to Type 1 diabetes in subjects with other islet autoantibodies. *Pediatric Diabetes*, Vol.6, pp.184-192, ISSN 1399-543X

Poirot, L.; Benoist, C. & Mathis, D. (2004). Natural killer cells distinguish innocuous and destructive forms of pancreatic islet autoimmunity. *Proc Natl Acad Sci U S A*, Vol.101, (21), pp.8102-8107, ISSN 0027-8424

Pozzilli, P.; Pitocco, D.; Visalli, N.; Cavallo, M.G.; Buzzetti, R.; Crino, A.; Spera, S.; Suraci, C.; Multari, G.; Cervoni, M.; Manca Bitti, M.L.; Matteoli, M.C.; Marietti, G.; Ferrazzoli, F.; Cassone Faldetta, M.R.; Giordano, C.; Sbriglia, M.; Sarugeri, E. & Ghirlanda, G. (2000). No effect of oral insulin on residual beta-cell function in recent-onset type I diabetes (the IMDIAB VII). IMDIAB Group. *Diabetologia*, Vol.43, (8), pp.1000-1004, ISSN 0012-186X

Rabinovitch, A.; Sumoski, W.; Rajotte, R.V. & Warnock, G.L. (1990). Cytotoxic effects of cytokines on human pancreatic islet cells in monolayer culture. *J Clin Endocrinol Metab*, Vol.71, (1), pp.152-156, ISSN 0021-972X

Raz, I.; Elias, D.; Avron, A.; Tamir, M.; Metzger, M. & Cohen, I.R. (2001). Beta-cell function in new-onset type 1 diabetes and immunomodulation with a heat-shock protein peptide (DiaPep277): a randomised, double-blind, phase II trial. *Lancet*, Vol.358, (9295), pp.1749-1753, ISSN 0140-6736

Roberts, T.L.; Sweet, M.J.; Hume, D.A. & Stacey, K.J. (2005). Cutting edge: species-specific TLR9-mediated recognition of CpG and non-CpG phosphorothioate-modified oligonucleotides. *J Immunol*, Vol.174, (2), pp.605-608, ISSN 0022-1767

Roep, B.O. (2003). The role of T-cells in the pathogenesis of Type 1 diabetes: from cause to cure. *Diabetologia*, Vol.46, (3), pp.305-321, ISSN 0012-186X

Saudek, F.; Havrdova, T.; Boucek, P.; Karasova, L.; Novota, P.&Skibova, J. (2004). Polyclonal anti-T-cell therapy for type 1 diabetes mellitus of recent onset. *Rev Diabet Stud*, Vol.1, (2), pp.80-88, ISSN 1614-0575

Saxena, V.; Ondr, J.K.; Magnusen, A.F.; Munn, D.H. & Katz, J.D. (2007). The countervailing actions of myeloid and plasmacytoid dendritic cells control autoimmune diabetes in the nonobese diabetic mouse. *J Immunol*, Vol.179, (8), pp.5041-5053, ISSN 0022-1767

Schloot, N.C.; Meierhoff, G.; Lengyel, C.; Vandorfi, G.; Takacs, J.; Panczel, P.; Barkai, L.; Madacsy, L.; Oroszlan, T.; Kovacs, P.; Suto, G.; Battelino, T.; Hosszufalusi, N. & Jermendy, G. (2007). Effect of heat shock protein peptide DiaPep277 on beta-cell function in paediatric and adult patients with recent-onset diabetes mellitus type 1: two prospective, randomized, double-blind phase II trials. *Diabetes Metab Res Rev*, Vol.23, (4), pp.276-285, ISSN 1520-7552

Simon, G.; Parker, M.; Ramiya, V.; Wasserfall, C. & Huang, Y. (2008). Murine antithymocyte globulin therapy alters disease progression in NOD mice by a time-dependent induction of immunoregulation. *Diabetes* Vol.57, pp.405–414, ISSN1939-327X

Tang, Q. & Bluestone, J.A. (2006). Regulatory T-cell physiology and application to treat autoimmunity. *Immunol Rev*, Vol.212, pp.217-237, ISSN 0105-2896

Tarbell, K.V.; Yamazaki, S.; Olson, K.; Toy, P. & Steinman, R.M. (2004). CD25+ CD4+ T cells, expanded with dendritic cells presenting a single autoantigenic peptide, suppress autoimmune diabetes. *J Exp Med*, Vol.199, (11), pp.1467-1477, ISSN 0022-1007

Thomas, H.E.; Irawaty, W.; Darwiche, R.; Brodnicki, T.C.; Santamaria, P.; Allison, J. & Kay, T.W. (2004). IL-1 receptor deficiency slows progression to diabetes in the NOD mouse. *Diabetes*, Vol.53, (1), pp.113-121, ISSN 0012-1797

Tian, J.; Clare-Salzler, M.; Herschenfeld, A.; Middleton, B.; Newman, D.; Mueller, R.; Arita, S.; Evans, C.; Atkinson, M.A.; Mullen, Y.; Sarvetnick, N.; Tobin, A.J.; Lehmann, P.V. & Kaufman, D.L. (1996). Modulating autoimmune responses to GAD inhibits disease progression and prolongs islet graft survival in diabetes-prone mice. *Nat Med*, Vol.2, (12), pp.1348-1353, ISSN 1078-8956

Tisch, R.; Liblau, R.S.; Yang, X.D.; Liblau, P. & McDevitt, H.O. (1998). Induction of GAD65-specific regulatory T-cells inhibits ongoing autoimmune diabetes in nonobese diabetic mice. *Diabetes*, Vol.47, (6), pp.894-899, ISSN 0012-1797

Tisch, R.; Yang, X.D.; Singer, S.M.; Liblau, R.S.; Fugger, L. & McDevitt, H.O. (1993). Immune response to glutamic acid decarboxylase correlates with insulitis in non-obese diabetic mice. *Nature*, Vol.366, (6450), pp.72-75, ISSN 0028-0836

Todd, J.A.; Walker, N.M.; Cooper, J.D.; Smyth, D.J.; Downes, K.; Plagnol, V.; Bailey, R.; Nejentsev, S.; Field, S.F.; Payne, F.; Lowe, C.E.; Szeszko, J.S.; Hafler, J.P.; Zeitels, L.; Yang, J.H.; Vella, A.; Nutland, S.; Stevens, H.E.; Schuilenburg, H.; Coleman, G.; Maisuria, M.; Meadows, W.; Smink, L.J.; Healy, B.; Burren, O.S.; Lam, A.A.; Ovington, N.R.; Allen, J.; Adlem, E.; Leung, H.T.; Wallace, C.; Howson, J.M.; Guja, C.; Ionescu-Tirgoviste, C.; Simmonds, M.J.; Heward, J.M.; Gough, S.C.; Dunger, D.B.; Wicker, L.S. & Clayton, D.G. (2007). Robust associations of four new chromosome regions from genome-wide analyses of type 1 diabetes. *Nat Genet*, Vol.39, (7), pp.857-864, ISSN 1061-4036

Trucco, M. (1992). To be or not to be Asp 57, that is the question. *Diabetes Care*, Vol.15, (5), pp.705-715, ISSN 0149-5992

Trucco, M. & Giannoukakis, N. (2007). Immunoregulatory dendritic cells to prevent and reverse new-onset Type 1 diabetes mellitus. *Expert Opin Biol Ther*, Vol.7, (7), pp.951-963, ISSN 1744-7682

Turley, S.; Poirot, L.; Hattori, M.; Benoist, C. & Mathis, D. (2003). Physiological beta cell death triggers priming of self-reactive T cells by dendritic cells in a type-1 diabetes model. *J Exp Med*, Vol.198, (10), pp.1527-1537, ISSN 0022-1007

Ueno, H.; Klechevsky, E.; Morita, R.; Aspord, C.; Cao, T.; Matsui, T.; Di Pucchio, T.; Connolly, J.; Fay, J.W.; Pascual, V.; Palucka, A.K. & Banchereau, J. (2007). Dendritic cell subsets in health and disease. *Immunol Rev*, Vol.219, pp.118-142, ISSN 0105-2896

van Belle, T.L.; Coppieters, K.T. & von Herrath, M.G. (2011). Type 1 diabetes: etiology, immunology, and therapeutic strategies. *Physiol Rev*, Vol.91, (1), pp.79-118, ISSN 1522-1210

von Herrath, M.; Sanda, S. & Herold, K. (2007). Type 1 diabetes as a relapsing-remitting disease? *Nat Rev Immunol*, Vol.7, (12), pp.988-994, ISSN 1474-1741

von Herrath, M.G.; Fujinami, R.S. & Whitton, J.L. (2003). Microorganisms and autoimmunity: making the barren field fertile? *Nat Rev Microbiol*, Vol.1, (2), pp.151-157, ISSN 1740-1526

Weber, S.E.; Harbertson, J.; Godebu, E.; Mros, G.A.; Padrick, R.C.; Carson, B.D.; Ziegler, S.F. & Bradley, L.M. (2006). Adaptive islet-specific regulatory CD4 T cells control autoimmune diabetes and mediate the disappearance of pathogenic Th1 cells in vivo. *J Immunol*, Vol.176, (8), pp.4730-4739, ISSN 0022-1767

Wegmann, D.R.; Gill, R.G.; Norbury-Glaser, M.; Schloot, N. & Daniel, D. (1994). Analysis of the spontaneous T cell response to insulin in NOD mice. *J Autoimmun*, Vol.7, (6), pp.833-843, ISSN 0896-8411

Wenzlau, J.M.; Juhl, K.; Yu, L.; Moua, O.; Sarkar, S.A.; Gottlieb, P.; Rewers, M.; Eisenbarth, G.S.; Jensen, J.; Davidson, H.W. & Hutton, J.C. (2007). The cation efflux transporter ZnT8 (Slc30A8) is a major autoantigen in human type 1 diabetes. *Proc Natl Acad Sci U S A*, Vol.104, (43), pp.17040-17045, ISSN 0027-8424

Xiu, Y.; Wong, C.P.; Bouaziz, J.D.; Hamaguchi, Y.; Wang, Y.; Pop, S.M.; Tisch, R.M. & Tedder, T.F. (2008). B lymphocyte depletion by CD20 monoclonal antibody prevents diabetes in nonobese diabetic mice despite isotype-specific differences in Fc gamma R effector functions. *J Immunol*, Vol.180, (5), pp.2863-2875, ISSN 0022-1767

Yanaba, K.; Bouaziz, J.D.; Haas, K.M.; Poe, J.C.; Fujimoto, M. & Tedder, T.F. (2008). A regulatory B cell subset with a unique CD1dhiCD5+ phenotype controls T cell-dependent inflammatory responses. *Immunity*, Vol.28, (5), pp.639-650, ISSN 1097-4180

11

Immunogenetics of Type 1 Diabetes

Rajni Rani
National Institute of Immunology, New Delhi, India

1. Introduction

Type 1 diabetes (T1D), also known as Insulin dependent diabetes mellitus (IDDM) is an incurable multi-factorial autoimmune disorder. The disease is characterized by the loss of insulin producing beta cells of the pancreas resulting in abnormal metabolism of glucose which may lead to ketoacidosis and several other complications like retinopathy, nephropathy and even cardio-vascular diseases and pre-mature deaths (Pociot & Mcdermott, 2002). World-wide disease affects 1 in 300-400 children (Todd, 1995). Population based data from South India shows the incidence of T1D for four year period to be 10.5/100,000/ year (Ramachandran et al., 1996). Similar prevalence of type 1 diabetes has been observed in North India. A study from district of Karnal in North India reported the prevalence to be 10.20/100,000 population, with a higher prevalence in urban (26.6/100,000) as compared to rural areas (4.27/100,000) (Kalra et al. 2010). T1D develops as a result of complex interaction of many genetic and environmental factors leading to autoimmune destruction of the insulin producing pancreatic beta cells. While 20 genomic intervals have been implicated for the manifestation of the disease (Pociot & Mcdermott, 2002), role of an intricate network of the products of these genes cannot be ruled out. However, unravelling different factors involved and how they interact in integrated networks is like solving a jig-saw puzzle which is the aim of our studies. Basic problem with T1D patients is that by the time they first report to the physician, most of their pancreatic beta cells are already destroyed which leaves the clinicain with no option but to give daily insulin injections. So, there is a need to identify the prediabetics before the onset of the disease and device ways to inhibit autoimmunity in them. Following sections will show the work done in our laboratory to understand the intricate networks in which the genes involved in immune responses interact and their implications.

2. Role of Major Histocompatibility Complex (IDDM1)

The Major Histocompatibility Complex (MHC) region on chromosome 6p21.31 has been shown to have major role in predisposition to get type 1 diabetes. It is also called IDDM1.

2.1 Genes and proteins of the Major Histocompatibility Complex (MHC)

The human MHC, Human Leukocyte Antigen (HLA) system is the most polymorphic system of the human genome with more than 5000 alleles. The alleles of HLA loci are co-dominant i.e. both the alleles at a particular locus are equally expressed. The genes of HLA code for

glycoprotein molecules which are expressed on nucleated cells and are responsible for the recognition of non-self from self. The function of MHC molecules is to present exogenous and endogenous antigens in the form of peptides to the T cells for subsequent immune response to take place. The gene map of the MHC region of man on chromosome 6p21.3 shows that it spans about 4 megabases (3,838,986 bp to be precise). It is the most gene-dense region of the human genome with 224 genes of which 128 are known to be expressed. 40% of the expressed genes in this region have immune related functions (Horton et al., 2004).
There are two types of MHC molecules : MHC Class-I and Class-II which differ from each other in their constituents as well as their functions.

2.1.1 MHC class-I genes and proteins

MHC class-I genes are expressed on all nucleated cells in the form of cell surface glycoproteins. Function of MHC class-I molecules is to present antigenic peptides to $CD8^+$ cytotoxic T cells (CTLs). The classical class-I genes in humans are HLA-A, HLA-B and HLA-C. All these genes are very polymorphic with 1519 alleles for HLA-A locus, 2069 alleles for B-locus and 1016 alleles for C-locus and these numbers are increasing with the discovery of new alleles everyday.
The MHC class-I molecule is a hetero-dimer of a heavy alpha chain (about 40-45 KDa) and the light chain, beta 2 microglobulin (β_2m) of 12 KDa (Bjorkman et al., 1987). While the genes for the heavy chains i.e. the alpha chains are encoded on chromosome 6, the gene for β_2m is encoded on human chromosome 15. The alpha chain of the MHC class-I molecule has three domains alpha 1 (α1), alpha 2 (α2)and alpha 3 (α3). Alpha 1 (α1) and alpha 2 (α2) domains are the most polymorphic domains since they constitute the peptide binding groove of the MHC molecule. The genes encoding MHC class-I alpha chain have 8 exons with second and the third exons of the alpha chain gene being most polymorphic since they code for the α1 and α2 domains. The peptides that are presented by the MHC molecules have allele specific motifs, which means that certain peptides can be presented by certain MHC molecules. The affinity of the peptide to bind to the peptide binding groove is determined by the anchors present on the peptide binding groove where the peptides go and bind through hydrogen bonds. Specific motifs on the peptides determine which peptides would bind to which MHC molecule (Falk et al., 1991, Garrett et al., 1989).

2.1.2 MHC class-II genes and proteins

MHC class-II glycoproteins in humans are HLA-DR, -DP and –DQ. The MHC class-II molecule is a heterodimer of two polypeptide chains: an alpha (25-33 KDa) and a beta chain (24-29KDa) (Brown et al., 1993, De Vries & Van Rood, 1985). Unlike MHC class-I, both alpha and beta chains of the class-II molecule are encoded on chromosome 6. DRB1 gene encodes DR beta chain while DRA1 encodes DR alpha chain with 966 DRB1 alleles and 3 DRA1 alleles. Similarly DQB1 and DPB1 encode beta chains of DQ and DP molecules with 144 and 145 alleles respectively and DQA1 and DPA1 encode the alpha chains of DQ and DP molecules with 35 and 28 alleles respectively (Robinson et al., 2009).
While HLA class-I molecules are expressed on all nucleated cells, HLA class-II molecules are expressed on antigen presenting cells like macrophages, dendritic cells, B cells, thymic epithelium and activated T cells (Holling et al., 2004). The function of MHC class-II molecules is to present antigenic peptides to the $CD4^+$ T helper cells (Th cells) which in turn initiate a cascade of immunological events resulting in activation of $CD8^+$ cytotoxic T cells

(Horton et al., 2004). When a non-self antigen is presented to CD4+ T helper cells, they get activated and secrete certain cytokines like Interferon gamma and TNF-alpha in case of Th1 cells and IL-4, IL-5 and/or IL-6 in case of Th2 cells. While the cytokines secreted by Th1 cells activate the cytotoxic T cells which have already seen the antigen in the context of HLA class-I, Th2 cytokines activate the B cells to become plasma cells which make the antibodies against antigen they have seen. Thus an immune response takes place which varies in strength depending on the host factors and the peptides being presented.

There are about 50,000-100,000 MHC molecules on each cell. Most MHC molecules are occupied by self peptides and the T cells are tolerized against them during thymic education so that auto-immune responses do not take place, however, some times something goes awry and there is a break in the tolerance resulting in recognition of self as non-self by the immune system resulting in an auto-immune response. This could be due to low expression of some antigens in the thymus which may result in self-reactive T cells to reach the peripheral circulation. Or it could be due to escape of self-reactive T cells from clonal deletion during T cell development.

2.2 MHC and Type 1 diabetes

Despite so much polymorphism, significant increase of one or more alleles of HLA in a disease population as compared to healthy controls, suggests functional implications due to their role in antigen presentation. We observed a significant increase of *DRB1*03:01* ($p<10^{-6}$, Odds Ratio (OR) =11.0), *DRB1*04:01* ($p<0.01$, OR=6.4) and *DRB1*04:05* ($p<0.03$, OR=5) in the patients (Figure 1a) using high resolution typing method of polymerase chain reaction followed by hybridization with sequence specific oligonucleotide probes(PCR-SSOP) (Rani et al., 2004, Rani et al., 1999).

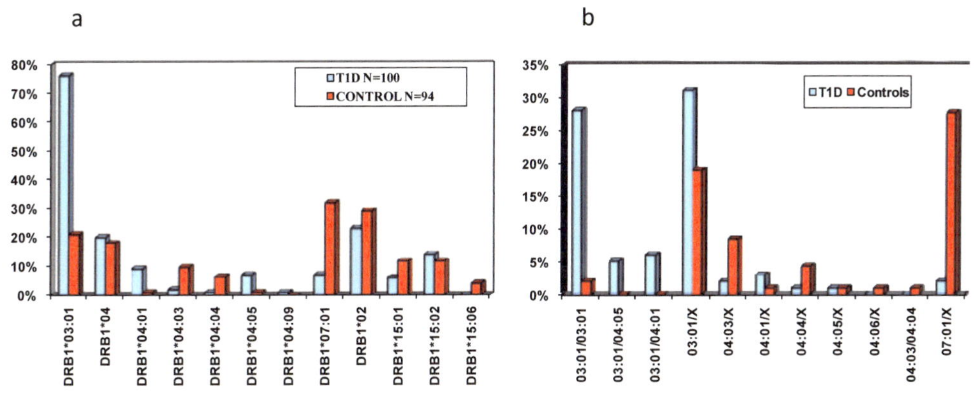

Rani et al., Tissue Antigens : 64:145-155, 2004

Fig. 1. Distribution of *HLA-DRB1* alleles significantly increased in Type 1 diabetes. **a.** *DRB1*03:01, DRB1*04:01, DRB1*04:05* showing significant increase and *DRB1*04:03, DRB1*04:04 and DRB1*07:01* showing significant reduction in T1D patients as compared to healthy controls. **b**. shows the homozygosity and heterozygosity of predisposing and protective alleles significantly increased or reduced in the T1D patients. Homozygous *DRB1*03:01/03:01,* heterozygous *DRB1*03:01/04:05, DRB1*03:01/04:01* and *DRB1*03:01/X* were significantly increased and *DRB1*04:03/X* and *DRB1*07:01 X* were significantly reduced in the T1D patients as compared to controls.

Our results were in concordance with earlier studies in North Indians (Gupta et al., 1991, Kanga et al., 2004, Mehra et al., 2002, Sanjeevi et al., 1999, Witt et al., 2002). However, we also observed *DRB1*07:01*($p<7x10^{-6}$, OR= 0.16), *DRB1*04:03* (p< 0.02, OR=0.25) and *DRB1*04:04* (p< 0.05, OR= 0.2) to be significantly decreased in the patients as compared to controls. We did not find any significant reduction of HLA-DR2 haplotype *DRB1*15:01-DQB1*06:02* which has been shown to confer strong protection from T1D in most ethnic groups (Baisch et al., 1990, Pugliese et al., 1995), probably because this haplotype has been found with a low frequency of only 1.06% in North Indians (Rani et al., 1998). On the other hand, we observed a marginally reduced frequency of *DRB1*15:06* in patients as compared to controls, which did not remain significant when *p* was corrected for the number of alleles tested for DRB1 locus (Rani et al., 2004).

Figure 1b shows the homozygosity and heterozygosity of *DRB1*03:01* and *DRB1*04* alleles significantly increased in T1D. Homozygous *DRB1*03:01* ($p<10^{-7}$, OR=14.54), heterozygous *DRB1*03:01/*04:05* (p<0.03, OR =10.9) and *DRB1*03:01/*04:01* (p<0.01, OR = 13) were significantly increased in the patients as compared to controls who lacked this heterozygous combination. Heterozygous *03:01*/X (i.e. any other allele) (p<0.04, OR = 1.89) was also significantly increased in the patients as compared to controls. Heterozygous *DRB1*04:03/X* (p<0.04, OR = 0.22) and *DRB1*07:01/X* ($p < 10^{-7}$, OR = 0.066) were significantly reduced in the T1D patients as compared to controls suggesting their protective role. **S**ignificant protection has been shown to be associated with *DRB1*04:03* allele in a Belgian study of diabetes (Van Der Auwera et al., 1995). *DRB1*03:01, DRB1*04:01* and *DRB1*04:05* have also been shown to be associated with T1D patients in Sardinians, black population from Zimbabwe, Lithuanians, Czecks, Lebanese, Brazilians and African Americans (Alves et al., 2009, Cucca et al., 1995, Ei Wafai et al., , Fernandez-Vina et al., 1993, Garcia-Pacheco et al., 1992, Skrodeniene et al., , Tait et al., 1995, Weber et al.).

Cucca et al suggested that amino acid position β74 and β86 in DR beta chain are the key residues in the P4 and P1 pockets of the peptide binding groove of HLA-DR molecules (Cucca et al., 2001). A combined presence of Asp, Glu and Val in positions β57 (P9), β74 (P4) and β86 (P1) in protective *DRB1*04:03* has been shown to be different from high risk *DRB1*04:05* which has Ser, Ala and Gly at these positions. However, in the North Indians we observed *DRB1*03:01* to be at highest risk and this allele has Asp, Arg, and Val in the three positions (Figure 2). A less predisposing allele in North Indians, *DRB1*04:01* has Asp, Ala, Gly and the protective *DRB1*04:04* and *DRB1*07:01* have Asp, Ala, Val and Val, Gln and Gly in the three positions respectively. Thus, Asp, Arg and Val in *DRB1*03:01* is entirely different from Val, Gln, and Gly in *DRB1*07:01* which seems to be important in our study since all the four DR4 alleles are present in less than 10% of the patients or control samples. In essence, these data suggest that it is probably not β74 and β86 alone, rather an integration of all the pockets of the peptide binding groove that determines which peptide of an auto-antigen would bind to the MHC molecule and result in auto-aggression based on the thymic education.

We also studied the alleles of *DQB1 locus*. *DQB1*02:01* which is linked to *DRB1*03:01* was significantly increased ($p<1x10^{-8}$, OR=5.08) in patients (Figure 3a). However *DQB1*03:02* and *DQB1*03:07*, alleles linked with *DRB1*04:01*, *DRB1*04:03*, *DRB1*04:04* and *DRB1*04:05* were not significantly increased in the patients because two of these alleles *DRB1*04:01* and *DRB1*04:05* were increased in the patients and the other two DR4 alleles *DRB1*04:03* and *DRB1*04:04* were significantly reduced in the patients. *DQB1*03:01* ($p<6x10^{-4}$, OR=0.27) and

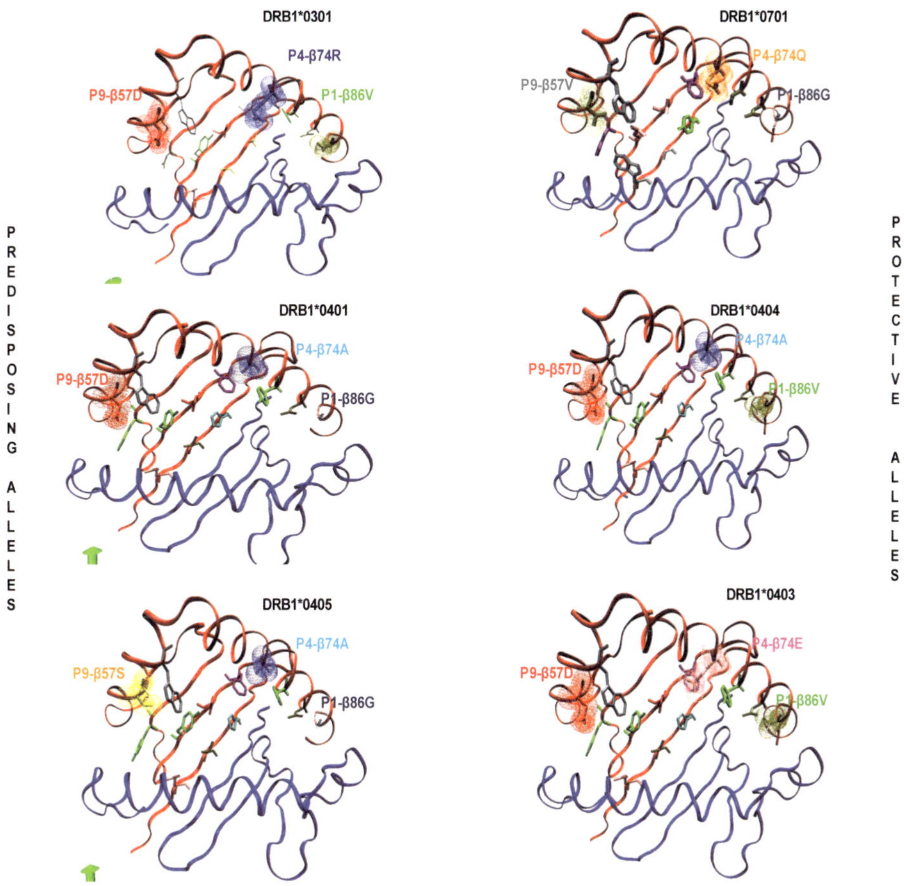

Fig. 2. Peptide binding groove of the predisposing and protective HLA-DRB1 alleles showing positions β57 (P9), β74 (P4) and β86 (P1) for predisposing *DRB1*03:01, DRB1*04:01* and *DRB1*04:05* and protective *DRB1*07:01, DRB1*04:04* and *DRB1*04:03* alleles.

*DQB1*05:03* ($6x10^{-4}$, OR=0.28) were significantly reduced in the patients. Homozygosity of *DQB1*02:01* was significantly ($p<1x10^{-5}$, OR=5.4) increased in the patients (Figure 3b). *DQB1*03:02* which was not significantly increased in the patients, showed a significant increase in heterozygous combination with *DQB1*0201* ($p<2x10^{-5}$, OR=34.16). In fact none of the controls had *DQB1*0201/*0302* heterozygous combination. In a Swedish study, *DQA1*0301/DQB1*0302* and heterozygous combinations of *DQA1*0301/DQB1*0302* and *DQA1*0201/DQB1*0501* have been shown to confer the highest susceptibility (Sanjeevi et al., 1995).

Some critical residues within the peptide binding sites of HLA-DQ beta chain have been proposed to play a crucial role in conferring predisposition to and protection from the diseases (Nepom & Kwok, 1998, Sheehy, 1992, Todd et al., 1987). Several studies have suggested that aspartic acid at DQβ residue 57 confers protection while DQB1 alleles with alanine at that position (*DQB1*02:01* and *DQB1*03:02*) and DQA1 with arginine at position 52 (R^{52}) confer susceptibility (Badenhoop et al., 1995, Chauffert et al., 1995, Todd et al., 1987). However, an individual can be either homozygous or heterozygous for alleles carrying

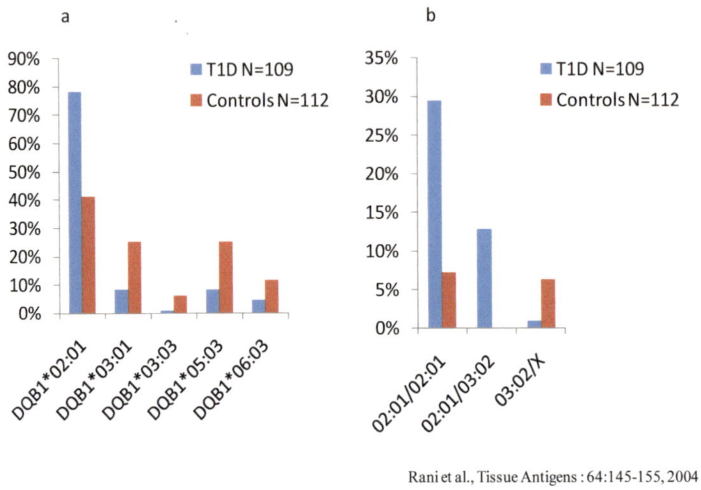

Fig. 3. Distribution of *HLA-DQB1* alleles in T1D patients and controls. **a** shows *DQB1*02:01* was significantly increased and *DQB1*03:01* and *DQB1*05:03* were significantly reduced in T1D patients as compared to controls. **b**. Homozygous and heterozygous DQB1 alleles in T1D. Homozygous *DQB1*02:01/*02:01* and heterozygous *DQB1*02:01/*03:02* were significantly increased and *DQB1*03:02/X* were significantly reduced in T1D patients as compared to controls (Rani et al., 2004).

Asp^{57} in DQB1 or Arg^{52} in DQA1. Our in-depth investigation revealed that when DR3 homozygosity was considered along with codon 57 of *DQB1* and codon 52 of *DQA1*, the only combination that was significantly increased in the patients group as compared to the controls was *DRB1*03:01,03:01-DQB1*XX-DQA1*RR*, suggesting that *DRB1*03:01* association is primary since the *DQB1* and *DQA1* alleles which are in linkage disequilibrium with *DRB1*03:01* have non-Asp57 (DQB1*X) and Arg52 (DQA1*R), respectively(Rani et al., 1999).

3. Insulin linked polymorphic region in T1D (IDDM2)

Insulin linked polymorphic region *(IDDM2)* consists of a highly polymorphic stretch of 14-15 base pair repeats of DNA lying 365 bp upstream of the initiation of transcription of the *insulin (INS)* gene. *IDDM2* has been shown to have a role in transcription of insulin in thymus. Several forms of IDDM2 have been reported based on the number of repeats (Bell et al., 1981, Kennedy et al., 1995). These *INS-variable number of tandem repeats (VNTR)* are divided into three different classes based on their sizes: *class-I* (26-63 repeats), *Class II* (about 85 repeats) and *class III* (141-209 repeats) (Bell et al., 1982, Bennett et al., 1995, Rotwein et al., 1986). T1D is associated with class I homozygosity (Bell et al., 1981, Bennett et al., 1995, Kennedy et al., 1995, Lucassen et al., 1993). We studied *INS-VNTR Class-I* and *Class-III* alleles based on typing for *Insulin gene 1127 Pst I* site (3'end) by PCR-RFLP as described by Pugliese et al (Pugliese et al., 1997)
Table 1 shows the frequencies of *Insulin VNTR* in T1D patients and healthy controls. While the frequency of *class-I VNTR* was increased significantly in the patients, *class-III VNTR* was decreased in them as compared to the controls. However, when the genotypes were studied, *class I* homozygosity was considerably increased in the patients as compared to controls,

giving an Odds ratio of 7.8. *Class I, III* heterozygosity was significantly reduced in the patients (Rani et al., 2004).

INS-VNTR	DIABETES		CONTROLS		p value	OR
	No.	%	No.	%		
Class I	108	98.2	85	89.47	0.008	6.35
Class III	64	58.2	87	91.57	2×10^{-8}	0.13
Genotypes						
Class I, I	46	41.8	8	8.42	2×10^{-8}	7.8
Class I, III	62	56.4	77	81.05	10^{-5}	0.301
Class III, III	2	1.8	10	10.52	0.008	0.157

Table 1. INS-VNTR allele frequencies and Genotype frequencies in T1D patients and controls.

3.1 Simultaneous presence of predisposing *HLA-DRB1* and *INS-VNTR* alleles

MHC and *VNTR* are encoded on two different chromosomes. However, they may have integrated roles in manifestation of T1D due to the functional implications of these genes. So, we studied if simultaneous presence of the predisposing alleles of the two genes had any role to play in manifestation of T1D.

Our investigation revealed that homozygous *Class-I INS-VNTR* along with homozygous or heterozygous *DRB1*03:01* were significantly increased in the T1D patients ($p<1\times10^{-8}$) with a Relative Risk of 70.81 (Rani et al., 2004). In fact, none of the controls had homozygous *Class-I INS-VNTR* along with *DRB1*03:01* in homozygous or heterozygous state. This combination gives a positive predictive value (PPV) of 100% with a specificity of 100% and sensitivity of 32.63% since only 32.63% of the patients showed this combination. Since *DRB1*03:01* homozygosity is significantly increased in the patients, homozygous *DRB1*03:01* and heterozygous *DRB1*03:01* only with *DRB1*04:01* and *DRB1*04:05* along with heterozygous *I, III-INS-VNTR* may also be considered as predisposing since it gives a relative risk of 10.55 (Rani et al., 2004).

If we add all these predisposing combinations i.e. simultaneous presence of homozygous or heterozygous *HLA-DRB1*03:01* along with homozygous (Class-I, I) or heterozygous (I, III) VNTR class-I and III, 50.53% of the patients as compared to only 1.4% of the controls had these combinations giving a relative risk of 48.67. This combination gives a PPV of 97.96% with a specificity of 98.6% and sensitivity of 50.5% since only 50.5% of the patients showed this combination. Thus, our results showed that: (1) homozygous or heterozygous *DRB1*03:01* along with homozygous Class-I INS-VNTR and (2) homozygous *DRB*03:01* and heterozygous *DRB1*03:01* only with *DRB1*04:01* or *DRB1*04:05* with heterozygous *Class-I/III* INS-VNTR may be used to predict a pre-diabetic before the onset of the disease in North Indian high risk group (Rani et al., 2004). However, typing a larger cohort may be required to confirm such a major increase in risk.

Pathogenesis of T1D is extremely complex. Significant association with *HLA-DRB1*03:01* and *INS-VNTR Class-I* may have functional implications. Increase in frequency of particular MHC allele suggests that these molecules may be preferentially presenting certain auto-peptides to the T cells resulting in subsequent autoimmune responses. Studies on *INS-VNTR,* however, have shown that *class-III* alleles are associated with 2 to 3 fold higher mRNA levels of insulin than *Class-I* in thymii of fetuses, suggesting poor expression of thymic INS expression resulting in poor thymic education for insulin in people with homozygous *Class-I,I* and *class-I,III VNTRs* resulting in break of tolerance in predisposed individuals. However, higher expression of insulin in the thymii of individuals with homozygous *class-III, III* may be able to facilitate immune tolerance induction, as a mechanism for dominant protective effect of *Class-III* alleles (Pugliese et al., 1997, Vafiadis et al., 1997).

Our results are contrary to that of Veijola et al. (Veijola et al., 1995) on Finnish children who showed that both 5' and 3' INS loci showed an association with T1D in *non-DR3/non-DR4* patients (Veijola et al., 1995). However, in our studies only 9.47% of the non-*DR3/DR4* patients were homozygous for *Class-I INS-VNTR* as compared to 4.2% controls and this difference was not significant statistically. Julier et al. (Julier et al., 1991), on the other hand, had reported that the risk contributed by the INS region was increased in *DR4*-positive patients. Again, in our study only 6.32% of the patients as compared to 1.39% of controls had *INS-VNTR class-I* homozygosity with *DRB1*04:01* and *DRB1*04:05* alleles and this difference was not significant statistically.

4. Cytokine genes

Cytokines are the coordinators of the immune system that interact in integrated networks and functions of one cytokine may be modulated or substituted by another (Bidwell et al., 1999). A cascade of cytokines are involved in pro-inflammatory auto-immune responses in T1D. Single nucleotide polymorphisms (SNPs) in different pro-inflammatory and anti-inflammatory cytokine genes at certain defined regions have been shown to be associated with differential amount of their production (Asderakis et al., 2001, Awad et al., 1998, Bittar et al., 2006, Burzotta et al., 2001, Fishman et al., 1998, Louis et al., 1998, Pociot et al., 1993). Pro-inflammatory cytokines and their integrated influences are known to regulate complex immune responses during autoimmune destruction of tissues (Rabinovitch, 1994). Hence it is necessary that they are studied and analysed in context of each other and not in isolation from each other. We had reported for the first time the integration and interaction of *TNF-α* gene with other cytokine genes and *HLA-DRB1* and *B* loci alleles (Kumar et al., 2007).

We studied the cytokine gene polymorphism using XIIIth International Histocompatibility Workshop's (IHWC, Heidelberg kit) and One lambda's cytokine typing kits (Canoga Park, CA, USA) based on Polymerase Chain reaction (PCR) with sequence specific primers (PCR-SSP). PCR-SSPs were done for *IFN-γ* ($A^{+874}T$) (14), *TNF-α* ($G^{-308}A$) (15), *IL-6* ($G^{-174}C$) (9), *IL-10* ($A^{-1082}G$, $T^{-819}C$, $C^{-592}A$) (16), and *TGFβ1* ($T^{cdn10}C$, $G^{cdn25}C$) (11). *T→C* substitution in nucleotide 29, codon 10 of the first exon of TGFβ1, changes the amino acid Leu → Pro. Similarly *G→ C* substitution in nucleotide 74, codon 25 of first exon of *TGFβ1*, changes the amino acid Arg → Pro. However, since we are studying the SNPs in the two codons, we will refer to the SNPs in codons 10 and 25 hereafter. and not the resultant amino acids to avoid any confusion and to maintain consistency with the other SNPs.

Our results showed that the high producing genotype of *TNF-α-308GA* and *AA* were significantly increased and low producing genotype *GG* was significantly reduced in T1D patients as compared to controls ($p < 7 \times 10^{-6}$). None of the other cytokine genes showed any significant difference between the patients and controls.

4.1 Simultaneous presence of TNF-α genotypes with IFN-γ, IL-6, IL-10 and TGF-β1 genotypes and haplotypes

TNF-α, IFN-γ, IL-10, IL-6 and *TGF-β1* genes are localized on different chromosomes. *TNF-α* is encoded on chromosome 6p21.3, *IFN-γ* is encoded on 12q14, *IL-10* is encoded on 1q31-q32, *IL-6* is encoded on 7p21 and *TGF-β1* is encoded on 19q13.2. However, the products of these genes interact in integrated networks. Since only *TNF-α* showed a significant association with T1D, we studied whether simultaneous presence of *TNF-α* genotypes with different genotypes of the other cytokines in an individual could suggest an interaction between these cytokine genes.

Other cytokines	TNF-α GA/AA				TNF-α GG			
Genotype / haplotype	T1D No. (%)	Controls No. (%)	p	OR (95% CI)	T1D No. (%)	Controls No. (%)	p	OR (95% CI)
IFN-γ Int +874	N=235	N=128			N=235	N=128		
AA (L)	41 (17.4)	9 (7.0)	0.003@	2.79 (1. 25-6.42)	46 (19.6)	44 (34.4)	0.001@	0.465 (0.28-0.77)
TA+TT (H)	56 (23.8)	15 (11.07)	0.003@	2.39 (1.24-4.66)	92 (39.1)	60 (46. 9)	0.188	0.729 (0.461-1.15)
IL-6 -174	N=235	N=127$			N=235	N=127$		
CC (L)	11 (4.7)	1 (0.78)	0.03#	4.3 (1. 21-14.56)	14 (5.95)	8 (6.29)	0.531	0.919 (0.357-2.53)
GG+GC (H)	86 (36.6)	23 (18.1)	0.0001@	2.61 (1.5-4.56)	124 (52.75)	95 (74.8)	0.000004@	0.76 (0.227-0.621)
IL-10 Haplotypes*	N=235	N=128			N=235	N=128		
Low secretor	45 (19.2)	16 (12.7)	0.068	1.65 (0.86-3.22)	77 (32.76)	57 (44.5)	0.03#	0. 607 (0. 38-0.96)
High Secretor	52 (22.1)	8 (6. 25)	0.0001@	4.26 (1.9-10.1)	61 (25.95)	47 (36.7)	0.04#	0.6 (0.37-0.98)
TGF-β1 Haplotypes*	N=235	N=128			N=235	N=128		
Low secretor	8 (3.4)	1 (0.8)	0.11	3.17 (0.87-12.11)	7 (2.98)	3 (2.3)	0.506	1.17 (0.443-3.23)
High Secretor	89 (37.8)	23 (18.0)	0.00004@	2.8 (1.6-4.86)	131 (55.7)	101 (78.9)	0.000006@	0. 336 (0.198-0.568)

N=Total number of samples studied, $Number of control samples studied for IL-6 were 127, one sample could not be typed due to PCR failure. TNF-α GA/AA have been combined as high secretor genotypes.
# Corrected p value (pc) not significant, @ Corrected p value (pc) significant,
*IL-10 : halpotype combinations -1082/-819/-590 : GCC,GCC; GCC,ACC; GCC,ATA= high secretors; ACC,ACC; ACC,ATA = Low secretors.
TGF- β1 halpotype combinations Cdn10/Cdn25 : TG,TG; TG,CG; TG,CC; CG,CG =High secretors, CG,CC, CC,CC = Low secretors.

Table 2. Simultaneous presence of *TNF-α* genotypes with *IFN-γ, IL-6, IL-10* and *TGF-β1* genotypes and haplotypes (Kumar et al., 2007).

Table 2 shows the simultaneous presence of high and low secreting genotypes of *TNF-α,* along with *IFN-γ, IL-6, IL-10* and *TGF-β1* genotypes and haplotypes. When *IFN-γ* was studied by itself, it did not show any significant difference between patients and controls. However, when studied in the context of *TNF-α -308G/A,* both low and high secretor genotypes, *IFN-γ (+874AA* and *TA+TT* respectively) along with high secretor genotypes of *TNF-α -308 GA+AA* were significantly increased in patients as compared to controls, suggesting its effect is rather neutral. However, low producer genotypes of *TNF-α -308GG* along with low producer genotype of *IFN-γ +874 AA* seems to be protective. Interestingly, 66. 7% of the patients who had low producer genotype of *TNF-α -308GG* had high producer genotype of *IFN-γ +874 TA+TT*. Hence, in the absence of high secretor genotype of *TNF-α, IFN-γ* may have a role in autoimmune destruction of pancreatic beta cells. *IFN-γ* acts singularly as well as synergistically with other inflammatory stimuli to induce NO production which can be cytotoxic and thus has been implicated in pathogenesis of certain autoimmune and inflammatory diseases (Mccartney-Francis et al., 1993).
Similarly, promoter SNPs of *IL-6 -174G/C* did not show any significant difference between patients and controls, but when studied in the context of *TNF-α -308G/A,* high producer genotypes, *IL-6 -174 GG+GC* (Fishman et al., 1998) were increased in patients with *TNF-α -308 GA+AA.* Kristiansen and Mandrup-Poulsen (Kristiansen & Mandrup-Poulsen, 2005) have shown that IL-6 promotes islet inflammation but is unable to promote β-cell destruction for which other pro-inflammatory cytokines are needed. The other pro-inflammatory cytokine playing a role in destruction β-cells in the present scenario could be

HLA-B-DRB1-haplotypes	Patients N=210		Controls N=91.		p	OR (95% C.I.)
	No*	%	No*	%		
*B*8-DRB1*03*	69	32.85	3	3.3	10^{-8}	14.35 (4.19 -37.93)
*B*8- Non DRB1*03*	2	0.95	1	1.1	0.662	0.865 (0.498-1.5)
*B*50 – DRB1*03*	41	19.5	3	3.3	$6x10^{-5}$	7.11 (2.04-21.47)
*B*50 – Non-DRB1*03*	6	2.86	4	4.4	0.355	0.639 (0.155-2.77)
*B*58 – DRB1*03*	36	17.1	5	5.5	0.003	3.55 (1.27-10.72)
*B*58 – Non DRB1*03*	3	1.4	8	8.8	0.003	0.165 (0.06-0.433)
*NonB8/B50/58-DRB1*03*	35	16.7	6	6.6	0.01	2.83 (1.09-7.82)
*NonB8/B50/B58/non DRB1*03*	38	18.1	59	64.8	10^{-8}	0.12 (0.06-0.216)

* No. of patients /Controls with the haplotypes shown in the first column.

Table 3. Comparison of HLA-B-DRB1 haplotypes showing significant association, between patients and controls (Kumar et al., 2007)

TNF- α in patients with *GA* and *AA* genotypes and IFN-γ in patients with *TNF-α GG* genotype. High producer genotype *IL-6 -174 GG+GC* along with low producer genotype of *TNF-α -308GG* seems to be protective.
Different haplotypes of *IL-10* based on SNPs in the promoter region have been shown to be associated with quantity of IL-10 production in-vitro (Asderakis et al., 2001, Stanilova et al., 2006). The frequency of low producer haplotype of *IL-10 ATA* (haplotype with positions -1082/-819/-590) has been shown to be increased in the adult onset patients in Japan, with no significant differences between T1D patients and controls (Ide et al., 2002). Reynier et al (Reynier et al., 2006) did not see any significant association of *IL-10-1082G/A* with T1D in French population. However, they did observe a significant association of *IL-10 -1082* polymorphism to be associated with GAD and IA-2 antibody at clinical onset. In our study also, we did not observe any significant difference between TID patients and controls when *IL-10* was studied by itself. However, simultaneous presence of high producer genotypes of *TNF-α -308 GA+AA* and high producer haplotypes of *IL-10* in the patients may have a role in recruitment of islet specific CD8$^+$ T cells and thus may have a role in insulitis through ICAM-1 dependent pathway. In non-obese diabetic (NOD) mice (animal model for human Type 1 diabetes) pancreatic IL-10 has been shown to hyper-induce ICAM-1 expression on vascular endothelium. However, in the absence of ICAM-1, insulitis and diabetes could be prevented, thus providing evidence that IL-10 is sufficient to drive pathogenic autoimmune responses and accelerated diabetes via an ICAM-1 dependent pathway (Balasa et al., 2000). Presence of IL-10 during early stages of IDDM has also been shown to favor the generation of effector CD8$^+$ T cells leading to accelerated diabetes in NOD mice (Balasa et al., 2000). Treatment of young mice with anti-TNF-α and anti-IL-10 mAb has also been shown to prevent diabetes and insulitis (Lee et al., 1996, Yang et al., 1994).
Similarly, when *TGF-β1* was studied by itself, no significant difference was observed between patients and controls. A significant increase of high producer haplotypes of *TGF-β1* with *TNF-α -308 GA+AA* and a significant decrease of high producer haplotypes of *TGF-β*1 with *TNF-α -308GG* in T1D patients as compared to controls was observed. These results show that different cytokines work in concert with each other and may alter or modulate their functions depending on the milieu. TGF-β1 has been shown to be an extremely potent chemotactic factor in-vitro which influences monocyte recruitment and accumulation via increased expression of α and β integrins (Wahl et al., 1993). It has been shown to rapidly and transiently up-regulate α-4 integrin dependent adhesion of leukocyte cell lines and peripheral blood lymphocytes (Bartolome et al., 2003). α-4 integrin, in turn, has been shown to play a prominent role in the spontaneous development of insulitis and diabetes in NOD mice (Yang et al., 1997). Increased levels of TGF-β1 have been associated with destruction of pancreatic beta cells and pathogenesis of diabetic complications (Korpinen et al., 2001). Hence, in the presence of high secretors of *TNF-α*, the high secretor genotypes of *TGF-β1* may have a role both in destruction of pancreatic beta cells as well as in migration of CD4$^+$ and CD8$^+$ T cells into the pancreas (Insulitis) through α-4 integrin, which act against pancreatic beta cells along with Nitric oxide mediated cytotoxicity. Under these circumstances, TGF-β1 may not be able to arrest the pro-inflammatory functions of TNF-α and IFN-γ.
So, our data provides circumstantial evidence justifying the presence of high secretor genotypes of T*NF-α -308GA* and *AA* along with high secretor genotypes of *IL-6, IL-10* and *TGF-β1* and provide an immunogenetic basis for the autoimmune responses in T1D. The data suggest that the beta cell destruction in T1D may be mediated by both CD4$^+$ T helper

cells and CD8+ cytotoxic T cells recruited through Integrins and ICAM-1 dependent pathways in the pancreas for which cytokine genes seem to play a pivotal role.

4.2 *TNF-* α and *HLA* genes

TNF-α gene is very closely linked to the MHC. Deng et al (Deng et al., 1996) observed that the *TNF-α* associations in Caucasians and Chinese of Taiwan, may be due to its being in linkage disequilibrium with *DR3-DQB1*0201* haplotype. We too had observed *DRB1*03:01, DRB1*04:01* and *DRB1*04:05* to be associated with T1D in North Indians (Rani et al., 2004). Hence, we wanted to study if the *TNF-α* association was independent of these alleles or due to linkage disequilibrium (LD) between *TNF-α -308A* and the predisposing *DRB1* alleles. Interestingly, the LD analysis showed that both *TNF-α -308A* as well as *TNF-α -308G* alleles are in LD with *DRB1*03:01,* the most predisposing *HLA-DRB1* allele, suggesting that the effect of *TNF-α -308A* is not because of its being in LD with *HLA-DRB1*03:01,* the predisposing MHC allele.
Since *TNF-α* locus is very closely linked to *HLA-B* locus, we also studied the alleles of B-locus for a possibility of *TNF-α -308A* allele being in LD with one of the B-locus alleles . Surprisingly we observed LD between *TNF-α -308G* with *B*08* and *TNF-α -308A* allele with *HLA B*50:01* and *B*58:01*. All the three B-locus alleles *B*08:01, B*50:01* and *B*58:01* were in linkage disequilibrium with *DRB1*03:01* (Table 3). Because of *HLA-B*08* being in LD with *TNF-α -308G, B*08:01-DRB1*03:01* haplotype was also in LD with *TNF-α -308G* (Table 4).

HLA-B-TNF-α-DRB1-haplotypes	Number of haplotypes observed 2N=418	Haplotype frequencies	D_{abc}#
*B*8- TNF-α -308A-DRB1*03*	19	0.045	-0.013
*B*8- TNF-α -308G-DRB1*03*	75	0.179	0.015
*B*50- TNF-α -308A-DRB1*03*	42	0.1	0.0329
*B*50- TNF-α -308G-DRB1*03*	32	0.076	-0.0023
*B*58- TNF-α -308A-DRB1*03*	33	0.079	0.0141
*B*58- TNF-α -308G-DRB1*03*	28	0.067	-0.0032

Table 4. Linkage disequilibrium analysis of *HLA-B- TNF-a -DRB1* haplotypes prevalent in T1D patients from North India (Kumar et al., 2007).

However, B*50:01-DRB1*03:01 and B*58:01-DRB1*03:01 haplotypes were in LD with TNF-α -308A allele. We observed 48.8 % of the patients had B*08/non-B*08/non-B*50:01/non-B*58:01-**TNF-α-308G**-DRB1*03:01 haplotypes as compared to 34 % with B*50:01/ B*58:01-**TNF-α -308A**-DRB1*03:01 haplotypes. With this in-depth analysis, it becomes clear that the effect of TNF-α -308A allele is not because of its being in LD with DRB1*03:01, B*08:01, B*50:01 or B*58:01, but due its functional implications and its integrated effect with other cytokines. In conclusion, while the MHC may be involved in auto-antigen presentation, TNF- alpha and other cytokines play an integrated role in destruction of the pancreatic beta cells though enrichment and recruitment of autoantigen specific CD4+ and CD8+ T cells which have immunogenetic bases (Figure 6).

5. Vitamin D receptor

Vitamin D Receptor (VDR) is a ligand dependent transcription factor that belongs to the super family of the Nuclear Hormone Receptors (Evans, 1988). The ligand for VDR is

Vitamin D3 i.e., 1,25-$(OH)_2D_3$ which mediates its biological actions through VDR. When 1,25-$(OH)_2D_3$ binds to VDR, it induces conformational changes in VDR promoting its hetero-dimerization with Retinoid X Receptor (RXR), followed by translocation of this complex into the nucleus. The RXR-VDR heterodimer in turn binds to the vitamin D_3 responsive elements (VDRE) in promoter regions of vitamin D responsive genes (Boonstra et al., 2001). This results in the regulatory function of Vitamin D3. In the absence of classical responsive elements, 1,25-$(OH)_2D_3$ may controls the expression of some genes like cytokine genes by targeting inducible transcription factors like NFAT in IL-2 in a sequence specific manner (Takeuchi et al., 1998). 1,25-$(OH)_2D_3$ has been shown to have an important immuno-modulatory role since it represses transcription of Th1 cytokines like *IL-2* (Alroy et al., 1995, Bhalla et al., 1984), *IFN-γ* (Cippitelli & Santoni, 1998) and *IL-12* (D'ambrosio et al., 1998) and up regulates the production of Th2 cytokines IL-4 and TGF-β1 (Cantorna et al., 1998). It has been shown to enhance the development of TH2 cells via a direct effect on naive $CD4^+$ cells (Boonstra et al., 2001). Besides, 1,25-$(OH)_2D_3$ has also been shown to modulate the expression of *HLA* class-II alleles on monocytes and human bone cells (Rigby et al., 1990, Skjodt et al., 1990)

Studies have shown that administration of Vitamin D3 in NOD mice, before the onset of Insulitis, can effectively prevent the disease progression. However, when administered after the establishment of insulitis, vitamin D3 was not as effective. Similarly, in humans too, vitamin D supplementation in early childhood has been shown to reduce the incidence of T1D (Hypponen et al., 2001, Jones et al., 1998). Since 1,25-$(OH)_2D_3$ mediatesi its effect through VDR, we studied the *VDR* gene polymorphisms and their interaction with the most predisposing *MHC* alleles to investigate their role, if any, in the pathophysiology of T1D.

The VDR SNPs studied include the T>C SNP in exon2 initiation codon detected with *FokI* restriction enzyme (Gross et al., 1996), the A>G SNP detected with *BsmI* (Morrison et al., 1992) and G>T SNP detected with *ApaI* (Faraco et al., 1989) located in Intron 8, and a silent C>T SNP (Durrin et al., 1999) detected with *TaqI,* located in Exon 9. These SNPS were studied using PCR amplification and restriction digestion by the aforesaid enzymes as described earlier (Faraco et al., 1989, Hustmyer et al., 1993). We also studied the interaction between *VDR* alleles and predisposing *HLA* alleles using LD based statistics (Zhao et al., 2006) and subsequently sequenced the promoter region of the predisposing *MHC* allele to detect the VDRE sequence which has been shown to modulate the expression of the HLA alleles (Ramagopalan et al., 2009), suggesting the functional implications of the statistically significant interaction (Israni et al., 2009). We further provided documentary evidence that expression of HLA class-II molecules was being modulated by vitamin D3.

5.1 VDR *FokI, BsmI, ApaI* and *TaqI* genotypes and haplotypes in T1D patients

While there were no significant differences in the genotypes of *ApaI* and *TaqI* in patients and controls. *FokI 'ff'* was significantly increased in the patient group as compared to controls and *BsmI 'bb'* was significantly decreased in the patient group. However, these differences did not remain significant after Boneferroni's correction (Israni et al., 2009).

Haplotype analysis was carried out for the four restriction sites studied in the VDR gene in patients and controls using SHEsis program (http://202.120.7.14/analysis/myAnalysis.php) (Shi & He, 2005). Additionally, Famhap (http://famhap.meb.uni-bonn.de) was used to confim the frequencies of the haplotypes. Haplotype *FBAt* and *fBAT* were significantly increased in T1D patients and *fBAt* was significantly reduced in them as compared to controls.

5.2 Gene to gene interaction of *VDR* haplotypes with predisposing *HLA* alleles

Simulateneous presence of different VDR haplotypes along with the predisposing *HLA* alleles was studied in patients. Interestingly, simultaneous presence of haplotypes *FBAT* and *FbaT* along with the predisposing *DRB1* alleles was significantly increased while the same haplotypes were protective when associated with non-predisposing alleles of *DRB1*. Similar results were obtained with other haplotypes like *FBAt, fBAT and fbaT* in association with the predisposing *HLA-DRB1* alleles (Israni et al., 2009).

To study the interaction between two unlinked loci i.e., *VDR* and the predisposing *HLA-DRB1* alleles, we used LD based statistics as described by Zhao et al (Zhao et al., 2006). The analysis revealed that *F* and *T* alleles in the exons 2 and 9 for *FokI* and *TaqI* restriction sites respectively showed significant interactions with predisposing *HLA-DRB1* allele *DRB1*03:01* (Israni et al., 2009).

```
                          S-BOX                            X-BOX
Reference    TTTCAGAAGAGGACCTTCATACAGCATCTCTGACCAGCAACTGATGATGCTATTGAACTC
ID007        TTTCAGAAGAGGACCTTCATACAGCATTTCTGACCAGCAACTGATGATGCTATTGAACTC
ID059        TTTCAGAAGAGGACCTTCATACAGCATTTCTGACCAGCAACTGATGATGCTATTGAACTC
ID090        ---------------TCATACAGCATCTCTGACCAGCAACTGATGATGCTATTGAACTC
A217         TTTCAGAAGAGGACCTTCATACAGCATTTCTGACCAGCAACTGATGATGCTATTGAACTC
A177         ----------------TCATACAGCATCTCTGACCAGCAACTGATGATGCTATTGAACTC
A212         ----------------TCATACAGCATCTCTGACCAGCAACTGATGATGCTATTGAACTC
             *************************** ********************************

                    Y-BOX                      CCAAY BOX
Reference    AGATGCTGATTGGTTCTCCAACACGAGATTACCCAATCCAGGAGCAAGGAAATCAGTAA
ID007        AGATGCTGATTGGTTTTCCAACACTAGATTACCCAATCCAGGAGCAAGGAAATCAGTAA
ID059        AGATGGGGATTCGTTTTCCACCACTAGATTACCCAATCCAGGAGCAAGGAAATCAGTAA
ID090        AGATGCTGATTCGTTCTCCAACACTAGATTACCCAATCCAGGAGCAAGGAAATCAGTAA
A217         AGATGCTGATTGGTTCTCCAACACTAGATTACCCAATCCAGGAGCAAGGAAATCAGTAA
A177         AGATGCTGATTCGTTCTCCAACACTAGATTACCCAATCCAGGAGCAAGGAAATCAGTAA
A212         AGATGCTGATTCGTTCTCCAACACTAGATTACCCAATCCAGGAGCAAGGAAATCAGTAA
             *****  **** *** **** *** **********************************

                      TATA BOX             VDRE     Transcriptional start site
Reference    CTTCCTCCCTATAACTTGGAATGTGGGTGGAGGGGTTCATAGTTCTCCCTGAGTGAGACT
ID007        CTTCCTCCCTATAACTTGGAATGTGGGTGGAGGGGTTCATAGTTCTCCCTGAGTGAGACT
ID059        CTTCCTCCCTATAACTTGGAATGTGGGTGGAGGGGTTCATAGTTCTCCCTGAGTGAGACT
ID090        CTTACTCCCTATAACTTGGAATGTGGGTGGAGGGGTTCATAGTTCTCCCTGAGTGAGACT
A217         CTTCCCCCCTATAACTTGGAATGTGGGTGGAGGGGTTCATAGTTCTCCCTGAGTGATACT
A177         CTTACTCCCTATAACTTGGAATGTGGGTGGAGGGGTTCATAGTTCTCCCTGAGTGAGACT
A212         CTTACTCCCTATAACTTGGAATGTGGGTGGAGGGGTTCATAGTTCTCCCTGAGTGAGACT
             *** * ***************************************************** ***

Reference    TGCCTGCTTCTCTGGCCCCTGGTCCTGTCCTGTTCTCCAGCATGGTGTGTCTGAAGCTCC
ID007        TGCCTGCTGCTCTGGCCCCTGGTCCTGTCCTGTTCTCCAGCATGGTGTGTCTGAGGCTCC
ID059        TGCCTGCTGCTCTGGCCCCTGGTCCTGTCCTGTTCTCCAGCATGGTGTGTCTGAGGCTCC
ID090        TGCCTGCTGCTCTGGCCCCTGGTCCTGTCCTGTTCTCCAGCATGGTGTGTCTGATGCTCC
A217         TGCCTGCTGCTCTGGCCCCTGGTCCTGTCCTGTTCTCCAGCATGGTGTGTCTGAGGCTCC
A177         TGCCTGCTGCTCTGGCCCCTGGTCCTGTCCTGTTCTCCAGCATGGTGTGTCTGATGCTCC
A212         TGCCTGCTGCTCTGGCCCCTGGTCCTGTCCTGTTCTCCAGCATGGTGTGTCTGATGCTCC
             ******** ********************************************* *****
```

Fig. 4. *HLA- DRB1*03:01* promoter sequence from 3 subjects suffering from T1D and 3 normal healthy individuals homozygous for *DRB1*03:01*. Important regulatory elements like S-box, X-box, Y-box, CCAAY-box, TATA-box and VDRE are highlighted. Star (*) in the last row shows homology and dots (.) shows nucleotide substitution in one or more samples at that particular site and dashes(-) represent gaps inserted to maximize the homology. (Israni et al., 2009).

5.3 Sequence analysis of HLA DRB1*0301 promoter region

Amongst the predisposing *HLA-DRB1* alleles, majority of the patients (85.9%) had *DRB1*03:01*. Thus, we sought to look for the VDRE in the promoter region of the allele. The promoter regions of 3 T1D subjects and 3 healthy controls homozygous for *HLA-DRB1*03:01* were amplified and sequenced to determine the VDRE variants in the North Indian population. Sequences were aligned using ClustalW2, and the presence of a VDRE was confirmed in-silico using JASPAR_CORE version 3.0 database using default conditions (Sandelin et al., 2004). Figure 4 shows the *HLA- DRB1*03:01* promoter sequences showing the localization of vitamin D response element (VDRE) in the promoter region of HLA-*DRB1*0301* from the 6 subjects.

Interestingly, the alignment showed exactly the same sequence of VDRE in the promoter region of *HLA-DRB1*03:01* which has been shown to influence the expression of *HLA* allele *DRB1*15:01* by Ramagopalan et al (Ramagopalan et al., 2009) suggesting the bases for interaction of VDR with *HLA-DRB1*03:01*

5.4 Altered expression of *HLA-DRB1*03:01* by 1,25-$(OH)_2D_3$ (Calcitriol)

5.4.1 Flow cytometry

To study if vitamin D3 administartion would alter the expression of MHC class-II, we stimulated *HLA-DRB1*03:01* homozygous B-lymphoblastoid cell (B-LCL) line VAVY (International Histocompatibility Workshop cell line Number IHW09023) with 100nM of calcitriol (Sigma) for 24 hours and stained with anti-HLA DR-PE antibody (BD Biosciences) and acquired on BD-LSR to study the expression of HLA-DR on stimulated and unstimulated B-LCL The data was analysed using WinMDI 2.9 software. The results showed significantly higher expression of HLA-DR in the B-LCL stimulated with calcitriol as compared to the unstimulated one (Figure 5A and B).

5.4.2 Real time PCR

We also studied the levels of transcripts for *HLA-DRB1* in B-LCL VAVY after 24 hour stimulation with calcitriol and compared it to unstimulated B-LCL using real time PCR. The data shows 1.89 fold increase in the *HLA-DRB1* transcripts from B-LCL stimulated with calcitriol as compared to the unstimulated one. These results were confirmed on perpheral blood mononuclear cells (PBMCs) derived from a normal healthy control homozygous for *HLA-DRB1*03:01.*

Our results showed enhanced expression of HLA-DR on the B-LCLs stimulated with calcitriol as compared to the unstimulated one confirming that indeed the interaction of VDR with *HLA-DRB1*03:01* is occurring through the VDRE present in the promoter region of the gene. Based on the earlier studies and the present data one can speculate that in the absence of required amount of Vitamin D in early life in the predisposed individuals with *HLA-DRB1*03:01*, the expression of the allele may be impaired in the thymus (Ramagopalan et al., 2009) resulting in escape from thymic deletion of autoreactive T cells leading to T1D manifestations.

6. Conclusions

Our studies show that simultaneous presence of *DRB1*03:01* along with homozygous *INS-VNTR* class-I was significantly increased ($p < 10^{-8}$) in T1D patients, giving a relative risk of 70.81 (Rani et al., 2004). *INS-VNTR* class-I has been shown to be associated with lower

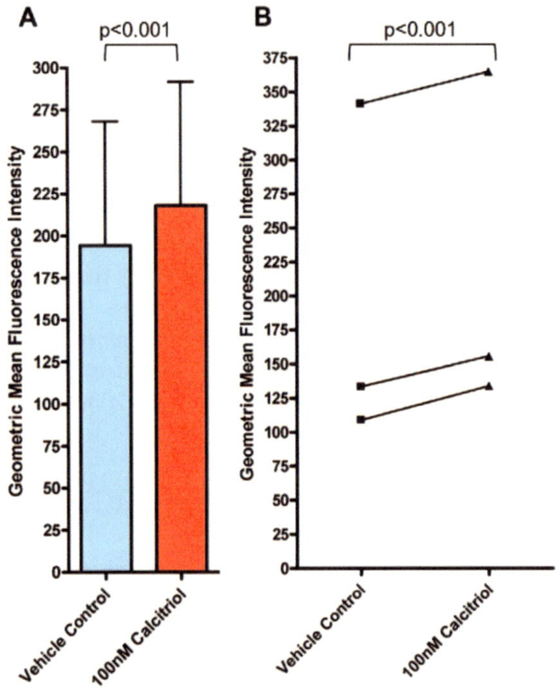

Fig. 5. Flow cytometric analysis of HLA-DR expression. A: Histogram of HLA-DR-PE staining of B-LCL-VAVY cells treated with and without 100nM calcitriol. The figure shows enhanced expression of HLA-DR in stimulated B-LCL as compared to unstimulated one. B: VAVY cells show a significant increase in surface HLA-DR expression as determined by the geometric mean fluresence intensity of antibody staining (Israni et al., 2009).

expression of Insulin in thymii of fetuses as compared to Class-III alleles (Pugliese et al., 1997, Vafiadis et al., 1997) which may be responsible for poor thymic education for insulin resulting in autoimmunity against pancreatic beta cells. Our studies provide additional evidence based on the statistically significant interaction between the predisposing *HLA* allele and high producer alleles of *VDR* which may be detrimental for the manifestation of T1D in the absence of 1,25-$(OH)_2D_3$ in early childhood and/or *in-utero* and this interaction is mediated by VDRE present in the promoter region of *DRB1*03:01*(Israni et al., 2009). With poor thymic education for insulin and *HLA-DRB1*03:01* protein, environmental factors like viral infections, vitamin D deficiency and some milk proteins may be involved in initiation of the autoimmune responses against the pancreatic beta cells. While HLA class-II molecules may be involved in auto-antigen presentation to T helper cells, higher producing genotypes of pro-inflammatory cytokines like *IFN-gamma* and *TNF-alpha* may be involved in enhancing the cell mediated immune responses through proliferation of $CD4^+$ and $CD8^+$ T cells, while higher producing genotypes of *IL-10* and *TGF-beta* may have a role in recruitment of these autoreactive T cells in the pancreas through ICAM-1 and Integerin dependent pathways. Final destruction of pancreatic beta cells may occur through $CD4^+$ and $CD8^+$ T cells and nitric oxide production since IFN-γ may act singularly as well as synergistically with other inflammatory stimuli to induce NO production which can be cytotoxic and thus may have a role in pathogenesis of T1D (Figure 6). Future studies should focus on developing approaches to inhibit autoimmunity before the onset of the disease.

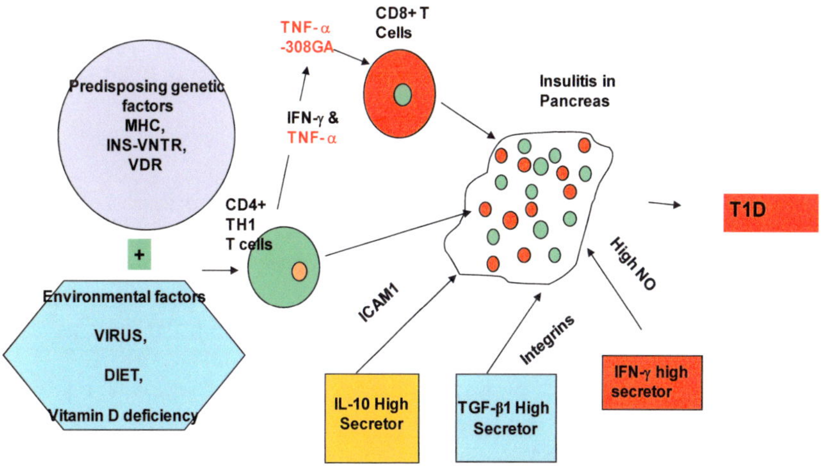

Fig. 6. Conclusions of our studies. Predisposing genetic factors like MHC, INS-VNTR and VDR may be involved in poor thymic education for insulin and *HLA-DRB1*03:01* protein resulting in recognition of self proteins as non-self by T cells . These genetic factors along with environmental factors like viral infections, vitamin D deficiency and some milk proteins may be involved in initiation of the autoimmune responses against the pancreatic beta cells. While HLA class-II molecules may be involved in auto-antigen presentation to T helper cells, higher producing genotypes of pro-inflammatory cytokines like *IFN-γ* and *TNF-α* may be involved in the cell mediated immune responses. Higher producing genotypes of *IL-10* and *TGF-beta,* may have a role in recruitment of the autoreactive $CD4^+$ and $CD8^+$ T cells in the pancreas through ICAM-1 and Integerin dependent pathways respectively. Final destruction of pancreatic beta cells may occur through $CD4^+$ and $CD8^+$ T cells and nitric oxide production since IFN-γ may act singularly as well as synergistically with other inflammatory stimuli to induce NO production which can be cytotoxic and thus may have a role in pathogenesis of T1D.

7. Acknowledgment

The studies were funded in part by grants from Department of Science and Technology (DST), Department of Biotechnology (DBT), Ministry of Science and Technology, Government of India and partly by Core funds of National Institute of Immunology, New Delhi, India. The patient sample for this work came from All India Institute of Medical Sciences (AIIMS), New Delhi and I would like to acknowledge Dr. Ravinder Goswami, the endocrinologist from AIIMS for the same. I would like to acknowledge the students and project fellows who have been involved in doing this work: Avinash Kumar, Rashmi Kumar, Shruti Agarwal, Neetu Israni, Shailendra Kumar Singh. I am thankful to Dr. Alberto Pugliese for valuable suggestions and INS-VNTR protocol. I would like to thank Dr. Joannis Mytilineos and the technical staff of Heidelberg University for the cytokine typing kit supplied for cytokine gene polymorphism component of XIIIth International Histocompatibility Workshop. We are thankful to Yong Yong Shi for providing the SHEsis program (http://202.120.7.14/analysis/myAnalysis.php) for haplotype analysis. We are thankful to the Fred Hutchinson Cancer Research Center IHWG Cell and Gene Bank for providing *HLA-DRB1*03:01* homozygous lymphoblastoid Cell lines for studies showing effect of vitamin D on HLA-DR expression. Mr. Kapoor Chand's technical support is acknowledged. Help of Dr. Narendra Kumar, Georgia Institute of Technology, USA, in making the ribbon diagrams for HLA-DRB1 peptide binding pockets is acknowledged.

8. References

Alroy, I., Towers, T.L. & Freedman, L.P. (1995). Transcriptional repression of the interleukin-2 gene by vitamin D3: direct inhibition of NFATp/AP-1 complex formation by a nuclear hormone receptor. *Mol Cell Biol*, 15, 10,(Oct, 1995) 5789-99.

Alves, C., Toralles, M.B. & Carvalho, G.C. (2009). HLA class II polymorphism in patients with type 1 diabetes mellitus from a Brazilian racially admixtured population. *Ethn Dis*, 19, 4,(Autumn, 2009) 420-4.

Asderakis, A., Sankaran, D., Dyer, P., Johnson, R.W., Pravica, V., Sinnott, P.J., Roberts, I. & Hutchinson, I.V. (2001). Association of polymorphisms in the human interferon-gamma and interleukin-10 gene with acute and chronic kidney transplant outcome: the cytokine effect on transplantation. *Transplantation*, 71, 5,(Mar 15, 2001) 674-7.

Awad, M.R., El-Gamel, A., Hasleton, P., Turner, D.M., Sinnott, P.J. & Hutchinson, I.V. (1998). Genotypic variation in the transforming growth factor-beta1 gene: association with transforming growth factor-beta1 production, fibrotic lung disease, and graft fibrosis after lung transplantation. *Transplantation*, 66, 8,(Oct 27, 1998) 1014-20.

Badenhoop, K., Walfish, P.G., Rau, H., Fischer, S., Nicolay, A., Bogner, U., Schleusener, H. & Usadel, K.H. (1995). Susceptibility and resistance alleles of human leukocyte antigen (HLA) DQA1 and HLA DQB1 are shared in endocrine autoimmune disease. *J Clin Endocrinol Metab*, 80, 7,(Jul, 1995) 2112-7.

Baisch, J.M., Weeks, T., Giles, R., Hoover, M., Stastny, P. & Capra, J.D. (1990). Analysis of HLA-DQ genotypes and susceptibility in insulin-dependent diabetes mellitus. *N Engl J Med*, 322, 26,(Jun 28, 1990) 1836-41.

Balasa, B., La Cava, A., Van Gunst, K., Mocnik, L., Balakrishna, D., Nguyen, N., Tucker, L. & Sarvetnick, N. (2000). A mechanism for IL-10-mediated diabetes in the nonobese diabetic (NOD) mouse: ICAM-1 deficiency blocks accelerated diabetes. *J Immunol*, 165, 12,(Dec 15, 2000) 7330-7.

Bartolome, R.A., Sanz-Rodriguez, F., Robledo, M.M., Hidalgo, A. & Teixido, J. (2003). Rapid up-regulation of alpha4 integrin-mediated leukocyte adhesion by transforming growth factor-beta1. *Mol Biol Cell*, 14, 1,(Jan, 2003) 54-66.

Bell, G.I., Karam, J.H. & Rutter, W.J. (1981). Polymorphic DNA region adjacent to the 5' end of the human insulin gene. *Proc Natl Acad Sci U S A*, 78, 9,(Sep, 1981) 5759-63.

Bell, G.I., Selby, M.J. & Rutter, W.J. (1982). The highly polymorphic region near the human insulin gene is composed of simple tandemly repeating sequences. *Nature*, 295, 5844,(Jan 7, 1982) 31-5.

Bennett, S.T., Lucassen, A.M., Gough, S.C., Powell, E.E., Undlien, D.E., Pritchard, L.E., Merriman, M.E., Kawaguchi, Y., Dronsfield, M.J., Pociot, F. & et al. (1995). Susceptibility to human type 1 diabetes at IDDM2 is determined by tandem repeat variation at the insulin gene minisatellite locus. *Nat Genet*, 9, 3,(Mar, 1995) 284-92.

Bhalla, A.K., Amento, E.P., Serog, B. & Glimcher, L.H. (1984). 1,25-Dihydroxyvitamin D3 inhibits antigen-induced T cell activation. *J Immunol*, 133, 4,(Oct, 1984) 1748-54.

Bidwell, J., Keen, L., Gallagher, G., Kimberly, R., Huizinga, T., McDermott, M.F., Oksenberg, J., McNicholl, J., Pociot, F., Hardt, C. & D'Alfonso, S. (1999). Cytokine gene polymorphism in human disease: on-line databases. *Genes Immun*, 1, 1,(Sep, 1999) 3-19.

Bittar, M.N., Carey, J.A., Barnard, J.B., Pravica, V., Deiraniya, A.K., Yonan, N. & Hutchinson, I.V. (2006). Tumor necrosis factor alpha influences the inflammatory response after coronary surgery. *Ann Thorac Surg*, 81, 1,(Jan, 2006) 132-7.

Bjorkman, P.J., Saper, M.A., Samraoui, B., Bennett, W.S., Strominger, J.L. & Wiley, D.C. (1987). Structure of the human class I histocompatibility antigen, HLA-A2. *Nature*, 329, 6139,(Oct 8-14, 1987) 506-12.

Boonstra, A., Barrat, F.J., Crain, C., Heath, V.L., Savelkoul, H.F. & O'Garra, A. (2001). 1alpha,25-Dihydroxyvitamin d3 has a direct effect on naive CD4(+) T cells to enhance the development of Th2 cells. *J Immunol*, 167, 9,(Nov 1, 2001) 4974-80.

Brown, J.H., Jardetzky, T.S., Gorga, J.C., Stern, L.J., Urban, R.G., Strominger, J.L. & Wiley, D.C. (1993). Three-dimensional structure of the human class II histocompatibility antigen HLA-DR1. *Nature*, 364, 6432,(Jul 1, 1993) 33-9.

Burzotta, F., Iacoviello, L., Di Castelnuovo, A., Glieca, F., Luciani, N., Zamparelli, R., Schiavello, R., Donati, M.B., Maseri, A., Possati, G. & Andreotti, F. (2001). Relation of the -174 G/C polymorphism of interleukin-6 to interleukin-6 plasma levels and to length of hospitalization after surgical coronary revascularization. *Am J Cardiol*, 88, 10,(Nov 15, 2001) 1125-8.

Cantorna, M.T., Woodward, W.D., Hayes, C.E. & DeLuca, H.F. (1998). 1,25-dihydroxyvitamin D3 is a positive regulator for the two anti-encephalitogenic cytokines TGF-beta 1 and IL-4. *J Immunol*, 160, 11,(Jun 1, 1998) 5314-9.

Chauffert, M., Cisse, A., Chevenne, D., Parfait, B., Michel, S. & Trivin, F. (1995). HLA-DQ beta 1 typing and non-Asp57 alleles in the aborigine population of Senegal. *Diabetes Care*, 18, 5,(May, 1995) 677-80.

Cippitelli, M. & Santoni, A. (1998). Vitamin D3: a transcriptional modulator of the interferon-gamma gene. *Eur J Immunol*, 28, 10,(Oct, 1998) 3017-30.

Cucca, F., Lampis, R., Congia, M., Angius, E., Nutland, S., Bain, S.C., Barnett, A.H. & Todd, J.A. (2001). A correlation between the relative predisposition of MHC class II alleles to type 1 diabetes and the structure of their proteins. *Hum Mol Genet*, 10, 19,(Sep 15, 2001) 2025-37.

Cucca, F., Lampis, R., Frau, F., Macis, D., Angius, E., Masile, P., Chessa, M., Frongia, P., Silvetti, M., Cao, A., De Virgiliis, S. & Congia, M. (1995). The distribution of DR4 haplotypes in Sardinia suggests a primary association of type I diabetes with DRB1 and DQB1 loci. *Hum Immunol*, 43, 4,(Aug, 1995) 301-8.

D'Ambrosio, D., Cippitelli, M., Cocciolo, M.G., Mazzeo, D., Di Lucia, P., Lang, R., Sinigaglia, F. & Panina-Bordignon, P. (1998). Inhibition of IL-12 production by 1,25-dihydroxyvitamin D3. Involvement of NF-kappaB downregulation in transcriptional repression of the p40 gene. *J Clin Invest*, 101, 1,(Jan 1, 1998) 252-62.

de Vries, R.R. & van Rood, J.J. (1985). Immunobiology of HLA class-I and class-II molecules. Introduction. *Prog Allergy*, 36, 1985) 1-9.

Deng, G.Y., Maclaren, N.K., Huang, H.S., Zhang, L.P. & She, J.X. (1996). No primary association between the 308 polymorphism in the tumor necrosis factor alpha promoter region and insulin-dependent diabetes mellitus. *Hum Immunol*, 45, 2,(Feb, 1996) 137-42.

Durrin, L.K., Haile, R.W., Ingles, S.A. & Coetzee, G.A. (1999). Vitamin D receptor 3'-untranslated region polymorphisms: lack of effect on mRNA stability. *Biochim Biophys Acta*, 1453, 3,(Mar 30, 1999) 311-20.

Ei Wafai, R.J., Chmaisse, H.N., Makki, R.F. & Fakhoury, H. Association of HLA class II alleles and CTLA-4 polymorphism with type 1 diabetes. *Saudi J Kidney Dis Transpl*, 22, 2,(Mar, 273-81.

Evans, R.M. (1988). The steroid and thyroid hormone receptor superfamily. *Science*, 240, 4854,(May 13, 1988) 889-95.

Falk, K., Rotzschke, O., Stevanovic, S., Jung, G. & Rammensee, H.G. (1991). Allele-specific motifs revealed by sequencing of self-peptides eluted from MHC molecules. *Nature*, 351, 6324,(May 23, 1991) 290-6.

Faraco, J.H., Morrison, N.A., Baker, A., Shine, J. & Frossard, P.M. (1989). ApaI dimorphism at the human vitamin D receptor gene locus. *Nucleic Acids Res*, 17, 5,(Mar 11, 1989) 2150.

Fernandez-Vina, M., Ramirez, L.C., Raskin, P. & Stastny, P. (1993). Genes for insulin-dependent diabetes mellitus (IDDM) in the major histocompatibility complex (MHC) of African-Americans. *Tissue Antigens*, 41, 2,(Feb, 1993) 57-64.

Fishman, D., Faulds, G., Jeffery, R., Mohamed-Ali, V., Yudkin, J.S., Humphries, S. & Woo, P. (1998). The effect of novel polymorphisms in the interleukin-6 (IL-6) gene on IL-6 transcription and plasma IL-6 levels, and an association with systemic-onset juvenile chronic arthritis. *J Clin Invest*, 102, 7,(Oct 1, 1998) 1369-76.

Garcia-Pacheco, J.M., Herbut, B., Cutbush, S., Hitman, G.A., Zhonglin, W., Magzoub, M., Bottazzo, G.F., Kiere, C., West, G., Mvere, D. & et al. (1992). Distribution of HLA-DQA1, -DQB1 and DRB1 alleles in black IDDM patients and controls from Zimbabwe. *Tissue Antigens*, 40, 3,(Sep, 1992) 145-9.

Garrett, T.P., Saper, M.A., Bjorkman, P.J., Strominger, J.L. & Wiley, D.C. (1989). Specificity pockets for the side chains of peptide antigens in HLA-Aw68. *Nature*, 342, 6250,(Dec 7, 1989) 692-6.

Gross, C., Eccleshall, T.R., Malloy, P.J., Villa, M.L., Marcus, R. & Feldman, D. (1996). The presence of a polymorphism at the translation initiation site of the vitamin D receptor gene is associated with low bone mineral density in postmenopausal Mexican-American women. *J Bone Miner Res*, 11, 12,(Dec, 1996) 1850-5.

Gupta, M.M., Raghunath, D., Kher, S.K. & Radhakrishnan, A.P. (1991). Human leucocyte antigen and insulin dependent diabetes mellitus. *J Assoc Physicians India*, 39, 7,(Jul, 1991) 540-3.

Holling, T.M., Schooten, E. & van Den Elsen, P.J. (2004). Function and regulation of MHC class II molecules in T-lymphocytes: of mice and men. *Hum Immunol*, 65, 4,(Apr, 2004) 282-90.

Horton, R., Wilming, L., Rand, V., Lovering, R.C., Bruford, E.A., Khodiyar, V.K., Lush, M.J., Povey, S., Talbot, C.C., Jr., Wright, M.W., Wain, H.M., Trowsdale, J., Ziegler, A. & Beck, S. (2004). Gene map of the extended human MHC. *Nat Rev Genet*, 5, 12,(Dec, 2004) 889-99.

Hustmyer, F.G., DeLuca, H.F. & Peacock, M. (1993). ApaI, BsmI, EcoRV and TaqI polymorphisms at the human vitamin D receptor gene locus in Caucasians, blacks and Asians. *Hum Mol Genet*, 2, 4,(Apr, 1993) 487.

Hypponen, E., Laara, E., Reunanen, A., Jarvelin, M.R. & Virtanen, S.M. (2001). Intake of vitamin D and risk of type 1 diabetes: a birth-cohort study. *Lancet*, 358, 9292,(Nov 3, 2001) 1500-3.

Ide, A., Kawasaki, E., Abiru, N., Sun, F., Takahashi, R., Kuwahara, H., Fujita, N., Kita, A., Oshima, K., Sakamaki, H., Uotani, S., Yamasaki, H., Yamaguchi, Y. & Eguchi, K. (2002). Genetic association between interleukin-10 gene promoter region polymorphisms and type 1 diabetes age-at-onset. *Hum Immunol*, 63, 8,(Aug, 2002) 690-5.

Israni, N., Goswami, R., Kumar, A. & Rani, R. (2009). Interaction of vitamin D receptor with HLA DRB1 0301 in type 1 diabetes patients from North India. *PLoS One*, 4, 12,(2009) e8023.

Jones, G., Strugnell, S.A. & DeLuca, H.F. (1998). Current understanding of the molecular actions of vitamin D. *Physiol Rev*, 78, 4,(Oct, 1998) 1193-231.

Julier, C., Hyer, R.N., Davies, J., Merlin, F., Soularue, P., Briant, L., Cathelineau, G., Deschamps, I., Rotter, J.I., Froguel, P. & et al. (1991). Insulin-IGF2 region on chromosome 11p encodes a gene implicated in HLA-DR4-dependent diabetes susceptibility. *Nature*, 354, 6349,(Nov 14, 1991) 155-9.

Kalra, S., Kalra, B. & Sharma, A. (2010) Prevalence of type 1 diabetes mellitus in Karnal district, Haryana state, India. *Diabetol Metab Syndr*, 2, 14.

Kanga, U., Vaidyanathan, B., Jaini, R., Menon, P.S. & Mehra, N.K. (2004). HLA haplotypes associated with type 1 diabetes mellitus in North Indian children. *Hum Immunol*, 65, 1,(Jan, 2004) 47-53.

Kennedy, G.C., German, M.S. & Rutter, W.J. (1995). The minisatellite in the diabetes susceptibility locus IDDM2 regulates insulin transcription. *Nat Genet*, 9, 3,(Mar, 1995) 293-8.

Korpinen, E., Groop, P.H., Fagerudd, J.A., Teppo, A.M., Akerblom, H.K. & Vaarala, O. (2001). Increased secretion of TGF-beta1 by peripheral blood mononuclear cells from patients with Type 1 diabetes mellitus with diabetic nephropathy. *Diabet Med*, 18, 2,(Feb, 2001) 121-5.

Kristiansen, O.P. & Mandrup-Poulsen, T. (2005). Interleukin-6 and diabetes: the good, the bad, or the indifferent? *Diabetes*, 54 Suppl 2, Dec, 2005) S114-24.

Kumar, R., Goswami, R., Agarwal, S., Israni, N., Singh, S.K. & Rani, R. (2007). Association and interaction of the TNF-alpha gene with other pro- and anti-inflammatory cytokine genes and HLA genes in patients with type 1 diabetes from North India. *Tissue Antigens*, 69, 6,(Jun, 2007) 557-67.

Lee, M.S., Mueller, R., Wicker, L.S., Peterson, L.B. & Sarvetnick, N. (1996). IL-10 is necessary and sufficient for autoimmune diabetes in conjunction with NOD MHC homozygosity. *J Exp Med*, 183, 6,(Jun 1, 1996) 2663-8.

Louis, E., Franchimont, D., Piron, A., Gevaert, Y., Schaaf-Lafontaine, N., Roland, S., Mahieu, P., Malaise, M., De Groote, D., Louis, R. & Belaiche, J. (1998). Tumour necrosis factor (TNF) gene polymorphism influences TNF-alpha production in lipopolysaccharide (LPS)-stimulated whole blood cell culture in healthy humans. *Clin Exp Immunol*, 113, 3,(Sep, 1998) 401-6.

Lucassen, A.M., Julier, C., Beressi, J.P., Boitard, C., Froguel, P., Lathrop, M. & Bell, J.I. (1993). Susceptibility to insulin dependent diabetes mellitus maps to a 4.1 kb segment of DNA spanning the insulin gene and associated VNTR. *Nat Genet*, 4, 3,(Jul, 1993) 305-10.

McCartney-Francis, N., Allen, J.B., Mizel, D.E., Albina, J.E., Xie, Q.W., Nathan, C.F. & Wahl, S.M. (1993). Suppression of arthritis by an inhibitor of nitric oxide synthase. *J Exp Med*, 178, 2,(Aug 1, 1993) 749-54.

Mehra, N.K., Kaur, G., Kanga, U. & Tandon, N. (2002). Immunogenetics of autoimmune diseases in Asian Indians. *Ann N Y Acad Sci*, 958, Apr, 2002) 333-6.

Morrison, N.A., Yeoman, R., Kelly, P.J. & Eisman, J.A. (1992). Contribution of trans-acting factor alleles to normal physiological variability: vitamin D receptor gene polymorphism and circulating osteocalcin. *Proc Natl Acad Sci U S A*, 89, 15,(Aug 1, 1992) 6665-9.

Nepom, G.T. & Kwok, W.W. (1998). Molecular basis for HLA-DQ associations with IDDM. *Diabetes*, 47, 8,(Aug, 1998) 1177-84.

Pociot, F., Briant, L., Jongeneel, C.V., Molvig, J., Worsaae, H., Abbal, M., Thomsen, M., Nerup, J. & Cambon-Thomsen, A. (1993). Association of tumor necrosis factor (TNF) and class II major histocompatibility complex alleles with the secretion of TNF-alpha and TNF-beta by human mononuclear cells: a possible link to insulin-dependent diabetes mellitus. *Eur J Immunol*, 23, 1,(Jan, 1993) 224-31.

Pociot, F. & McDermott, M.F. (2002). Genetics of type 1 diabetes mellitus. *Genes Immun*, 3, 5,(Aug, 2002) 235-49.

Pugliese, A., Gianani, R., Moromisato, R., Awdeh, Z.L., Alper, C.A., Erlich, H.A., Jackson, R.A. & Eisenbarth, G.S. (1995). HLA-DQB1*0602 is associated with dominant protection from diabetes even among islet cell antibody-positive first-degree relatives of patients with IDDM. *Diabetes*, 44, 6,(Jun, 1995) 608-13.

Pugliese, A., Zeller, M., Fernandez, A., Jr., Zalcberg, L.J., Bartlett, R.J., Ricordi, C., Pietropaolo, M., Eisenbarth, G.S., Bennett, S.T. & Patel, D.D. (1997). The insulin gene is transcribed in the human thymus and transcription levels correlated with allelic variation at the INS VNTR-IDDM2 susceptibility locus for type 1 diabetes. *Nat Genet*, 15, 3,(Mar, 1997) 293-7.

Rabinovitch, A. (1994). Immunoregulatory and cytokine imbalances in the pathogenesis of IDDM. Therapeutic intervention by immunostimulation? *Diabetes*, 43, 5,(May, 1994) 613-21.

Ramachandran, A., Snehalatha, C. & Krishnaswamy, C.V. (1996). Incidence of IDDM in children in urban population in southern India. Madras IDDM Registry Group Madras, South India. *Diabetes Res Clin Pract*, 34, 2,(Oct, 1996) 79-82.

Ramagopalan, S.V., Maugeri, N.J., Handunnetthi, L., Lincoln, M.R., Orton, S.M., Dyment, D.A., Deluca, G.C., Herrera, B.M., Chao, M.J., Sadovnick, A.D., Ebers, G.C. & Knight, J.C. (2009). Expression of the multiple sclerosis-associated MHC class II Allele HLA-DRB1*1501 is regulated by vitamin D. *PLoS Genet*, 5, 2,(Feb, 2009) e1000369.

Rani, R., Fernandez-Vina, M.A. & Stastny, P. (1998). Associations between HLA class II alleles in a North Indian population. *Tissue Antigens*, 52, 1,(Jul, 1998) 37-43.

Rani, R., Sood, A. & Goswami, R. (2004). Molecular basis of predisposition to develop type 1 diabetes mellitus in North Indians. *Tissue Antigens*, 64, 2,(Aug, 2004) 145-55.

Rani, R., Sood, A., Lazaro, A.M. & Stastny, P. (1999). Associations of MHC class II alleles with insulin-dependent diabetes mellitus (IDDM) in patients from North India. *Hum Immunol*, 60, 6,(Jun, 1999) 524-31.

Reynier, F., Cazalis, M.A., Lecoq, A., Paye, M., Rosa, A., Durand, A., Jhumka, U., Mougin, B., Miossec, P., Bendelac, N., Nicolino, M. & Thivolet, C. (2006). Lack of association of IL-10 promoter gene variants with type 1 diabetes in a French population. *Hum Immunol*, 67, 4-5,(Apr-May, 2006) 311-7.

Rigby, W.F., Waugh, M. & Graziano, R.F. (1990). Regulation of human monocyte HLA-DR and CD4 antigen expression, and antigen presentation by 1,25-dihydroxyvitamin D3. *Blood*, 76, 1,(Jul 1, 1990) 189-97.

Robinson, J., Waller, M.J., Fail, S.C., McWilliam, H., Lopez, R., Parham, P. & Marsh, S.G. (2009). The IMGT/HLA database. *Nucleic Acids Res*, 37, Database issue,(Jan, 2009) D1013-7.

Rotwein, P., Yokoyama, S., Didier, D.K. & Chirgwin, J.M. (1986). Genetic analysis of the hypervariable region flanking the human insulin gene. *Am J Hum Genet*, 39, 3,(Sep, 1986) 291-9.

Sandelin, A., Alkema, W., Engstrom, P., Wasserman, W.W. & Lenhard, B. (2004). JASPAR: an open-access database for eukaryotic transcription factor binding profiles
10.1093/nar/gkh012. *Nucl. Acids Res.*, 32, suppl_1,(January 1, 2004, 2004) D91-94.

Sanjeevi, C.B., Kanungo, A., Shtauvere, A., Samal, K.C. & Tripathi, B.B. (1999). Association of HLA class II alleles with different subgroups of diabetes mellitus in Eastern India identify different associations with IDDM and malnutrition-related diabetes. *Tissue Antigens*, 54, 1,(Jul, 1999) 83-7.

Sanjeevi, C.B., Landin-Olsson, M., Kockum, I., Dahlquist, G. & Lernmark, A. (1995). Effects of the second HLA-DQ haplotype on the association with childhood insulin-dependent diabetes mellitus. *Tissue Antigens*, 45, 2,(Feb, 1995) 148-52.

Sheehy, M.J. (1992). HLA and insulin-dependent diabetes. A protective perspective. *Diabetes*, 41, 2,(Feb, 1992) 123-9.

Shi, Y.Y. & He, L. (2005). SHEsis, a powerful software platform for analyses of linkage disequilibrium, haplotype construction, and genetic association at polymorphism loci. *Cell Res*, 15, 2,(Feb, 2005) 97-8.

Skjodt, H., Hughes, D.E., Dobson, P.R. & Russell, R.G. (1990). Constitutive and inducible expression of HLA class II determinants by human osteoblast-like cells in vitro. *J Clin Invest*, 85, 5,(May, 1990) 1421-6.

Skrodeniene, E., Marciulionyte, D., Padaiga, Z., Jasinskiene, E., Sadauskaite-Kuehne, V., Sanjeevi, C.B. & Ludvigsson, J. HLA class II alleles and haplotypes in Lithuanian children with type 1 diabetes and healthy children (HLA and type 1 diabetes). *Medicina (Kaunas)*, 46, 8,(505-10.

Stanilova, S.A., Miteva, L.D., Karakolev, Z.T. & Stefanov, C.S. (2006). Interleukin-10-1082 promoter polymorphism in association with cytokine production and sepsis susceptibility. *Intensive Care Med*, 32, 2,(Feb, 2006) 260-6.

Tait, B.D., Drummond, B.P., Varney, M.D. & Harrison, L.C. (1995). HLA-DRB1*0401 is associated with susceptibility to insulin-dependent diabetes mellitus independently of the DQB1 locus. *Eur J Immunogenet*, 22, 4,(Aug, 1995) 289-97.

Takeuchi, A., Reddy, G.S., Kobayashi, T., Okano, T., Park, J. & Sharma, S. (1998). Nuclear factor of activated T cells (NFAT) as a molecular target for 1alpha,25-dihydroxyvitamin D3-mediated effects. *J Immunol*, 160, 1,(Jan 1, 1998) 209-18.

Todd, J.A. (1995). Genetic analysis of type 1 diabetes using whole genome approaches. *Proc Natl Acad Sci U S A*, 92, 19,(Sep 12, 1995) 8560-5.

Todd, J.A., Bell, J.I. & McDevitt, H.O. (1987). HLA-DQ beta gene contributes to susceptibility and resistance to insulin-dependent diabetes mellitus. *Nature*, 329, 6140,(Oct 15-21, 1987) 599-604.

Vafiadis, P., Bennett, S.T., Todd, J.A., Nadeau, J., Grabs, R., Goodyer, C.G., Wickramasinghe, S., Colle, E. & Polychronakos, C. (1997). Insulin expression in human thymus is modulated by INS VNTR alleles at the IDDM2 locus. *Nat Genet*, 15, 3,(Mar, 1997) 289-92.

Van der Auwera, B., Van Waeyenberge, C., Schuit, F., Heimberg, H., Vandewalle, C., Gorus, F. & Flament, J. (1995). DRB1*0403 protects against IDDM in Caucasians with the high-risk heterozygous DQA1*0301-DQB1*0302/DQA1*0501-DQB1*0201 genotype. Belgian Diabetes Registry. *Diabetes*, 44, 5,(May, 1995) 527-30.

Veijola, R., Vahasalo, P., Tuomilehto-Wolf, E., Reijonen, H., Kulmala, P., Ilonen, J., Akerblom, H.K. & Knip, M. (1995). Human leukocyte antigen identity and DQ risk alleles in autoantibody-positive siblings of children with IDDM are associated with reduced early insulin response. Childhood Diabetes in Finland (DiMe) Study Group. *Diabetes*, 44, 9,(Sep, 1995) 1021-8.

Wahl, S.M., Allen, J.B., Weeks, B.S., Wong, H.L. & Klotman, P.E. (1993). Transforming growth factor beta enhances integrin expression and type IV collagenase secretion in human monocytes. *Proc Natl Acad Sci U S A*, 90, 10,(May 15, 1993) 4577-81.

Weber, P., Meluzinova, H., Kubesova, H., Ambrosova, P., Polcarova, V., Cejkova, P. & Cerna, M. Type 1 diabetes and LADA--occurrence of HLA-DRB1 *03 and DRB1 *04 alleles in two age different groups of diabetics. *Adv Gerontol*, 23, 2,(243-8.

Witt, C.S., Price, P., Kaur, G., Cheong, K., Kanga, U., Sayer, D., Christiansen, F. & Mehra, N.K. (2002). Common HLA-B8-DR3 haplotype in Northern India is different from that found in Europe. *Tissue Antigens*, 60, 6,(Dec, 2002) 474-80.

Yang, X.D., Sytwu, H.K., McDevitt, H.O. & Michie, S.A. (1997). Involvement of beta 7 integrin and mucosal addressin cell adhesion molecule-1 (MAdCAM-1) in the development of diabetes in obese diabetic mice. *Diabetes*, 46, 10,(Oct, 1997) 1542-7.

Yang, X.D., Tisch, R., Singer, S.M., Cao, Z.A., Liblau, R.S., Schreiber, R.D. & McDevitt, H.O. (1994). Effect of tumor necrosis factor alpha on insulin-dependent diabetes mellitus in NOD mice. I. The early development of autoimmunity and the diabetogenic process. *J Exp Med*, 180, 3,(Sep 1, 1994) 995-1004.

Zhao, J., Jin, L. & Xiong, M. (2006). Test for interaction between two unlinked loci. *Am J Hum Genet*, 79, 5,(Nov, 2006) 831-45.

12

Graves' Disease - The Interaction of Lymphocytes and Thyroid Cells

Ben-Skowronek Iwona
Medical University in Lublin,
Poland

1. Introduction

Human autoimmune thyroid disorders (AITD), Graves' disease (GD) and Hashimoto's thyroiditis, are characterized by reactivity to self-thyroid antigens. Graves' disease is the archetype for organ-specific autoimmune disorders, very important to our understanding the mechanisms responsible for progression of autoimmunity.

It has been known for years that hyperthyroidism in Graves'disease is induced by immunological reaction, in which TSH receptor antibodies bind to the receptors on the surface of thyrocytes, activate them and initiate thyroid hormone production independent of the hypothalamic-hypophyseal control. It is known nowadays that, probably for environmental or endogenous reasons, Graves'disease may develop in genetically predisposed individuals [Weetman, 2004].

2. Antigen presentation

A small number of antigen presenting cells (APCs) as CD1a+ presenting dendritic cells (DC) were observed in the thyroids without AITD, but their number was significantly higher in the thyroids from Graves' disease patients [Ben-Skowronek et al., 2007, 2008]. There are indications that such DCs are able to proliferate, which indicates that not all of the thyroid DCs need to have recently immigrated with the blood stream [Quadbeck et al. 2002]. CD1a antigen has the structure of an α-chain connected with β-microglobulins and is characteristic for immature APCs [Brigl & Brenner, 2004]. Thyroidal DCs are often in close contact with thyrocytes; they are clearly in an immature state and often show monocyte marker characteristics. The presence of positive reaction to CD1a protein in the granules of the apical part of some thyrocytes suggested that the thyrocytes may probably be antigen presenting cells in the thyroid autoimmune reactivity [Ben-Skowronek et al., 2007,2008]. The investigations of transgenic mice by Kimura et al. [Kimura et al., 2004] indicated that expression of class II MHC molecules on epithelial thyroid cells is not required for the initiation of an autoimmune attack to the thyroid. The initiation, then, seems to be mainly mediated by the professional antigen presenting cells in the lymphoid tissue. The antigen can be presented to CD4+ cells by conventional antigen presenting cells, particularly dendritic cells and also by B-cells and activated T-cells, and less effectively by thyrocytes. The antigen presentation by thyroid epithelial cells sustains the autoimmune reaction.

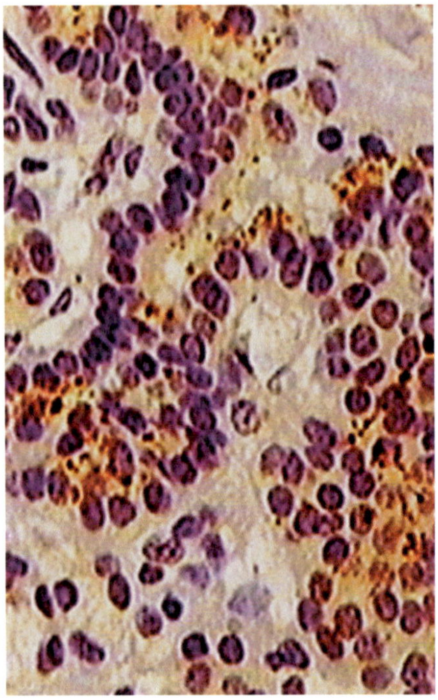

Fig. 1. The thyrocytes are antigen presenting cells and show reaction with the CD1a monoclonal antibody. Magn. 400x

While analyzing the process of antigen presentation in thyroids sampled from patients, the treatment process should be taken into account. Metimazole and carbimazole change the presentation of antigens by thyrocytes. Thionamides have been reported to influence the expression the antigens of the major histocompatibility complex class I, IL-1 (interleukin-1), IL-6 (interleukin- 6), prostaglandins E2 produced by thyrocytes [Zantut-Wittmann et al., 2001]. The expression of major histocompatibility complex class II is unchanged by thionamides [Dedecjus et al. 2010].

Numerous investigations indicate that adhesion molecules are engaged in the process of migration of lymphocytes to the thyroid and lymphocyte adhesion [Arao et al., 2000]. Adhesion molecule ICAM-1 (Inter-Cellular Adhesion Molecule 1) belonging to the superfamily IgG is a natural ligand of antigen located on lymphocytes LFA-1 (Lymphocytic function-associated antigen - 1). This antigen belongs to the integrin-β2 superfamily [Springer, 1990]. ICAM-1 is located on different cells: fibroblasts, endotheliocytes, and thymocytes. It was identified on thyrocytes as well [Weetman et al., 1989, Martin et al., 1990, Springer,1990].The expression of ICAM-1 is regulated by proinflammatory cytokines: interferon γ, interleukin 1β (IL 1β) and TNF-α (Tumor Necrosis Factor -1) [Dustin et al., 1986, Martin et al., 1990, Springer 1990, Bagnasco et al., 1991]. In Graves' disease, the ICAM-1/LFA-1 pathway plays a key role in migration and settlement of lymphocytes in the thyroid, and particularly in the process of adhesion of lymphocytes to thyrocytes [Arao et al.,2000]. In vitro experiments have shown that thyrocytes behave like antigen presenting cells and can induce lymphocyte migration [Estienne et al., 2002].

Expression of HLA DR II and the immunoglobulin Fc receptor (FcγRIIB2) has been found on the basal and apical surfaces of thyrocytes [Botazzo et al., 1983, Wu et al., 1999]. The presentation of the latter antigen is dependent on the low level of androgens, which is probably connected with higher prevalence of AITD in women [Estienne et al., 2002]. Presentation of antigens by thyrocytes without the costimulatory molecule B7 does not lead to activation of T-cells [Marelli-Berg et al., 1997]. The expression APC characteristic antigens are dependent on TSH [Todd et al., 1987, Estienne et al., 2004]. Thyrocytes may produce HLA I under the influence of cytokines of lymphocytes present in the thyroid. In this way, the autoimmunologic reaction is sustained [Catalfamo et al., 1999].

3. The development of autoimmune reaction

When immune tolerance to thyroid antigens is broken, the endothelial cells of regional postcapillary venules are activated, allowing extravasation of blood leukocytes. In Graves' disease, the lymphatic tissue arranged in lymphoid follicles containing T- cells may be formed in the thyroid. T-cells form infiltrations and lymphatic follicles but do not damage thyrocytes [Kuby et al., 2007].

Graves' disease patients seem to have mixed Th1/Th2 profiles. The lymphocyte subsets produce signal interleukin: Th1 – IL2 and Th2- IL4.The immunological response proceeds via T-cell receptor (TCR) antigen recognition, followed by activation of the T- cell through a combined effect of antigen recognition and co-stimulatory signals, including interleukin -1 (IL-1) action leading to T- cell IL 2 secretion and IL-2 receptor expression and, subsequently, to proliferation of the T- cell into an active clone. [Janeway et al., 2001 Janeway & Medzhitov 2002]

In Graves' disease, the increased percentage of CD4+ T helper cells, in comparison to non-AITD, leads to development of humoral autoimmune response. Antigens of self-thyrocytes are presented in such a way that they are recognized by self – T-helper CD4+ lymphocytes. T-helper cells CD4+ sporadic occurred in thyroids of children from the control group, seldom in the simple goiter and slightly more often in the nontoxic nodular goiter. The number of T-helper cells in Graves' disease was the largest [Ben-Skowronek et al., 2007, 2008].

The subset of CD4+cells includes the regulatory lymphocytes - Tregs, which play a fundamental role in modulation of immunological response through their inhibitive effect on autoreactive T-cells [Piccirillo & Shevach,2004, Piccirillo & Thornton, 2004, Shewach, 2006]. The mechanism of this suppression is unknown, but many investigators consider it to be dependent on the contact between lymphocytes and independent of secretion of IL-10 and TGFβ [Piccirillo et.al. 2002,2003]. In the remission phase during thyrotoxic treatment, the subsets of lymphocytes were not different from the control group and from children with the simple goiter and nontoxic goiter [Bossowski et al. 2003]. The cells were characterized by expression of CD25 (the α-chain of IL2) and intracellular expression of FoxP3 (Forkhead winged helix box3). Only the subset of CD4+cells with maximal expression of CD25 (CD4+CD25+high) is responsible for the suppressor – regulatory effect of these lymphocytes [Cao et al., 2003, Baecher-Allan et al., 2001, 2003, Bossowski 2010]. The CD4+CD25+ cells can occur natural or can be induced – they are generated in the lymphatic tissue from CD4+CD25+ cells by different stimulant agents: by immature dendritic cells, IL-10, TGFβ, supply of vitamin D3 or dexamethasone, anti-lymphatic treatment or small doses of antigens. The Treg cells not need costimulation of CD28-B7 for their development or activity. They play a pivotal role in sustenance of immunologic tolerance [Piccirillo & Shewach, 2004, Piccirillo & Thornton, 2004]. TGF-β is assumed to be necessary for the regulatory function of Treg cells; it also prevents activation of lymphocytes and autoimmune reactions [Bommireddy et al., 2008]. The quantity of lymphocytes in this subset is decreased in Graves' disease [Deshun et al., 2009].

An increase in T-helper lymphocytes, especially in Th1 lymphocytes, results in activation of B lymphocytes and their transformation into plasma cells which produce thyroid antibodies, predominantly TRAB (TSH receptor antibody), TSI (TSH stimulated immunoglobulin), and also TPO Ab (Antithyroperoxidase antibody) and TG Ab (Antithyroglobulin antibody).

T cells CD8+ are observed in the thyroid more often in Graves' disease than in non-AITD; they have a regulatory T-cell function. Electron microscopy examinations did not demonstrate any damage to thyrocytes, but CD8+ lymphocytes frequently entered the thyroid follicles through the basal membrane [Ben-Skowronek et al., 2009].

The T-suppressor-cytotoxic CD8+ cells were observed in thyroid follicles between thyrocytes, in mononuclear infiltrations and in lymphatic follicles in the mantle zone. In light microscopy, CD8+ T-cells and adherent normal thyrocytes were visible in high magnifications. Bossowski et al. have found a correlation between expression of costimulatory molecules CTLA-4 and CD28 on T-cells and the level of antibodies against the TSH receptor [Bossowski et al., 2005]. The investigations of Negrini et al. [Negrini et al., 2006] indicate a possibility of presentation of GITR receptors on the surface T-cells CD8+ characteristic for Treg cells. Own observations have confirmed this character of CD8+ T-cells, because they are located between thyrocytes and do not cause apoptosis.

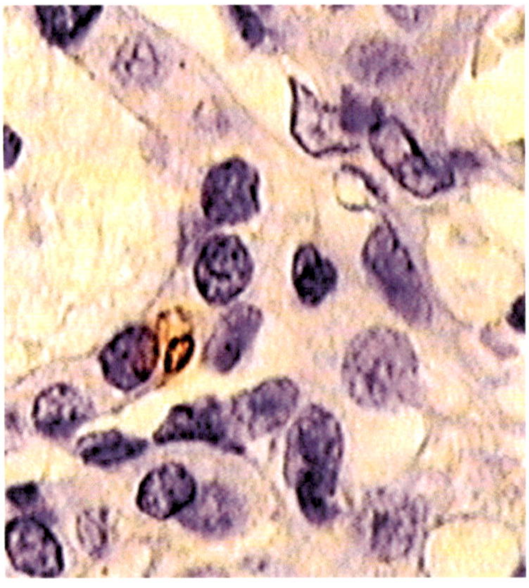

Fig. 2. The CD8+ T-cell between thyrocytes in thyroid follicle wall. The thyrocytes are active and present no signs of apoptosis or cell damage. Magn. 400x.

In vitro investigations and observations of the thyroid tissue in electron microscopy indicate the possibility of formation of the so-called immunological synapse of a character of a tight junction between lymphocytes and thyrocytes with participation of adhesive proteins. This physical contact may result in establishment of an immunological synapse able to stimulate intra thyroid T lymphocyte proliferation and differentiation.

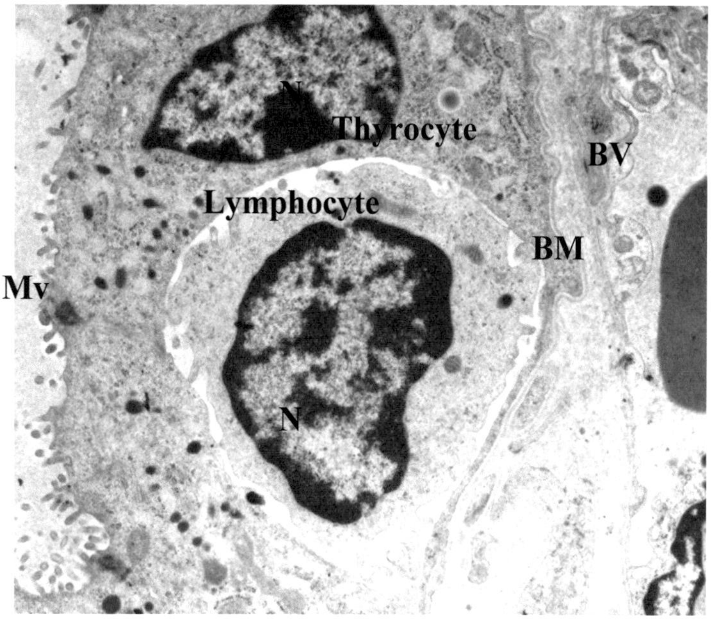

Fig. 3. T cells among thyrocytes in the thyroid epithelium. The thyrocytes are active without destruction signs. N- nucleus, Mv – microvilli, BM – basal membrane, BV – blood vessel. Transmission Electron Microscopy Magn. 15 000x.

Recent investigations have suggested that a crucial role in peripheral tolerance or autoreactive T- cells is played by T regulatory subsets (Tregs) divided into two populations: naturally occurring and inducible [Wieczorek *et al.*, 2009]. Tregs so far identified as participating in the pathogenesis of Graves' disease include naturally occurring CD4+,CD25+T cells , C8+CD122+T cells and natural killer cells [Bossowski et al., 2010]. Comparison of immunohistochemical localization of CD4+ T cells in ultrastructural investigations has shown that lymphocytes CD4+T were small cells with large nuclei and a small amount of cytoplasm in contact with thyrocytes and other lymphocytes [Ben-Skowronek et al., 2009].

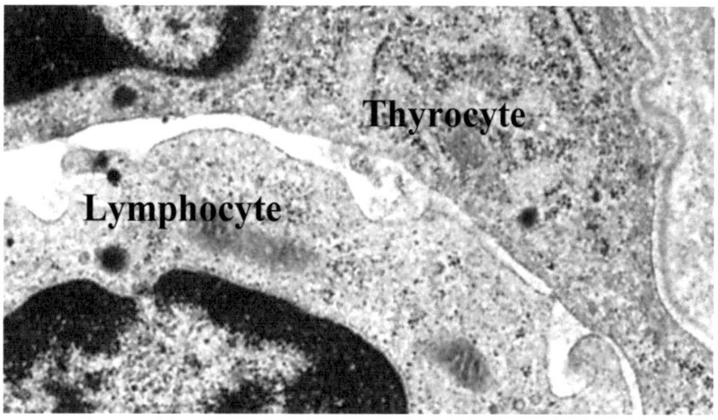

Fig. 4. The immunological synapse between T-cells and thytrocytes in Graves' disease. Transmission Electron Microscopy Magn. 20 000x

Rifa'i et al. [Rifa'i et al., 2004] have described subsets of naturally occurring Tregs CD8+CD25+. It is possible that CD8+T cells in contact with thyrocytes play the role of Tregs in the pathogenesis of Graves' disease. The investigations of Negrini et al. [Negrini et al. 2006] have characterized a subpopulation of CD8 T suppressor lymphocytes able to inhibit both cell proliferation and cytotoxicity; they have observed that glucocorticoid-induced TNF-like receptor (GITR) is expressed on such CD8 T suppressor cells. The papers of Nakano et al. [Nakano et al., 2006] and Nagayama [Nagayama et al., 2007] suggest a preventive role of Tregs in autoimmune reaction in the thyroid with AITD.

Patients with Graves' disease have an increased number of circulating B-cells but plasma cells predominate in the thyroid. The close contact with T-cells (probably Th2 cells) and plasma cells has been frequently observed only in Graves' disease and sporadically in the non-AITD and suggested the regulation function of the T-cells stimulating plasma cells to produce autoantibodies [Ben-Skowronek et al., 2008].

The plasma cells in Graves' disease penetrate between thyreocytes; nevertheless, they caused no destruction of thyroid follicles and epithelial cells. Ultrastructural changes in plasma cells were observed in patients with Graves' disease: a large, active nucleus with a nucleolus, a well-developed rough endoplasmic reticulum in which antibodies were

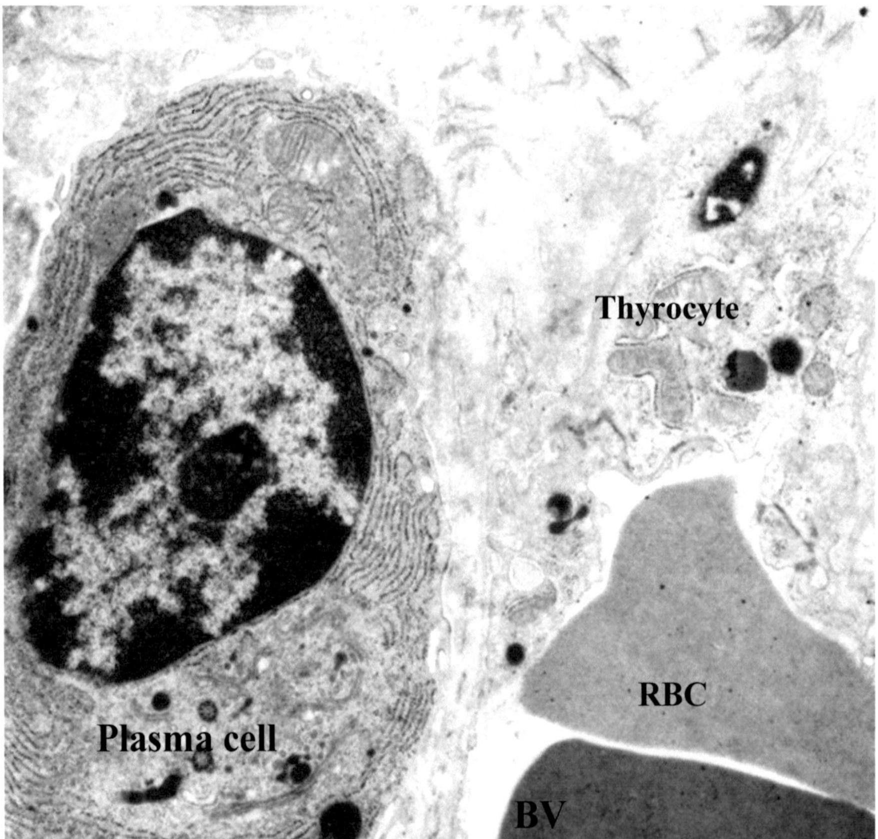

Fig. 5. The plasma cell producing antibodies in contact with thyrocytes. RBC-red blood cell, BV- Blood vessel. Transmission Electron Microscopy Magn. 15.00x

produced. The number of plasma cells in the thyroid was inversely proportional to time of treatment, which proved the immunomodulant activity of thyrostatic drugs [Ben-Skowronek et al., 2009].

In Graves' disease, the immunological deposits observed in the basal membrane of the thyroid follicles lead to thickening of this membrane and probably to changes in polarization of cell membranes. The thyrocytes in this region are columnar, with signs of increased activity (big nuclei; active, enlarged mitochondria; a big number of granules in the apical pole; long microvilli). [Ben-Skowronek et al., 2008,2009]. The antibody deposits do not damage thyrocytes but enhance their activity and metabolism by activation of the THS receptors, and lead to hyperthyroidism.

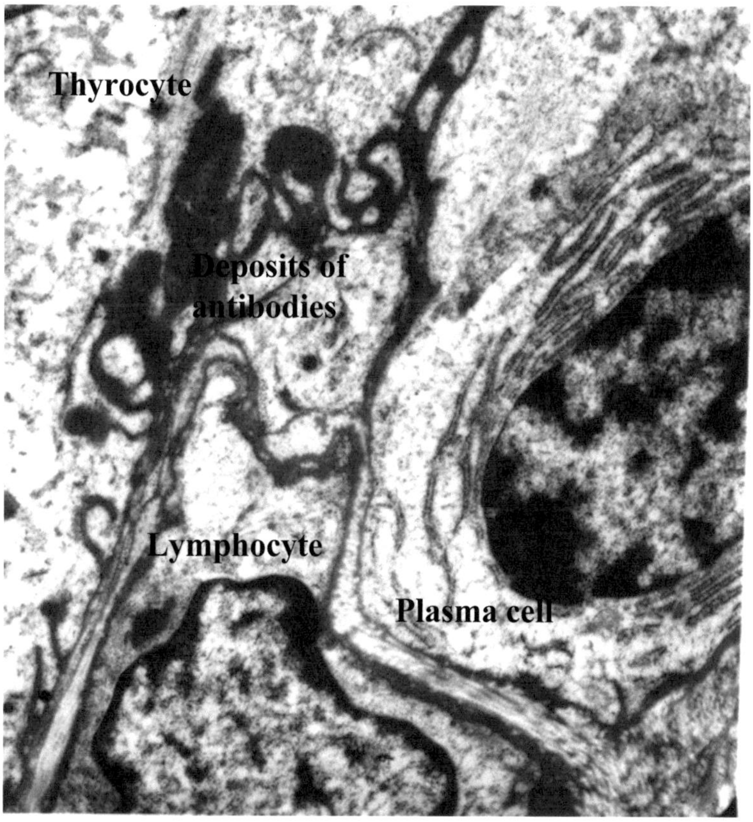

Fig. 6. The late phase of development of antibodies deposits in the basal membrane of the thyrocytes. Transmission Electron Microscopy Magn. 20 00x

Numerous reports have shown that Th-1 cell activating the antibody-dependent cellular cytotoxicity (ADCC) can be detected in Graves' disease, although the response is usually weak and not present in many patients [Guo et al., 1997, Metcalfe et al., 1997]. ADCC of thyroid cells is induced by anti TPO antibody positive sera, but other unknown antibody-antigen systems and methimazole therapy also contribute. Large granular lymphocytes – phenotypic NK cells - are rarely present in the lumen of the thyroid follicle. Here, degenerative changes in the thyrocytes were observed by electron microscopy [Ben-Skowronek et al., 2009].

Antibodies may be produced against the TSH receptor (TSH receptor stimulating antibodies - TS Ab, TSH binding inhibiton immunoglobulins - TBII, TSH stimulation blocking antibodies - TSBAb), against thyroperoxidase (TPO Ab), against thyroglobulin (TG Ab), against megalin [Marino et al., 1999], against the iodine symporter, against thyroid's DNA, against components of external eye muscles and fibroblasts, against parietal cells and against platelets [Weetmann, 2004].
The stimulating antibodies (TSAb) react with the TSH receptor and initiate activity of adenyl cyclase and phospholipase A2of the receptor, thus stimulating production of thyroid hormones and growth and division of thyrocytes [Orgiazzi et al.,1976, DiCerbo et al., 1999, Ewans et al.,1999, Morshed et al., 2009]. The blocking antibodies act like weak agonists of the TSH receptor [Lenzner et al., 2003, Schwarz-Lauer et al., 2002].

4. References

Arao T, Morimoto I, Kukinuma A, Ishida O, Zeki K, Tanaka Y, Ishikawa N, Ito K, Ito K, Eto S. (2000) Thyrocytes proliferation by cellular adhesion to infiltrating lymphocytes through the intercellular adhesion molekule-1/lymphocyte function-associated antygen-1 pathway in Graves'disease. J Clin Endocrinol Metab, 85,1: 382-389

Baecher-Allan C, Brown JA, Freeman GJ, Hafler DA. (2001) CD4+CD25 high regulatory cells in human peripheral blood. J Immunol., 167:1245–53.

Baecher-Allan C, Wolf E, Hafler DA. (2005) Functional analysis of highly defined, FACS-isolated populations of human regulatory CD4 + CD25 + T cells. Clin Immunol 115:10-18

Bagdi E, Krenacs l, Miller K, Isaacson PG. (2001) Follicular dendritic cells in reactive and neoplastic lymphoid tissues: a reevaluation of staining patterns of CD21, CD23, and CD35 antibodies in paraffin sections after wet heat-induced epitope retrieval. Appl Immunohistochem Mol Morphol 9:117-124.

Bagnasco M, Caretto A, Olive D, Pedini B, Canonica GW, and Betterle C. (1991) Expression of intercellular adhesion molecule-1 (ICAM-1) on thyroid epithelial cell in Hashimoto's thyroiditis but not in Graves' disease or papillary thyroid cancer. Clin Exp Immunol. 83:309–313.

Ben-Skowronek I, Szewczyk L., Sierocinska-Sawa J, Korobowicz E. (2007) The subsets of lymphocytes in autoimmunological and non-autoimmunological thyroid diseases in children. Endokrynol Ped 6 nr 3, s. 9-20.

Ben-Skowronek I, Sierocinska-Sawa J, Korobowicz E, Szewczyk L. (2008) Lymphocytes in peripheral blood and thyroid tissue in children with Graves' disease. World Journal of Pediatrics 4:274-282.

Ben-Skowronek I, Sierocinska-Sawa J, Korobowicz E, Szewczyk L. (2009), Interaction of Lymphocytes and Thyrocytes in Graves' Disease and Nonautoimmune Thyroid Diseases in Immunohistochemical and Ultrastructural Investigations. Horm Res 71,6 : 350-358

Bommireddy R, Babcock G, Singh RR, Doetschman T. (2008) TGFβ1 deficiency does not affect the generation and maintenance of CD4+CD25+FOXP3+ putative Treg cells, but causes the numerical inadequacy and loss of regulatory function. Clin Immunol, 127(2):206-213

Brigl M, Brenner MB. (2004). CD1: antigen presentation and T cell function. Annu. Rev. Immunol. 22 (1): 817–90.]

Bossowski A, Moniuszko M, Mrugasz M, Sawicka B, Dąbrowska M, Bodzenta-Łukaszczyk A. (2010). The assessment o CD4+CD25high, CD4+CD25+CD127low and CD4+FoxP3+ T cell n th peripheral blood of children with autoimmune thyroid diseases. Horm Res 73 (sppl 3): 47

Bossowski A, Stasiak –Barmuta A, Urban M. (2005). Relationship between CTLA-4 and CD28 Molecule expression on T Lymphocytes and Stimulating and Blocking Autoantibodies to the TSH-Receptor in children with Graves'disease. Horm.Res. 64,4: 189-197

Bossowski A, Urban M, Stasiak-Barmuta A. (2003). Analysis of changes in the percentage of B (CD19) and T (CD3) lymphocytes, subsets CD4, CD8 and their memory (CD45RO), and naive (CD45RA) T cells in children with immune and non-immune thyroid diseases. J Pediatr Endocrinol Metab, 16(1):63-70.

Bottazzo GF, Pujol-Borrell R, Hanafusa T, and Feldmann M. (1983). Role of aberrant HLA-DR expression and antigen presentation in induction of endocrine autoimmunity. Lancet 2: 1115–1119.

Cao D, Malmstrom V, Baecher-Allan C, Hafler D, Klareskog L, Trollmo C. (2003). Isolation and functional characterization of regulatory CD25brightCD4+ Tcells from target organ of patients with rheumatoid arthritis. Eur J Immunol , 33:215-223.

Catalfamo M, Seradell L, Roura - Mir C, Kolkowi E, Sospedra M, Vives-Pi M, Vargas-Nieto F, Pujol-Borrel R, Jaraquemada D. (1999). HLA-DM and invariant chain are expressed by thyroid folliocular cells, enabling the expression of compact DR molecules. Int Immunol, 11,2: 269-277.

Dedecjus M, Stasiołek M, Brzeziński J Selmaj K, Lewiński A (2010). Hormones Influence Human Dendritic Cells'Phenotype, Function, and Subsets Distribution. Thyroid 2010 Dec. 29[Epub ahead of print]

Deshun P, Shin YH, Gopalakrishnan G, Hennessey J, De Groot L. (2009). Regulatory T-cells in Graves-Disease. Clin Enocrinol, 71 (4) 587-593.

DiCerbo A, Di Paola R, Menzaghi C, Fillips VD, Tahara K, Corda D, et al. (1999). Graves'immunoglobulins activate phospholipase A by recognizing specific epitopes on thyrotropin receptor. J Clin Endocrinol Metab;84:3283-3292

Dustin ML, Rothlein R, Bhan AK, Dinarello CA, Springer TA. (1986). Induction of IL-1 and interferon, tissue distribution, biochemistry, and function of a natural adherence molecule (ICAM-1). J Immunol. 137:245–254.

Estienne V. Bisbarre N, Blanchin S, Durand-Gorde JM, Carayon P, Ruf J. (2004). An In vitro model based on cell monolayers grown on the underside of large-pore filters In bicameral chambers for studying thyrocyte-lymphocyte interactions. Am J Physiol Cell Physiol 287: C1763-C1768.

Estienne V, Duthoit C, Blanchin S , Montserret R, Durand-Gorde J-M, Chartier M, Baty D, Carayon P, and Ruf J. (2002) Analysis of a conformational B cell epitope of human thyroid peroxidase: identification of a tyrosine residue at a strategic location for immunodominance. Int. Immunol., 14(4): 359 - 366.

Estienne V, Duthoit C, Reichert M, Praetor A, Carayon P, Hunziker W, and Ruf J. (2002). Androgen-dependent expression of Fc RIIB2 by thyrocytes from patients with autoimmune Graves' disease: a possible molecular clue for sex dependence of autoimmune disease. FASEB J 16: 1087–1092.

Ewans C, Morgenthaler NG, Lee S, Llewellyn DH, Clinton-Bligh R, John R, Lazarus JH, Chatterjee VKK, Ludgate M. (1999). Development of a luminescent bioassay for thyroid stimulating antibodies. J Clin Endocrinol Metab; 84: 374

Guo J, Jaume JC, Rapoport B, Mc Lachlan SM. (1997). Recombinant thyroid peroxidase-specific Fab converted to immunoglobulin G (IgG) molecules: evidence for thyroid cell damage by IgG1, but not IgG4, autoantibodies. J Clin Endocrinol Metab 82:925-931

Janeway C.A, Jr Travers P, Walport M, and Shlomchik M.J. (2001). The Immune System in Health and Disease in: Immunobiology, 5th edition, New York: Garland Science.

Janeway CA, Medzhitov R. (2002) Innate immune recognition. Annu Re Immunol , 20:197

Kimura, H., M. Kimura, S. C. Tzou, Y. C. Chen, K. Suzuki, N. R. Rose, P. Caturegli. (2004). Expression of class II MHC molecules on thyrocytes does not cause spontaneous thyroiditis, but mildly increases its severity after immunization. Endocrinology 146: 1154-1162.

Kuby J., Kindt TJ.,Goldsby RA., Osborne BA. (2007). Kuby Immunology. New York: W.H. Freeman. , Janeway, Charles (2005). Immunobiology: the immune system in health and disease. New York: Garland Science. ISBN 0-8153-4101-6.

Lenzner C, Morgenthaler NG (2003) The effect of thyrotropin-receptor blocking antibodies on stimulating autoantibodies from patients with Graves' disease. Thyroid 13:1153–1161

Marelli-Berg FM, Weetman A, Frasca L, Deacock SJ, Imami N, Lombardi G, and Lechler RI. (1997) Antigen presentation by epithelial cells induces anergic immunoregulatory CD45RO+ T cells and deletion of CD45RA+ T cells. J Immunol 159: 5853–5861.

Marino M, Chiovato L, Friedlander JA, Latrofa F, Pinchera A and McCluskey RT. (1999). Serum antibodies against megalin (GP330) in patients with autoimmune thyroiditis. J Clin Endocrinol Metab. Jul;84(7):2468-74.

Martin A, Huber GK, and Davies TF. (1990). Induction of human thyroid cell ICAM-1 (CD54) antigen expression and ICAM-1-mediated lymphocyte binding. Endocrinology. 127:651–657.

Metcalfe RA, Oh YS, Stround C, Arnold K, Weetman AP. (1997). Analysis of antibody - dependent cell mediated cytotoxicuty in autoimmune thyroid disease. Autoimmunity 25:65-72

Morshed S.A, Latif R, Davies TF. (2009). Characterization of thyrotropin Receptor Antibody-Induced nSignaling Cascades. Endocrinol, 150(1):519-529

Nagayama Y, Horie I, Saitoh O, Nakahara M, Abiru N. (2007). CD4+CD25+ naturally occurring regulatory T cells and not lymphopenia play a role in the pathogenesis of iodide-induced autoimmune thyroiditis in NOD-H2h4 mice. J Autoimmun.29(2-3):195-202. Epub 2007 Sep 10.

Nakano A, Watanabe M, Iida T, Kuoda S, Matsuzuka F, Miyauschi A, Witani Y, (2007). Apoptosis induced decrease of intrathyroidal CD4+CD25+ regulatory T cells in autoimmune thyroid diseases.Thyroid ,17(1):25-31

Negrini, S., Fenoglio, D., Balestra, P., Fravega, M., Filaci, G. and Indiveri, F. (2006) Endocrine Regulation of Suppressor Lymphocytes. Ann Ny Acad Sci 1069: 377-385.

Orgiazzi J, Williams DE, Chora IJ, Solomon DH. (1976) Human thyroid adenyl cyclase stimulating activity in immunoglobulin G of patients with Graves'disease. J. Clin Endocrinol Metab 42:341

Piccirillo CA, Letterio JJ, Thornton AM, et al. (2002). CD4(+)CD25(+) regulatory T cells can mediate suppressor function in the absence of transforming growth factor beta1 production and responsiveness. J Exp Med. 196:237–246.

Piccirillo CA., Shevach E. (2003). CD4+CD25+Treg cells: naturally occurring but adaptable. Nature Revievs Immunology 3,3 online only (access 20.04.2011)

Piccirillo CA, Shevach EM. (2004). Naturalny occurring CD4+CD25+ immunoregulatory cells: central players In the arena of peripheral tolerance. Seminars in Immunoloy , 16:81-88.

Piccirillo CA, Thornton AM. (2004). Cornerstone of periferal tolerance naturally occurring CD4+CD25+ Tregulatory cells. Trends Immunol 25: 374-380.

Quadbeck B, Eckstein AK , Tews S, Walz M, Hoermann R,. Mann K, Gieseler M .(2002). Maturation of Thyroidal Dendritic Cells in Graves' Disease .Scand.J Immunol 55(6)612-620.

Rifa'i M, Kawamoto Y, Nakashima I, Suzuki H. (2004). Essential roles of CD8+CD122+ regulatory T cells in the maintenance of T cell homeostasis. J Exp Med; 200:1123-34.

Schwarz-Lauer L, Chazenbalk GD, McLachlan SM, Ochi Y, Nagayama Y, Rapoport B. (2002). Evidence for a simplified view of autoantibody interactions with the thyrotropin receptor. Thyroid 12:115–120

Shewach EM. (2006). From vanilla to 28 flavors: multiple varietes of T regulatory cells. Immunity 25: 195-201.

Springer TA. (1990). Adhesion receptors of the immune system. Nature. 346:425–434

Todd I, Pujol-Borrell R, Hammond LJ, McNally JM, Feldmann M, and Bottazzo GF. (1987). Enhancement of thyrocyte HLA class II expression by thyroid stimulating hormone. Clin Exp Immunol 69: 524–531.

Weetman AP. (2004). Autoimmune thyroid disease. Autoimmunity 37: 337-340

Weetman AP. (2010). Diseases associated with thyroid autoimmunity: explanations for the expanding spectrum. Clin Endocrinol (Oxf). [Epub ahead of print]

Wieczorek G., Asemissen A, Model F, Turbachova I, Floess S, Liebenberg V, Baron U, Stauch D. (2009). Quantitative DNA methylation analysis of FOXP3 as a new method for counting regulatory T cells in peripheral blood and solid tissue. Cancer Res 69 (2): 599–608.

Wu Z, Biro PA, Mirakian R, Hammond L, Curcio F, Ambesi-Impiobato FS, and Bottazzo GF. (1999). HLA-DMB expression by thyrocytes: indication of the antigen-processing and possible presenting capability of thyroid cells. Clin Exp Immunol 116: 62-69.

Zantut-Wittmann DE, Tambascia MA, da Silva Trevisan MA, Pinto GA, Vassallo J. (2001). Antithyroid drugs inhibit in vivo HLA-DR expression in thyroid follicular cells in Graves' disease. Thyroid 11:575-580

13

Hashimoto's Thyroiditis – Interactions of Lymphocytes, Thyroid Cells and Fibroblasts

Ben-Skowronek Iwona
Medical University Lublin
Poland

1. Introduction

Autoimmune Hashimoto's thyroiditis involves painless enlargement of the thyroid, which, in histopathological analysis, is characterised by diffuse lymphocytic infiltrations, fibrosis, and atrophic changes. It is a diffuse process, a combination of epithelial cell destruction, lymphocyte infiltrations, and fibrosis. The incidence of Hashimoto's thyroiditis ranges between 0,3 and 1,5 per 1000 persons. It is diagnosed 15-20 times more frequently in females than in males. The forms of Hashimoto's thyroiditis include: euthyroid goitre, and goitre in subclinical or clinical hypothyroidism, hypothyroidism without goitre, silent thyroiditis, postpartum thyroiditis, alternating hyperthyroidism and hypothyroidism [Weetman &McGregor 1994].

Hashimoto's thyroiditis is often associated with type I diabetes, coeliac disease and other autoimmune diseases. It is one of the components of the autoimmune polyglandular syndrome.

In histopathological investigations of Hashimoto's thyroiditis, the follicular epithelial cells in the thyroid are large and often eosinophilic; they are the so-called Hurthle or Askenazy cells packed with mitochondria. Lymphocyte clusters present between the follicles form typical lymphoid follicles in some sites. Infiltrations contain numerous plasma cells. In Hashimoto's thyroiditis, the immunological attack appears to be destructive, rather than stimulating, as in Graves' disease. Two variants of Hashimoto's thyroiditis have been reported so far: atrophic - related to gene HLA-DR3 inheritance, and hypertrophic - involving goitre enlargement associated with HLA-DR5 [Weetman, 2004]. A study of autoimmune thyroiditis in monozygotic twins demonstrated environmental factors inducing development of the disease [Brix et al., 2000]: high iodine intake, selenium deficiency, smoking, infectious diseases, e.g. hepatitis C, and some drugs [Duntas, 2008]. Prolonged exposure to iodine leads to enhanced iodination of thyroglobulin, which increases its antigenicity and initiates autoimmune processes in genetically predisposed individuals. Selenium deficiency causes a decrease in the activity of selenoproteins, including glutathione peroxidise, which leads to an increase in the concentration of hydrogen peroxide and development of inflammatory processes.

Classical histopathological descriptions of the thyroid in Hashimoto's thyroiditis emphasise the fact that the changes include destruction of thyrocytes, lymphocytic infiltration, and fibrosis.

2. The course of the immune response in Hashimoto's thyroiditis

2.1 Antigen presentation

Stimulation of the immune system depends on maturity of dendritic cells. Immature dendritic cells are characterized by expression of small numbers of co-stimulatory molecules and proinflammatory cytokines; they may also cause anergy. Maturing dendritic cells display significantly higher expression of MHC class II and co-stimulatory molecules, but low levels of proinflammatory cytokines. Only mature dendritic cells can induce regulatory T cells [Jonuleit et al., 2001; Menges et al., 2002; Gad et al., 2003; Wakkach et al., 2005]. Antigen presenting cells are more frequently found in Hashimoto's thyroiditis than in healthy thyroid glands or individuals with non-autoimmune thyroid diseases (simple goitre, non-toxic nodular goitre) [Ben-Skowronek et al., 2008, 2011]. No mature dendritic cells presenting MHC class II antigens have been found in thyroid preparations. The investigations conducted by Kimura et al. have indicated that MHC class II antigens may be expressed on thyrocytes in the autoimmune thyroid inflammation. Our own research has shown a positive reaction with the monoclonal antibody CD1a specific for dendritic cells in some thyrocytes. This is not sufficient to initiate the autoimmune response, but sufficient to sustain it [Kimura et al., 2004].

2.2 Development of immunological reaction in the thyroid gland

Lymphatic follicles appear inside the thyroid gland in the course of Hashimoto's thyroiditis. The study of Armengol et al. has demonstrated higher levels of lymphokines and their ligands responsible for lymphocyte migration, settlement, and formation of lymphoid follicles (lymphotoxin α, lymphotoxin β, CC chemokine ligand (CCL)), and CXC (CXCL 12, CXCL13) chemokine ligands). Moreover, in response to inflammatory cytokines, thyrocytes can produce CXCL12. Tissue stress caused by viral or bacterial inflammation is likely to lead to formation of lymphoid follicles in the thyroid [Armengol, et al., 2003]. Production of cytokine ligands for CXCL21, CXCL 22, and CXCL 13 by thyrocytes is correlated with the level of anti-thyroid antibodies, and thus, directly with the inflammatory response in the thyroid [Armengol et al., 2003].

From the physiological point of view, lymphoid follicles are small structures in which processes of somatic hypermutation, maturation of immune affinity receptors, switching of antibody isotypes (e.g. from IgM to IgG), and receptor control take place. Autoreactive T cells arise de novo in the germinal centres; here operates the mechanism sustaining tolerance - apoptosis of autoreactive lymphocytes [Pulendrav et al., 1997, Janevay et al., 2002]. In autoimmune diseases of the thyroid, muscles, and joints as well as in Sjögren's syndrome and autoimmune alveolitis, the ectopic lymphoid tissue is arranged in lymphoid follicles in non-lymphatic organs, which do not contain physiological, growing lymphoid tissue [Crawford et al.1983, Schroeder et al., 1996, Wallace et al.1996, Shione et al 1997, Stott et al 1998, Itoh et. al 2000, Sims et al,. 2001]. The function of this lymphoid tissue, sometimes defined as tertiary lymphoid tissue (primary tissues - thymus and bone marrow, secondary - lymphatic glands and organs), is unclear [Weetman et al. 1994, Ruddle et al. 1999, Armengol et al , 2001]. The structure of the ectopic lymphoid follicles in the thyroid is similar to that of typical lymphoid follicles in lymphoid organs: they consist of a germinal centre and a peripheral zone (mantle zone) containing lymphocytes B and T, and dendritic cells. An analysis of immunoglobulin gene rearrangement (RAG1 and RAG2) has confirmed the possibility of formation of high endothelial venules in lymphoid follicles and production of cytokines responsible for lymphocyte migration and settlement, which would trigger an autoimmune reaction [Armengol et al., 2001]. TG Ab, TPO Ab and TRAK anti-thyroid antibodies are produced in B cells in the lymphoid follicles [Armengol et al., 2001]. High levels of antibodies against thyroglobulin (TG Ab) and thyroperoxidase (TPO Ab) are detected in the serum of patients with Hashimoto's thyroiditis. These antibodies are regarded to have cytotoxic activity. However, investigations of thyroids of foetuses from mothers with Hashimoto's thyroiditis did not show the expected damage. Hypothyroidism was observed only in some children.

T cells originating from mice immunized with TPO strongly react with sequence 540-559; immunisation of mice with this peptide results in development of hypothyroidism and thyroiditis. Peptide 540-559 is probably a key factor in the immune response against TPO [Kawakami et al. 1992]. Natural *HLA-DR-associated peptides* have also been identified; they are present in the colloid, and some of them derive from thyroglobulin [Ng et al., 2006]. A larger proportion of lymphocytes binding to thyroglobulin are present in the thyroid than in peripheral blood [Heuer et al., 1996]. Being the major stimulatory antigen, thyroglobulin is indispensable for T cell response [Sugihara et al., 1993]. The severity of autoimmune reactions following immunization with thyroglobulin has been observed in transgenic mice producing IL-12 [Kimura et al.,2005].

Immune reactions involving T cells are controlled by certain T lymphocyte subpopulations: CD4 + Treg and natural killer lymphocytes are employed in the control of the magnitude and class of the immune response, while lymphocytes CD8 + are responsible for recognition for self- and non-self- antigens [Jang et al., 2006].

A slightly larger number of CD4 + cells have been observed in Hashimoto's thyroiditis than in non-autoimmune thyroid diseases; however, the number was statistically significantly lower than in Graves' disease [Ben-Skowronek et al., 2007,2008]. The studies of McLachlan suggest that the reduction in the number of Treg cells (particularly CD25) induces lymphocyte infiltration in the thyroid accompanied by transient or permanent hypothyroidism [Mc Lachlan et al., 2007].

Animal studies have shown that depletion of CD4 + CD25 + Treg in mice increases susceptibility to thyroiditis by enhancement of the immune reaction against thyroglobulin and exacerbates the existing thyroiditis, whereas an increase in the number of CD4 + CD25 + T cells restores resistance to thyroiditis [Morris et al., 2006,2007, Nagayama ey al. 2007]. It appears that an insufficient percentage of CD4 + T cells in Hashimoto's disease is the cause of the destructive autoimmune reaction in the thyroid.

Suppressor/cytotoxic lymphocytes CD8 + have been found among thyrocytes in thyroid follicles, in lymphatic infiltrations and in the lymphoid follicles of the mantle zone. Glycoprotein CD8 present on the surface of cytotoxic lymphocytes may bind to the class I MHC molecule, which leads to activation of T cells CD8+. This activation is also dependent on co-stimulatory proteins binding to antigen CD28 (the so-called two-signal model). Once activated, cytotoxic lymphocytes may secrete cytotoxins, and granzymes and granulysins. They perforate the cell membrane and form pores, which induces apoptosis of the target cell. Another pathway leading to apoptosis is activation of the Fas ligand [Iannacone et al., 2005,2006, Subramanian et. al., 2005]. Hypothyroidism in patients with autoimmune thyroiditis is associated with apoptosis of alveolar epithelial cells induced by cytokines. Expression of Fas ligand on thyrocytes of patients with Hashimoto thyroiditis and a weak reaction for Bcl-2 have been detected, which suggests cytokine-induced apoptosis [Kawakami et al., 1996, Mitsiiades et al.,1998, Stassi et al., 2002]. TPO-specific T cells cause destruction through cytotoxic mechanisms involving CD4+ and CD8 + cells or programmed Fas- TNF-alpha-induced apoptosis [Stassi et al., 2002]. In Hashimoto's disease, damaged thyrocytes in contact with CD8 + T lymphocytes may be observed in the light microscope. The electron microscopy has shown contact sites of lymphocytes with thyrocytes located in the thyroid follicular epithelium. Polarization of endolysosomes near the site of contact has been detected in the lymphocytes which displayed the T-cell phenotype of and CD8 + location. Similar observations of cultured CD8 + and dendritic cells in experimental conditions were conducted by Gardella et al. [Gardella et al., 2001]. The studies of Negrini et al. [Negrini et al.,2006] have indicated possible presence of the GITR (Glucocorticoid-Induced TNF-Like Receptor) antigen on the surface of CD8 + T cells, which would render them as regulatory Treg cells. Therefore, it is believed that cytotoxic T cells, K (killer) lymphocytes, NK (natural killer) cells, and regulatory (Treg) or suppressor T cells may play an important role in autoimmune thyroid damage. Some studies indicate the ability of T cells to transfer thyroid autoimmune processes, both in animals with experimental autoimmune thyroiditis and patients who have undergone bone marrow transplantation [Kawakami et al.,, 1992, Ng et al., 2006, Drabko et. al., 2006].

Active lymphocytes B CD79alfa+ and antibody-producing plasma cells were found in a small percentage of thyroids from healthy children (4,11%), in the colloid goitre (1,83%) and the nodular goitre (5,22%). The largest number of CD79 alpha+ lymphocytes was observed in thyroid specimens from patients with Hashimoto's thyroiditis (average 31,65%) In lymphatic infiltrates, plasma cells constituted almost half of the cells (46,67%), and amounted to 17,23% in the thyroid parenchyma. Foci of damaged thyroid follicles and numerous fibroblasts and collagen bands have been observed at the plasma cell accumulation sites. The thyroid glands in children with Hashimoto's thyroiditis displayed characteristics of lymphocyte activation, the so-called blastic transformation, consisting in an increase in the volume of the cell and, particularly, of the nucleus, appearance of nucleoli and an increase in the cytoplasm volume through enlargement of the rough endoplasmic reticulum, in which antibody production takes place [Ben-Skowronek et al., 2007].

Thyrocytes in Hashimoto's thyroiditis are cuboidal or flat. The thyroid cells exhibit damage. Cell nuclei are often folded; secretory vesicles are sporadically present in the apical pole (sometimes there are no vesicles); and swollen mitochondria are present in the basal pole. The swollen part of thyrocytes without microvilli or with single microvilli projects into the lumen of the follicle. The basal membrane is thickened. Plasma cells, lymphocytes and fibroblasts are visible among the thyroid follicles. At the lymphoid infiltration sites, the lymphoid cells separate the thyroid epithelium from the basal membrane of the capillary blood vessels. Lymphocytes are often in direct contact with plasma cells. Plasma cells filled with concentrically arranged layers of the rough endoplasmic reticulum adhere to the basal membrane of the thyroid follicle and the surrounding thyrocytes. The thick, electron dense basal membrane contains numerous collagen fibres. The adjacent cytoplasmic membrane does not exhibit characteristic folds. The fibrous basal membrane hinders blood flow in the capillary blood vessels and deformed erythrocytes can be seen in their lumen. The exchange of nutrients and oxygen between thyrocytes, the interstitium, and blood vessels is impeded [Fig. 1].

3. Apoptosis in autoimmune thyroid diseases

Apoptosis is a physiological form of cell death resulting from the need of multicellular organisms to maintain balance between dividing and dying cells. Typical morphological

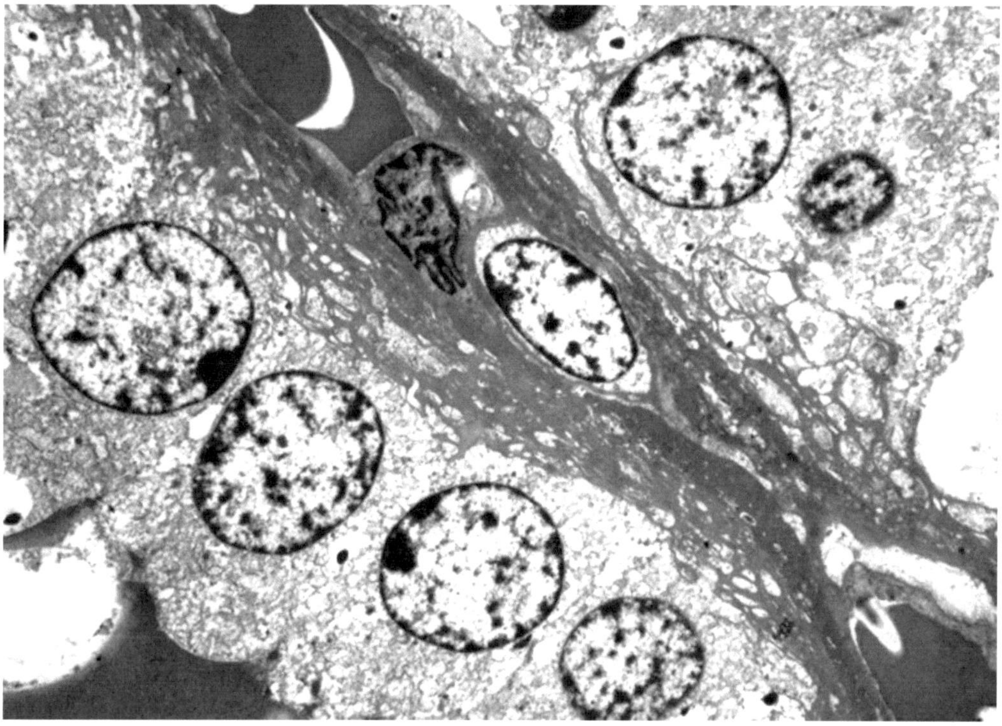

Fig. 1. A markedly thickened basal membrane of the thyroid follicle containing collagen fibres impedes thyrocyte contact with the capillary vessel lumen. In the basal membrane is present lymphocyte (phenotype lymphocyte T). The thyrocytes exhibit signs of damage of thyroid follicular cells- swollen mitochondria, dilated cisterns of the rough endoplasmic reticulum, absence of secretory granules, and atrophy of microvilli. Transmission Electron Microscope Magn. 10 000x.

changes in cells that received the signal to begin the apoptotic process include folding of the cell membrane, condensation of cytoplasm and cellular organelles, disappearance of the mitochondrial membrane, shrinkage of the nucleus, and condensation of chromatin [Yamazaki et al., 2000, Lorenz et al., 2005].

Apoptosis can be initiated by T cells through two pathways:

- by perforins secreted by lymphocytes into the junctions between lymphocytes and target cells; they perforate the cell membrane and form pores thus inducing osmotic lysis of the cell; simultaneously, granzymes B activate the caspase cascade, which leads to cell apoptosis;
- the Fas ligand and TNF-related apotosis induced ligand (TRAIL) secreted by lymphocytes stimulate the so-called death receptors on the cell surface causing activation of caspase cascade through caspase 8 and 10.

Lymphocytic infiltration and antibodies secreted by plasma cells lead to destruction of thyrocytes, but actively stimulate the production of collagen by fibroblasts. As a result, large amounts of collagen accumulate in the follicular and vascular basal membranes. In the final stage of the process, thyrocytes are destroyed via apoptosis. Typical signs of cell apoptosis are visible: chromatin condensation in the nuclei of thyroid epithelial cells, condensation of the cytosol and swelling of the mitochondria [Fig.2].

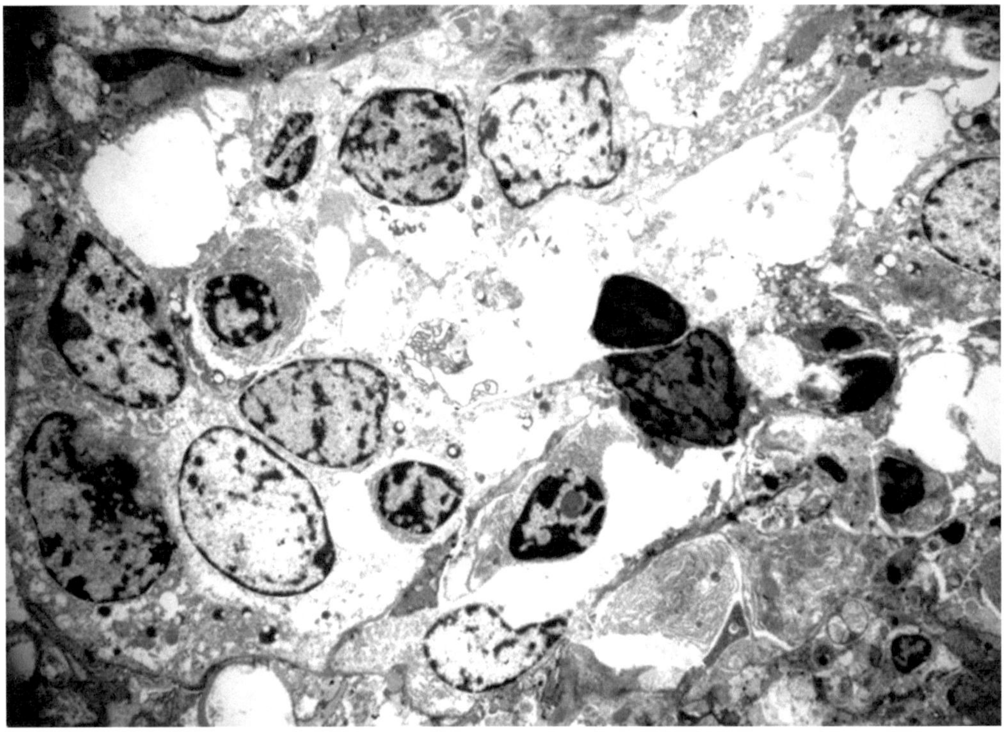

Fig. 2. The last phase of destruction of the thyroid in Hashimoto's thyroiditis. The thyrocytes are damaged due to apoptotic processes. Plasma cells and lymphocytes predominate in the interstitium. The fibroblast migrates to this place and produces collagen fibres. Transmission Electron Microscope. magn. 5000x.

Various phases of thyrocyte death were visible at the lymphocyte infiltration sites; apoptosis was caused by active plasma cells and lymphocytes of the large granular lymphocyte phenotype (LGL) [Fig.2] Ultrastructural investigations have revealed that the reaction between lymphocytes and plasma cells producing antibody results in thyrocyte damage, which, in turn, changes the permeability of cell membranes and intracellular membranes and leads to accumulation of water in the endoplasmic reticulum cisterns in the mitochondria and cytoplasm. Consequently, the cell is enlarged, microvilli disappear, and swollen mitochondria occupy the basal pole of thyroid cells causing cell staining with acidic dyes. At the same time, electron-dense substances (probably antibodies) are deposited in the follicular basal membrane. In response, large amounts of collagen are secreted around the damaged follicles. Communication between the lumen of capillary vessels and thyrocytes is impeded; hence, the transport of oxygen, nutrients, and substrates for production of thyroid hormones is inhibited. The thyrocyte metabolism is decelerated, and production of hormone and protein colloid is disrupted. Thyrocytes gradually die and exfoliate into the follicle lumen. Lymphocytes migrate to replace them and form lymphoid follicles. Fibroblast bands producing collagen fibres penetrate the site as well.

The contact between lymphocytes and thyrocytes in Hashimoto's thyroiditis forms an immunological synapse, which has been described as a specialized intercellular connection between T cells and antigen presenting cells [Paul et al., 1994, Dustin et al., 1999, Grakoui et al., 1999].

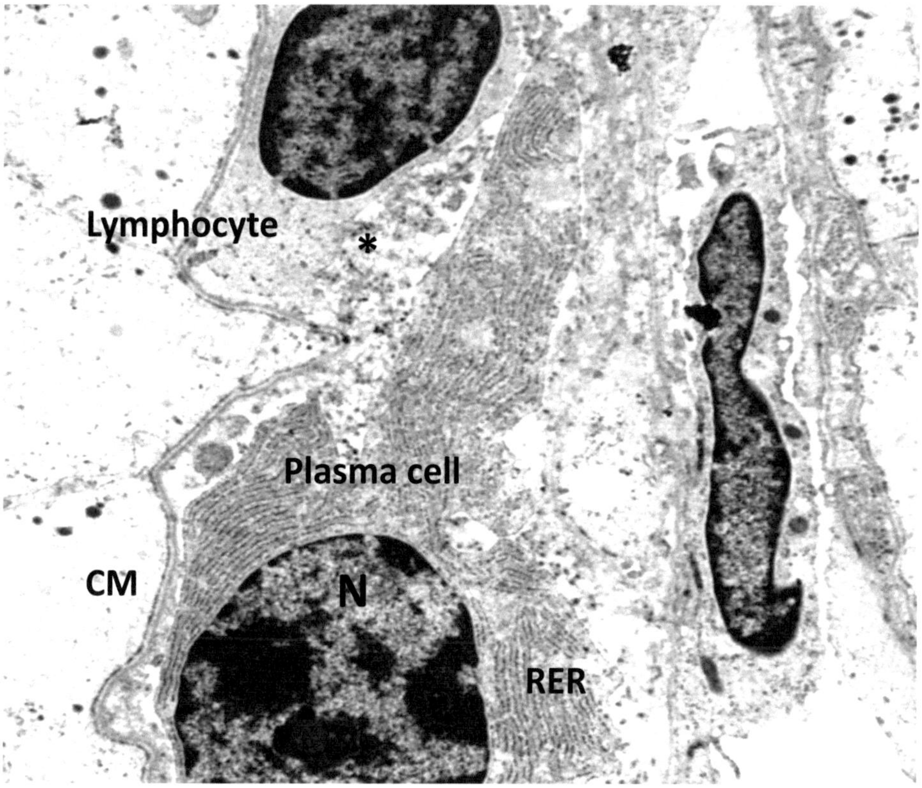

Fig. 3. Junction between the lymphocyte and plasma cell in Hashimoto's thyroiditis. Electron-dense (probably protein) substance is visible in the intercellular space. N - cell nucleus, RER - rough endoplasmic reticulum, L - lysosome, CM - cell membrane. Transmission Electron Microscope magnification 25 000x

The immunological synapse consists of a central zone containing antigen receptors and a surrounding ring of adhesion molecules [Dustin, 2002]. Lymphocytes form projections - lamellipodia - and form junctions with the cell membrane of thyrocytes. Presumably, it is at these sites that antigen presentation by thyrocytes occurs [Bromley et al., 2001]. Recent studies demonstrate different types of immunological synapses: cytotoxic [Dustin et al., 2010] and transitory (the so-called kinapses) [Dustin et al. 2007, 2010]. Observations of the interaction between lymphocytes and other thyroid cells in the course of AITD indicate possible formation of analogous junctions between thyrocytes and lymphocytes, i.e. cytotoxic synapses in Hashimoto's thyroiditis. This implies that lymphocytes secrete granzymes and other cytotoxic substances leading to cell damage.

The junctions of plasma cells with thyrocytes are large adhesion zones with thyrocyte apoptosis visible nearby [Fig.3]. The junctions between plasma cells and fibroblasts, however, are associated with production of collagen fibres. In Hashimoto's thyroiditis, numerous junctions between lymphocytes and plasma cells in the form of adhesion zones and spaces have been detected, into which medium electron-density substances (probably proteins) were secreted [Fig.3]; there are also synapses between young and mature lymphocytes T and B in the lymphoid follicles.

Such cell junctions occur mainly in the lymphoid nodes. Very tight junctions are visible between lymphoblasts and B cells, which are phenotypically similar to plasma cells. Immunological synapses have been found also between lymphocytes [Ben-Skowronek in press]

In Hashimoto's disease, activation of apoptotic processes is also associated with activation of Th1 cells, which enhance the activity of caspase and apoptosis through production of IFN-γ. While reduction in the number of CD4 + cell subsets in the thyroid parenchyma has been reported both in our own study and in animal models of the disease [Sugihara et al., 1993], an increase in the number of active CD4 + IL-4 + was observed in the peripheral blood [Maziotti et al., 2003]. However, no correlation has been found between the number of CD4 + T cells in the thyroid and the antiperoxidase antibody levels in serum [Watanabe et al., 2002, Pandit et al., 2003].

Antibody-dependent cell-mediated cytotoxicity (ADCC) plays an important role in development of Hashimoto's thyroiditis, whereas complement-dependent cytotoxicity (CDC) exerts a lesser effect. The thyroid peroxidase antigen evokes the reaction [Czarnocka et al., 1985, Estienne et al., 2002, Guo et al., 2005 Rebuffat et al., 2006, Ng et al., 2004, 2006]. TPO Ab has been detected in 90% of Hashimoto's thyroiditis patients [Rappaport et al., 2001]. Anti-TPO antibodies are various isotypes of the IgG antibodies. Anti-peroxidase antibodies TPOAb can damage thyrocytes through the ADCC and CDC mechanisms. The cytotoxic ADCC mechanism depends on the interaction between the target cell, antibody and effector cell. Monocytes, which due to FcγRI receptors are effector cells activated by TPOAb, can affect T cells and lead to destruction of thyrocytes [Rebuffat et al.,2008]. FcγRIII are present on Natural Killer cells and FcγRII on monocytes and neutrophils. All FcγR fragments are involved in the ADCC reaction [Rebuffat et al., 2008]. The investigations of Giancotti and Williams et al. suggest that integrins β2 may participate in cytotoxic reactions involving FcγR [Giancotti et al., 1999, Williams et al., 1999]. The study of Rebufatt et al. [Rebuffat et al., 2008], however, indicates involvement of two monocytic cell lines in this process.

It has not been sufficiently documented yet whether specific IgG antibody subclasses take part in thyrocyte damage [Metcalfe 1997, Guo 1997]. Xie L-D et al. investigated the occurrence of anti-TPO IgG subclasses and found that IgG1 was present in 70.2%, IgG2 in 35.1%, IgG3 in 19.6%, and IgG4 in 66.1% of patients; increased proportion of IgG2 predisposes to thyroid damage and hypothyroidism [Xie et al., 2008].

Metcalfe et al. found no correlation between the IgG subclasses and thyrocyte damage in vitro [Metcalfe et al., 1997], whereas Guo et al. demonstrated that thyrocyte damage is associated with subclass IgG1 [Guo et al., 1997]. Recent studies conducted by Rebuffat et al. [Rebuffat et al., 2010, Pappenwali et al., 2010] indicate that anti-TPO antibodies exhibit moderate activity in the ADCC process and can be used in the new methods of treatment of papillary thyroid cancer, the cells of which show expression of TPO.

Thyrocyte damage continues and is potentialized by the CDC reaction [Rebuffat et al., 2008]. Complement component C4, hyperexpressed on the surface of thyrocytes in Hashimoto's thyroiditis, participates in this reaction [Blanchin et al., 2003]. The key antigen here is thyroid peroxidase. The TPO ectodomain consists of a long module similar to myeloperoxidase, followed by a module similar to the complement control protein (CCP) and a module similar to the epidermal growth factor (EGF). The CCP contains a fragment that activates the complement. Therefore, TPO can activate the complement cascade without the help of immunoglobulins. Tg Ab antibodies do not fix the complement [Weetmann et al.,

2004] and probably are not directly involved in the CDC reaction, which is related to the fact that thyroglobulin is not expressed on the surface of thyrocytes.

Reduction or loss of intercellular communication in the final phase of Hashimoto's thyroiditis may lead to destruction of thyrocytes and hypothyroidism [Greek et al., 1996, Green et al., 1997, DiMatola et al., 2000]

- Fibrocytes and fibroblasts in autoimmune thyroid diseases

Fibrocytes and fibroblasts are frequently disregarded in analyses of autoimmune reactions in the thyroid. Ultrastructural studies have revealed significant participation of fibroblasts in the pathogenetic processes in Hashimoto's disease. They enter the space between the basal membrane and thyrocytes and produce substantial amounts of collagen, thus leading to thickening of the basal membrane and impeded contact between the capillary vessel lumen and thyrocytes [Fig. 1,2].

Influx and proliferation of lymphocytes in the thyroid as well as production of collagen is a response to inflammation processes and a stimulus for further thyrocyte damage through isolation thereof from oxygen and nutrients in the blood vessels. Progressive damage of thyrocytes leads to release of large amounts of autoantigen and triggers the inflammatory response. Own observations indicate a possible direct impact of plasma cells, lymphocytes and fibroblasts, since thyroids of Hashimoto's thyroiditis patients exhibit close contact between the groups of lymphocytes, plasma cells and fibroblasts.

4. References

Armengol MP, Cardoso-Smith CB, Fernandez M, Ferrer X, Pujol-Borrel R, Manel J. 2003 Chemokines determine local lymphogenesis and a reduction circulating CXCR4+T andCCR7B an T lymphocytes in thyroid autoimmune Diseases. J Immunol, 170:6320-6328

Armengol MP; Juan M; Lucas-Martin A; Fernandez-Figueras MT; Jaraquemada D; Gallart T; Pujol-Borrell R. 2001 Thyroid autoimmune disease: demonstration of thyroid antigen-specific B cells and recombination-activating gene expression in chemokine-containing active intrathyroidal germinal centers. Am J Pathol , 159(3): 861-73

Armengol, M. P., M. Juan, A. Lucas-Martín, M. T. Fernández-Figueras, D. Jaraquemada, T. Gallart, R. Pujol-Borrell. 2001. Ectopic lymphoid follicles in thyroid autoimmune glands are sites of active B cell expansion and maturation: relevance to pathogenesis. Am. J. Pathol. 159:861.

Ben-Skowronek I, Szewczyk L., Sierocinska-Sawa J, Korobowicz E. 2007 The subsets of lymphocytes in autoimmune and non-autoimmune thyroid diseases in children. Endokrynol Ped 6 (3), 9-20.

Ben-Skowronek I, Sierocinska-Sawa J, Korobowicz E, Szewczyk L. 2008 Lymphocytes in peripheral blood and thyroid tissue in children with Graves' disease. World Journal of Pediatrics 4:274-282.

Ben-Skowronek I, Szewczyk L, Ciechanek R, Korobowicz E. The interactions of lymphocytes, thyrocytes and fibroblasts in Hashimoto's thyroiditis - immunohistochemical and ultrastructural study. In press

Brix TH, Kyvik KO, Hegedus L. 2000 A population-based study of chronic autoimmune hypothyroidism in Danish twins. J Clin Endocrinol Metab. 85, 2 536-539.

Bromley SK, Burack WR, Johnson KG, Somersalo K, Sims TN, Sumen C, Davis MM , Shaw AS, Allen PM, and Dustin ML. 2001 The immunological synapse. Annual Review of Immunology Vol. 19: 375.

Crawford, D. H., S. M. McLachlan. 1983. The relationship between the Epstein-Barr virus and rheumatoid arthritis. Br. J. Rheumatol. 22:129.

Czarnocka B, Ruf J, Fernand M, Carayon P, Lissitzky S.1985 Purification of the human thyroid peroxidase and its identification as the microsomal antigen involved in autoimmune thyroid disease. FEBS lett. , 190,147-152

DiMatolaT, Mueller F, Fenzi G, Rosi G, Bifulco , Marzano LA, Vitale M. 2000 Serum withdrawal-induced apoptosis in thyroid cells is caused by loss of fibronectin-integrin interaction. J Clin Endocrinol Metab 85: 1188-1193.

Drabko K, Winnicka D, Gaworczyk A, Ben-Skowronek I, Skomra D, Kowalczyk JR. 2006 Donor origin of Graves' disase i BMT recipient: evidence from FISH studies of thyroid tissue. Bone Marrow Transplantation 37, 789-91.

Duntas LH 2008. Environmental factors and autoimmune thyroiditis. Nat Clin Pract Endocrinol Metab. 4(8):454-60.

Dustin ML, 2007 Cell adhesion molecules and actin cytoskeleton at immune synapses and kinapses . Curr Opin Cell Biol. 19(5): 529–533.

Dustin ML, Long EO, 2010 Cytotoxic immunological synapses .Immunological Reviews Special Issue: Cytotoxic CellsVolume 235, 1: 24–34. Dustin ML, Rothlein R, Bhan AK, Dinarello CA, Springer TA. 1986 Induction of IL-1 and interferon, tissue distribution, biochemistry, and function of a natural adherence molecule (ICAM-1). J Immunol. 137:245–254.

Dustin ML and Shaw AS. 1999 Perspectives Immunology. Costimulation: Building an Immunological Synapse Science . 283, 5402, 649 – 650.

Dustin ML, 2002 The immunological synapse . Arthritis Res Therapy 4 (Suppl3): 119-125.

Estienne V, Bisbarre N, Blanchin S, Durand-Gorde JM, Carayon P, Ruf J. 2004 An In vitro model based on cell monolayers grown on the underside of large-pore filters In bicameral chambers for studying thyrocyte-lymphocyte interactions. Am J Physiol Cell Physiol 287: C1763-C1768.

Estienne V, Duthoit C, BlanchinS , Montserret R, Durand-Gorde J-M, Chartier M, Baty D, Carayon P, and Ruf J. 2002 Analysis of a conformational B cell epitope of human thyroid peroxidase: identification of a tyrosine residue at a strategic location for immunodominance. Int. Immunol., 14(4): 359 - 366.

Gad, M., M. H. Claesson, A. E. Pedersen. 2003. Dendritic cells in peripheral tolerance and immunity. APMIS 111: 766-775.

Gardella S, Andrei C, Lotti L, Poggi A, Torrisi R, Zocchi R, Rubartelli A.2001 CD8+ T lymphocytes induct polarized exocytosis of secretory lysosomes by dendritic cells with release of interleukin 1β and cathepsin D. Blood, 90(7):2152-2159

Grakoui A, Bromley SK, Sumen C, Davis MM, Shaw AS, Allen PM, Dustin ML 1999 The immunological synapse: A molecular machine controlling T cell activation .Science 285:221-227.

Greek LM, LaBue M, Lazarus JP, Jennings JC. 1996 Reduced cell-cell communication in experimentally induced autoimmune thyroid disease. Endocrinol 137: 2823-2832.

Green LM, Lazarus JP, Song ,Stagg RB, LaBue M, Hilliker S. 1997 Elevation of protein kinase C in thyrocytes isolated from a Lews Rat model of autoimmune thyroiditis

prevents assembly of immunodetecteable connexin 43 gap junction and reduces intercellular communication. Thyroid 7: 913-921.
Guo J, Jaume JC, Rapoport B, Mc Lachlan SM. 1997 Recombinant thyroid peroxidase-specific Fab converted to immunoglobulin G (IgG) molecules: evidence for thyroid cell damage by IgG1, but not IgG4, autoantibodies. J Clin Endocrinol Metab 82:925-931.
Guo J, McLachlan S. M., Pichurin P. N., Chen C.R., Pham N., Aliesky H. A., David C. S., and Rapoport B. 2005 Relationship between Thyroid Peroxidase T Cell Epitope Restriction and Antibody Recognition of the Autoantibody Immunodominant Region in Human Leukocyte Antigen DR3 Transgenic Mice. Endocrinology, 146(11): 4961 - 4967.
Heuer M, Aust G, Ode-Hakim S, Scherbaum WA. 1996 Different Cytokine mRNA Profiles in Graves' Disease, Hashimoto's Thyroiditis, and Nonautoimmune Thyroid Disorders Determined by Quantitative Reverse Transcriptase Polymerase Chain Reaction (RT-PCR) Thyroid., 6(2): 97-106.
Iannacone, M, Sitia, G,; Guidotti, L G. 2006 Pathogenetic and antiviral immune responses against hepatitis B virus. Future Virology 1: 189–96.
Iannacone, M, Sitia, G, Isogawa, M, Marchese, P, Castro, M G, Lowenstein, PR; Chisari, FV, Ruggeri V, Zaverio M et al. 2005 Platelets mediate cytotoxic T lymphocyte–induced liver damage. Nature Medicine 11 (11): 1167–9.
Itoh M, Takahashi T, Sakaguchi N, Kuniyasu Y, Shimizu J, Otsuka F, Sakaguchi S 1999 Thymus and Autoimmunity: Production of CD25+CD4+ naturally anergic and suppressive T Cells as a key function of the thymus in maintaining immunologic self-tolerance. J Immunol 162: 5317-5326.
Itoh, K., E. Meffre, E. Albesiano, A. Farber, D. Dines, P. Stein, S. E. Asnis, R. A. Furie, R. I. Jain, N. Chiorazzi. 2000. Immunoglobulin heavy chain variable region gene replacement as a mechanism for receptor revision in rheumatoid arthritis synovial tissue B lymphocytes. J. Exp. Med. 192:1151.
Janeway C.A, Jr Travers P, Walport M, and Shlomchik M.J. 2001 The Immune System in Health and Disease in: Immunobiology, 5th edition, New York: Garland Science.
Janeway CA, Medzhitov R. 2002 Innate immune recognition. Annu Re Immunol , 20:197
Jang H, Hess L. 2006 Regulation of immune response by T- cells . NEJM 354; 1166-1176.
Jonuleit, H., E. Schmitt, K. Steinbrink, A. H. Enk. 2001. Dendritic cells as a tool to induce anergic and regulatory T cells. Trends Immunol. 22: 394-400.
Karandikar NJ, Vanderlugt CL, Walunas TL, Miller SD, Bluestone JA. 1996 CTLA4: A negative regulator of autoimmune disease. J Exp Med 184:783-788.
Kawakami A, Eguchi K, Matsuoka N, Tsuboi M, Kawabe Y, Ishikawa N, Ito K, Nagataki S. 1996 Thyroid-stimulating hormone inhiibits Fas antigen-mediated apoptosis ofhuman thyrocytes in vitro. Endocrinology 137:316.
Kawakami Y, Fisfalen M-E, DeGroot LJ. 1992 Proliferative responses of peripheral blood mononuclear cells from patients with autoimmune thyroid diseases. J Immunol *148*:2084–2089.
Kimura H., Tzou S.C, Rocci R, Kimura M, Suzuki K, Parlow A.F, Noel R. 2005 Interleukin12 driver primary hypothyroidism: the contrasting role sof two Th1 cytokines (IL-12 and IFN γ. Endocrinol 8; 3642-3651.
Kimura, H., M. Kimura, S. C. Tzou, Y. C. Chen, K. Suzuki, N. R. Rose, P. Caturegli. 2004. Expression of class II MHC molecules on thyrocytes does not cause spontaneous

thyroiditis, but mildly increases its severity after immunization. Endocrinology 146: 1154-1162.

Lorenz M, Hermann M, Winkler T, Gaipl U, Kalden JR. 2000 Role of apoptosis in autoimmunity. Apoptosis 5:443-449.

Maziotti G., Sorvillo F., Naclerio C., Tarzati A., Cioffi M., Perna R., Valentini G., Farziati B., Amato G., Carella C. 2003 Type-1 response in peripheral CD4+ and CD8+ T-cells from patients with Hashimoto's thyroiditis; Eur. J. Endocrinol.:148(4), 383-388.

McLachlan SM, Nagayama Y, Pichurin PN, Mizutori Y, Chen CR, Misharin A, Aliesky Rapoport B. 2007 The link between Graves' disease and Hashimoto's thytroiditis: a role for regulatory T-cells. Endocrinology 148:5724-5733.

Menges, M., S. Rossner, C. Voigtlander, H. Schindler, N. A. Kukutsch, C. Bogdan, K. Erb, G. Schuler, M. B. Lutz. 2002. Repetitive injections of dendritic cells matured with tumor necrosis factor αinduce antigen-specific protection of mice from autoimmunity. J. Exp. Med. 195: 15-21.

Metcalfe RA, Oh YS, Stround C, Arnold K, Weetman AP.1997 Analysis of antibody - dependent cell mediated cytotoxicuty in autoimmune thyroid disease. Autoimmunity 25:65-72.

Mitsiiades N, Poulaki V, Kotoula V, Mastorakos G, Balafouta S, Koutras DA, Tsokos 1998 Fas/Fas ligand up-regulation and BCL-2 down-regulation may be significant in the pathogenesis of Hashimoto' thyroiditis. J Clin Endo Metab 83:2199

Morris GP, Chen L, Kong YC 2007 CD137 signaling function of CD4+CD25+ regulatory T-cells in induced tolerance to experimental immune thyroiditis. Cell Immunol 226:20-29.

Morris, G.P. and Kong, Y.M. 2006 Interference with $CD4^{+}CD25^{+}$ T cell-mediated tolerance to experimental autoimmune thyroiditis by glucocorticoid-induced tumor necrosis factor receptor monoclonal antibody. J. Autoimmunity, 26:24-31.

Nagayama Y, Horie I, Saitoh O, Nakahara M, Abiru N. 2007 CD4+CD25+ naturally occurring regulatory T cells and not lymphopenia play a role in the pathogenesis of iodide-induced autoimmune thyroiditis in NOD-H2h4 mice. J Autoimmun.29(2-3):195-202. Epub 2007 Sep 10.

Negrini S, Fenoglio D, Balestra P, Fravega M, Filaci G and Indiveri F. 2006 Endocrine Regulation of Suppressor Lymphocytes. Ann Ny Acad Sci 1069: 377-385.

Ng HP, Kung AWC 2006 Induction of Autoimmune Thyroiditis and Hypothyroidism by Immunization of Immunoactive T Cell Epitope of Thyroid Peroxidase Endocrinology, 147(6): 3085 - 3092.

Ng HP, BangaJP, and Kung AWC 2004 Development of a Murine Model of Autoimmune Thyroiditis Induced with Homologous Mouse Thyroid Peroxidase. Endocrinology, 145(2): 809 - 816.

Pandit AA, Vijay Warde M, Menon PS. 2003 Correlation of number of intrathyroid lymphocytes with antimicrosomal antibody titer in Hashimoto's thyroiditis. Diagn Cytopathol 28 (2):63-65.

Pappenwali C, Ehlers M, Schott M.2010 Advances in cellular therapy for the treatment of thyroid cancer. J Oncol ID 179491 in press

Paul WE, Seder RA 1994 Lymphocyte responses and cytokines. Cell 76:241-251.

Pulendrav B, van Driel R, Nossal GJ. 1997 Immunologicl toleranc in germinal centres. Immunol Today, 18:27.

Rapaport B, McLachlan SM 2001 Thyroid autoimmunity. Clin Invest 108:1253-1259.
Rebuffat SA, Bresson D, Nguyen B, and Peraldi-Roux S. 2006 The key residues in the immunodominant region 353-363 of human thyroid peroxidase were identified. Int. Immunol., 18(7): 1091 - 1099.
Rebuffat SA, Morin M, Nguyen B Castex F, Robert B, Peraldi-Roux S. 2010 Human recombinant anti-thyroperoxidase autoaibodies: in vitro cytotoxic activity on papillary thyroid cancer expressing TPO. Br J Cancer 102: 852-861.
Rebuffat SA, Nguyen B,Robert B, Castex F, Peraldi Roux S. 2008 Antiperoxidase Antibody-Dependent Cytotoxicity in Autoimmune Thyroid Disease. J Clin Endocrinol Metab, 93;3: 929-934
Ruddle, N. H.. 1999. Lymphoid neo-organogenesis: lymphotoxin's role in inflammation and development. Immunol. Res. 19:119.
Schroeder A, Greiner EA, Seyfert, A. Berek C. 1996. Differentiation of B cells in the nonlymphoid tissue of the synovial membrane of patients with rheumatoid arthritis. Proc. Natl. Acad. Sci. USA 93:221.
Shione H, Fujii Y, Okumura Y, Yakeuchi M, Inoue M, Matsuda H. 1997. Failure to down-regulate Bcl-2 protein in thymic germinal center B cells in myasthenia gravis. Eur. J. Immunol. 27:805.
Sims GP, Shiono H, Willcox N, Stott DI. 2001. Somatic hypermutation and selection of B cells in thymic germinal centers responding to acetylcholine receptor in myasthenia gravis. J. Immunol. 167:1935.
Stassi G, De Maria R 2002 Autoimmune thyroid disease: New model of cell health in autoimmunity. Nat Rev Immunol 2: 198-204
Stassi G, Di Liberto D, Todaro M, Zeuner A, Ricci-Vitiani L, Stoppacciaro A, Ruco L, Farina F, Zummo G and De Maria G. 2000 Control of target cell survival in thyroid autoimmunity by T helper cytokines via regulation of apoptotic proteins Nature Immunology 1, 483 - 488.
Stott D, Hiepe, M, Hummel, Steinhauser C. Berek. A. 1998. Antigen-driven clonal proliferation of B cell within the target tissue of an autoimmune disease. J. Clin. Invest. 102:938.
Subramanian S, Ramalingam K. 2005 Electron microscopic evidence on the participation Cytotoxic T Lymphocytes and Macrophages in Mtb adjuvant induced connective tissue inflammation and arthritogenesis in Rattus norvegicus. Asian Journal of Microbiology, Biotechnology and Environmental Sciences 7 (2): 227–233.
Sugihara S, Fuiwara H, Sherarer GM. 1993 Autoimmune thyroiditis In mice depleted of particular T cell subsets. Characterization of thyroiditis- inducing T cell lines and clones derived from thyroid lesions. J Immunol 150 (2),:683-694.
Wakkach, A., N. Fournier, V. Brun, J. P. Breittmayer, F. Cottrez, H. Groux. 2003. Characterization of dendritic cells that induce tolerance and T regulatory 1 cell differentiation in vivo. Immunity 18: 605-617.
Wallace, WEH, Howie SEM, Krajewaki AS. 1996. The immunological architecture of B-lymphocytes aggregates in cryptogenic fibrosing alveolitis. J. Pathol. 178:323.
Watanabe M, Yamamoto N, Maruoka H, Tamai H, Matsuzuka F, Miyauchi A, Iwatani Y. 2002 Independent involvement of CD8+CD25+ cells and thyroid autoantibodies in disease severity of Hashimoto's disease. Thyroid 12 (9):801-808
Weetman AP 2004 Autoimmune thyroid disease. Autoimmunity 37: 337-340

Weetman AP, McGregor AM. 1994. Autoimmune thyroid disease: further developments in our understanding. Endocr. Rev. 15:788.

Xie LD, Gao MR, Lu GZ,Guo XH.2008 Distribution of immunoglobulin G subclasses of anti-thyroid peroxidase antibody in sera from patients with Hashimoto's thyroiditis with different thyroid functional status. Clin Exp Immunol 154: 172-177.

Yamazaki H, Bretz J, Arscott PL, Baker JR. 2000 Apoptosis and the thyroid: the biology and potential implications for thyroid disease. Curr Opinion in Endocrinology and Diabetes;7(5):260-264.

14

Autoimmunity in Vitiligo

E. Helen Kemp[1], Sherif Emhemad[1],
David J. Gawkrodger[2] and Anthony P. Weetman[1]
[1]Department of Human Metabolism, The Medical School, University of Sheffield, Sheffield,
[2]Department of Dermatology, Royal Hallamshire Hospital, Sheffield,
United Kingdom

1. Introduction

Vitiligo is an idiopathic disorder of pigmentation characterised by the presence of depigmented skin macules due to the chronic and progressive loss of melanocytes from the cutaneous epidermis. Large population surveys have shown a worldwide incidence of 1-2% (Boisseau-Garsaud et al., 2000; Howitz et al., 1977; Majumder et al. 1993; Mehta et al., 1973), although a prevalence of 8.8% has been reported in India (Sehgal & Srivastava, 2007). The disease occurs independently of age and race, and both sexes are equally affected (Behl et al., 2003; Cho et al., 2000; Handa & Dogra, 2003; Hann & Lee, 1996; LePoole & Boissy, 1997; Zaima & Koga, 2002). In approximately half of all cases, vitiligo appears before the age of 20 years, and 70-80% of patients develop the disease by the age of 30 years (Behl et al., 2003; Herane, 2003). Frequently, patients with vitiligo also suffer from other autoimmune conditions (Alkhateeb et al., 2003; Laberge et al., 2005).

Usually, vitiligo is viewed as a minor disease, but the impact on patients' psychological well-being and social interactions is often underestimated (Kent & Al' Abadie, 1996; Ongenae et al., 2006; Porter et al., 1986). The treatment of choice in vitiligo is dependent upon factors which include vitiligo type (non-segmental, segmental), patient age, and location and stability of depigmented lesions (Taieb & Picardo, 2010). However, despite the many available therapeutic modalities (Abu Tahir et al., 2010; Olsson, 2010), repigmentation in the majority of vitiligo patients is rarely complete or long-lasting, so a better understanding of the precise aetiology and pathogenesis of the disease is crucial to improving the efficacy of treatment regimens.

Currently, the exact aetiology of vitiligo remains obscure, but many factors have been implicated in the development of the disease including infections (Grimes et al., 1996; Shegan, 1971), stress (Al'Abadie et al., 1994a), neural abnormalities (Al'Abadie et al., 1994b), defective melanocyte adhesion (Gauthier et al., 2003), and genetic susceptibility (Spritz, 2010). The biochemical hypothesis argues that melanocyte destruction is due to the accumulation of toxic metabolites from melanogenesis, the break-down of free-radical defence and an excess of hydrogen peroxide (Dell'Anna & Picardo, 2006; Schallreuter et al., 1991; Schallreuter et al., 2001; Schallreuter et al., 2005). In addition, many studies have indicated a role for both cellular (Ogg et al., 1998; Van den Boorn et al., 2009; Wankowicz-Kalinska et al., 2003) and humoral (Gilhar et al., 1995; Naughton et al., 1983a; Norris et al., 1988a) immunity in the pathogenesis of vitiligo. Ultimately, these different factors may act independently or together to yield the same effect, namely the disappearance of melanocytes from the skin and this is proposed in the convergence theory (Le Poole et al., 1993a). For example, autoimmunity might arise as a secondary phenomenon following the self-destruction of pigment cells and this might then amplify the damage to melanocytes. In addition, different pathogenic mechanisms could account for the various clinical types of vitiligo: the possible neural mechanisms are usually related to segmental vitiligo, whereas autoimmunity is most often associated with the non-segmental (generalised) form (Taieb, 2000).

2. Immunological factors in vitiligo aetiology and pathogenesis

The evidence for the role of autoimmunity in the aetiology and pathogenesis of vitiligo will be discussed in the next sections.

2.1 Immuno-genetic factors

The majority of cases of vitiligo are sporadic without a family history of the disease. Nevertheless, 15-20% of patients report at least one affected first-degree relative (Alkhateeb et al., 2003), lending evidence for a genetic role in the aetiology of vitiligo. Furthermore, among Caucasians, the risk of vitiligo developing in a patient's sibling is approximately 6.1% (Alkhateeb et al., 2003), an increase of 16-fold compared to the general Caucasian population where the prevalence of the disease is 0.38% (Howitz et al., 1977). Similarly, an increased risk among first-degree relatives is found in Indian-Pakistanis at 6.1% (Alkhateeb et al., 2003), in American Hispanic-Latinos at 4.8% (Alkhateeb et al., 2003) and in Han Chinese at 2.6% (Sun et al., 2006). A simple Mendelian inheritance pattern is not displayed in these familial aggregations of vitiligo cases (Alkhateeb et al., 2003; Bhatia et al., 1992; Carnevale et al., 1980; Das et al., 1985; Hafez et al., 1983; Laberge et al., 2005; Majumder et al., 1988; Majumder et al., 1993; Mehta et al., 1973; Nath et al., 1994; Sun et al., 2006), suggesting that the disease is probably transmitted as a polygenic trait. Indeed, earlier disease onset in familial cases (Alkhateeb et al., 2003; Laberge et al., 2005) and reduced risk of vitiligo with increasing genetic distance from the patient (Alkhateeb et al. 2003) are indicative of a polygenic disorder. Formal genetic segregation analyses of vitiligo have also suggested that multiple loci contribute to vitiligo susceptibility (Majumder et al., 1993; Nath et al., 1994; Sun et al., 2006). Seldomly have large multi-generation families been reported where vitiligo segregates in an autosomal dominant pattern (Alkhateeb et al., 2005). Twin studies have also provided evidence of a genetic component to vitiligo aetiology. For vitiligo in monozygotic twins, the concordance is 23% (Alkhateeb et al. 2003), a disease risk that is 60-fold greater than that in the general population (Howitz et al., 1977) and 4-fold higher than that for a patient's sibling (Alkhateeb et al., 2003).

The genetic epidemiological evidence has prompted the search for genes which predispose an individual to vitiligo. Investigations have included families with vitiligo as well as cohorts of patients without a familial history of the disease (Cantón et al., 2005; Fain et al., 2003). In addition, different approaches have been employed to identify genes which confer susceptibility to vitiligo including candidate gene association studies (Blomhoff et al., 2005; Cantón et al., 2005), genome-wide linkage studies (Chen et al., 2005; Fain et al., 2003; Liang et al., 2007; Spritz et al., 2004), and genome-wide association studies (Birlea et al., 2010; Jin et al., 2010a; Quan et al., 2010). The majority of genes and genetic loci so far identified have a role in the function of the immune system (Spritz, 2010), and these are summarised in the following sections.

2.1.1 Human leukocyte antigen alleles of the major histocompatibility complex

Initial case-control analyses demonstrated an association between predisposition to vitiligo and several different human leukocyte antigen (HLA) alleles of the major histocompatibility complex (MHC), and these are summarised in Table 1. Although these studies showed weak and variable associations, a significant association of HLA-DR4 and vitiligo was demonstrated in several populations (Dunston et al. 1990; Foley et al. 1983; Venneker et al. 1992) and a subsequent meta-analysis of a series of case-control studies reported association of vitiligo with HLA-A2 (Liu et al., 2007).

Population	Associated HLA Allele	Reference
American (Caucasian)	DR4	Foley et al., 1983
American (African)	DR4, DQw3	Dunston et al., 1990
American and British (European-derived, Caucasian)	DRB1A*04-DQB1*0301	Fain et al., 2006
American and British (European-derived, Caucasian)	Class I (specifically A*0201) and II antigens	Jin et al., 2010a
Chinese (Han)	DQA1*0302, DQB1*0303, DQB1*0503	Yang et al., 2005
Chinese (Han)	A25-Cw*0602-DQA1*0302	Xia et al., 2006
Chinese (Han and Uygar)	Class I and II antigens	Quan et al., 2010
Dutch	DR4, DR6, Cw6	Venneker et al., 1993; Venneker et al., 1992
Dutch	DRB4*0101, DQB1*0303	Zamani et al., 2001
German (Northern)	A2	Schallreuter et al., 1993
Hungarian	DR1, DR3	Poloy et al., 1991
Italian	A30, B27, Cw6, DQw3	Finco et al., 1991
Italian (Northern)	A3	Lorini et al., 1992
Italian (Northern)	A30, Cw6, DQw3	Orecchia et al., 1992
Japanese	A31, Bw46, Cw4	Ando et al., 1993
Kuwaiti	B21, Cw6	Al-Fouzan et al., 1995
Moroccan (Jewish)	B13	Metzker et al., 1980
Omani	Bw6, DR7	Venkataram et al., 1995
Slovak	A2, Dw7	Buc et al., 1996
Turkish	DRB1*03, DRB1*04, DRB1*07	Tastan et al., 2004
Yemeni	Bw35	Metzker et al., 1980

Table 1. Association of human leukocyte antigen (HLA) alleles with vitiligo susceptibility

More recently, the use of better analytical and statistical methods has revealed associations of vitiligo with HLA-DRB1*04, HLA-DRB1*03 and HLA-DRB1*07 alleles in Turkish patients (Tastan et al., 2004), with HLA-DRB4*0101 and HLA-DQB1*0303 in Dutch patients (Zamani et al., 2001), and HLA-A25-Cw*0602-DQA1*0302, HLA-DQA1*0302, HLA-DQB1*0303 and HLA-DQB1*0503 in Han Chinese patients (Xia et al., 2006; Yang et al., 2005). Furthermore, a study of 76 Caucasian multiplex vitiligo families found the HLA-DRB1A*04-DQB1*0301 haplotype to be associated with a higher risk of developing vitiligo and with an earlier onset of the disease (Fain et al., 2006). Finally, two genome-wide association studies undertaken on populations of vitiligo patients have reported that predisposition of vitiligo is associated with HLA class I and II antigens (Jin et al., 2010a; Quan et al., 2010).

2.1.2 Immune-response genes and loci

Variations in several immune-response genes, including CCR6, FOXP1, FOXP3, TSLP and XBP1, have a confirmed association with predisposition to vitiligo and these are summarised in Table 2 (Birlea et al., 2011; Cheong et al., 2009; Jin et al., 2010a; Jin et al., 2010b; Quan et al., 2010; Ren et al., 2009). Of particular note, the allelic variation R620W of the PTPN22 gene, which encodes lymphoid protein tyrosine phosphatase, a molecule involved in T cell signalling, has been shown to confer vitiligo susceptibility in several independent reports (Cantón et al., 2005; Jin et al., 2010a; Laberge et al., 2008a; Laberge et al., 2008b). In addition, allelic variants in the NLRP1 gene (previously NALP1 or SLEV1), which encodes a key regulator of the innate immune system, have been reproducibly associated with an increased risk of vitiligo in different populations (Jin et al., 2007a; Jin et al., 2007b; Nath et al., 2001; Spritz et al., 2004).

The study of variations in the cytotoxic T lymphocyte antigen 4 (CTLA4) gene has yielded conflicting results with respect to vitiligo susceptibility (Birlea et al., 2011; Birlea et al., 2009; Blomhoff et al., 2005; Deeba et al., 2010; Itirli et al., 2005; Kemp et al., 1999; Laberge et al., 2008a; Pehlivan et al., 2009). Presently, allelic differences in CTLA4 appear to be predominantly associated with vitiligo occurring together with other autoimmune diseases (Blomhoff et al., 2005), and it has been suggested, therefore, that the association of CTLA4 with vitiligo is probably secondary to its primary association with disorders such as autoimmune thyroid disease (Spritz, 2010).

2.2 Associated autoimmune disease

Vitiligo is frequently associated with other autoimmune disorders, particularly autoimmune thyroid disease (Boelaert et al., 2010; Ochi & DeGroot, 1969), autoimmune polyendocrine syndromes (Ahonen et al., 1990; Neufeld et al., 1990), pernicious anaemia (Dawber, 1970), Addison's disease (Zelissen et al., 1995), and alopecia areata (Ahmed et al., 2007). Furthermore, patients with vitiligo are more likely to suffer from autoimmune conditions than those in the general population (Birlea et al., 2008; Cunliffe et al., 1968; Liu et al., 2005; Turnbridge et al., 1977). In a survey of more than 2,600 unselected Caucasian vitiligo patients, elevated frequencies of autoimmune thyroid disease, Addison's disease, systemic lupus erythematosus and pernicious anaemia were found, with approximately 30% of patients being affected with at least one additional autoimmune disorder (Alkhateeb et al., 2003). Moreover, these same autoimmune diseases occurred at an increased frequency in the first-degree relatives of the patients studied (Alkhateeb et al., 2003). Similarly, in multiplex generalised vitiligo families, higher frequencies of psoriasis, rheumatoid arthritis and type 1 diabetes mellitus were noted in addition to autoimmune thyroid disease, Addison's disease, systemic lupus erythematosus and pernicious anaemia (Laberge et al., 2005). Such data indicate that individuals can be genetically predisposed to a specific group of autoimmune diseases that includes vitiligo, and are also evidence for an autoimmune aetiology for this depigmenting disorder.

Gene or Locus	Function/Comment	Reference
AIS2	Autoimmune susceptibility locus 2. Function undefined. Associated with autoimmune disease.	Spritz et al., 2004
CCR6	Cytokine-chemokine receptor for CCL20. Recruits immune cells on binding of ligand. Associated with inflammatory bowel disease.	Jin et al., 2010a; Jin et al., 2010b; Quan et al., 2010
C1QTNF6	C1q and tumour necrosis factor-related protein- 6. Associated with rheumatoid arthritis and type 1 diabetes mellitus.	Jin et al., 2010a
FOXP1	Forkhead box P1. Transcription factor which regulates development of immune cells.	Jin et al., 2010a; Jin et al., 2010b
FOXP3	Forkhead box P3. Transcription factor which regulates regulatory T cell development. Causes autoimmune IPEX syndrome.	Birlea et al., 2011
GZMB	Granzyme B. Regulates cell-mediated immune responses.	Jin et al., 2010a
IL2RA	Interleukin (IL)-2 receptor alpha chain. Receptor for cytokine IL2 which induces T and B cell proliferation. Associated with many autoimmune diseases.	Jin et al., 2010a
LPP	LIM domain-containing preferred translocation partner in lipoma. Function unknown. Associated with celiac disease and rheumatoid arthritis.	Jin et al., 2010a
NLRP1 (NALP1; SLEV1)	NACHT leucine-rich-repeat protein 1. Functions in the innate immune response. Associated with many autoimmune diseases.	Jin et al., 2007a; Jin et al., 2007b; Nath et al., 2001; Spritz et al., 2004
PTPN22	Lymphoid protein tyrosine phosphatase. Negatively regulates T cell activation. Associated with many autoimmune diseases.	Cantón et al., 2005; Jin et al., 2010a; Laberge et al., 2008a; Laberge et al., 2008b
TSLP	Thymic stromal lymphopoietin. Cytokine which induces naïve CD4+ T cells to produce T helper cell 2 cytokines.	Birlea et al., 2011; Cheong et al., 2009
UBASH3A	Ubiquitin-associated and SH3 domain-containing A gene. Regulates T cell receptor signalling. Associated with type 1 diabetes mellitus.	Jin et al., 2010a
XBP1	X-box binding protein 1. Transcription factor which regulates MHC class II gene expression. Associated with inflammatory bowel disease.	Birlea et al., 2011; Ren et al., 2009

Table 2. Confirmed associations of immune-response gene variants with vitiligo susceptibility

2.3 Animal models

The study of animal models has added credence to the theory that immune mechanisms play a part in the development of vitiligo. Several spontaneous animal models of vitiligo exist, although the exact relevance of such models to the equivalent human disorder remains to be established (Boissy & Lamoreux, 1988). The well-documented Smyth chickens express a genetically inherited form of vitiligo-like depigmentation resulting from the loss of melanocytes in feather and ocular tissues (Smyth, 1989). In this avian model, vitiligo begins with an inherent melanocyte defect that is followed by an autoimmune response involving both humoral and cellular reactions that eliminate abnormal pigment cells (Boissy et al., 1984; Boyle et al., 1987; Lamont & Smyth, 1981; Pardue et al., 1988). An increase in T cells in the feather pulp and circulating inflammatory leukocytes has been shown in Smyth chickens prior to the onset, and during the development of, vitiligo (Erf & Smyth, 1996; Erf et al., 1995). Antibodies to chicken melanocytes have also been detected in the sera of 100% of Smyth chicks but not in the sera of normally pigmented birds (Austin et al., 1992). These antibodies were found to be present both before and during the presentation of vitiligo (Searle et al., 1991), and the primary target antigen was identified as the melanogenic enzyme tyrosinase-related protein-1 (Austin & Boissy, 1995). In other animals with vitiligo including horses, cats and dogs, antibody reactivity occurs against a similar pattern of melanocyte antigens to that found in patients with the disease (Naughton et al., 1983b; Naughton et al., 1986a), suggesting that similar immunological responses occur in both animals and humans.

2.4 Vitiligo melanocytes

Several studies have shown abnormal expression of MHC class II antigen HLA-DR and increased expression of intercellular adhesion molecule-1 by perilesional melanocytes in vitiligo compared with melanocytes from normal skin (Al Badri et al., 1993a; Hedley et al., 1998; Van den Wijngaard et al., 2000). Since these molecules have important roles in antigen presentation and in the activation of helper T cells, their expression by melanocytes could contribute to the anti-melanocyte cellular immune responses that are seen in vitiligo (Ogg et al., 1998; Van den Boorne et al., 2009). Both vitiligo and normal melanocytes are also capable of expressing MHC class I molecules (Hedley et al., 1998), which could allow interaction with destructive cytotoxic T cells. Furthermore, melanocytes have an antigen processing and presenting capability which can make them target cells for T cell-mediated cytotoxicity (Le Poole et al., 1993b). In perilesional vitiligo biopsies, melanocytes express macrophage markers CD68 and CD36 (Van den Wijngaard et al., 2000) and reduced levels of membrane regulators of complement activation, including decay acceleration factor and membrane cofactor protein (Van den Wijngaard et al., 2002), which suggests a vulnerability of these cells to attack by macrophages and the complement system, respectively.

2.5 Vitiligo treatments

Repigmentation in vitiligo patients receiving treatment with immunosuppressive agents indirectly supports the theory that immune-mediated processes are involved in vitiligo pathogenesis. Topically applied tacrolimus (FK506), a therapeutic agent which exerts a potent immunosuppressive effect on T cells by blocking the action of the cytokine gene-activating cofactor calcineurin (Homey et al., 1998), has resulted in successful repigmentation responses in vitiligo patients (Boone et al., 2007; Hartmann et al., 2008).

Topical corticosteroids, which have anti-inflammatory and immunosuppressive actions, are considered to be an effective first-line treatment in children and adults with segmental or non-segmental vitiligo of recent onset (Abu Tahir et al., 2010; Gawkrodger et al., 2010), and, indeed, following treatment of vitiligo patients with systemic steroids, a reduction in anti-melanocyte antibody levels and in antibody-mediated anti-melanocyte cytotoxicity has been demonstrated (Hann et al., 1993; Takei et al., 1984).

Psoralen with ultraviolet radiation (PUVA) is used as a second-line therapy for vitiligo (Alomar, 2010; Gawkrodger et al., 2010). Following PUVA treatment, a reduction in the number of Langerhans cells and a decrease in the expression of vitiligo-associated melanocyte antigens, which could lead to a blocking of antibody-dependent cell-mediated cytotoxicity against melanocytes, have been noted in vitiligo patients (Kao & Yu, 1992; Viac et al., 1997). In addition, ultraviolet radiation can induce the expression of anti-inflammatory cytokines, modulate the expression of intercellular adhesion molecule-1, and induce apoptosis of skin-infiltrating T lymphocytes (Duthie et al., 1999; Krutmann & Morita, 1999).

2.6 Humoral immune responses

2.6.1 Melanocyte antibodies

Antibodies to melanocytes occur at a significantly increased frequency in the sera of vitiligo patients compared with healthy individuals (Cui et al., 1992; Cui et al., 1995; Farrokhi et al., 2005; Hann et al., 1996a; Hann et al., 1996b; Naughton et al., 1983a; Naughton et al., 1983b; Rocha et al., 2002). As well as circulating antibodies, antibody deposits have been noted in the basement membrane zones of depigmented areas in patients with vitiligo (Uda et al., 1984). However, no B cells or antibody has yet been isolated from vitiligo lesions. Interestingly, correlations can also exist between the incidence and level of melanocyte antibodies and both the activity and extent of vitiligo (Aronson & Hashimoto, 1987; Harning et al., 1991; Kemp et al., 2011; Naughton et al., 1986b; Yu et al., 1993), indicating that melanocyte antibodies are possible markers of disease progression.

Predominantly, melanocyte antibodies have been characterised as IgG (Cui et al., 1992; Cui et al., 1995; Farrokhi et al., 2005; Hann et al., 1996a; Hann et al., 1996b; Naughton et al., 1983a; Naughton et al., 1983b; Rocha et al., 2002; Uda et al., 1984) and as belonging to subclasses IgG1, IgG2 and IgG3 (Xie et al., 1991), although anti-melanocyte IgA antibodies have also been reported (Aronson & Hashimoto, 1987). Initial immunoprecipitation studies using melanoma cell extracts revealed that antibodies in vitiligo patients were most commonly directed against antigens with molecular weights of 35, 40-45, 75, 90 and 150 kDa (Cui et al., 1992). Several of the proteins (40-45, 75 and 150 kDa) appeared to be common tissue antigens, while others (35 and 90 kDa) were preferentially expressed on melanocytes (Cui et al., 1992). In immunoblotting studies with melanocyte extracts, antigens of 45, 65, and 110 kDa have been identified (Hann et al., 1996b; Park et al., 1996), while vitiligo-associated antibodies have been demonstrated to recognise melanoma cell proteins of 68, 70, 88, 90, 110 and 165 kDa (Hann et al., 1996a; Rocha et al., 2002).

The identity of several vitiligo-associated antibody targets has been reported and these are summarised in Table 3. Included are the melanogenic enzymes tyrosinase (Baharav et al., 1996; Kemp et al., 1997a; Song et al., 1994) and tyrosinase-related protein-2 (Kemp et al., 1997b; Okamoto et al., 1998), and the melanosomal matrix protein gp100 (Pmel17) (Kemp et al., 1998a). The technique of peptide phage-display has identified the melanin-concentrating hormone receptor 1 (MCHR1) and tyrosine hydroxylase as targets of vitiligo patient antibodies (Kemp et al., 2002). Recent proteomic analysis has also revealed lamin A is a vitiligo-associated antigen (Li et al., 2010).

Antigen	Number of Patients with Antibodies (%)	Number of Controls with Antibodies (%)	Reference
Lamin A	24/84 (28.6)	2/64 (3.1)	Li et al., 2010
MCHR1	9/55 (16.4)	0/28 (0)	Kemp et al., 2002
MCHR1	12/84 (14.3)	Not reported	Li et al., 2010
Pmel17	3/53 (5.9)	0/20 (0)	Kemp et al., 1998a
SOX10	3/93 (3.2)	0/65 (0)	Hedstrand et al., 2001
SOX9	1/93 (1.1)	0/65 (0)	Hedstrand et al., 2001
Tyrosinase	16/26 (61)	0/31 (0)	Song et al., 1994
Tyrosinase	7/18 (39)	0/12 (0)	Baharav et al., 1996
Tyrosinase	5/46 (10.9)	0/20 (0)	Kemp et al., 1997a
TRP-1	3/53 (5.9)	0/20 (0)	Kemp et al., 1998b
TRP-1	8/84 (9.5)	Not reported	Li et al., 2010
TRP-2	3/53 (5.9)	0/20 (0)	Kemp et al., 1997b
TRP-2	10/15 (67)	0/21 (0)	Okamoto et al., 1998
TRP-2	20/30 (67)	1/35 (2)	Okamoto et al., 1998
Tyrosine hydroxylase	18/79 (23)	0/28 (0)	Kemp et al., 2011

Table 3. Defined antibody targets in patients with vitiligo

2.6.2 Pathogenic mechanisms

With respect to pathogenic effects, vitiligo-associated antibodies are able to destroy melanocytes and melanoma cells *in vitro* and *in vivo* by complement-mediated damage and antibody-dependent cellular cytotoxicity (Fishman et al., 1993; Gottumukkala et al., 2006; Norris et al., 1998a). Complement-mediated cytolysis of melanocytes by vitiligo patient antibodies appears to be cell selective and more common in individuals with active disease (Cui et al., 1993). Passive immunisation of nude mice grafted with human skin has also indicated that IgG from vitiligo patients can induce melanocyte destruction (Gilhar et al., 1995). Furthermore, IgG melanocyte antibodies from individuals with vitiligo can induce HLA-DR and intercellular adhesion molecule-1 expression on and release of interleukin-8 from melanocytes (Yi et al., 2000). Such changes that may enhance the antigen-presenting activity of melanocytes allowing antigen-specific immune effector cell attack resulting in melanocyte destruction.

Antibodies against MCHR1 have been shown to block the function of the receptor in a heterologous cell line (Gottumukkala et al., 2006). Stimulation of MCHR1 in cultured melanocytes with melanin-concentrating hormone (MCH) can down regulate the actions of α-melanocyte-stimulating hormone, including the production of melanin, suggesting that the MCH/MCHR1 signalling pathway has a role with the melanocortins in regulating melanocyte function (Hoogduijn et al., 2002). Any adverse effects of MCHR1 antibodies upon the functioning of the receptor in melanocytes could potentially disrupt normal melanocyte behaviour, a feature that could precede the clinical manifestation of vitiligo. However, this has not yet been reported and is still the object of study. More recent work has found that 69% (9/13) of vitiligo patient sera tested induced melanocyte detachment in a reconstructed epidermis model, although this was unrelated to either the extent or the activity of the disease (Cario-Andre et al., 2007). Further studies are needed to confirm that this serum effect is antibody mediated and, if so, that the antibody activity is specific to vitiligo patient sera.

2.6.3 Other antibodies

Circulating organ-specific autoantibodies, particularly to the thyroid, adrenal glands, gastric parietal cells, and pancreatic islet cells are commonly detected in the sera of vitiligo patients (Brostoff, 1969; Betterle et al., 1976; Mandry et al., 1996; Zauli et al., 1986). Moreover, antinuclear antibody and IgM-rheumatoid factor have been detected at a significant frequency in vitiligo patients (Farrokhi et al., 2005). Anti-keratinocyte intracellular antibodies that correlate with disease extent and activity have also been detected in vitiligo patients (Yu et al., 1993).

2.7 Cellular immune responses

2.7.1 Cytokines

An imbalance of cytokines, which can affect melanocyte activity and survival, has been shown in vitiligo lesional skin (Moretti et al., 2002). The level of granulocyte-macrophage colony-stimulating factor is reduced in patients with active vitiligo compared with healthy controls (Yu et al., 1997; Moretti et al., 2002). This cytokine has been found to act as a growth factor for melanocytes and a decrease in its production slows down the proliferation of surviving melanocytes in vitiligo lesions (Imokawa et al., 1996). Other melanogenic cytokines, including stem cell factor and endothelin-1, are also lowered in depigmented lesions (Moretti et al., 2002).

Serum levels of soluble interleukin-2 receptor can be used to monitor *in vivo* immune activation, and its elevation has been correlated with T cell-mediated immune disease. Indeed, the level of the soluble interleukin-2 receptor level in vitiligo patients is significantly increased compared with that of controls, indicating that the activation of T cells is a component in the pathogenesis of vitiligo (Tu et al., 1999; Yeo et al., 1999). The production of interleukin-6 by mononuclear cells is also elevated in vitiligo patients (Yu et al., 1997). This cytokine can induce the expression of intercellular adhesion molecule-1 on melanocytes thereby facilitating leukocyte-melanocyte interactions and consequently cause immunological damage (Kirnbauer et al., 1992). Increased production of interleukin-8, which can attract neutrophils to vitiligo lesions amplifying destructive inflammatory reactions, has also been reported in the mononuclear cells of vitiligo patients (Yu et al., 1997). Furthermore, the expression of tumour necrosis factor-alpha, an inflammatory mediator involved in the pathogenesis of autoimmune disease, is significantly elevated in vitiligo skin (Moretti et al., 2002). However, the exact roles in vitiligo pathogenesis of these inflammatory cytokines, which can also act as paracrine inhibitors of melanocyte proliferation and of melanogenesis, remain to be determined.

2.7.2 Macrophages

Macrophage infiltration has been demonstrated in vitiligo lesions, with increased numbers present in perilesional skin (Le Poole et al., 1996; Van den Wijngaard et al., 2000). It is possible that macrophages are involved in clearing melanocytes that have been induced to apoptose by cytotoxic T lymphocytes. Additional evidence for the active involvement of macrophages in vitiligo pathogenesis is demonstrated by their expression of immunoglobulin receptors: in a mouse model, it has been shown that macrophages, expressing the common gamma chain of the activating Fc gamma receptors, can mediate vitiligo in the presence and absence of complement C3 fraction (Trcka et al., 2002)

2.7.3 Dendritic cells

The density of Langerhans cells in vitiliginous skin has been variously reported as normal, increased and decreased compared with pigmented skin from the same patients and from control subjects (Claudy & Rouchouse, 1984; Hatchcome et al., 1987; Riley, 1967; Searle et al., 1991). The differences in the documented Langerhans cells densities may be due to the type of vitiligo, the sampling techniques used or the site of skin biopsies. An increase in the number of Langerhans cells could contribute to the immunological processes that damage melanocytes. However, although degenerative changes in Langerhans cells have been observed in vitiligo skin lesions, their role in vitiligo still remains unclear. More recently, dendritic cell-mediated destruction of melanocytes has been demonstrated *in vivo* and *in vitro* (Kroll et al., 2005). This process is related to the release of heat-shock protein 70 by stressed melanocytes, which induces an immune response against the cells from which it is produced, and to the increased expression of tumour-necrosis factor-related apoptosis inducing ligand receptors on stressed melanocytes making them more prone to killing by dendritic cells (Denman et al., 2008; Kroll et al., 2005).

2.7.4 T cells

Autoimmune disorders are often associated with an expansion of peripheral helper T cells. However, with respect to vitiligo, inconsistent data regarding abnormalities in circulating helper T cells have been reported. An increase in the number of activated helper T cells was detected in patients with stable vitiligo as well as in their first-degree relatives when compared with healthy individuals (Abdel-Naser et al., 1992; D'Amelio et al., 1990; Soubiran et al., 1985). In contrast, a decrease in the helper T cell population has also been observed in individuals with vitiligo (Grimes et al., 1986; Halder et al., 1986). No simple explanation exists for these differences but they could be attributable to the factors such as the population of patients under study, disease characteristics and received treatments.
Circulating melanocyte-specific cytotoxic T lymphocytes that target melanocyte-specific antigens, including Melan-A (MART-1), gp100 (Pmel17) and tyrosinase, have been detected in vitiligo patients (Lang et al., 2001; Ogg et al., 1998; Palermo et al., 2001). They express high levels of the skin-homing receptor cutaneous lymphocyte-associated antigen and their frequency correlates with both the extent and activity of the disease (Lang et al., 2001). In addition, melanocyte-specific T cells have cytotoxic reactivity towards melanocytes (Ogg et al., 1998). Such findings are consistent with a role for skin-homing, autoreactive, melanocyte-specific T cells in causing the destruction of melanocytes in vitiligo.
Histological studies of skin biopsies from vitiligo patients have demonstrated that infiltrating cytotoxic and helper T cells are most prominent at the periphery of vitiligo lesions (Al Badri et al., 1993b; Van den Wijngaard et al., 2000). Many of the inflammatory cells are activated, as indicated by the expression of the MHC class II antigen HLA-DR, and a significant number also exhibit high levels of the receptor cutaneous lymphocyte-associated antigen, typical of skin-homing T cells (Al Badri et al., 1993b; Van den Wijngaard

et al., 2000). Local activation of cytotoxic T cells at the perilesional epidermal/dermal junction of vitiliginous skin is also suggested by the presence of granzyme B+ and perforin+ cells (Van den Wijngaard, et al., 2000). There is evidence for interleukin-2 receptor and interferon-gamma receptor expression by the lymphocytic infiltrate (Abdel-Naser et al., 1994), and also for down-regulation of the helper T cell 2-dependent CDw60 molecule in the vitiliginous epidermis suggesting that infiltrating T cells may exhibit a helper T cell 1-type cytokine production pattern which is consistent with cell-mediated organ-specific autoimmunity (Le Poole et al., 2003). In addition, perilesional T cell clones exhibit a predominant type-1-like cytokine secretion profile (Wankowicz-Kalinska et al., 2003). More recently it has been demonstrated that T lymphocytes obtained from perilesional skin biopsies are enriched for cytotoxic T cells that recognise melanocyte antigens tyrosinase, gp100 and MelanA (Van den Boorn et al., 2009). Moreover, upon infiltration of autologous pigmented skin, isolated perilesional T lymphocytes efficiently kill melanocytes, providing direct evidence that cytotoxic T cells can cause the depigmentation seen in vitiligo (Van den Boorn et al., 2009). Additional to this, are findings that regulatory T cells occur at a reduced level in the skin of vitiligo patients (Klarquist et al., 2010). This may allow the unchecked destruction of melanocytes by cytotoxic T cells in vitiligo lesions (Klarquist et al., 2010).

3. Conclusion

Autoimmunity is one hypothesis forwarded to explain the development of vitiligo due to the evidence presented in this review. However, it is most likely that interacting mechanisms, of which immune responses are a part, are responsible for the clinical manifestations of the disease (Le Poole et al., 1993a). In addition, although the evidence for the role of immune-related genes in the aetiology of vitiligo is clear, the limited concordance in identical twins (Alkhateeb et al., 2003) indicates that other factors, probably environmental, are also involved in its development, making the disease complex, polygenic, and multi-factorial. Notably, *in vitro* studies have provided a link and a temporal sequence connecting cellular oxidative stress (Dell'Anna & Picardo, 2006; Schallreuter et al., 1991; Schallreuter et al., 2001; Schallreuter et al., 2005) and the immune response in vitiligo: stressed melanocytes were found to mediate dendritic cell-activation with the consequent dendritic cell effector functions playing a role in the destruction of melanocytes (Kroll et al., 2005). This work suggests that intrinsic damage to melanocytes could be the initiating event in vitiligo development followed by a secondary immune response by cytotoxic T cells which exacerbates the destruction of melanocytes and progresses the disease (Hariharan et al., 2010; Le Poole & Luiten, 2008; Van den Boorn et al., 2011). Indeed, 50% of vitiligo patients experience a Koebner phenomenon, whereby depigmented lesions develop at a site previously exposed to a physical stress (Le Poole & Luiten, 2008).

As indicated, it is most likely that immune responses in vitiligo are of a secondary nature following melanocyte damage. Indeed, several vitiligo-associated autoantigens such as tyrosinase and gp100 are located intracellularly, and it has been suggested that either the formation of neo-antigens due to haptenation, the exposure of cryptic epitopes or the modification of proteins during apoptosis could account for immune responses to these molecules (Namazi, 2007; Westerhof & d'Ischia, 2007). Following processing by mature Langerhans cells, antigenic peptides could be presented to T cells which have escaped clonal deletion or to naïve T lymphocytes which have not been tolerised against cryptic epitopes (Namazi, 2007; Westerhof & d'Ischia, 2007). Antibodies could then be produced following the stimulation of B lymphocytes by activated helper T cells (Namazi, 2007), and activated cytotoxic T cells could directly attack melanocytes expressing antigenic peptides on their surface in the context MHC class I molecules (Hedley et al., 1998; Le Poole et al., 1993b). In the case of immune reactivities against common cellular antigens, the selective destruction of melanocytes in vitiligo might occur because they are intrinsically more sensitive to immune-mediated injury than other skin cells (Norris et al., 1988b).

4. References

Abdel-Naser, M.B., Ludwig, W.D., Gollnick, H. & Orfanos, C.E. (1992). Non-segmental vitiligo: decrease of the CD45R+ T cell subset and evidence for T cell activation. *Int J Dermatol*, Vol.31, pp. 321-326

Abdel-Naser, M.B., Kruger-Krasagakes, S., Krasagakis, K., Gollnick, H., Abdel-Fattah, A. & Orfanos, C.E. (1994). Further evidence for involvement of both cell mediated and humoral immunity in generalized vitiligo. *Pigment Cell Res*, Vol.7, pp. 1-8

Abu Tahir, M., Pramod, K., Ansari, S.H. & Ali, J. (2010). Current remedies for vitiligo. *Autoimmun Rev*, Vol.9, pp. 516-520

Ahmed, I., Nasreen, S. & Bhatti, R. (2007). Alopecia areata in children. *J Coll Physicians Surg Pak,* Vol.17, pp. 587-590

Ahonen, P., Myallarniemi, S., Sipila, I. & Perheentupa, J. (1990). Clinical variation of autoimmune endocrinopathy-candidiasis-ectodermal dystrophy (APECED) in a series of 68 patients. *N Eng J Med*, Vol.322, pp. 1829-1836

Al'Abadie, M.S., Kent, G.G. & Gawkrodger, D.J. (1994a). The relationship between stress and the onset and exacerbation of psoriasis and other skin conditions. *Br J Dermatol*, Vol.130, pp. 199-203

Al'Abadie, M.S., Senior, H.J., Bleehen, S.S. & Gawkrodger, D.J. (1994b). Neuropeptide and neuronal marker studies in vitiligo. *Br J Dermatol,* Vol.131, pp. 160-165

Al Badri, A.M., Fouli, A.K., Todd, P.M., Gariouch, J.J., Gudgeon, J.E., Stewart, D.G., Gracie, J.A. & Goudie, R.B. (1993a). Abnormal expression of MHC class II and ICAM-1 by melanocytes in vitiligo. *J Pathol*, Vol.169, pp. 203-206

Al Badri, A.M.T., Todd, P.M., Garioch, J.J., Gudgeon, J.E., Stewart, D.G. & Goudie, R.B. (1993b). An immunohistological study of cutaneous lymphocytes in vitiligo. *J Pathol*, Vol.170, pp. 149-155

Al-Fouzan, A., Al-Arbash, M., Fouad, F., Kaaba, S.A., Mousa, M.A. & Al-Harbi, S.A. (1995). Study of HLA class I/IL and T lymphocyte subsets in Kuwaiti vitiligo patients. *Eur J Immunogenet*, Vol.22, pp. 209-213

Alomar, A. (2010). PUVA and related treatment. In: *Vitiligo*, M. Picardo & A. Taïeb (Eds.), pp. 345-350, Springer–Verlag, Berlin, Germany

Alkhateeb, A., Fain, P.R., Thody, A., Bennett, D.C. & Spritz, R.A. (2003). Epidemiology of vitiligo and associated autoimmune diseases in Caucasian probands and their relatives. *Pigment Cell Res*, Vol.16, pp. 208-214

Alkhateeb, A., Fain, P.R. & Spritz, R.A. (2005). Candidate functional promoter variant in the FOXD3 melanoblast developmental regulator gene in autosomal dominant vitiligo. *J Invest Dermatol*, Vol.125, pp. 388-391

Ando, I., Chi, H.I., Nakagawa, H. & Otsuka, F. (1993). Difference in clinical features and HLA antigens between familial and non-familial vitiligo of non-segmental type. *Br J Dermatol*, Vol.129, pp. 408-410

Aronson, P.J. & Hashimoto, K. (1987). Association of IgA anti-melanoma antibodies in the sera of vitiligo patients with active disease. *J Invest Dermatol*, Vol.88, 475

Austin, L.M., Boissy, R.E., Jacobsen, B.S. & Smyth, J.R. (1992). The detection of melanocyte autoantibodies in the Smyth chicken model for vitiligo. *Clin Immunol Immunopathol*, Vol.64, pp. 112-120

Austin, L.M. & Boissy, R.E. (1995). Mammalian tyrosinase-related protein-1 is recognised by autoantibodies from vitiliginous Smyth chickens. *Am J Pathol*, Vol.146, 1529-1541

Baharav, E., Merimski, O., Shoenfeld, Y., Zigelman, R., Gilbrud, B., Yecheskel, G., Youinou, P. & Fishman, P. (1996). Tyrosinase as an autoantigen in patients with vitiligo. *Clin Exp Immunol*, Vol.105, pp. 84–88

Behl, P.N., Aggarwal, A. & Srivastava, G, (2003). Vitiligo, In: *Practice of Dermatology*, P.N. Behl & G. Srivastava (Eds.), pp. 238-241, CBS Publishers, New Delhi, India

Betterle, C., Del Prete, G.F., Peserico, A., Bersani, G., Caracciolo, F., Trisotto, A. & Poggi, F. (1976). Autoantibodies in vitiligo. *Arch Dermatol*, Vol.112, pp. 1328

Bhatia, P.S., Mohan, L., Pandey, O.N., Singh, K.K., Arora, S. K. & Mukhija, R.D. (1992). Genetic nature of vitiligo. *J Dermatol Sci*, Vol.4, pp. 180-184

Birlea, S.A., Fain, P.R. & Spritz, R.A. (2008). A Romanian population isolate with high frequency of vitiligo and associated autoimmune diseases. *Arch Dermatol*, Vol.144, pp. 310-316

Birlea, S.A., Labergem G.S., Procopciucm, L.M., Fain, P.R. & Spritz, R.A. (2009). CTLA4 and generalized vitiligo: two genetic association studies and a meta-analysis of published data. *Pigment Cell Melanoma Res*, Vol.22, pp. 230-234

Birlea, S.A., Gowan K., Fain, P.R. & Spritz, R.A. (2010). Genome-wide association study of generalized vitiligo in an isolated European founder population identifies SMOC2, in close proximity to IDDM8. *J Invest Dermatol*, Vol.130, pp. 798-803

Birlea, S.A., Jin, Y., Bennett, D.C., Herbstman, D.M., Wallace, M.R., McCormack, W.T., Kemp, E.H., Gawkrodger, D.J., Weetman, A.P., Picardo, M., Leone, G., Taïeb, A., Jouary, T., Ezzedine, K., Van Geel, N., Lambert, J., Overbeck, A., Fain, P.R. & Spritz, R.A. (2011). Comprehensive association analysis of candidate genes for generalized vitiligo supports XBP1, FOXP1, and TSLP. *J Invest Dermatol*, Vol.131, pp. 371-381

Blomhoff, A., Kemp, E.H., Gawkrodger, D.J., Weetman, A.P, Husebye, E.S., Akselsen, H.E., Lie, B.A. & Undlien, D.E. (2005). CTLA4 polymorphisms are associated with vitiligo, in patients with concomitant autoimmune diseases. *Pigment Cell Res*, Vol.18, pp. 55-58

Boelaert, K., Newby, P.R., Simmonds, M.J., Holder, R.L., Carr-Smith, J.D., Heward, J.M., Manji, N., Allahabadia, A., Armitage, M., Chatterjee, K.V., Lazarus, J.H., Pearce, S.H., Vaidya, B., Gough, S.C. & Franklyn, J.A. (2010). Prevalence and relative risk of other autoimmune diseases in subjects with autoimmune thyroid disease. *Am J Med*, Vol.123, pp. 183.e1-183.e9

Boisseau-Garsaud, A.M., Garsaud, P., Cales-Quist, D., Helenon, R., Queneherve, C. & Claire, R.C. (2000). Epidemiology of vitiligo in the French West Indies (Isle of Martinique). *Int J Dermatol*, Vol.39, pp. 18-20

Boissy, R.E., Lamont, S.J. & Smyth, J.R. (1984). Persistence of abnormal melanocytes in immunosuppressed chickens of the autoimmune "DAM" line. *Cell Tissue Res*, Vol.235, pp. 663-668

Boissy, R.E. & Lamoreux, M.L. (1988). Animal models of an acquired pigmentary disorder: vitiligo. In: *Advances in Pigment Cell Research,* J. Bagnara J, (Ed.), pp. 207-218, Alan R. Liss Inc., New York, USA

Boone, B., Ongenae, K., Van Geel, N., Vernijns, S., De Keyser, S. & Naeyaert, J.M. (2007). Topical pimecrolimus in the treatment of vitiligo. *Eur J Dermatol,* Vol.17, pp. 55-61

Boyle, M.L., Pardue, S.L., Smyth, J.R. Effect of corticosterone on the incidence of amelanosis in Smyth delayed amelanotic line chickens. (1987). *Poultry Sci,* Vol.66, pp. 363-367

Brostoff, J. (1969). Autoantibodies in patients with vitiligo. *Lancet,* Vol.2 pp. 177-178

Buc, M., Busová, B., Hegyi, E. and Kolibásová, K. (1996). Vitiligo is associated with HLA-A2 and HLA-Dw7 in the Slovak populations. *Folia Biol (Praha),* Vol.42, pp. 23-25

Cario-Andre, M., Pain, C., Gauthier, Y. & Taieb A. (2007). The melanocytorrhagic hypothesis of vitiligo tested on pigmented, stressed, reconstructed epidermis. *Pigment Cell Res,* Vol.20, pp. 385-393

Cantón, I., Akhtar. S., Gavalas, N.G., Gawkrodger, D.J., Blomhoff, A., Watson, P.F., Weetman, A.P. & Kemp, E.H. (2005). A single nucleotide polymorphism in the gene encoding lymphoid protein tyrosine phosphatase (PTPN22) confers susceptibility to generalised vitiligo. *Genes Immunol,* Vol.6, pp. 584-587

Chen, J.J., Huang, W., Gui, J.P., Yang, S., Zhou, F.S., Xiong, Q.G., Wu, H.B., Cui,Y., Gao, M., Li, W., Li, J. X., Yan, K.L., Yuan, W.T., Xu, S.J., Liu, J.J. & Zhang, X.J. (2005). A novel linkage to generalized vitiligo on 4q13-q21 identified in a genomewide linkage analysis of Chinese families. *Am J Hum Genet,* Vol.76, pp. 1057-1065

Cheong, K.A., Chae, S.C., Kim, Y.S., Kwon, H.B., Chung, H.T. & Lee, A.Y. (2009). Association of thymic stromal lymphopoietin gene -847C>T polymorphism in generalized vitiligo. *Exp Dermatol,* Vol.18, pp. 1073-1075

Cho, S., Kang, H.C. & Hahm, J.H. (2000). Characteristics of vitiligo in Korean children. *Pediatr Dermatol,* Vol.17, pp. 189-193

Claudy, A. & Rouchouse, B. (1984). Langerhans cells and vitiligo: quantitative study of T6 and HLA-DR-antigen expressing cells. *Acta Dermatol Venereol,* Vol.64, pp. 334-336

Cui, J., Harning, R., Henn, M. & Bystryn, J.-C. (1992). Identification of pigment cell antigens defined by vitiligo antibodies. *J Invest Dermatol,* Vol.98, pp. 162-165

Cui, J., Arita, Y. & Bystryn, J.-C. (1993). Cytolytic antibodies to melanocytes in vitiligo. *J Invest Dermatol,* Vol.100, pp. 812-815

Cui, J., Arita, Y. & Bystryn, J.-C. (1995). Characterisation of vitiligo antigens. *Pigment Cell Res,* Vol.8, pp.53-59

Cunliffe, W.J., Hall, R., Newell, D.J. & Stevenson, C.J. (1968). Vitiligo, thyroid disease and autoimmunity. *Br J Dermatol,* Vol.80, pp. 135-139

D'Amelio, R., Frati, C., Fattorossi, A. & Aiuti, F. (1990). Peripheral T cell subset imbalance in patients with vitiligo and their apparently healthy first-degree relatives. *Ann Allergy,* Vol.65, pp. 143-145

Das, S.K., Majumder, P.P., Majumdar, T.K. & Haldar, B. (1985). Studies on vitiligo. II. Familial aggregation and genetics. *Genet Epidemiol,* Vol.2, pp. 255-262

Dawber, R.P. (1970). Integumentary association of pernicious anaemia. *Br J Dermatol,* Vol.82, pp. 221-222

Deeba, F., Syed, R., Quareen, J., Waheed, M.A., Jamil, K. & Rao, H. (2010). CTLA-4 A49G gene polymorphism is not associated with vitiligo in South Indian population. *Indian J Dermatol,* Vol.55, 29-32

Dell'Anna, M.L. & Picardo, M. (2006). A review and a new hypothesis for non-immunological pathogenetic mechanisms in vitiligo. *Pigment Cell Res*, Vol.19, pp. 406-411

Denman, C.J., McCracken, J., Hariharan, V., Klarquist, J., Oyarbide-Valencia, K., Guevara-Patiño, J.A. & Le Poole, I.C. (2008). HSP70i accelerates depigmentation in a mouse model of autoimmune vitiligo. *J Invest Dermatol*, Vol.128, pp. 2041-2048

Dunston, G.M & Halder, R.M. (1990). Vitiligo is associated with HLA-DR4 in black patients. A preliminary report. *Arch Dermatol*, Vol.126, pp. 56-60

Duthie, M.S., Kimber, I., Norval, M. (1999). The effects of ultraviolet radiation on the immune system. *Br J Dermatol*, Vol.140, pp. 995-1009

Erf, G.F., Trejo-Skalli, A.V. & Smyth, J.R. (1995). T cells in regenerating feathers of Smyth line chickens in vitiligo. *Clin Immunol Immunopathol*, Vol.76, pp. 120-126

Erf, G.F. & Smyth, J.R. (1996). Alterations in blood leukocyte populations in Smyth line chickens with autoimmune vitiligo. *Poultry Sci*, Vol.75, pp. 351-356

Fain, P.R., Gowan, K., LaBerge, G.S., Alkhateeb, A., Stetler, G.L., Talbert, J., Bennett, D.C. & Spritz, R.A. (2003). A genome-wide screen for generalized vitiligo: confirmation of AIS1 on chromosome 1p31 and evidence for additional susceptibility loci. *Am J Hum Genet*, Vol.72, pp. 1560–1564

Fain, P.R., Babu, S.R., Bennett, D.C. & Spritz, R.A. (2006). HLA class II Haplotype DRB1*04-DQB1*0301 contributes to risk of familial generalized vitiligo and early disease onset. *Pigment Cell Res*, Vol.19, pp. 51-57

Farrokhi, S., Farsangi-Hojjat, M., Noohpisheh. M.K., Tahmasbi, R. & Rezaei, N. (2005). Assessment of the immune system in 55 Iranian patients with vitiligo. *J Eur Acad Dermatol Venereol*, Vol.19, pp. 706-711

Finco, O., Cuccia, M., Martinetti, M., Ruberto, G., Orecchia, G. & Rabbiosi, G. (1991). Age of onset in vitiligo: relationship with HLA supratypes. *Clin Genet*, Vol.39, pp. 448-454

Fishman, P., Azizi, E., Shoenfeld, Y., Sredni, B., Yecheskel, G., Ferrone, S., Zigelman, R., Chaitchik, S., Floro, S. & Djaldetti, M. (1993). Vitiligo autoantibodies are effective against melanoma. *Cancer*, Vol.72, pp. 2365-2369

Foley, L.M, Lowe, N.J., Misheloff, E. & Tiwari, J.L. (1983). Association of HLA-DR4 with vitiligo. *J Am Acad Dermatol*, Vol.8, pp. 39-40

Gauthier, Y., Cario-Andre, M. & Taieb, A. (2003). A critical appraisal of vitiligo etiologic theories. Is melanocyte loss a melanocytorrhagy? *Pigment Cell Res*, Vol.16, pp. 322-332

Gawkrodger, D. J., Ormerod, A. D., Shaw, L., Mauri-Sole, I., Whitton, M. E., Watts, M. J., Anstey, A. V., Ingham, J. & Young, K. (2010). Vitiligo: concise evidence based guidelines on diagnosis and management. *Postgrad Med J*, Vol.86, pp. 466-471

Gilhar, A., Zelickson, B., Ulman, Y. & Etzioni, A. (1995). In vivo destruction of melanocytes by the IgG fraction of serum from patients with vitiligo. *J Invest Dermatol*, Vol.105, pp. 683-686

Gottumukkala, R.V.S.R.K., Gavalas, N.G., Akhtar, S., Metcalfe, R.A., Gawkrodger, D. J., Haycock, J.W., Waston, P.F., Weetman, A.P. & Kemp, E. H. (2006). Function blocking autoantibodies to the melanin-concentrating hormone receptor in vitiligo patients. *Lab Invest*, Vol.86, pp. 781-789

Grimes, P.E., Ghoneum, M., Stockton, T., Payne, C., Kelly, A.P. & Alfred, L. (1986). T cell profiles in vitiligo. *J Am Acad Dermatol*, Vol.14, pp. 196-201

Grimes, P.E., Sevall, J.S. & Vojdani, A. (1996). Cytomegalovirus DNA identified in skin biopsy specimens of patients with vitiligo. *J Am Acad Dermatol*, Vol.35, pp. 21-26

Halder, R.M., Walters, C.S., Johnson, B.A., Chakarabarti, S.G. & Kenney, J.A. (1986). Aberrations in T lymphocytes and natural killer cells in vitiligo: a flow cytometric study. *J Am Acad Dermatol*, Vol.14, pp. 733-737

Handa, S. & Dogra, S. (2003). Epidemiology of childhood vitiligo: a study of 625 patients from north India. *Pediatr Dermatol*, Vol.20, pp. 207-210

Hann, S.K., Kim, H.I., Im, S., Park, Y.K., Cui, J. & Bystryn, J.-C. (1993). The change of melanocyte cytotoxicity after systemic steroid treatment in vitiligo patients. *J Dermatol Sci*, Vol.6, pp. 201-205

Hann, S.K. & Lee, H.J. (1996). Segmental vitiligo: clinical findings in 208 patients. *J Am Acad Dermatol*, Vol.35, pp. 671-674

Hann, S.K., Koo, S.W., Kim, J.B. & Park, Y.K. (1996a). Detection of antibodies to human melanoma cells in vitiligo and alopecia areata by Western blot analysis. *J Dermatol*, Vol.23, pp. 100-103

Hann, S.K., Shin, H.K., Park, S.H., Reynolds, S.R. & Bystryn, J.-C. (1996b). Detection of antibodies to melanocytes in vitiligo by western blotting. *Yonsei Med J*, Vol.37, pp. 365-370

Hariharan, V., Klarquist, J., Reust, M.J., Koshoffer, A., McKee, M.D., Boissy, R.E. & Le Poole, I.C. (2010). Monobenzyl ether of hydroquinone and 4-tertiary butyl phenol activate markedly different physiological responses in melanocytes: relevance to skin depigmentation. *J Invest Dermatol*, Vol.130, pp. 211-220

Harning, R., Cui, J. & Bystryn, J.-C. (1991). Relation between the incidence and level of pigment cell antibodies and disease activity in vitiligo. *J Invest Dermatol*, Vol.97, 1078-1080

Hartmann, A., Brocker, E.B. & Hamm, H. (2008). Occlusive treatment enhances efficacy of tacrolimus 0.1% ointment in adult patients with vitiligo: results of a placebo-controlled 12-month prospective study. *Acta Derm Venereol*, Vol.88, pp. 474-479

Hatchome, N., Aiba, S., Kato, T., Torinuki, W. & Tagami, H. (1987). Possible functional impairment of Langerhans' cells in vitiliginous skin. Reduced ability to elicit dinitrochlorobenzene contact sensitivity reaction and decreased stimulatory effect in the allogeneic mixed skin cell lymphocyte culture reaction. *Arch Dermatol*, Vol.123, pp. 51-54

Hedley, S.J., Metcalfe, R., Gawkrodger, D.J., Weetman A.P. & MacNeil, S. (1998). Vitiligo melanocytes in long-term culture show normal constitutive and cytokine-induced expression of intercellular adhesion molecule-1 and major histocompatibility complex class I and class II molecules. *Br J Dermatol*, Vol.139, pp. 965-973

Hedstrand, H., Ekwall, O., Olsson, M.J., Landgren, E., Kemp, E.H., Weetman, A.P., Perheentupa, J., Husebye, E., Gustafsson, J., Betterle, C., Kämpe, O. & Rorsman, F. (2001). The transcription factors SOX9 and SOX10 are vitiligo autoantigens in autoimmune polyendocrine syndrome type I. *J Biol Chem*, Vol.276, pp. 35390-35395

Herane, M.I. (2003). Vitiligo and leukoderma in children. *Clin Dermatol*, Vol.21, pp. 283-295

Homey, B., Assmann, T., Vohr, H.W., Ulrich, P., Lauerma, A.I., Ruzicka, T., Lehmann, P. & Schuppe, H.C. (1998). Topical FK506 suppresses cytokine and costimulatory molecule expression in epidermal and local draining lymph node cells during primary skin immune responses. *J Immunol*, Vol.160, pp. 5331-5340

Hoogduijn, M.J., Ancans, J., Suzuki, I., Estdale, S. & Thody, A.J. (2002). Melanin-concentrating hormone and its receptor are expressed and functional in human skin. *Biochem Biophys Res Commun*, Vol.296, pp. 698-701

Howitz, J., Brodthagen, H., Schwartz, M. & Tomsen, K. (1977). Prevalence of vitiligo: Epidemiological survey on the Isle of Bornholm, Denmark. *Arch Dermatol*, Vol.113, pp. 47-52

Imokawa, G., Yada, Y., Kimura, M. & Morisaki, N. (1996). Granulocyte/macrophage colony-stimulating factor is an intrinsic keratinocyte-derived growth factor for human melanocytes in UVA-induced melanosis. *Biochem J*, Vol.313, pp. 625-631

Itirli, G., Pehlivan, M., Alper, S., Yuksel, S.E., Onay, H., Ozkinay, F. & Pehlivan, S. (2005). Exon-3 polymorphism of CTLA-4 gene in Turkish patients with vitiligo. *J Dermatol Sci*, Vol.38, pp. 225-227

Jin, Y., Birlea, S.A., Fain, P.R. & Spritz, R.A. (2007a). Genetic variations in NALP1 are associated with generalized vitiligo in a Romanian population. *J Invest Dermatol*, Vol.127, pp. 2558-2562

Jin, Y., Mailloux, C.M., Gowan, K., Riccardi, S.L., LaBerge, G., Bennett, D.C., Fain, P.R. & Spritz, R.A. (2007b). NALP1 in vitiligo-associated multiple autoimmune disease. *N Engl J Med*, Vol.356, pp. 1216-1225

Jin, Y., Birlea, S.A., Fain, P.R., Gowan, K., Riccardi, S.L., Holland, P.J., Mailloux C.M., Sufit, A.J., Hutton, S.M., Amadi-Myers, A., Bennett, D.C., Wallace, M.R., McCormack, W.T., Kemp, E.H., Gawkrodger, D.J., Weetman, A.P., Picardo, M., Leone, G., Taieb, A., Jouary, T., Ezzedine, K., van Geel, N., Lambert, J., Overbeck, A. & Spritz, R.A. (2010a). Variant of TYR and autoimmunity susceptibility loci in generalized vitiligo. *N Engl J Med*, Vol.362, pp. 1686-1697

Jin, Y., Birlea, S.A., Fain, P.R., Mailloux, C.M., Riccardi, S.L., Gowan, K., Holland, P.J., Bennett, D.C., Wallace, M.R., McCormack, W.T., Kemp, E.H., Gawkrodger, D.J., Weetman, A.P., Picardo, M., Leone, G., Taieb, A., Jouary, T., Ezzedine, K., van Geel, N., Lambert, J., Overbeck, A. & Spritz, R.A. (2010b). Common variants in FOXP1 are associated with generalized vitiligo. *Nat Genet*, Vol.42, pp. 576-578

Kao, C.H. & Yu, H.S. (1992). Comparison of the effect of 8-Methoxypsoralen (8-MOP) plus UVA (PUVA) on human melanocytes in vitiligo vulgaris and *in vitro*. *J Invest Dermatol*, Vol.98, pp. 734-740

Kemp, E.H., Gawkrodger, D.J., MacNeil, S., Watson, P.F. & Weetman, A.P. (1997a). Detection of tyrosinase autoantibodies in patients with vitiligo using ^{35}S-labeled recombinant human tyrosinase in a radioimmunoassay. *J Invest Dermatol*, Vol.109, pp. 69-73.

Kemp, E.H., Gawkrodger, D.J., Watson, P.F. & Weetman, A.P. (1997b). Immunoprecipitation of melanogenic enzyme autoantigens with vitiligo sera: evidence for cross-reactive autoantibodies to tyrosinase and tyrosinase-related protein-2 (TRP-2). *Clin Exp Immunol*, Vol.109, pp. 495–500

Kemp, E.H., Gawkrodger, D.J., Watson, P.F. & Weeman, A.P. (1998a). Autoantibodies to human melanocyte-specific protein Pmel17 in the sera of vitiligo patients: a sensitive and quantitative radioimmunoassay (RIA). *Clin Exp Immunol*, Vol.114, pp. 333-338

Kemp, E.H., Waterman, E.A., Gawkrodger, D.J., Watson, P.F. & Weetman, A.P. (1998b). Autoantibodies to tyrosinase-related protein-1 detected in the sera of vitiligo patients using a quantitative radiobinding assay. *Br J Dermatol*, Vol.139, pp. 798-805

Kemp, E.H., Ajjan, R.A., Waterman, E.A., Gawkrodger, D.J., Cork, M.J., Watson, P.F. & Weetman, A.P. (1999). Analysis of a microsatellite polymorphism of the cytotoxic T-lymphocyte antigen-4 gene in patients with vitiligo. *Br J Dermatol*, Vol.140, pp. 73-78

Kemp, E.H., Waterman, E.A., Hawes, B.E., O'Neill, K., Gottumukkala, R.V., Gawkrodger, D.J., Weetman, A.P. & Watson, P.F. (2002). The melanin-concentrating hormone receptor 1, a novel target of autoantibody responses in vitiligo. *J Clin Invest*, Vol.109, pp. 923-930

Kemp, E.H., Emhemad, S., Akhtar, S., Watson, P.F., Gawkrodger, D.J. & Weetman, A.P. (2011). Autoantibodies against tyrosine hydroxylase in patients with non-segmental (generalised) vitiligo. *Exp Dermatol*, Vol.20, pp. 35-40

Kent, G. & Al' Abadie, M.S.K. (1996). Psychologic effects of vitiligo: a critical incident analysis. *J Am Acad Dermatol*, Vol.35, pp. 895-898

Kirnbauer, R., Charvat, B., Schauer, E., Kock, A., Urbanshi, A., Forster, E., Neuner, P., Assmann, I., Luger, T.A. & Schwarz, T. (1992). Modulation of intercellular adhesion molecule-1 expression on human melanocytes and melanoma cells: evidence for a regulatory role of IL-6, IL-7, TNF beta, and UVB light. *J Invest Dermatol*, Vol.98, pp. 320-326

Klarquist, J., Denman, C.J., Hernandez, C., Wainwright, D.A., Strickland, F.M., Overbeck, A. Mehrotra, S., Nishimura, M.I. & Le Poole, I.C. (2010). Reduced skin homing by functional Treg in vitiligo. *Pigment Cell Melanoma Res*, Vol.23, pp. 276-286

Kroll, T.M., Bommiasamy, H., Boissy, R.E., Hernandez, C., Nickoloff, B.J., Mestril, R. & Le Poole, I.C. (2005). 4-tertiary butyl phenol exposure sensitizes human melanocytes to dendritic cell-mediated killing: relevance to vitiligo. *J Invest Dermatol*, Vol.124, pp. 798–806

Krutmann, J. & Morita, A. (1999). Mechanisms of ultraviolet (UV) B and phototherapy. *J Invest Dermatol Symp Proc*, Vol.4, pp. 70-72

Laberge, G., Mailloux, C.M., Gowan, K., Holland, P., Bennett, D.C., Fain, P.R. & Spritz, R.A. (2005). Early onset and increased risk of other autoimmune diseases in familial generalized vitiligo. *Pigment Cell Res*, Vol.18, pp. 300-305

Laberge, G.S., Bennett, D.C., Fain, P.R. & Spritz, R.A. (2008a). PTPN22 is genetically associated with risk of generalized vitiligo, but CTLA4 is not. *J Invest Dermatol*, Vol.128, pp. 1757-1762

Laberge, G. S., Birlea, S.A., Fain, P.R. & Spritz, R.A. (2008b). The PTPN22-1858C>T (R620W) functional polymorphism is associated with generalized vitiligo in the Romanian population. *Pigment Cell Melanoma Res*, Vol.21, pp. 206-208

Lamont, S.J. & Smyth, J.R. (1981). Effect of bursectomy on development of a spontaneous postnatal amelanosis. *Clin Immunol Immunopathol*, Vol.21, pp. 407-411

Lang, K.S., Caroli, C.C., Muhm, D., Wernet, D., Moris, A., Schittek, B., Knauss-Scherwitz, E., Stevanovic, S., Rammensee, H.-G. & Garbe, C. (2001). HLA-A2 restricted, melanocyte-specific CD8+ T lymphocytes detected in vitiligo patients are related to disease activity and are predominantly directed against MelanA/MART1. *J Invest Dermatol*, Vol.116, pp.891-897

Le Poole, I.C. & Boissy, R.E. (1997). Vitiligo. *Semin Cutan Med Surg*, Vol.16, pp. 3-14

Le Poole, I.C. & Luiten, R.M. (2008). Autoimmune etiology of generalized vitiligo. *Curr Dir Autoimmun*, Vol.10, pp. 227-243

Le Poole, I.C., Das, P.K., van den Wijngaard, R.M., Bos, J.D. & Westerhof, W. (1993a). Review of the etiopathomechanism of vitiligo: a convergence theory. *Exp Dermatol*, Vol.2, pp. 145-153

Le Poole, I.C., Mutis, T., van den Wijngaard, R.M., Westerhof, W., Ottenhoff, T., de Vries, R.R. & Das, P.K. (1993b). A novel, antigen-presenting function of melanocytes and its possible relationship to hypopigmentary disorders. *J Immunol*, Vol.151, pp. 7284-7292

Le Poole, I.C., van den Wijngaard, R.M.J.G.J., Westerhof, W. & Das, P.K. (1996). Presence of T cells and macrophages in inflammatory vitiligo skin parallels melanocyte disappearance. *Am J Pathol*, Vol.148, 1219-1228

Le Poole, I.C., Stennett. L.S., Bonish, B.K., Dee L., Robinson, J.K., Hernandez, C., Hann, S.K., & Nickoloff, B.J. (2003). Expansion of vitiligo lesions is associated with reduced epidermal CDw60 expression and increased expression of HLA-DR in perilesional skin. *Br J Dermatol*, Vol.149, pp. 739-748

Li, Q., Lv, Y., Li, C., Yi, X., Long, H.A., Qiao, H., Lu, T., Luan, Q., Li, K., Wang, X., Wang, G. & Gao, T. (2010). Vitiligo autoantigen VIT75 is identified as lamin A in vitiligo by serological proteome analysis based on mass spectrometry. *J Invest Dermatol*, Vol.131, pp. 727-734

Liang, Y., Yang S., Zhou, Y., Gui, J., Ren, Y., Chen, J., Fan, X., Sun, L., Xiao, F., Gao, M., Du, W., Fang, Q., Xu, S., Huang, W. & Zhang, X. (2007). Evidence for two susceptibility loci on chromosomes 22q12 and 6p21-p22 in Chinese generalized vitiligo families. *J Invest Dermatol*, Vol.127, pp. 2552-2557

Liu, J. B., Li, M., Yang, S., Gui, J. P., Wang, H. Y., Du, W. H., Zhao, X. Y., Ren, Y. Q., Zhu, Y. G. & Zhang, X. J. (2005). Clinical profiles of vitiligo in China: an analysis of 3742 patients. *Clin Exp Dermatol*, Vol.30, pp. 327-331

Liu, J.B., Li, M., Chen, H., Zhong, S. Q., Yang, S., Du, W.D., Hao, J. H., Zhang, T.S., Zhang, X.J. & Zeegers, M.P. (2007). Association of vitiligo with HLA-A2: a meta-analysis. *J Eur Acad Dermatol Venereol*, Vol.21, pp. 205-213

Lorini, R., Orecchia, G., Martinetti, M., Dugoujon, J.M. & Cuccia, M. (1992). Autoimmunity in vitiligo: relationship with HLA, Gm and Km polymorphisms. *Autoimmunity*, Vol.11, 255-260

Majumder, P.P., Das, S.K. & Li, C.C. (1988). A genetical model for vitiligo. *Am J Hum Genet*, Vol.43, pp. 119-125

Majumder, P.P., Nordlund, J.J. & Nath, S.K. (1993). Pattern of familial aggregation of vitiligo. *Arch Dermatol*, Vol.129, pp. 994-998

Mandry, R.C., Ortiz, L.J., Lugo-Somolinos, A. & Sanchez J.L. (1996). Organ-specific autoantibodies in vitiligo patients and their relatives. *Int J Dermatol*, Vol.35 pp. 18-21

Mehta, N.R., Shah, K.C., Theodore, C., Vyas, V.P . & Patel, A.B. (1973). Epidemiological study of vitiligo in Surat area, South Gujarat. *Indian J Med Res*, Vol.61, pp. 145-154

Metzker, A., Zamir, R., Gazit, E., David, M. & Feuerman, E.J. (1980). Vitiligo and the HLA system. *Dermatologica*, Vol.160, pp. 100-105

Moretti, S., Spallanzani, A., Amato, L., Hautmann, G., Gallerani, I., Fabiani, M. & Fabbri, P. (2002). New insights into the pathogenesis of vitiligo: imbalance of epidermal cytokines at sites of lesions. *Pigment Cell Res,* Vol.15, pp. 87-92

Namazi, M.R. (2007). Neurogenic dysregulation, oxidative stress, and melanocytorrhagy in vitiligo: can they be interconnected? *Pigment Cell Res*, Vol.20, pp. 360-363

Nath, S.K., Majumder, P.P. & Nordlund, J.J. (1994). Genetic epidemiology of vitiligo: multilocus recessivity cross-validated. *Am J Hum Genet*, Vol.55 pp. 981-990

Nath, S.K., Kelly, J.A., Namjou, B., Lam, T., Bruner, G.R., Scofield, R.H., Aston, C.E. & Harley, J.B. (2001). Evidence for a susceptibility gene, SLEV1, on chromosome 17p13 in families with vitiligo-related systemic lupus erythematosus. *Am J Hum Genet,* Vol.69, pp. 1401-1406

Naughton, G.K., Eisinger, M. & Bystryn, J.C. (1983a). Detection of antibodies to melanocytes in vitiligo by specific immunoprecipitation. *J Invest Dermatol,* Vol.81, pp. 540-542

Naughton G.K., Eisinger, M. & Bystryn, J.-C. (1983b). Antibodies to normal human melanocytes in vitiligo. *J Exp Med*, Vol.158, pp. 246-251

Naughton, G.K., Mahaffey, M. & Bystryn, J.-C. (1986a). Antibodies to surface antigens of pigmented cells in animals with vitiligo. *Proc Soc Exp Biol Med,* Vol.181, pp. 423-426

Naughton, G.K., Reggiardo, M.D. & Bystryn, J.-C. (1986b). Correlation between vitiligo antibodies and extent of depigmentation in vitiligo. *J Am Acad Dermatol,* Vol.15, pp. 978-981

Neufeld, M., Maclaren, N.K. & Blizard, R.M. (1981). Two types of autoimmune Addison's disease associated with different polyglandular autoimmune (PGA) syndrome. *Medicine,* Vol.60, pp. 355-362

Norris, D.A., Kissinger, R.M., Naughton, G.M. & Bystryn, J.-C. (1988a). Evidence for immunologic mechanisms in human vitiligo: patients' sera induce damage to human melanocytes in vitro by complement-mediated damage and antibody-dependent cellular cytotoxicity. *J Invest Dermatol*, Vol.90, pp.783-789

Norris, D.A., Capin, L., Muglia, J.J., Osborn, R.L., Zerbe, G.O., Bystryn J.-C. & Tonnesen, M.G. (1988b) Enhanced susceptibility of melanocytes to different immunologic effector mechanisms in vitro: potential mechanisms for post-inflammatory hypopigmentation and vitiligo. *Pigment Cell Res,* Vol.1 (Supplement), pp. 113-123

Ochi, Y. & DeGroot, L.J. (1969). Vitiligo in Graves' disease. *Ann Intern Med,* Vol.71, pp. 935-940

Ogg, G.S., Dunbar P.R., Romero P., Chen, J.L. & Cerundolo, V. (1998). High frequency of skin-homing melanocyte-specific cytotoxic T lymphocytes in autoimmune vitiligo. *J Exp Med,* Vol.188, pp. 1203–1208

Okamoto, T., Irie, R.F., Fujii, S., Huang, S., Nizze, A.J., Morton, D.L. & Hoon, D.S. (1998). Anti-tyrosinase-related protein-2 immune response in vitiligo and melanoma patients receiving active-specific immunotherapy. *J Invest Dermatol,* Vol.111, pp. 1034-1039

Olsson, M.J. (2010). Surgical therapies. In: *Vitiligo,* M. Picardo & A. Taïeb (Eds.), pp. 394-406, Springer-Verlag, Berlin, Germany

Ongenae, K., Beelaert, L., van Geel, N. & Naeyaert, J.M. (2006). Psychosocial effects of vitiligo. *J Eur Acad Dermatol Venereol,* Vol.20, pp. 1-8

Orecchia, G., Perfetti, L., Malagoli, P., Borghini, F. & Kipervarg, Y. (1992). Vitiligo is associated with a significant increase in HLA-A30, Cw6 and Dqw3 and a decrease in C4AQ0 in northern Italian patients. *Dermatology,* Vol.185, pp. 123-127

Palermo, B., Campanelli, R., Garbelli, S., Mantovani, S., Lantelme, E., Brazzelli, V., Ardigo, M., Borroni, G., Martinetti, M., Badulli, C., Necker, A. & Giachino, C. (2001). Specific cytotoxic T lymphocyte responses against Melan-A/MART1, tyrosinase and gp100 in vitiligo by the use of major histocompatibility complex/peptide tetramers: the role of cellular immunity in the etiopathogenesis of vitiligo. *J Invest Dermatol,* Vol.117, pp. 326-332

Pardue, S.L., Fite, K.V., Bengston, L., Lamont, S.J., Boyle, M.L. & Smyth J.R. (1988). Enhanced integumental and ocular amelanosis following the termination of cyclosporin administration. *J Invest Dermatol,* Vol.88, pp. 758-761

Park, Y.K., Kim, N.S., Hann, S.K. & Im, S. (1996). Identification of autoantibody to melanocytes and characterisation of vitiligo antigen in vitiligo patients. *J Dermatol Sci,* Vol.11, pp. 111-120

Pehlivan, S., Ozkinay, F., Alper, S., Onay, H., Yuksel, E., Pehlivan, M. & Ozkinay, C. (2009). Association between IL4 (-590), ACE (I)/(D), CCR5 (Delta32), CTLA4 (+49) and IL1-RN (VNTR in intron 2) gene polymorphisms and vitiligo. *Eur J Dermatol,* Vol.19, pp. 126-128

Poloy, A., Tibor, L., Kramer, J., Anh-Tuan, N., Kraszits, E., Medgyessy, I., Füst, G., Stenszky, V. & Farid, N.R. (1991). HLA-DR1 is associated with vitiligo. *Immunol Lett,* Vol.27, pp. 59-62

Porter, J.R., Beuf, A.H., Lerner, A. & Nordlund, J. (1986). Psychosocial effect of vitiligo: a comparison of vitiligo patients with "normal" control subjects, with psoriasis patients, and with patients with other pigmentary disorders. *J Am Acad Dermatol,* Vol.15, pp. 220-224

Quan, C., Ren, Y.Q., Xiang, L.H., Sun, L.D., Xu, A.E., Gao, X.H., Chen, H.D., Pu, X.M., Wu, R.N., Liang, C.Z., Li, J.B., Gao, T.W., Zhang, J.Z., Wang, X.L., Wang, J., Yang, R.Y., Liang, L., Yu, J.B., Zuo, X.B., Zhang, S.Q., Zhang, S.M., Chen, G., Zheng, X.D., Li, P., Zhu, J., Li, Y.W., Wei, X.D., Hong. W.S., Ye, Y., Zhang, Y., Wu, W.S., Cheng, H., Dong, P.L., Hu, D. Y., Li, Y., Li, M., Zhang, X., Tang, H.Y., Tang, X.F., Xu, S.X., He, S. M., Lv, Y. M., Shen, M., Jiang, H.Q., Wang, Y., Li, K., Kang, X.J., Liu, Y. Q., Sun, L., Liu, Z.F., Xie, S.Q., Zhu, C.Y., Xu, Q., Gao, J.P., Hu, W.L., Ni, C., Pan, T.M., Yao, S., He, C.F., Liu, Y.S., Yu, Z.Y., Yin, X.Y., Zhang, F.Y., Yang, S., Zhou, Y. & Zhang, X.J. (2010). Genome-wide association study for vitiligo identifies susceptibility loci at 6q27 and the MHC. *Nat Genet,* Vol.42, pp. 614-618

Ren, Y., Yang, S., Xu, S., Gao, M., Huang, W., Gao, T., Fang, Q., Quan, C., Zhang, C., Sun, L., Liang, Y., Han, J., Wang, Z., Zhang, F., Zhou, Y., Liu, J. & Zhang, X. (2009). Genetic variation of promoter sequence modulates XBP1 expression and genetic risk for vitiligo. *PLoS Genet,* Vol.5, e1000523

Riley, P. (1967). A study of the distribution of epidermal dendritic cells in pigmented and unpigmented skin. *J Invest Dermatol,* Vol.48, pp. 28-38

Rocha, I.M., Oliveira, L.J., De Castro, L.C., ., De Araujo Pereira, L.I., Chaul, A., Guerra, J.G., Silvestre, M.C., Batista, K.M., Pereira, F.A., Gomide, M.A. & Guillo, L.A. (2002). Recognition of melanoma cell antigens with antibodies present from patients with vitiligo. *Int J Dermatol,* Vol.39, pp. 840-843

Schallreuter, K.U., Wood, J.M. & Berger, J. (1991). Low catalase levels in the epidermis of patients with vitiligo. *J Invest Dermatol,* Vol.97, pp. 1081-1085

Schallreuter, K.U, Levenig, C., Kühnl, P., Löliger, C., Hohl-Tehari, M. & Berger, J. (1993). Histocompatibility antigens in vitiligo: Hamburg study on 102 patients from northern Germany. *Dermatology,* Vol.187, pp. 186-192

Schallreuter, K.U., Moore, J., Wood, J.M., Beazley, W.D., Peters, E.M.J., Marles, L.K., Behrens-Williams, S.C., Dummer, R., Blau, N. & Thony, B. (2001). Epidermal H2O2 accumulation alters tetrahydrobiopterin (6BH4) recycling in vitiligo: identification of a general mechanism in regulation of all 6BH4-dependent processes? *J Invest Dermatol,* Vol.116, pp. 167–174

Schallreuter, K.U., Chavan, B., Rokos, H., Hibberts, N., Panske, A. & Wood, J.M. (2005). Decreased phenylalanine uptake and turnover in patients with vitiligo. *Mol Genet Metabol,* Vol.86, pp. S27-S33

Searle, E.A., Boissy, R.E., Austin, L.M. & Nordlund, J.J. (1991). Smyth chicken melanocyte autoantibodies: cross-reactivity, in vivo binding, and plasma membrane location of the antigen(s). *J Invest Dermatol,* Vol.96, pp. 631

Sehgal, V.N. & Srivastava, G. (2007). Vitiligo: compendium of clinico-epidemiological features. *Indian J Dermatol Venereol Leprol,* Vol.73, pp. 149-156

Shegan, V.N. (1971). Hypopigmented lesions in leprosy. *Br J Dermatol,* Vol.4, pp. 91-93

Smyth, J.R. The Smyth chicken: a model for autoimmune amelanosis. (1989). *CRC Crit Rev Poultry Biol,* Vol.2, pp. 1-19

Song, Y.H., Connor, E., Li, Y., Zorovich, B., Balducci, P. & Maclaren, N. (1994). The role of tyrosinase in autoimmune vitiligo. *Lancet,* Vol.344, pp. 1049-1052

Soubiran, P., Bezaken, S., Bellet, C., Lacour, J.P. & Ortonne, J.-P. (1985). Vitiligo: peripheral T cell subset imbalance as defined by monoclonal antibodies. *Br J Dermatol,* Vol.113, pp. 124-127

Spritz, R.A. (2010). Shared genetic relationships underlying generalized vitiligo and autoimmune thyroid disease. *Thyroid,* Vol.20, pp. 745-754

Spritz, R.A., Gowan, K., Bennett, D.C. & Fain, P.R. (2004). Novel vitiligo susceptibility loci on chromosomes 7 (AIS2) and 8 (AIS3), confirmation of SLEV1 on chromosome 17, and their roles in an autoimmune diathesis. *Am J Hum Genet,* Vol.74, pp. 188-191

Sun, X., Xu, A., Wei, X., Ouyang, J., Lu, L., Chen, M. & Zhang, D. (2006). Genetic epidemiology of vitiligo: a study of 815 probands and their families from south China. *Int J Dermatol,* Vol.45, 1176-1181

Taïeb, A. (2000). Intrinsic and extrinsic pathomechanisms in vitiligo. *Pigment Cell Res,* Vol.13, pp. 41-47

Taïeb, A. & Picardo, M. (2010). Epidemiology, definitions and classification. In: *Vitiligo,* M. Picardo & A. Taïeb (Eds.), pp. 13-24, Springer–Verlag, Berlin, Germany

Takei, M., Mishima, Y. & Uda, H. (1984). Immunopathology of vitiligo vulgaris, Sutton's leukoderma and melanoma-associated vitiligo in relation to steroid effects. I. Circulating antibodies for cultured melanoma cells. *J Cutan Pathol,* Vol.11, pp. 107-113.

Tastan, H.B., Akar, A., Orkunoglu, F.E., Arca, E. & Inal, A. (2004). Association of class I HLA antigens and class II HLA alleles with vitiligo in a Turkish population. *Pigment Cell Res,* Vol.17, pp. 181-184

Trcka J., Moroi, Y., Clynes, R.A., Goldberg, S.M., Bergtold, A., Perales, M.A., Ma, M., Ferrone, C.R., Carroll, M.C., Ravetch, J.V. & Houghton, A.N. (2002). Redundant and alternative roles for activating Fc receptors and complement in an antibody-dependent model of autoimmune vitiligo. *Immunity*, Vol.16, pp. 861-868

Tu, C.X., Fu, H.W. & Lin, X.R. (1999). Levels of soluble interleukin-2 receptor in the sera and skin tissue fluids of patients with vitiligo. *J Dermatol Sci*, Vol.21, pp. 59-62

Turnbridge, W.M., Evered, D.C., Hall, R., Appleton, D., Brewis, M., Clark, F., Evans, J.J., Young, E., Bird, T. & Smith, P.A. (1977). The spectrum of thyroid disease in a community: the Whickham survey. *Clin Endocrinol*, Vol.7, pp. 481-492

Uda, H., Takei, M. & Mishima, Y. (1984). Immunopathology of vitiligo vulgaris, Sutton's leukoderma and melanoma-associated vitiligo in relation to steroid effects. II. The IgG and C3 deposits in the skin. *J Cut Pathol*, Vol.11, pp. 114-124

Van den Boorn, J.G., Konijnenberg, D., Dellemijn, T.A., van der Veen, J.P., Bos, J.D., Melief, C. J., Vyth-Dreese, F.A. & Luiten, R.M. (2009). Autoimmune destruction of skin melanocytes by perilesional T cells from vitiligo patients. *J Invest Dermatol*, Vol.129, pp. 2220-2232

Van den Boorn, J.G., Picavet, D.I., van Swieten, P.F., van Veen, H.A., Konijnenberg, D., van Veelen, P.A., van Capel, T., Jong, E.C., Reits, E.A., Drijfhout, J.W., Bos, J.D., Melief, C.J. & Luiten, R.M. (2011). Skin-depigmenting agent monobenzone induces potent T-cell autoimmunity toward pigmented cells by tyrosinase haptenation and melanosome autophagy. *J Invest Dermatol*, in press

Van den Wijngaard, R., Wankowicz-Kalinska, A., Le Poole, C., Tigges, A.J., Westerhof, W. & Das, P. (2000). Local immune response in skin of generalised vitiligo patients. Destruction of melanocytes is associated with the prominent presence of CLA+ T cells at the perilesional site. *Lab Invest*, Vol.80, pp. 1299-1309

Van den Wijngaard, R.M., Asghar, S.S., Pijnenborg, AC., Tigges, A.J., Westerhof, W. & Das, P. (2002). Aberrant expression of complement regulatory proteins, membrane cofactor protein and decay accelerating factor, in the involved epidermis of patients with vitiligo. *Br J Dermatol*, Vol.146, pp. 80-87

Venkataram, M.N., White, A.G., Leeny, W.A., al Suwaid, A.R. & Daar, A.S. (1995). HLA antigens in Omani patients with vitiligo. *Clin Exp Dermatol*, Vol.20, pp. 35-37.

Venneker, G.T., Westerhof, W., de Vries, I.J., Drayer, N.M., Wolthers, B.G., de Waal, L.P., Bos, J.D. & Asghar, S.S. (1992). Molecular heterogeneity of the fourth component of complement (C4) and its genes in vitiligo. *J Invest Dermatol*, Vol.99, pp. 853-858.

Venneker, G.T., de Waal, L.P., Westerhof, W., D'Amaro, J., Schreuder, G.M. & Asghar, S.S. (1993). HLA associations in vitiligo patients in the Dutch population. *Dis Markers*, Vol.11, pp. 187-190

Viac, J., Groujon, C., Misery, L., Staniek, V., Faure, M., Schmitt, D. & Claudy, A. (1997). Effect of UVB 311 mm irradiation on normal human skin. *Photodermatol Photoimmunol Photomed*, Vol.13, pp. 103-108

Wankowicz-Kalinska, A., Van Den Wijngaard, R.M., Tigges, B.J., Westerhof, W., Ogg, G.S., Cerundolo, V., Storkus, W.J. & Das, P.K. (2003). Immunopolarization of CD4+ and CD8+ T cell to type-1-like is associated with melanocyte loss in human vitiligo. *Lab Invest*, Vol.83, pp. 683–695

Westerhof, W. & d'Ischia, M. (2007). Vitiligo puzzle: the pieces fall in place. *Pigment Cell Res*, Vol.20, pp. 345-359

Xia, Q., Zhou, W.M,, Liang, Y.H., Ge, H.S., Liu, H.S., Wang, J.Y., Gao, M., Yang, S. & Zhang, X.J. (2006). MHC haplotypic association in Chinese Han patients with vitiligo. *J Eur Acad Dermatol Venereol,* Vol.20, pp. 941-946

Xie, P., Geohegan, W.D. & Jordan, R.E. (1991). Vitiligo autoantibodies. Studies of subclass distribution and complement activation. *J Invest Dermatol,* Vol.96, pp. 627

Yang, S., Wang, J.Y., Gao, M., Liu, H.S., Sun, L.D., He, P.P., Liu, J.B., Zhang, A.P., Cui, Y., Liang, Y.H., Wang, Z.X. & Zhang, X.J. (2005). Association of HLA-DQA1 and DQB1 genes with vitiligo in Chinese Hans. *Int J Dermatol,* Vol.44, pp. 1022-1027

Yeo, U.C., Yang, Y.S., Park, K.B., Sung, H.T., Jung, S.Y., Lee, E.S. & Shin, M.H. (1999). Serum concentration of the soluble interleukin-2 receptor in vitiligo patients. *J Dermatol Sci,* Vol.19, pp. 182-188

Yi, Y.L., Yu, C.H. & Yu, H.S. (2000). IgG anti-melanocyte antibodies purified from patients with active vitiligo induce HLA-DR and intercellular adhesion molecule-1 expression and an increase in interleukin-8 release by melanocytes. *J Invest Dermatol,* Vol.115, 969-973

Yu, H.S., Kao, C.H. & Yu, C.L. (1993). Coexistence and relationship of antikeratinocyte and antimelanocyte antibodies in patients with non-segmental-type vitiligo. *J Invest Dermatol,* Vol.100, pp. 823-828

Yu, H.S., Chang, K.L., Yu, C.L., Li, H.F., Wu, M.T., Wu, C.S. & Wu, C.S. (1997). Alterations in IL-6, IL-8, GM-CSF, TNF-alpha, and IFN-gamma release by peripheral mononuclear cells in patients with active vitiligo *J Invest Dermatol,* Vol.108, pp. 527-529

Zaima, H. & Koga, M. (2002). Clinical course of 44 cases of localized type vitiligo. *J Dermatol,* Vol.29, pp. 15-19

Zamani, M., Spaepen, M., Sghar, S.S., Huang, C., Westerhof, W., Nieuweboer-Krobotova, L. & Cassiman, J.J. (2001). Linkage and association of HLA class II genes with vitiligo in a Dutch population. *Br J Dermatol,* Vol.145, pp. 90-94

Zauli, D., Tosti, A., Biasco, G., Miserocchi, F., Patrizi, A., Azzaroni, D., Andiani, G., Di Febo, G. & Callegari, C. (1986). Prevalence of autoimmune atrophic gastritis in vitiligo. *Digestion,* Vol.34, pp. 169-172

Zelissen, P.M., Bast, E.J. & Croughs, R.J. (1995). Associated autoimmunity in Addison's disease. *J Autoimmun,* Vol.8, pp. 121-130

Part 3

Comorbidities of Autoimmune Disorders

15

Subclinical Atherosclerosis in Systemic Autoimmune Disorders

Giannelou M.[1], Gravani F.[1], Papadaki I.[1], Ioakeimidis D.[1] and Mavragani C.P.[2]
[1]*Department of Rheumatology, Athens General Hospital "G. Gennimatas," Athens,*
[2]*Department of Experimental Physiology, School of Medicine, University of Athens, Athens, Greece*

1. Introduction

Over the last years, accelerated atherosclerosis with consequent increased prevalence of cardiovascular disease (CV) in autoimmune patients, especially rheumatoid arthritis (RA) and systemic lupus erythematosus (SLE) has been well established (Toloza, Uribe et al. 2004). However, traditional risk factors associated with atherosclerosis including among others smoking, dyslipidemia, diabetes mellitus (DM), hypertension (HT) and increased body mass index (BMI), do not fully account for the high rates of subclinical atherosclerosis in these patients (Meune, Touze et al. 2009). In the present review, traditional and disease related risk factors of CV disease in the setting of chronic autoimmune disorders with special focus in RA, SLE and Sjogren's syndrome (SS) will be discussed.

2. Epidemiology of CV disease in systemic autoimmune disorders

RA

RA, a chronic systemic inflammatory disease affecting 0.5–1% of the adult population is associated with a two fold increase of CV disease. In a recent study by Evans et al, in 636 RA patients, the incidence of acute coronary syndromes (ACS) including myocardial infarction, unstable angina, cardiac arrest or death due to ischemic heart disease was 3.5 per 100 patient-years with the presence of carotid plaque, CV risk factors (particularly diabetes or hypertension), active polyarticular disease, high cumulative dose of glucocorticoids and male sex, being high risk contributors (Evans, Escalante et al. 2011). In patients with early RA, higher intima media thickness (IMT) scores- a surrogate marker of subclinical atherosclerosis- have been detected compared to healthy controls (Sodergren, Karp et al. 2010) (Georgiadis, Voulgari et al. 2008). Of interest, treatment with methotrexate and prednisolone led to significant reduction of IMT scores compared to baseline after one year of treatment. Several studies so far have demonstrated the independent relationship of elevated inflammatory markers (Myasoedova and Gabriel 2010), with the effects of the atherosclerotic process being reversed, after disease activity and chronic inflammation in RA patients are controlled (Bisoendial, Stroes et al. 2011).

SLE

SLE is a highly heterogeneous autoimmune disease, affecting women of childbearing age, with substantial mortality and morbidity. The effect of SLE on atherosclerotic disease has been recognised since the 70s, when Urowitz et al displayed a bimodal mortality peak; the first was attributed to disease activity and infections and the second to CV disease (Urowitz, Bookman et al. 1976). The prevalence of ischemic heart disease in SLE patients is estimated between 8% and 16% (Badui, Garcia-Rubi et al. 1985; Gladman and Urowitz 1987; Petri, Perez-Gutthann et al. 1992; Borchers, Keen et al. 2004) conferring a 50fold risk (Manzi, Meilahn et al. 1997). In regard to subclinical coronary artery disease, the rates seem to be even higher, reaching the percentage of 28%-40% (Manzi, Selzer et al. 1999; Svenungsson, Jensen-Urstad et al. 2001; Asanuma, Oeser et al. 2003; Manger, Kusus et al. 2003; Roman, Shanker et al. 2003; Vlachoyiannopoulos, Kanellopoulos et al. 2003). Esdaile et al revealed that even after statistical correction for the effects of all classical CV risk factors, patients with SLE still had a 7.9-fold increase in the risk of stroke and a 10.1-fold increase in risk of non-fatal myocardial infarction (Esdaile, Abrahamowicz et al. 2001). Given that standard Framingham scores cannot fully account for the rate of ischemic events, lupus is now regarded as an independent risk factor for the development of CV comorbidity (Manzi, Meilahn et al. 1997; Manzi 2000).

SS

SS or autoimmune epithelitis a slowly progressive autoimmune disease is characterized by salivary and lacrimal gland dysfunction and shares many common clinical and serologic features with other immune mediated autoimmune diseases especially SLE (Mavragani and Moutsopoulos 2010). SS has been recently associated with increased rates of subclinical CV disease in a limited number of studies. Vaudo et al, revealed higher carotid and femoral IMT scores in 37 untreated white women with primary SS compared to age and sex matched healthy counterparts, in association with leukopenia and the presence of anti-SSA antibodies (Vaudo, Bocci et al. 2005). In a subsequent study by Satish et al, patients with long standing disease demonstrated abnormal ankle brachial index (ABI) values compared to controls (Rachapalli, Kiely et al. 2009). While endothelium dependent flow mediated vasodilation (FMD) -a marker of endothelial function- did not differ significantly between primary SS patients and controls as a whole, the subset of patients with articular involvement or parotid gland enlargement had lower values of FMV than controls and patients without such characteristics.

On the other hand, nitrate mediated vasodilation (NMV) values -detecting smooth muscle relaxation independently of endothelial contribution- were lower in primary SS patients and particularly in those characterized by leukopenia, rheumatoid factor (RF), anti-SSB antibodies, and articular involvement. Of interest, NMV values, were directly correlated to the number of the circulating white blood cells and inversely correlated to vascular cell adhesion molecule 1 (VCAM-1) levels (Gerli, Vaudo et al. 2010).

3. Traditional CV risk factors in autoimmune diseases

3.1 Metabolic syndrome

The metabolic syndrome (MetS) describes a constellation of major risk factors for CV disease including dyslipidemia, obesity, hypertension and insulin resistance. Several studies so far have documented the increased frequency of MetS in patients with chronic rheumatic diseases compared to healthy control populations; the higher proinflammatory cytokine burden impairs insulin sensitivity and promotes the adverse lipoprotein profile seen in MetS (Pereira, de Carvalho et al. 2009; Santos and Fonseca 2009).

RA

The relationship between the BMI and overall CV mortality in patients with RA is well recognised (Kitas and Gabriel 2011). Quiet unexpectedly, compared to the general population, the risk of CV disease in RA patients is increased in younger females with low body mass index (<20kg/m^2), most likely due to the excess of inflammatory cytokines (Gabriel 2010; Ozbalkan, Efe et al. 2010; Kitas and Gabriel 2011). In accord with the previous observation, obesity is linked to hypertension and dyslipidemia, but with lower RA disease activity and consequently less CV mortality (Summers, Metsios et al. 2010). In contrast, in the study of Kallinoglou et al, multivariate analysis revealed an association of obesity with CV disease in patients with RA mainly due to concomitant presence of risk factors such as HT, high-density lipoprotein (HDL), insulin resistance and Mets (Stavropoulos-Kalinoglou, Metsios et al. 2009). On the other hand, a recent study has shown that in patients with established RA, both very low and very high BMI and BF associate independently with increased disease activity and physical dysfunction but not with the presence of erosions or joint surgery (Stavropoulos-Kalinoglou, Metsios et al. 2009). While the long-term use of glucocorticoids in RA may collectively contribute to the development of Mets syndrome and atherosclerosis, no association with long term low dose glucocorticoid has been detected in this population (Toms, Panoulas et al. 2008). Furthermore, Ku et al showed that RA patients have high basal levels of insulin and increased insulin resistance and that the degree of severity correlates with inflammatory indices (Ku, Imboden et al. 2009). Finally, in a study of a group of 105 Vietnamese women with early RA, a higher prevalence of MetS compared with healthy controls was demonstrated with disease activity, high inflammatory indices, disability score and less use of DMARDs being independent predictors (Dao, Do et al. 2010).
The link between obesity and inflammation has recently attracted particular attention. Adipocytokines -a newly identified cytokine subset- have been associated with adipose tissue and include among others leptin, adiponectin, resistin and visfatin. Leptin is essential for the regulation of appetite and body weight, as well as the modulation of immune responses (Rho, Chung et al. 2010). While resistin and visfatin are associated with inflammation, insulin resistance and subclinical atherosclerosis, adiponectin is mainly anti-inflammatory, and inversely associated with obesity, insulin resistance, CRP and CV risk (Fagerer and Kullich 2010; Yoshino, Kusunoki et al. 2011).

In patients with RA, higher levels of adipocytokines have been detected compared to control subjects. In a recent report, leptin and visfatin levels were associated with insulin resistance, but not with the presence of coronary calcification (Ozgen, Koca et al. 2010; Rho, Chung et al. 2010). As expected, in contrast to adiponectin, which was negatively associated with CRP, leptin and resistin levels were positively linked to CRP titers (Yoshino, Kusunoki et al. 2011).

While anti-tumor necrosis factor alpha (anti-TNF) treatment in RA patients does not change the levels of circulating visfatin and leptin (Popa, Netea et al. 2009; Gonzalez-Gay, Vazquez-Rodriguez et al. 2010), data on adiponectin is contradictory. In the largest so far study including 97 patients with RA, serum adiponectin was increased after 12 months of anti-TNF treatment (Nishida, Okada et al. 2008), an observation also confirmed in smaller reports with the same follow-up period, implying a potential underlying mechanism for CV risk reduction by anti-TNF agents (Komai, Morita et al. 2007; Serelis, Kontogianni et al. 2008; Engvall, Tengstrand et al. 2010). In contrast, with the exception of the Japanese study by Komai et al who revealed increased adiponectin levels as soon as 2 and 6 weeks, no changes or reduction in adiponectin levels have been reported by studies with a follow-up period of 6 months (Derdemezis, Filippatos et al. 2009; Popa, Netea et al. 2009).

SLE

In a large cohort of 250 patients with SLE and equal number of age-sex matched controls, increased waist-to-hip ratio and sedentary lifestyle in SLE patients was found (Bruce, Urowitz et al. 2003). The prevalence of obesity in SLE has been recently estimated in a cohort of 145 patients by two methods. Using the most common body composition measure (Body mass index, BMI), almost 30% were obese; using a more sensitive measure (by Dual X-ray absorptometry (DXA), the percentage rose to 50% (Katz, Gregorich et al. 2011). A higher prevalence of Mets was found in young lupus patients below 40 years compared to age matched controls (15.8% vs 4.2%) (Sabio, Zamora-Pasadas et al. 2008); the corresponding figures in the study of Chung et al were 32.4% versus 10.9% (using the WHO definition that requires direct determination of insulin resistance) and 29.4% versus 19.8% (using the National Cholesterol Education Program Adult Treatment Panel III definition -NCEP) and found to correlate with higher C-Reactive protein (CRP) levels and endothelial injury. In a subsequent study by Mok et al, the prevalence of Mets was 16.3% in lupus patients and correlated with coronary atherosclerosis (Mok, Poon et al. 2010). In another report, the presence of Mets was associated with higher aortic pulse wave velocity (PWV) –as an indicator of arterial stiffness- and increased biomarkers of subclinical atherosclerosis such as CRP, IL-6, C3, uric acid, homocysteine, fibrinogen and D-dimer (Sabio, Vargas-Hitos et al. 2009). Insulin resistance per se as defined by the WHO criteria was more prevalent in lupus patients compared to controls (44.1% versus 24.8%) (Chung, Avalos et al. 2007).
Similarly to RA, increased levels of adiponectin have been reported in SLE patients (Sada, Yamasaki et al. 2006; Chung, Long et al. 2009; Vadacca, Margiotta et al. 2009) and found to be associated with carotid plaque formation, as a physiologic attempt to limit endothelial damage (Sada, Yamasaki et al. 2006; Vadacca, Margiotta et al. 2009; Clancy and Ginzler 2010; Reynolds, Buyon et al. 2010). Opposite are the findings reported by Chung et al, where lower levels of adiponectin were associated with insulin resistance, BMI and CRP but not with coronary atherosclerosis (Chung, Long et al. 2009). In a murine lupus model, adiponectin has been recently shown to exert protective effects against lupus activity and concomitant atherosclerotic disease. The use of the peroxisome proliferator-activated receptor gamma (PPARgamma) agonist rosiglitazone reduces autoantibody production, renal disease, and atherosclerosis in mouse models of SLE possibly through adiponectin induction. At the same time, lupus mice that lack adiponectin develop more severe disease compared to adiponectin-sufficient lupus mice with the administration of exogenous adiponectin ameliorating disease (Aprahamian, Bonegio et al. 2009). Leptin levels were associated with insulin resistance, BMI and CRP but not with coronary or carotid atherosclerosis (Vadacca, Margiotta et al. 2009). Administration of leptin in lupus prone model led to increased pro-inflammatory HDL scores, atherosclerosis, and accelerated proteinuria, revealing its proatherogenic role (Hahn, Lourencco et al. 2010).

SS

In patients with SS, a higher prevalence of associated dyslipidemia, DM, and hyperuricemia compared to age and sex-matched controls has been observed. Hypercholesterolemia was associated with a lower frequency of immunological markers such as anti-Ro/SSA, anti-La/SSB antibodies, low C3, and C4 levels, while hypertriglyceridemia and DM were positively associated with the presence of extraglandular (renal, liver,vasculitic) involvement. A higher prevalence of DM was found in patients treated with corticosteroids (Ramos-Casals, Brito-Zeron et al. 2007).

3.2 Hypertension (HT)

RA

The prevalence of HT among patients with RA varies between different studies (Panoulas, Metsios et al. 2008). In the largest so far population study by Han et al. prevalence of HT was significantly higher in RA (34% vs 23.4%). However, a recent metaanalysis assessing the effect of traditional risk factors in the pathogenesis of CV disease in RA patients demonstrated similar rates of hypertension in RA patients compared to healthy controls (Gabriel 2010; Boyer, Gourraud et al. 2011).

HT has been found to be associated with subclinical atherosclerosis and CV morbidity in RA patients (Panoulas, Douglas et al. 2007). In a recent Greek cohort study of 325 RA patients, with late disease onset, inadequate early control of disease activity and leflunomide treatment, hypertension was clearly demonstrated to be an important risk factor for CV disease (Serelis, Panagiotakos et al. 2011).

HT and low grade inflammation have been previously linked in general population studies (Panoulas, Douglas et al. 2007; Kitas and Gabriel 2011). High CRP leads to vasoconstriction though reduction of endothelial nitric oxide production, increase in expression of endothelin-1 and upregulation of angiotensin type 1 receptor expression; furthermore, it induces platelet adherence, oxidation and thrombosis. Apart from systemic inflammation, physical inactivity due to articular involvement, genetic predisposition, various medications including NSAIDs, corticosteroids, leflunomide and cyclosporine might account for deregulated arterial pressure in patients with RA (Stavropoulos-Kalinoglou, Metsios et al. 2009; Kitas and Gabriel 2011).

Genetic contribution in occurrence of HT in RA patients was evidenced by the association of previously associated polymorphisms with HT in healthy populations. In RA patients, TGFB1 869T/C and endothelin gene polymorphisms have been shown to be linked with HT, with the latter found to be associated with raised endothelin-1 (ET-1) levels. In contrast to previous studies in healthy subjects, no associations between IL-6-174G/C and HT (Panoulas, Douglas et al. 2009) was detected. Furthermore, a cross-sectional study did not demonstrate significant associations between RA disease activity and hypertension (Panoulas, Metsios et al. 2008; Kitas and Gabriel 2011).

SLE

HT is a well recognised risk factor for CV disease development in SLE patients (Petri, Perez-Gutthann et al. 1992) as evidenced by several studies reporting its contribution in plaque formation (IMT measurement, coronary angiography) and arterial stiffening (Sella, Sato et al. 2003; Selzer, Sutton-Tyrrell et al. 2004; Maksimowicz-McKinnon, Magder et al. 2006; Cypiene, Dadoniene et al. 2010; Gallelli, Burdick et al. 2010). Several studies so far have confirmed the increased prevalence of arterial HT in these patients, ranging from 33% to 56% (de Leeuw, Freire et al. 2006; Bellomio, Spindler et al. 2009; Duarte, Couto et al. 2009; Boucelma, Haddoum et al. 2011; Sabio, Vargas-Hitos et al. 2011). In an effort to investigate

the contributors of HT in a cohort of 112 lupus patients, Sabio et al, reported that renal disease, insulin levels and disease activity indices such as Systemic Lupus Erythematosus Disease Activity Index (SLEDAI) were independent predictors of HT in these subjects. Of interest, in the younger age group (<40y), hypertension was also associated with higher non obesity-related insulin levels, while in the older group (>40y), with age and obesity (Sabio, Vargas-Hitos et al. 2011).
Arterial hypertension did not seem to influence subclinical atherosclerotic disease in patients with pSS (Vaudo, Bocci et al. 2005; Rachapalli, Kiely et al. 2009; Gerli, Vaudo et al. 2010).

3.3 Dyslipidemia

Increased levels of total cholesterol (TC), low-density-lipoprotein (LDL) cholesterol and decreased level of HDL cholesterol are associated with increased risk for CV disease in the general population (Nurmohamed 2009). Cholesterol is transported in the blood by LDL which contains esterified cholesterol and triglycerides surrounded by phospholipids, free cholesterol and apolipoprotein B100 (ApoB100). Circulating LDL particles can accumulate in the intima, where ApoB100 binds to proteoglycans of the extracellular matrix, they are oxidised (Hansson and Hermansson 2011) (oxLDLs), become proinflammatory and lead to endothelial activation. Monocytes are stimulated by macrophage colony-stimulating factor produced by activated endothelial cells and differentiate into macrophages. Macrophages upregulate their scavenger receptors that can take up oxLDL (Hahn, Grossman et al. 2008). Cholesterol accumulation in macrophages transforms them into foam cells that are characteristic of the atherosclerotic lesion. Dendritic cells (DCs) may take up LDL for antigen presentation in regional lymph nodes. In the normal artery wall, DCs promote antigen tolerization; however, atherogenesis leads to a switch from tolerance to the activation of adaptive immunity (Hansson and Hermansson 2011). Monocytes attract lymphocytes that recognize antigens and contribute to inflammation by releasing cytokines. As plaque matures, proteases and other proinflammatory molecules are produced, with hypertrophy of smooth muscle, damage to endothelial cells, bulging of plaque into the lumen of the artery, and formation of a fibrous cap over the plaque (Hahn, Grossman et al. 2008).

RA

Lipoprotein (α) (Lp(α)) is a cholesterol-rich modified form of LDL (Van Doornum, McColl et al. 2002) that is transformed in the liver by covalent attachment of ApoB to ApoA, a member of the plasminogen gene family (Tabas, Williams et al. 2007). Lp(α) has been identified as an independent risk factor for coronary heart disease and elevated levels have been demonstrated in RA patients with active disease (Van Doornum, McColl et al. 2002). Several studies suggest that Lp(α) is associated with early atherosclerosis in RA and possibly in other autoimmune disorders (Dursunoglu, Evrengul et al. 2005; Wang, Hu et al. 2008). In recent studies, complexes of β2-glycoprotein I with Lp(α) ((β2)-GPI-Lp(α)) are found in sera of active RA patients and associate with oxLDL, ox-Lpa and CRP levels (Zhang, Li et al. 2011).
On the other hand, low HDL levels have been previously associated with RA related atherosclerosis implying the potential link between HDL and autoimmunity. HDL possesses anti-inflammatory effects and inhibits the ability of antigen-presenting cells (APCs) to stimulate T cells (Yu, Wang et al. 2010). Given that inflammation has been shown to

suppress total and LDL cholesterol, active RA patients have lower total cholesterol, low LDL and depressed HDL resulting in a higher atherogenic index (total cholesterol/HDL-cholesterol ratio) (Nurmohamed 2009; Kitas and Gabriel 2011), although such alterations have been also observed 3-5 year prior to RA incidence (Myasoedova, Crowson et al. 2010). In a study of early RA patients higher levels of TC, LDL , triglycerides and very low levels in HDL have been observed compared to healthy controls resulting again in a significantly higher atherogenic ratio of TC/HDL as well as that of LDL/HDL (Georgiadis, Papavasiliou et al. 2006). Raised autoantibody titers against oxLDL and low lipoprotein-associated phospholipase A2 (Lp-PLA2) plasma activity have been also suggested as potential contributors in the pathogenesis of accelerated atherosclerosis in patients with early RA (Lourida, Georgiadis et al. 2007). Of interest, recent findings have revealed the contribution of several known RA susceptible genes such as TRAF1/C5, STAT4 and HLA-DRB1-SE in dyslipidemia observed in these patients (Toms, Panoulas et al. 2011).

Systemic inflammation, drug therapy, lifestyle and genetic factors can result not only in changes of overall lipid levels, but also can modify lipids structure and function (Toms, Symmons et al. 2010). Paraoxonase 1 (PON1) is an antiatherogenic enzyme with the ability to destroy biologically active oxLDL (Hahn, Grossman et al. 2008) and to protect LDL against oxidation (Zhao 2009). PON1 activity in RA patients is inversely related to CRP levels, suggesting that inflammation modulates PON activity (Ku, Imboden et al. 2009).

SLE

The classical pattern of dyslipoproteinemia in SLE is characterized by elevated levels of very-low-density lipoprotein cholesterol (VLDL), triglycerides and LDL and low levels of HDL (Borba, Bonfa et al. 2000), although HDL qualitative abnormalities such as peroxidation have been also described, often in association with active disease. Peroxidised HDLs (piHDLs) are unable to reverse cholesterol transport which normally clears oxLDL from the subendothelial space promoting endothelial injury. piHDLs occur in a larger proportion of patients with SLE compared to RA and are associated with carotid artery plaque formation, documented CV disease and low physical activity (McMahon, Grossman et al. 2006; McMahon, Grossman et al. 2009; Volkmann, Grossman et al. 2010).

Apart from HDL, LDL can be also modified in SLE; Frostergard et al disclosed higher levels of oxidized epitopes on LDL in lupus patients compared to controls, which were associated with arterial disease and renal manifestations (Frostegard, Svenungsson et al. 2005).

In a recent study, circulating lipoprotein remnant particles and the intermediate density lipoprotein (IDL) fraction have been strongly associated with IMT values in lupus patients (Gonzalez, Ribalta et al. 2010). Furthermore, reduced levels of apoA-I -the major apolipoprotein component of HDL- have been found in SLE patients with IgG anticardiolipin antibodies (Delgado Alves, Kumar et al. 2003) while antibodies to apoA-I have been previously documented in 32.5% of patients with SLE and 22.9% of patients with primary antiphospholipid syndrome (Dinu, Merrill et al. 1998).

Anti-HDL, anti-CRP anti-Apo A-I have been detected in SLE patients, with the latter found to be associated with persistent disease activity. In the subset of patients with lupus nephritis, anti-Apo A-I and anti-HDL levels correlated with serum anti-double-stranded DNA levels (O'Neill, Giles et al. 2010). Woo et al evaluated the effects of L-4F, (apolipoprotein A-1 mimetic peptide), alone or with pravastatin, in apoE-/-Fas-/-C57BL/6 female mice that spontaneously develop immunoglobulin G (IgG) autoantibodies, glomerulonephritis, osteopenia, and atherosclerotic lesions. As expected, L-4F treatment, significantly reduced IgG anti-dsDNA and IgG anti-oxPLs (anti-oxidised phospholipids), proteinuria, glomerulonephritis, and osteopenia in a murine lupus model of accelerated atherosclerosis (Woo, Lin et al. 2010).

SS

Low HDL cholesterol levels was a constant finding among SS patients in several studies (Vaudo, Bocci et al. 2005; Lodde, Sankar et al. 2006; Gerli, Vaudo et al. 2010). Of interest, HDL along with total cholesterol were found to be associated with immunoglobulin G levels. In particular, the presence of anti-SSA and anti-SSB antibodies have been linked to lower total cholesterol and reduced HDL cholesterol levels, respectively (Lodde, Sankar et al. 2006). Subsequently, Cruz et al, showed a trend to dyslipidemia defined as total cholesterol >200mg/dL, HDL cholesterol<40mg/dL, LDL cholesterol>130mg/dL or triglycerides > 150mg/dL in patients with pSS compared to controls (Cruz, Fialho et al. 2010).

3.4 Smoking

RA

Smoking is an important risk factor for the development of both RA and CVD. Smoking is associated with severe RA with more erosive disease and extra-articular involvement, as smokers are more likely to have positive RF and anti-CCP antibodies. It is not yet clear if smoking confers the same relative risk for CVD development in RA patients compared to the general population (Ozbalkan, Efe et al. 2010). Cigarette smoking is associated with reduced BMI and body fat (BF) in patients with RA, with heavy smoking particularly linked to lower muscle mass while smoking cessation appears to associate with increased BMI, BF, and waist circumference in these patients (Stavropoulos-Kalinoglou, Metsios et al. 2008). In a recent metaanalysis by Gabriel, the prevalence of smoking, but not of the other traditional CV risk factors appears to be increased in RA compared to non-RA patients, at the time of RA incidence (Gabriel 2010).

SLE

Cigarette smoking along with HT have been identified as the main predictors of extracranial carotid artery atherosclerosis, in an early study including 240 SLE patients (Homer, Ingall et al. 1991). While in the studies conducted by Asanuma and Roman, no association between smoking and carotid or coronary atherosclerosis was detected (Asanuma, Oeser et al. 2003; Roman, Shanker et al. 2003), in a subsequent multiethnic US cohort of 546 SLE patients, the role of smoking in the development of vascular events (cardiovascular, cerebrovascular and peripheral) has been suggested (Toloza, Uribe et al. 2004). Similarly, Selzer et al, compared risk factors for subclinical vascular disease in different vascular beds (carotid and aorta) in SLE female patients. Smoking was identified as a factor correlating with carotid plaque severity, together with older age, systolic hypertension and lower albumin levels. In regard to aortic stiffness, risk factors included older age and higher systolic blood pressure but not smoking (Selzer, Sutton-Tyrrell et al. 2004). Finally, a race-smoking interaction was also identified, as amongst black women with SLE, those with a history of smoking have higher IMT values than non smokers. This effect did not apply to white patients (Scalzi, Bhatt et al. 2009).

Smoking did not seem to influence subclinical atherosclerotic disease in patients with pSS (Vaudo, Bocci et al. 2005; Gerli, Vaudo et al. 2010).

3.5 Hyperomocysteinemia

Hyperhomocysteinemia is a recognised risk factor for arterial and venous disease in the general population. Homocysteine increases oxidative stress on the endothelium and causes modification of LDL, inhibition of nitric oxide synthesis, proliferation of smooth muscle cells, intimal hyperplasia, increased protease activity, activation of proinflammatory mediators and thrombosis (Durga, Verhoef et al. 2004). Hyperhomocysteinemia can originate either from a genetic polymorphism and/or a variety of factors including folic acid or vitamin B12 deficiency, corticosteroid or methotrexate treatment, and renal dysfunction. Hyperhomocysteinemia has been reported in 20%-42% of patients with RA and is related to treatment with antifolate agents and greater disease activity. Genetic investigations identified the C677T polymorphism in the gene coding for the MTHFR enzyme as a new candidate genetic risk factor for CV disease in the general population. The 677TT genotype is associated with higher plasma homocysteine levels than in heterozygotes or in individuals with wild-type C alleles (Palomino-Morales, Gonzalez-Juanatey et al. 2010). The increased levels of homocysteine caused by methotrexate therapy occur more often to patients heterozygous for the C677T mutation. Normal homocysteine levels are restored by folic acid supplementation (El Bouchti, Sordet et al. 2008).

RA

In a recent Spanish study of RA patients, the MTHFR A1298C rather the C677T was associated with increased risk of atherosclerosis, demonstrating that patients homozygous for the MTHFR 1298CC genotype had increased risk of CV events at 5 and 10 years follow up and more severe endothelial dysfunction (lower values of FMD %), when compared with those homozygous for the wild MTHFR 1298AA genotype (Palomino-Morales, Gonzalez-Juanatey et al. 2010). Interestingly an ongoing study from our group indicate that Greek RA patients with carotid or femoral plaque formation have a higher prevalence of MTHFR AC and CC genotypes compared with those without. The so far available results show that MTHFR 1298 A>C gene polymorphism confers an increased risk for plaque formation (Mavragani 2011).

SLE

Attention has been drawn over the past few years to the role of homocysteine concentration in the development of subclinical atherosclerosis in SLE patients. In a prospective study, Petri identified elevated homocysteine levels as a risk factor for the later development of CV disease in SLE patients (Petri 2000).

In the Toronto Risk Factor Study for coronary heart disease, SLE patients had homocysteine values>15μmoles/liter in a larger proportion compared to controls (11.6% versus 0.8%) despite having higher folate blood levels (Bruce, Urowitz et al. 2003). SLE patients with hyperhomocysteinemia have a threefold increase in odds ratio of thrombotic event (Refai, Al-Salem et al. 2002).

Several studies linked hyperhomocysteinemia to subclinical atherosclerosis (Svenungsson, Jensen-Urstad et al. 2001; Von Feldt, Scalzi et al. 2006; Von Feldt 2008). Roman et al prospectively studied a cohort of SLE patients with matched controls and determined carotid IMT scores as well as the presence of plaque. Over a period of approximately 3 years of follow-up, 28% of the patients had progressive atherosclerosis, defined as a higher plaque score (new plaque or more extensive plaque). Determinants of atherosclerotic progression after multivariate analysis were patient age at diagnosis, disease duration, and baseline homocysteine concentration. Lupus patients with stable plaque and progressive plaque were different only in baseline homocysteine concentration (Roman, Crow et al. 2007). A recent study by Perna et al implied a relationship of both asymmetric dimethylarginine and homocysteine to arterial stiffness, but not to the presence or extent of carotid atherosclerosis (Perna, Roman et al. 2010). In the Rho et al study, homocysteine levels in SLE patients were linked to macrophage activation, reflected by increased serum neopterin concentrations. Neopterin (marker of monocyte and macrophage activation associated with atherosclerosis and CV risk in the general population) was associated with atherogenic mediators of inflammation and homocysteine in SLE, but not with coronary atherosclerosis (Rho, Solus et al. 2011).

SS

No data to date regarding the role of homocysteine in the pathogenesis of CV disease in the setting of Sjogren's syndrome is available.

4. Disease related contributors of atherosclerosis in systemic autoimmune diseases

SLE

A number of studies evaluated specific disease parameters and their effect on atherosclerotic disease in SLE patients. Disease duration appears to be an important factor in CVD development. An inverse relationship between SLE activity and plaque size was reported by Manzi et al and longer disease duration was independently associated with carotid plaque (Manzi, Selzer et al. 1999) and coronary calcium scores (Von Feldt, Scalzi et al. 2006). In a cross-sectional and in a longitudinal study, Roman *et al.* found that longer disease duration and higher Systemic Lupus International Collaborative Clinics (SLICC) damage index were independent predictors of carotid plaque formation(Roman, et al. 2003; Roman, et al. 2007). In another report, SLE specific variables were associated with aortic stiffness and included older age, hypertension, higher C3 levels, lower white blood cell count, higher insulin levels, and renal disease (Selzer, Sutton-Tyrrell et al. 2004).

Rua-Figueroa et al who assessed the changes in carotid IMT and the associated risk factors in patients with lupus in a two year period, identified basal measurement IMT, age at diagnosis, homocysteine, C3 and C5a as risk factors for IMT progression (Rua-Figueroa, Arencibia-Mireles et al. 2010). In accord with the previous findings, Haque et al compared SLE patients with verified clinical CV disease (myocardial infarction or angina pectoris) to patients without clinical CV disease. Male sex, older age, increased SLICC damage index, prior use of corticosteroids and azathioprine and more exposure to all classic CV risk factors were positively correlated with clinical CV disease (Haque, Gordon et al. 2010). In our SLE cohort, IMT and the presence of plaque were both statistically significant associated with age, hypertension, triglyceridelevels and SLICC damage index score and only plaque with the levels of C3 and C4 (Giannelou 2011).

The role of SLE activity in the formation of non calcified coronary plaque (NCP) was investigated by Kiani et al.; unlike coronary calcium, which is not associated with SLE activity measures or with active serologies, NCP is more common in patients with active disease (Kiani, Vogel-Claussen et al. 2010). Additionally, the presence of lymphopenia and higher levels of serum creatinine and CRP seem to be disease related risk factors in the progression of carotid IMT in juvenile-onset SLE as demonstrated by Huang et al (Huang, Chung et al. 2009).

Although under normal conditions vascular damage is expected to be coupled by acceleration in repair of the endothelium, SLE patients have decreased numbers of circulating EPCs and aberrant function of cells involved in the vascular repair. In particular, lupus EPCs/CACs (myeloid circulating angiogenic cells) have decreased capacity to differentiate into mature ECs and synthesize decreased amounts of the molecules vascular endothelial growth factor and hepatic growth factor (Rajagopalan, Somers et al. 2004; Denny, Thacker et al. 2007; Lee, Li et al. 2007; Moonen, de Leeuw et al. 2007; Westerweel, Luijten et al. 2007). IFNα -a central mediator in lupus pathogenesis- has been recently suggested as a major player of impaired vasculogenesis and atherogenic risk in lupus patients through transcriptional repression of proangiogenic IL-1 pathways, enhancement of foam cell formation, and platelet activation (Lood, Amisten et al. 2010; Thacker, Berthier et al. 2010; Li, Fu et al. 2011).

Autoantibodies including antiOxLDL, AECAs (anti-endothelial cell antibodies) and antibodies against heat shock proteins and phospholipids (APLs) have been linked to lupus related CV disease. In regard to the role of the latter in the pathogenesis of CV disease in the setting of lupus, current evidence is rather conflicting. While in a multiethnic US cohort of patients with SLE, APLs were identified as an independent predictor of CV, cerebrovascular or peripheral vascular events (Toloza, Uribe et al. 2004), such an association has not been detected in three distinct large SLE cohorts (Manzi, Meilahn et al. 1997; Roman, Shanker et al. 2003; McMahon, Grossman et al. 2009). On the other hand, the presence of positive lupus anticoagulant or anti-β2glycoprotein-I antibodies have been also linked to development of myocardial infarction (Petri 2004). In lupus patients without previous CV history, the occurrence of a first ever CVE (defined as ischemic heart, cerebrovascular peripheral vascular disease or death due to CV disease) was dependent on the presence of positive APLs, markers of endothelial activation/damage advanced age and absence of thrombocytopenia (Gustafsson, Gunnarsson et al. 2009). Proposed mechanisms of APL related CV risk include inhibition of binding of annexin A5 (a protein shown to inhibit to plaque rupture) to the endothelium or reduction of the activity of the atheroprotective enzyme PON1 (Cederholm, Svenungsson et al. 2005) (Delgado Alves, Ames et al. 2002).

The role of anti-OxLDLs has not been yet clarified. In the general population, it is indicated that some aOxLDLs are decreased in the early stage of atherosclerosis development in non autoimmune disease but raised at later stages and in more advanced disease (Lopes-Virella, Virella et al. 1999; Wu, de Faire et al. 1999; Hulthe, Wiklund et al. 2001; Karvonen, Paivansalo et al. 2003). Anti-OxLDL antibodies have been detected in up to 80% of SLE patients with aPS (Vaarala, Alfthan et al. 1993), but no association with thrombosis has been identified (Aho, Vaarala et al. 1996).

In another report by Svenungsson et al anti-OxLDL antibodies were more common in SLE patients with a history of CV disease than in SLE controls or normal subjects (Svenungsson, Jensen-Urstad et al. 2001); titers of anti-OxLDL have been also found to be correlated with anti-double-stranded DNA antibody titres, complement activation and disease activity scores in patients with SLE (Gomez-Zumaquero, Tinahones et al. 2004). Of interest, increased atherosclerotic disease has been attributed to the presence of complexes of oxidized low-density liprotein/beta2 glycoprotein 1 (oxLDL/beta2GPI) and anti-complex IgG as well as IgM often in association with renal involvement and history of previous thromboembolic episodes (Bassi, Zampieri et al. 2009).

Finally, autoantibodies to endothelial cell (AECAs) and heat shock proteins have been proposed as potential mediators of atherosclerotic risk in lupus patients. (George, Harats et al. 1999; Mandal, Foteinos et al. 2005).AECAs are associated with lupus disease activity and vasculitis and can act directly on endothelial cells by promoting their activation (Margutti, Matarrese et al. 2008).

RA

Over the last decade, the inflammatory and immunologic mechanisms in the initiation and progression of atherosclerosis (Van Doornum, McColl et al. 2002) have become the focus of particular research interest. Pro-inflammatory cytokines such as TNF-α and IL-6 are released into the systemic circulation and have multiple effects on distant organs including the endothelium and the formation of the atherosclerotic plaque through upregulation of adhesion molecules such as vascular cellular adhesion molecule (VCAM), inhibiting of endothelial nitric oxide (eNOS) production and induction of formation of oxidized LDL (de Groot, Posthumus et al. 2010). Blockade of TNF-α in RA reduces cytokine levels, leucocyte trafficking and platelet levels which may all promote atherosclerotic complications (Full, Ruisanchez et al. 2009). A recently identified new player in atherosclerosis pathogenesis is the macrophage migration inhibitory factor (MIF) which induces the pro-inflammatory mediators TNF-α, IL-1, IL-6 and metalloproteinases (MMPs), activates T cells and promotes angiogenesis. In mice with advanced atherosclerosis, MIF blockade led to plaque regression and reduced monocyte and T-cell content in the plaques (de Groot, Posthumus et al. 2010). The increased arterial stiffness found in RA patients is significantly correlated with disease duration and inflammatory markers such as CRP and IL-6 (Tabas, Williams et al. 2007). As the atherosclerotic plaque matures, the apoptosis of cells in the plaque leads to extracellular lipid accumulation and cellular debris formation. Under the influence of macrophage proteinases, the fibrous cap of the plaques weakens, ruptures and secondary thrombosis may occur (de Groot, Posthumus et al. 2010).

In RA patients, genetic regulation of inflammation seems to be implicated in pathogenesis of accelerated atherosclerosis. Carriers of the allele IL-6-174 -found to be associated with higher IL-6 levels- demonstrated increased prevalence of CV disease (Panoulas, Douglas et al. 2009). In another study by Gabriel et al, inflammatory indicators such as high erythrocyte sedimentation rate (ESR), swelling of small and large joints, rheumatoid nodules, vasculitis and rheumatoid lung disease were all statistically significantly associated with an increased of CV death after adjusting for the above mentioned traditional CV risk factors (Gabriel 2010). Moreover, in patients with RA, the disease activity scale (DAS) was inversely correlated with the number of circulating EPCs, which are hematopoietic stem cells involved in vascular repair, suggesting an additional mechanism of atherogenesis in these patients (Pakozdi, Besenyei et al. 2009; Szekanecz and Koch 2010). Similarly, in patients with lupus, increased levels of circulating apoptotic ECs were correlated with lupus disease activity and endothelial dysfunction.

Serum concentration of autoantibodies in RA, specifically anti-modified citrullinated vimentin (anti-MCV) and anti-cyclic citrullinated peptide (anti-CCP) were found to be positively correlated with disease activity including hsCRP, IL-6, homeostasis model assessment for insulin resistance (HOMA-IR) index, serum levels of rheumatoid factors and IMT score. While anti-MCV and anti-CCP3 are equally sensitive in diagnosing early RA, the former appears to be very useful for monitoring associated subclinical atherosclerosis in early RA (El-Barbary, Kassem et al. 2011).

SS

Associations between signs of subclinical atherosclerosis with the presence of leukopenia, specific autoantibodies (RF, anti-SSA, anti-SSB), articular involvement and parotid gland enlargement, may suggest that immune dysregulation could contribute to the increased risk for atherosclerosis in pSS patients. In our SS cohort, subclinical atherosclerosis -detected by IMT determination- was associated with higher levels of salivary gland infiltration, reduced salivary flow as well as with the presence of SS specific autoantibodies (unpublished results)(Gravani et al, 2011), implying that SS related poor dental hygiene along with immune hyperactivity could contribute to the higher risk for atherosclerotic disease (Mattila, Nieminen et al. 1989)

Finally, circulating CD4+, CD28- cells -previously associated with atherosclerotic risk- did not differ between pSS patients and controls. However, pSS patients demonstrated higher levels of AECAs, (IgG and IgM), and sTM (soluble thrombomodulin), but lower levels of anti-Hsp60 (IgG and IgM) compared to their healthy counterparts, whereas anti-Hsp65 and anti-oxLDL antibody levels were similar in both groups (Vaudo, Bocci et al. 2005) (Gerli, Vaudo et al. 2010).

5. Conclusion

The increased prevalence of CV disease is well established in autoimmune diseases even after correction of the traditional risk factors. Several associations with disease related clinical or serological features, immunologic profile and proinflammatory cytokines are reported. Further investigation is needed to determine a yet unidentified, possibly disease specific mechanism in autoimmune patients.

6. Acknowledgements

We are indebted to Prof.Moutsopoulos, MD, FRCP, FACP for continuous inspiration, guidance and support.

7. References

Aho, K., O. Vaarala, et al. (1996). "Antibodies binding to anionic phospholipids but not to oxidized low-density lipoprotein are associated with thrombosis in patients with systemic lupus erythematosus." *Clin Exp Rheumatol.* 14(5): 499-506.

Aprahamian, T., R. G. Bonegio, et al. (2009). "The peroxisome proliferator-activated receptor gamma agonist rosiglitazone ameliorates murine lupus by induction of adiponectin." *J Immunol.* 182(1): 340-346.

Asanuma, Y., A. Oeser, et al. (2003). "Premature coronary-artery atherosclerosis in systemic lupus erythematosus." *N Engl J Med.* 349(25): 2407-2415.

Badui, E., D. Garcia-Rubi, et al. (1985). "Cardiovascular manifestations in systemic lupus erythematosus. Prospective study of 100 patients." *Angiology.* 36(7): 431-441.

Bassi, N., S. Zampieri, et al. (2009). "oxLDL/beta2GPI complex and anti-oxLDL/beta2GPI in SLE: prevalence and correlates." *Autoimmunity.* 42(4): 289-291.

Bellomio, V., A. Spindler, et al. (2009). "Metabolic syndrome in Argentinean patients with systemic lupus erythematosus." *Lupus.* 18(11): 1019-1025.

Bisoendial, R. J., E. S. Stroes, et al. (2011). "Critical determinants of cardiovascular risk in rheumatoid arthritis." *Curr Pharm Des.* 17(1): 21-26.

Borba, E. F., E. Bonfa, et al. (2000). "Chylomicron metabolism is markedly altered in systemic lupus erythematosus." *Arthritis Rheum.* 43(5): 1033-1040.

Borchers, A. T., C. L. Keen, et al. (2004). "Surviving the butterfly and the wolf: mortality trends in systemic lupus erythematosus." *Autoimmun Rev.* 3(6): 423-453.

Boucelma, M., F. Haddoum, et al. (2011). "Cardiovascular risk and lupus disease." *Int Angiol.* 30(1): 18-24.

Boyer, J. F., P. A. Gourraud, et al. (2011). "Traditional cardiovascular risk factors in rheumatoid arthritis: a meta-analysis." *Joint Bone Spine.* 78(2): 179-183. Epub 2010 Sep 2017.

Bruce, I. N., M. B. Urowitz, et al. (2003). "Risk factors for coronary heart disease in women with systemic lupus erythematosus: the Toronto Risk Factor Study." *Arthritis Rheum.* 48(11): 3159-3167.

Cederholm, A., E. Svenungsson, et al. (2005). "Decreased binding of annexin v to endothelial cells: a potential mechanism in atherothrombosis of patients with systemic lupus erythematosus." *Arterioscler Thromb Vasc Biol.* 25(1): 198-203. Epub 2004 Nov 2011.

Chung, C. P., I. Avalos, et al. (2007). "High prevalence of the metabolic syndrome in patients with systemic lupus erythematosus: association with disease characteristics and cardiovascular risk factors." *Ann Rheum Dis.* 66(2): 208-214. Epub 2006 Aug 2010.

Chung, C. P., A. G. Long, et al. (2009). "Adipocytokines in systemic lupus erythematosus: relationship to inflammation, insulin resistance and coronary atherosclerosis." *Lupus.* 18(9): 799-806.

Clancy, R. and E. M. Ginzler (2010). "Endothelial function and its implications for cardiovascular and renal disease in systemic lupus erythematosus." *Rheum Dis Clin North Am.* 36(1): 145-160, ix-x.

Cruz, W., S. Fialho, et al. (2010). "Is there a link between inflammation and abnormal lipoprotein profile in Sjogren's syndrome?" *Joint Bone Spine.* 77(3): 229-231. Epub 2010 Apr 2017.

Cypiene, A., J. Dadoniene, et al. (2010). "The influence of mean blood pressure on arterial stiffening and endothelial dysfunction in women with rheumatoid arthritis and systemic lupus erythematosus." *Medicina (Kaunas).* 46(8): 522-530.

Dao, H. H., Q. T. Do, et al. (2010). "Increased frequency of metabolic syndrome among Vietnamese women with early rheumatoid arthritis: a cross-sectional study." *Arthritis Res Ther.* 12(6): R218. Epub 2010 Dec 2023.

de Groot, L., M. D. Posthumus, et al. (2010). "Risk factors and early detection of atherosclerosis in rheumatoid arthritis." *Eur J Clin Invest* 40(9): 835-842.

de Leeuw, K., B. Freire, et al. (2006). "Traditional and non-traditional risk factors contribute to the development of accelerated atherosclerosis in patients with systemic lupus erythematosus." *Lupus.* 15(10): 675-682.

Delgado Alves, J., P. R. Ames, et al. (2002). "Antibodies to high-density lipoprotein and beta2-glycoprotein I are inversely correlated with paraoxonase activity in systemic lupus erythematosus and primary antiphospholipid syndrome." *Arthritis Rheum.* 46(10): 2686-2694.

Delgado Alves, J., S. Kumar, et al. (2003). "Cross-reactivity between anti-cardiolipin, anti-high-density lipoprotein and anti-apolipoprotein A-I IgG antibodies in patients with systemic lupus erythematosus and primary antiphospholipid syndrome." *Rheumatology (Oxford)*. 42(7): 893-899. Epub 2003 Apr 2016.

Denny, M. F., S. Thacker, et al. (2007). "Interferon-alpha promotes abnormal vasculogenesis in lupus: a potential pathway for premature atherosclerosis." *Blood*. 110(8): 2907-2915. Epub 2007 Jul 2916.

Derdemezis, C. S., T. D. Filippatos, et al. (2009). "Effects of a 6-month infliximab treatment on plasma levels of leptin and adiponectin in patients with rheumatoid arthritis." *Fundam Clin Pharmacol*. 23(5): 595-600. Epub 2009 Jun 2025.

Dinu, A. R., J. T. Merrill, et al. (1998). "Frequency of antibodies to the cholesterol transport protein apolipoprotein A1 in patients with SLE." *Lupus*. 7(5): 355-360.

Duarte, C., M. Couto, et al. (2009). "[Cardiovascular risk profile in a Portuguese cohort of SLE Portuguese patients]." *Acta Reumatol Port*. 34(2B): 349-357.

Durga, J., P. Verhoef, et al. (2004). "Homocysteine and carotid intima-media thickness: a critical appraisal of the evidence." *Atherosclerosis*. 176(1): 1-19.

Dursunoglu, D., H. Evrengul, et al. (2005). "Lp(a) lipoprotein and lipids in patients with rheumatoid arthritis: serum levels and relationship to inflammation." *Rheumatol Int*. 25(4): 241-245. Epub 2004 Jul 2031.

El-Barbary, A. M., E. M. Kassem, et al. (2011). "Association of Anti-Modified Citrullinated Vimentin with Subclinical Atherosclerosis in Early Rheumatoid Arthritis Compared with Anti-Cyclic Citrullinated Peptide." *J Rheumatol* 1: 1.

El Bouchti, I., C. Sordet, et al. (2008). "Severe atherosclerosis in rheumatoid arthritis and hyperhomocysteinemia: is there a link?" *Joint Bone Spine*. 75(4): 499-501. Epub 2008 May 2023.

Engvall, I. L., B. Tengstrand, et al. (2010). "Infliximab therapy increases body fat mass in early rheumatoid arthritis independently of changes in disease activity and levels of leptin and adiponectin: a randomised study over 21 months." *Arthritis Res Ther*. 12(5): R197. Epub 2010 Oct 2021.

Esdaile, J. M., M. Abrahamowicz, et al. (2001). "Traditional Framingham risk factors fail to fully account for accelerated atherosclerosis in systemic lupus erythematosus." *Arthritis Rheum*. 44(10): 2331-2337.

Evans, M. R., A. Escalante, et al. (2011). "Carotid atherosclerosis predicts incident acute coronary syndromes in rheumatoid arthritis." *Arthritis Rheum* 28(10): 30265.

Fagerer, N. and W. Kullich (2010). "[Adipocytokines in rheumatoid arthritis and obesity]." *Wien Med Wochenschr*. 160(15-16): 391-398.

Frostegard, J., E. Svenungsson, et al. (2005). "Lipid peroxidation is enhanced in patients with systemic lupus erythematosus and is associated with arterial and renal disease manifestations." *Arthritis Rheum*. 52(1): 192-200.

Full, L. E., C. Ruisanchez, et al. (2009). "The inextricable link between atherosclerosis and prototypical inflammatory diseases rheumatoid arthritis and systemic lupus erythematosus." *Arthritis Res Ther*. 11(2): 217. Epub 2009 Apr 2003.

Gabriel, S. E. (2010). "Heart disease and rheumatoid arthritis: understanding the risks." *Ann Rheum Dis*. 69(Suppl 1): i61-64.

Gallelli, B., L. Burdick, et al. (2010). "Carotid plaques in patients with long-term lupus nephritis." *Clin Exp Rheumatol*. 28(3): 386-392. Epub 2010 Jun 2023.

George, J., D. Harats, et al. (1999). "Atherosclerosis-related markers in systemic lupus erythematosus patients: the role of humoral immunity in enhanced atherogenesis." *Lupus.* 8(3): 220-226.

Georgiadis, A. N., E. C. Papavasiliou, et al. (2006). "Atherogenic lipid profile is a feature characteristic of patients with early rheumatoid arthritis: effect of early treatment--a prospective, controlled study." *Arthritis Res Ther.* 8(3): R82. Epub 2006 Apr 2028.

Georgiadis, A. N., P. V. Voulgari, et al. (2008). "Early treatment reduces the cardiovascular risk factors in newly diagnosed rheumatoid arthritis patients." *Semin Arthritis Rheum.* 38(1): 13-19. Epub 2008 Jan 2014.

Gerli, R., G. Vaudo, et al. (2010). "Functional impairment of the arterial wall in primary Sjogren's syndrome: combined action of immunologic and inflammatory factors." *Arthritis Care Res (Hoboken).* 62(5): 712-718.

Giannelou M, Mavragani C, et al (2011). "Inverse correlation of premature atherosclerosis and bone mass density in patients with systemic lupus erythematosus. EULAR meeting, London.

Gladman, D. D. and M. B. Urowitz (1987). "Morbidity in systemic lupus erythematosus." *J Rheumatol Suppl.* 14(Suppl 13): 223-226.

Gomez-Zumaquero, J. M., F. J. Tinahones, et al. (2004). "Association of biological markers of activity of systemic lupus erythematosus with levels of anti-oxidized low-density lipoprotein antibodies." *Rheumatology (Oxford).* 43(4): 510-513. Epub 2004 Feb 2010.

Gonzalez-Gay, M. A., T. R. Vazquez-Rodriguez, et al. (2010). "Visfatin is not associated with inflammation or metabolic syndrome in patients with severe rheumatoid arthritis undergoing anti-TNF-alpha therapy." *Clin Exp Rheumatol.* 28(1): 56-62.

Gonzalez, M., J. Ribalta, et al. (2010). "Nuclear magnetic resonance lipoprotein subclasses and the APOE genotype influence carotid atherosclerosis in patients with systemic lupus erythematosus." *J Rheumatol.* 37(11): 2259-2267. Epub 2010 Aug 2253.

Gravani F, Mavragani C, et al(2011). "Increased intimal media thickness scores in patients with primary Sjogren's syndrome- association with disease related risk factors. EULAR meeting, London.

Gustafsson, J., I. Gunnarsson, et al. (2009). "Predictors of the first cardiovascular event in patients with systemic lupus erythematosus - a prospective cohort study." *Arthritis Res Ther.* 11(6): R186. Epub 2009 Dec 2010.

Hahn, B. H., J. Grossman, et al. (2008). "Altered lipoprotein metabolism in chronic inflammatory states: proinflammatory high-density lipoprotein and accelerated atherosclerosis in systemic lupus erythematosus and rheumatoid arthritis." *Arthritis Res Ther* 10(4): 213.

Hahn, B. H., E. V. Lourencco, et al. (2010). "Pro-inflammatory high-density lipoproteins and atherosclerosis are induced in lupus-prone mice by a high-fat diet and leptin." *Lupus.* 19(8): 913-917. Epub 2010 Apr 2021.

Hansson, G. K. and A. Hermansson (2011). "The immune system in atherosclerosis." *Nat Immunol.* 12(3): 204-212.

Haque, S., C. Gordon, et al. (2010). "Risk factors for clinical coronary heart disease in systemic lupus erythematosus: the lupus and atherosclerosis evaluation of risk (LASER) study." *J Rheumatol.* 37(2): 322-329. Epub 2009 Dec 2001.

Homer, D., T. J. Ingall, et al. (1991). "Serum lipids and lipoproteins are less powerful predictors of extracranial carotid artery atherosclerosis than are cigarette smoking and hypertension." *Mayo Clin Proc.* 66(3): 259-267.

Huang, Y. L., H. T. Chung, et al. (2009). "Lymphopenia is a risk factor in the progression of carotid intima-media thickness in juvenile-onset systemic lupus erythematosus." *Arthritis Rheum.* 60(12): 3766-3775.

Hulthe, J., O. Wiklund, et al. (2001). "Antibodies to oxidized LDL in relation to carotid atherosclerosis, cell adhesion molecules, and phospholipase A(2)." *Arterioscler Thromb Vasc Biol.* 21(2): 269-274.

Karvonen, J., M. Paivansalo, et al. (2003). "Immunoglobulin M type of autoantibodies to oxidized low-density lipoprotein has an inverse relation to carotid artery atherosclerosis." *Circulation.* 108(17): 2107-2112. Epub 2003 Oct 2106.

Katz, P., S. Gregorich, et al. (2011). "Obesity and its measurement in a community-based sample of women with systemic lupus erythematosus." *Arthritis Care Res (Hoboken).* 63(2): 261-268. doi: 210.1002/acr.20343.

Kiani, A. N., J. Vogel-Claussen, et al. (2010). "Noncalcified coronary plaque in systemic lupus erythematosus." *J Rheumatol.* 37(3): 579-584. Epub 2010 Jan 2028.

Kitas, G. D. and S. E. Gabriel (2011). "Cardiovascular disease in rheumatoid arthritis: state of the art and future perspectives." *Ann Rheum Dis.* 70(1): 8-14. Epub 2010 Nov 2024.

Komai, N., Y. Morita, et al. (2007). "Anti-tumor necrosis factor therapy increases serum adiponectin levels with the improvement of endothelial dysfunction in patients with rheumatoid arthritis." *Mod Rheumatol.* 17(5): 385-390. Epub 2007 Oct 2019.

Ku, I. A., J. B. Imboden, et al. (2009). "Rheumatoid arthritis: model of systemic inflammation driving atherosclerosis." *Circ J* 73(6): 977-985.

Lee, P. Y., Y. Li, et al. (2007). "Type I interferon as a novel risk factor for endothelial progenitor cell depletion and endothelial dysfunction in systemic lupus erythematosus." *Arthritis Rheum.* 56(11): 3759-3769.

Li, J., Q. Fu, et al. (2011). "Interferon-alpha priming promotes lipid uptake and macrophage-derived foam cell formation: a novel link between interferon-alpha and atherosclerosis in lupus." *Arthritis Rheum.* 63(2): 492-502. doi: 410.1002/art.30165.

Lodde, B. M., V. Sankar, et al. (2006). "Serum lipid levels in Sjogren's syndrome." *Rheumatology (Oxford).* 45(4): 481-484. Epub 2005 Nov 2022.

Lood, C., S. Amisten, et al. (2010). "Platelet transcriptional profile and protein expression in patients with systemic lupus erythematosus: up-regulation of the type I interferon system is strongly associated with vascular disease." *Blood.* 116(11): 1951-1957. Epub 2010 Jun 1910.

Lopes-Virella, M. F., G. Virella, et al. (1999). "Antibodies to oxidized LDL and LDL-containing immune complexes as risk factors for coronary artery disease in diabetes mellitus." *Clin Immunol.* 90(2): 165-172.

Lourida, E. S., A. N. Georgiadis, et al. (2007). "Patients with early rheumatoid arthritis exhibit elevated autoantibody titers against mildly oxidized low-density lipoprotein and exhibit decreased activity of the lipoprotein-associated phospholipase A2." *Arthritis Res Ther.* 9(1): R19.

Maksimowicz-McKinnon, K., L. S. Magder, et al. (2006). "Predictors of carotid atherosclerosis in systemic lupus erythematosus." *J Rheumatol.* 33(12): 2458-2463. Epub 2006 Oct 2451.

Mandal, K., G. Foteinos, et al. (2005). "Role of antiheat shock protein 60 autoantibodies in atherosclerosis." *Lupus.* 14(9): 742-746.
Manger, K., M. Kusus, et al. (2003). "Factors associated with coronary artery calcification in young female patients with SLE." *Ann Rheum Dis.* 62(9): 846-850.
Manzi, S. (2000). "Systemic lupus erythematosus: a model for atherogenesis?" *Rheumatology (Oxford).* 39(4): 353-359.
Manzi, S., E. N. Meilahn, et al. (1997). "Age-specific incidence rates of myocardial infarction and angina in women with systemic lupus erythematosus: comparison with the Framingham Study." *Am J Epidemiol.* 145(5): 408-415.
Manzi, S., F. Selzer, et al. (1999). "Prevalence and risk factors of carotid plaque in women with systemic lupus erythematosus." *Arthritis Rheum.* 42(1): 51-60.
Margutti, P., P. Matarrese, et al. (2008). "Autoantibodies to the C-terminal subunit of RLIP76 induce oxidative stress and endothelial cell apoptosis in immune-mediated vascular diseases and atherosclerosis." *Blood.* 111(9): 4559-4570. Epub 2007 Nov 4559.
Mattila, K. J., M. S. Nieminen, et al. (1989). "Association between dental health and acute myocardial infarction." *Bmj.* 298(6676): 779-781.
Mavragani, C. P. and H. M. Moutsopoulos (2010). "The geoepidemiology of Sjogren's syndrome." *Autoimmun Rev.* 9(5): A305-310. Epub 2009 Nov 2010.
Mavragani, C. P., Papadaki I, et al(2011). "Association of subclinical atherosclerosis with disease activity and MTHFR polymorphisms in Greek patients with rheumatoid arthritis, EULAR meeting, London, 2011.
McMahon, M., J. Grossman, et al. (2006). "Proinflammatory high-density lipoprotein as a biomarker for atherosclerosis in patients with systemic lupus erythematosus and rheumatoid arthritis." *Arthritis Rheum.* 54(8): 2541-2549.
McMahon, M., J. Grossman, et al. (2009). "Dysfunctional proinflammatory high-density lipoproteins confer increased risk of atherosclerosis in women with systemic lupus erythematosus." *Arthritis Rheum.* 60(8): 2428-2437.
Meune, C., E. Touze, et al. (2009). "Trends in cardiovascular mortality in patients with rheumatoid arthritis over 50 years: a systematic review and meta-analysis of cohort studies." *Rheumatology (Oxford)* 48(10): 1309-1313.
Mok, C. C., W. L. Poon, et al. (2010). "Metabolic syndrome, endothelial injury, and subclinical atherosclerosis in patients with systemic lupus erythematosus." *Scand J Rheumatol.* 39(1): 42-49.
Moonen, J. R., K. de Leeuw, et al. (2007). "Reduced number and impaired function of circulating progenitor cells in patients with systemic lupus erythematosus." *Arthritis Res Ther.* 9(4): R84.
Myasoedova, E., C. S. Crowson, et al. (2010). "Total cholesterol and LDL levels decrease before rheumatoid arthritis." *Ann Rheum Dis.* 69(7): 1310-1314. Epub 2009 Oct 1323.
Myasoedova, E. and S. E. Gabriel (2010). "Cardiovascular disease in rheumatoid arthritis: a step forward." *Curr Opin Rheumatol* 22(3): 342-347.
Nishida, K., Y. Okada, et al. (2008). "Induction of hyperadiponectinemia following long-term treatment of patients with rheumatoid arthritis with infliximab (IFX), an anti-TNF-alpha antibody." *Endocr J.* 55(1): 213-216. Epub 2008 Feb 2013.
Nurmohamed, M. T. (2009). "Cardiovascular risk in rheumatoid arthritis." *Autoimmun Rev.* 8(8): 663-667. Epub 2009 Feb 2012.

O'Neill, S. G., I. Giles, et al. (2010). "Antibodies to apolipoprotein A-I, high-density lipoprotein, and C-reactive protein are associated with disease activity in patients with systemic lupus erythematosus." *Arthritis Rheum.* 62(3): 845-854.

Ozbalkan, Z., C. Efe, et al. (2010). "An update on the relationships between rheumatoid arthritis and atherosclerosis." *Atherosclerosis* 212(2): 377-382.

Ozgen, M., S. S. Koca, et al. (2010). "Serum adiponectin and vaspin levels in rheumatoid arthritis." *Arch Med Res.* 41(6): 457-463.

Pakozdi, A., T. Besenyei, et al. (2009). "Endothelial progenitor cells in arthritis-associated vasculogenesis and atherosclerosis." *Joint Bone Spine.* 76(6): 581-583. Epub .

Palomino-Morales, R., C. Gonzalez-Juanatey, et al. (2010). "A1298C polymorphism in the MTHFR gene predisposes to cardiovascular risk in rheumatoid arthritis." *Arthritis Res Ther.* 12(2): R71. Epub 2010 Apr 2026.

Panoulas, V. F., K. M. Douglas, et al. (2007). "Prevalence and associations of hypertension and its control in patients with rheumatoid arthritis." *Rheumatology (Oxford).* 46(9): 1477-1482. Epub 2007 Aug 1417.

Panoulas, V. F., K. M. Douglas, et al. (2009). "Transforming growth factor-beta1 869T/C, but not interleukin-6 -174G/C, polymorphism associates with hypertension in rheumatoid arthritis." *Rheumatology (Oxford).* 48(2): 113-118. Epub 2008 Dec 2023.

Panoulas, V. F., G. S. Metsios, et al. (2008). "Hypertension in rheumatoid arthritis." *Rheumatology (Oxford).* 47(9): 1286-1298. Epub 2008 May 1288.

Pereira, R. M., J. F. de Carvalho, et al. (2009). "Metabolic syndrome in rheumatological diseases." *Autoimmun Rev.* 8(5): 415-419. Epub 2009 Jan 2023.

Perna, M., M. J. Roman, et al. (2010). "Relationship of asymmetric dimethylarginine and homocysteine to vascular aging in systemic lupus erythematosus patients." *Arthritis Rheum.* 62(6): 1718-1722.

Petri, M. (2000). "Detection of coronary artery disease and the role of traditional risk factors in the Hopkins Lupus Cohort." *Lupus.* 9(3): 170-175.

Petri, M. (2004). "The lupus anticoagulant is a risk factor for myocardial infarction (but not atherosclerosis): Hopkins Lupus Cohort." *Thromb Res.* 114(5-6): 593-595.

Petri, M., S. Perez-Gutthann, et al. (1992). "Risk factors for coronary artery disease in patients with systemic lupus erythematosus." *Am J Med.* 93(5): 513-519.

Popa, C., M. G. Netea, et al. (2009). "Circulating leptin and adiponectin concentrations during tumor necrosis factor blockade in patients with active rheumatoid arthritis." *J Rheumatol.* 36(4): 724-730. Epub 2009 Feb 2027.

Rachapalli, S. M., P. D. Kiely, et al. (2009). "Prevalence of abnormal ankle brachial index in patients with primary Sjogren's syndrome." *Clin Rheumatol.* 28(5): 587-590. Epub 2009 Feb 2010.

Rajagopalan, S., E. C. Somers, et al. (2004). "Endothelial cell apoptosis in systemic lupus erythematosus: a common pathway for abnormal vascular function and thrombosis propensity." *Blood.* 103(10): 3677-3683. Epub 2004 Jan 3615.

Ramos-Casals, M., P. Brito-Zeron, et al. (2007). "High prevalence of serum metabolic alterations in primary Sjogren's syndrome: influence on clinical and immunological expression." *J Rheumatol.* 34(4): 754-761. Epub 2007 Feb 2015.

Refai, T. M., I. H. Al-Salem, et al. (2002). "Hyperhomocysteinaemia and risk of thrombosis in systemic lupus erythematosus patients." *Clin Rheumatol.* 21(6): 457-461.

Reynolds, H. R., J. Buyon, et al. (2010). "Association of plasma soluble E-selectin and adiponectin with carotid plaque in patients with systemic lupus erythematosus." *Atherosclerosis.* 210(2): 569-574. Epub 2009 Dec 2016.

Rho, Y. H., C. P. Chung, et al. (2010). "Adipocytokines, insulin resistance, and coronary atherosclerosis in rheumatoid arthritis." *Arthritis Rheum.* 62(5): 1259-1264.

Rho, Y. H., J. Solus, et al. (2011). "Macrophage activation and coronary atherosclerosis in systemic lupus erythematosus and rheumatoid arthritis." *Arthritis Care Res (Hoboken).* 63(4): 535-541. doi: 510.1002/acr.20365.

Roman, M. J., M. K. Crow, et al. (2007). "Rate and determinants of progression of atherosclerosis in systemic lupus erythematosus." *Arthritis Rheum.* 56(10): 3412-3419.

Roman, M. J., B. A. Shanker, et al. (2003). "Prevalence and correlates of accelerated atherosclerosis in systemic lupus erythematosus." *N Engl J Med.* 349(25): 2399-2406.

Rua-Figueroa, I., O. Arencibia-Mireles, et al. (2010). "Factors involved in the progress of preclinical atherosclerosis associated with systemic lupus erythematosus: a 2-year longitudinal study." *Ann Rheum Dis.* 69(6): 1136-1139. Epub 2009 Aug 1116.

Sabio, J. M., J. Vargas-Hitos, et al. (2009). "Metabolic syndrome is associated with increased arterial stiffness and biomarkers of subclinical atherosclerosis in patients with systemic lupus erythematosus." *J Rheumatol.* 36(10): 2204-2211. Epub 2009 Sep 2201.

Sabio, J. M., J. A. Vargas-Hitos, et al. (2011). "Prevalence of and Factors Associated with Hypertension in Young and Old Women with Systemic Lupus Erythematosus." *J Rheumatol* 16: 16.

Sabio, J. M., M. Zamora-Pasadas, et al. (2008). "Metabolic syndrome in patients with systemic lupus erythematosus from Southern Spain." *Lupus.* 17(9): 849-859.

Sada, K. E., Y. Yamasaki, et al. (2006). "Altered levels of adipocytokines in association with insulin resistance in patients with systemic lupus erythematosus." *J Rheumatol.* 33(8): 1545-1552.

Santos, M. J. and J. E. Fonseca (2009). "Metabolic syndrome, inflammation and atherosclerosis - the role of adipokines in health and in systemic inflammatory rheumatic diseases." *Acta Reumatol Port.* 34(4): 590-598.

Scalzi, L. V., S. Bhatt, et al. (2009). "The relationship between race, cigarette smoking and carotid intimal medial thickness in systemic lupus erythematosus." *Lupus.* 18(14): 1289-1297. Epub 2009 Oct 1227.

Sella, E. M., E. I. Sato, et al. (2003). "Coronary artery angiography in systemic lupus erythematosus patients with abnormal myocardial perfusion scintigraphy." *Arthritis Rheum.* 48(11): 3168-3175.

Selzer, F., K. Sutton-Tyrrell, et al. (2004). "Comparison of risk factors for vascular disease in the carotid artery and aorta in women with systemic lupus erythematosus." *Arthritis Rheum.* 50(1): 151-159.

Serelis, J., M. D. Kontogianni, et al. (2008). "Effect of anti-TNF treatment on body composition and serum adiponectin levels of women with rheumatoid arthritis." *Clin Rheumatol.* 27(6): 795-797. Epub 2008 Feb 2028.

Serelis, J., D. B. Panagiotakos, et al. (2011). "Cardiovascular disease is related to hypertension in patients with rheumatoid arthritis: a greek cohort study." *J Rheumatol.* 38(2): 236-241. Epub 2010 Nov 2015.

Sodergren, A., K. Karp, et al. (2010). "Atherosclerosis in early rheumatoid arthritis: very early endothelial activation and rapid progression of intima media thickness." *Arthritis Res Ther.* 12(4): R158. Epub 2010 Aug 2016.

Stavropoulos-Kalinoglou, A., G. S. Metsios, et al. (2008). "Cigarette smoking associates with body weight and muscle mass of patients with rheumatoid arthritis: a cross-sectional, observational study." *Arthritis Res Ther.* 10(3): R59. Epub 2008 May 2020.

Stavropoulos-Kalinoglou, A., G. S. Metsios, et al. (2009). "Underweight and obese states both associate with worse disease activity and physical function in patients with established rheumatoid arthritis." *Clin Rheumatol.* 28(4): 439-444. Epub 2008 Dec 2019.

Summers, G. D., G. S. Metsios, et al. (2010). "Rheumatoid cachexia and cardiovascular disease." *Nat Rev Rheumatol.* 6(8): 445-451. Epub 2010 Jul 2020.

Svenungsson, E., K. Jensen-Urstad, et al. (2001). "Risk factors for cardiovascular disease in systemic lupus erythematosus." *Circulation.* 104(16): 1887-1893.

Szekanecz, Z. and A. E. Koch (2010). "Vasculogenesis in rheumatoid arthritis." *Arthritis Res Ther.* 12(2): 110. Epub 2010 Mar 2018.

Tabas, I., K. J. Williams, et al. (2007). "Subendothelial lipoprotein retention as the initiating process in atherosclerosis: update and therapeutic implications." *Circulation.* 116(16): 1832-1844.

Thacker, S. G., C. C. Berthier, et al. (2010). "The detrimental effects of IFN-alpha on vasculogenesis in lupus are mediated by repression of IL-1 pathways: potential role in atherogenesis and renal vascular rarefaction." *J Immunol.* 185(7): 4457-4469. Epub 2010 Aug 4430.

Toloza, S. M., A. G. Uribe, et al. (2004). "Systemic lupus erythematosus in a multiethnic US cohort (LUMINA). XXIII. Baseline predictors of vascular events." *Arthritis Rheum.* 50(12): 3947-3957.

Toms, T. E., V. F. Panoulas, et al. (2008). "Lack of association between glucocorticoid use and presence of the metabolic syndrome in patients with rheumatoid arthritis: a cross-sectional study." *Arthritis Res Ther.* 10(6): R145. Epub 2008 Dec 2017.

Toms, T. E., V. F. Panoulas, et al. (2011). "Rheumatoid arthritis susceptibility genes associate with lipid levels in patients with rheumatoid arthritis." *Ann Rheum Dis* 11: 11.

Toms, T. E., D. P. Symmons, et al. (2010). "Dyslipidaemia in rheumatoid arthritis: the role of inflammation, drugs, lifestyle and genetic factors." *Curr Vasc Pharmacol.* 8(3): 301-326.

Urowitz, M. B., A. A. Bookman, et al. (1976). "The bimodal mortality pattern of systemic lupus erythematosus." *Am J Med.* 60(2): 221-225.

Vaarala, O., G. Alfthan, et al. (1993). "Crossreaction between antibodies to oxidised low-density lipoprotein and to cardiolipin in systemic lupus erythematosus." *Lancet.* 341(8850): 923-925.

Vadacca, M., D. Margiotta, et al. (2009). "Adipokines and systemic lupus erythematosus: relationship with metabolic syndrome and cardiovascular disease risk factors." *J Rheumatol.* 36(2): 295-297.

Van Doornum, S., G. McColl, et al. (2002). "Accelerated atherosclerosis: an extraarticular feature of rheumatoid arthritis?" *Arthritis Rheum.* 46(4): 862-873.

Vaudo, G., E. B. Bocci, et al. (2005). "Precocious intima-media thickening in patients with primary Sjogren's syndrome." *Arthritis Rheum.* 52(12): 3890-3897.

Vlachoyiannopoulos, P. G., P. G. Kanellopoulos, et al. (2003). "Atherosclerosis in premenopausal women with antiphospholipid syndrome and systemic lupus erythematosus: a controlled study." *Rheumatology (Oxford).* 42(5): 645-651.

Volkmann, E. R., J. M. Grossman, et al. (2010). "Low physical activity is associated with proinflammatory high-density lipoprotein and increased subclinical atherosclerosis in women with systemic lupus erythematosus." *Arthritis Care Res (Hoboken).* 62(2): 258-265.

Von Feldt, J. M. (2008). "Premature atherosclerotic cardiovascular disease and systemic lupus erythematosus from bedside to bench." *Bull NYU Hosp Jt Dis.* 66(3): 184-187.

Von Feldt, J. M., L. V. Scalzi, et al. (2006). "Homocysteine levels and disease duration independently correlate with coronary artery calcification in patients with systemic lupus erythematosus." *Arthritis Rheum.* 54(7): 2220-2227.

Wang, J., B. Hu, et al. (2008). "Native, oxidized lipoprotein(a) and lipoprotein(a) immune complex in patients with active and inactive rheumatoid arthritis: plasma concentrations and relationship to inflammation." *Clin Chim Acta.* 390(1-2): 67-71. Epub 2008 Jan 2011.

Westerweel, P. E., R. K. Luijten, et al. (2007). "Haematopoietic and endothelial progenitor cells are deficient in quiescent systemic lupus erythematosus." *Ann Rheum Dis.* 66(7): 865-870. Epub 2007 Feb 2028.

Woo, J. M., Z. Lin, et al. (2010). "Treatment with apolipoprotein A-1 mimetic peptide reduces lupus-like manifestations in a murine lupus model of accelerated atherosclerosis." *Arthritis Res Ther.* 12(3): R93. Epub 2010 May 2018.

Wu, R., U. de Faire, et al. (1999). "Autoantibodies to OxLDL are decreased in individuals with borderline hypertension." *Hypertension.* 33(1): 53-59.

Yoshino, T., N. Kusunoki, et al. (2011). "Elevated serum levels of resistin, leptin, and adiponectin are associated with C-reactive protein and also other clinical conditions in rheumatoid arthritis." *Intern Med.* 50(4): 269-275. Epub 2011 Feb 2015.

Yu, B. L., S. H. Wang, et al. (2010). "HDL and immunomodulation: an emerging role of HDL against atherosclerosis." *Immunol Cell Biol.* 88(3): 285-290. Epub 2010 Jan 2012.

Zhang, C., X. Li, et al. (2011). "Increased serum levels of beta(2)-GPI-Lp(a) complexes and their association with premature atherosclerosis in patients with rheumatoid arthritis." *Clin Chim Acta* 4: 4.

Zhao, Q. (2009). "Inflammation, autoimmunity, and atherosclerosis." *Discov Med.* 8(40): 7-12.

16

Chronic Periaortitis as a Systemic Autoimmune Disease

Chang-Hee Suh
Rheumatology, Ajou University School of Medicine
Korea

1. Introduction

Chronic periaortitis is an idiopathic disease whose hallmark is the presence of a fibro-inflammatory tissue arising from the adventitia of the abdominal aorta and the common iliac arteries and extending into the surrounding retroperitoneum and frequently encasing neighboring structures such as the ureters and the inferior vena cava (Mitchinson, 1984; Parums, 1990). It should be regarded as a generalized disease with three different pathophysiological entities, specifically idiopathic retroperitoneal fibrosis, inflammatory abdominal aortic aneurysms, and perianeurysmal retroperitoneal fibrosis (Vaglio et al., 2003; Jois et al., 2004).

Idiopathic retroperitoneal fibrosis is characterized by periaortic fibroinflammatory tissue, which often causes obstruction of the ureters and other adjacent abdominal structures by extending into the retroperitoneum (Mitchinson, 1970; Gilkeson & Allen, 1996). A dilated aorta is usually not present in idiopathic retroperitoneal fibrosis. Its initial signs and symptoms are often nonspecific, such as malaise, anorexia, weight loss, fever, and flank, back, or abdominal pain. Inflammatory abdominal aortic aneurysms characteristically develop the mass around a dilated aorta, but usually do not cause obstructions (Crawford et al., 1985; Pennell et al., 1985). It usually presents with typical symptoms and signs characterized by the triad of abdominal or back pain, a pulsatile and sometimes tender abdominal mass, and an elevated erythrocyte sedimentation rate. Perianeurysmal retroperitoneal fibrosis, which represents a link between these two diagnoses, involves an abdominal aortic aneurysms surrounded by fibroinflammatory tissue that encases other abdominal organs (Serra et al, 1980).

These definitions may be a little confusing, and it would probably be more appropriate to distinguish aneurysmal from nonaneurysmal forms of chronic periaortitis; idiopathic retroperitoneal fibrosis may be referred as non-aneurysmal chronic periaortitis, where as inflammatory abdominal aortic aneurysms and perianeurysmal retroperitoneal fibrosis as aneurysmal chronic periaortitis (Vaglio et al., 2006).

It is important to diagnose chronic periaortitis early in its course in order to attempt to prevent the severe secondary complication of renal failure due to ureteric obstruction and the potentially fatal consequence of aortic rupture (Jois et al., 2004). Although most studies have considered these entities separately, these conditions have common clinical and histopathologic findings, and thus probably represent different manifestations of the same disease.

2. Epidemiology

The prevalence of chronic periaortitis is not well known; the only available epidemiological data concern idiopathic retroperitoneal fibrosis and inflammatory abdominal aortic aneurysms. Reports from Duke University and the Mayo Clinic estimate that the incidence of idiopathic retroperitoneal fibrosis is less than 1 per 10,000 patients (Gilkeson & Allen 1996). A recent study conducted in Finland on idiopathic retroperitoneal fibrosis has demonstrated that its incidence and prevalence are 1/1,000,000 person-year and 1.38 cases/100,000 inhabitants (Uibu et al., 2004). On the other hand, data regarding the incidence of the aneurysmal forms of chronic periaortitis in the whole population are lacking, however they represent about 4% to 10% of all abdominal aortic aneurysms (Rasmussen et al, 1997; von Fritschen et al., 1999; Yusuf et al., 2007).

Chronic periaortitis frequently develops in middle-aged adults with a mean age of approximately 60 years, but it may also occur in children (Miller et al. 2003; Uibu et al., 2004; Vaglio et al., 2006). Men are affected two to three times as often as women and that is even more pronounced in the inflammatory abdominal aortic aneurysms (Gilkeson & Allen 1996; Uibu et al., 2004; Vaglio et al., 2006).

There is no evidence of a clear ethnic predisposition or familial clustering, and the disease has been reported in twins and siblings only in anecdotal cases (Duffy et al., 1984; Doolin et al. 1987). A few studies have addressed the question whether genetic factors may contribute to the development of chronic periaortitis. Recent studies have suggested that immunogenetic factors may be involved in the pathogenesis of the disease (Rasmussen et al., 1997; Martorana et al., 2006).

A case-control study evaluated the prevalence of HLA alleles in patients with inflammatory abdominal aortic aneurysms compared with healthy subjects found that in the inflammatory abdominal aortic aneurysms a genetic risk determinant mapping at the HLA-DRB1 locus (Rasmussen et al., 1997). Additionally, they identified HLA-DRB1*15 and B1*0404 as predisposing alleles.

Another recent case-control study on patients with chronic periaortitis and healthy controls in order to investigate the role of HLA in the susceptibility to chronic periaortitis revealed that the frequency of the HLA-DRB1*03 allele was markedly higher in patients with chronic periaortitis than in the controls (Martorana et al., 2006). The HLA-DRB1*03 allele is a well-known marker of autoimmunity, since it is associated with a number of autoimmune diseases, which include systemic lupus erythematosus and autoimmune thyroid disease (Davidson and Diamond, 2001). Also, the HLA-B*08 allele was significantly associated with chronic periaortitis and it is itself linked to a wide range of immune-mediated diseases. Furthermore, the comparison of the clinical and laboratory characteristics of HLA-DRB1*03-positive and HLA-DRB1*03-negative patients showed that the HLA-DRB1*03-positive patients with chronic periaortitis have higher acute-phase reactant levels at the time of diagnosis (Martorana et al., 2006). These results could imply that the HLA system not only confers susceptibility to the development of the disease but also plays a role in the modulation of the inflammatory response.

More recently, CC chemokine receptor 5 (CCR5) gene delta 32 polymorphism has been mapped in 100 patients with chronic periaortitis (Boiardi L et al., 2011). The distribution of the CCR5 gene delta 32 genotype differed between patients with chronic periaortitis and controls ($P = 0.01$). The CCR5 gene delta 32 allele was more frequent in patients with chronic periaortitis [$P = 0.02$, odds ratio (OR) 2.8 (95% CI 1.2, 6.4)]. Furthermore, CCR5 gene delta 32 allele occurred more frequently in patients with inflammatory abdominal aortic aneurysms than in patients with idiopathic retroperitoneal fibrosis [P = 0.001, OR 6.4 (95% CI 2.1, 19.1)]. The CCR5 gene delta 32 allele frequency was higher in inflammatory abdominal aortic aneurysms patients without established atherosclerotic disease compared with controls [66.7 vs 5.6%, P = 0.00001, OR 34.0 (95% CI 7.4, 156.3)].

The CC chemokine receptor 5 is expressed on many immune cells, particularly Th1 cells, and acts by binding to different chemokines, including RANTES, MIP-1α and MIP-1β. The CCR5 gene delta 32 polymorphism creates a truncated, nonfunctional receptor and probably shifts the immune response toward a Th2 pattern. Interestingly, the association between the CCR5 gene delta 32 polymorphism and aneurysmal chronic periaortitis is even stronger in patients without overt atherosclerotic disease, which suggests that immune mechanisms independent of atherosclerosis play a role in the pathogenesis of chronic periaortitis (Vaglio et al., 2011).

Additionally, environmental and occupational agents have been shown to contribute to susceptibility to chronic periaortitis. In a recent study, it has been demonstrated that asbestos exposure is associated with a markedly increased risk of developing the chronic periaortitis, and smoking is also a significant risk factor (Uibu et al., 2004; Hellmann et al., 2007). Although smoking is an established risk factor for classical atherosclerotic abdominal aortic aneurysms, its frequency is even higher in patients with inflammatory abdominal aortic aneurysms (Nitecki et al., 1996; Hellmann et al., 2007).

3. Pathology

Chronic periaortitis affects the aortic wall and the surrounding retroperitoneum. The classical macroscopic appearance of chronic periaortitis is grossly a whitish and hard periaortic mass which extends between the origin of the renal arteries and the bifurcation of the common iliac vessels and often distorting medially the ureters but histologically there is a continuum of lesions ranging from acute changes to chronic damage (Mitchinson, 1970).

In the early stages of chronic periaortitis, or in patients with a prominent acute-phase reaction, the tissue is highly inflammatory, with numerous lymphocytes, plasma cells, macrophages and scattered eosinophils and loose deposits of collagen matrix in thick, irregular bands (Mitchinson, 1970; Corradi et al., 2007). In late disease, these aspects evolve, either spontaneously or after glucocorticoid therapy, into a relatively acellular fibrous tissue. Perivascular involvement of the thoracic aorta is not uncommon, while rarely atypical localizations such as peri-duodenal, peri-pancreatic and pelvic sites have also been found (Hughes & Buckley, 1993; Corradi et al., 2007).

Microscopic examination shows signs of active mononuclear cell inflammation in a framework of fibrous tissue and fibroblasts (Serra et al, 1980; Gilkeson & Allen, 1996). The background of chronic periaortitis consists of varying degrees of fibrosis, characterized by a mild-to-moderate and mitotically inactive fibroblasts and myofibroblasts, which are immuno-histochemically positive for vimentin and, in the more cellular areas, for α-smooth muscle actin (Vaglio et al., 2006). The fibrous component is particularly abundant in the late stages when the tissue becomes relatively avascular and acellular; its distribution is usually diffuse, but sometimes perivascular and perineural.

The inflammatory infiltrate includes mononuclear cells such as T and B lymphocytes, macrophages and plasma cells, although scattered eosinophils can also be found

(Mitchinson, 1970). The majority of lymphocytes, macrophages and most vascular endothelial cells are HLA-DR-positive. The Ki67 and BerH2 staining is found in B cells and T-helper cells, indicating that these cells were proliferating and activated (Meier et al., 2007). Two main inflammatory patterns are usually seen, perivascular and diffuse. The perivascular aggregates consist mainly of B lymphocytes and a smaller component of plasma cells, macrophages, and T lymphocytes, most of which are CD4+ (Corradi et al., 2007). Sometimes, these follicular aggregates show a germinal center architecture. The sclerotic component consists of thick fascicles of type-I collagen, irregularly distributed along the lesion; a pathological hallmark is the presence of a regular circumferential fibrous bundle surrounding blood vessels and nerves. On the other hand, the diffuse infiltrate has an equal percentage of T cells and B cells. Scattered eosinophils are common, whereas neutrophils are rare (Mitchinson, 1970; Vaglio et al., 2003). In cases of severe inflammation, there may be focal infiltration of the small and medium-sized retroperitoneal vessels, with frank vasculitis and fibrinoid necrosis.

The aortic wall also shows particular changes, such as atherosclerotic degeneration of the intima, medial thinning, and marked adventitial inflammation and fibrosis. The composition of the inflammatory infiltrate in the aortic wall is similar to the retroperitoneal one, with diffuse and perivascular patterns. The adventitial inflammatory infiltrate is often organized in lymphoid follicles (Sakata et al., 2008), which are examples of ectopic lymphoneogenesis and expression of a highly structured inflammatory or immune-mediated response. Adventitial vasa vasorum in aortas of chronic periaortitis show inflammatory infiltration up to frank necrotizing vasculitis, endarteritis obliterans, or obliterative phlebitis (Vaglio et al., 2003; Sakata et al., 2008). These aortic wall changes are found in all chronic periaortitis disease entities, regardless of the presence of aneurysmal dilatation.

It is interesting to note that autopsy studies have documented the presence of adventitial inflammation in aortic sections lacking periaortic fibrosis, which may suggest that aortitis could precede the development of adventitial and periadventitial fibrosis (Mitchinson, 1970). Another autopsy studies have shown that moderate adventitial inflammation and fibrosis may not be limited to the abdominal aorta, but may also involve its thoracic aorta (Mitchinson, 1972).

Molecular analysis of aortic biopsies in patients with chronic periaortitis shows gene transcripts consistent with lymphocyte activation, such as IFN-γ, IL-1α, IL-2 and IL-4, in keeping with the concept that chronic periaortitis is an active inflammatory aortic disease (Ramshaw et al., 1994).

4. Pathogenesis

Chronic periaortitis is idiopathic in nature, and its pathogenesis remains a matter of debate. Initially, it was postulated to represent a local inflammatory reaction to antigens such as ceroid and oxidised low-density lipoproteins (LDL), which can be found in the atherosclerotic plaques of the abdominal aorta (Parums et al., 1986; Parums et al., 1990; Ramshaw & Parums, 1994). Since an intact media constitutes an immunoprivileged site, the capacity of lipids deposited in the intima and media to elicit an inflammatory reaction in the adventitia may depend on the thinning or breach of the media itself, with consequent transit of the lipids. These can be processed by adventitial macrophages and presented to B and T cells, thus eliciting a local inflammatory reaction which eventually leads to adventitial and peri-aortic inflammation and fibrosis.

Morphologic and experimental findings showed that adventitial inflammation also seems to be more marked where the media is thinner (Mitchinson, 1972; Mitchinson 1984; Parums et al., 1990). IgG has been detected in close apposition to extracellular ceroid, and serum antibodies to oxidized LDL and ceroid were more common in patients with chronic periaortitis than in healthy individuals (Parums et al., 1986; Parums et al., 1990). Furthermore, a wide spectrum of adhesion molecules and gene products for cytokines, such as interleukin-1α, interleukin-2, interleukin-4, and interferon-γ, have been detected in the aortic adventitia, thus strengthening the hypothesis that chronic periaortitis is associated with active adventitial chronic inflammation (Ramshaw & Parums, 1994; Ramshaw et al., 1994).

According to this hypothesis, advanced atherosclerosis is a *sine qua non* for the development of chronic periaortitis, which may be an exaggerated local immune response to plaque antigens. The notion that chronic periaortitis is secondary to atherosclerosis is challenged by several findings. There was no substantial difference in the incidence of advanced atherosclerosis between patients with chronic periaortitis and healthy controls (Uibu et al., 2004; Breems et al., 2000). Also, chronic periaortitis may affect patients without atherosclerosis, and it has been reported in pediatric patients (Miller et al., 2003). A recent study showed no significant differences in anti-ox-LDL antibody levels between patients with chronic periaortitis and controls (van Bommel et al., 2011).

Furthermore, a number of findings support the hypothesis that chronic periaortitis may be a manifestation of systemic disease rather than the result of a local reaction. These include its constitutional symptoms, the high acute-phase reactant levels, autoantibody positivity, and the frequent association with other autoimmune diseases (Gilkeson & Allen, 1996; Demko et al., 1997; Vaglio et al., 2003; Marcolongo et al., 2004). Additionally, the association with HLA-DRB1, a marker of autoimmune diseases, is an additional clue to its autoimmune origin (Martorana et al., 2006).

Chronic periaortitis also has histologic similarities to large vessel vasculitis such as giant cell arteritis and Takayasu's arteritis; prominent adventitial inflammation and the involvement of the vasa vasorum (Ramshaw et al., 1994; Vanoli et al., 2005; Vaglio et al., 2006; Salvarani et al., 2008), and sometimes extends beyond the abdominal aorta (Mitchinson 1972; Cid et al., 1998; Jois et al., 2004). In addition, in some patients with chronic periaortitis the disease involves not only the abdominal aorta and the iliac vessels, but also other vascular territories such as the thoracic aorta. This finding was already observed long time ago by autopsy studies (Mitchinson, 1972). Recently, in a study using 18F-fluorodeoxyglucose positron emission tomography, it have also shown that in some patients with chronic periaortitis the high 18F-fluorodeoxyglucose uptake in the abdominal aorta and in the common iliac arteries coexists with a pathologic uptake in the thoracic aorta and its main branches, which confirms the idea that chronic periaortitis is a systemic disease in some cases (Salvarani et al., 2005).

These findings strengthen the idea that chronic periaortitis may originate as a primary arteritis involving the aorta. The perivascular- and sometimes transmural-involvement of vasa vasorum may represent the initial event of the disease. Its centrifugal extension could induce a fibro-inflammatory periaortic reaction, whereas its centripetal spreading could promote atherosclerosis, medial thinning and aneurysm formation (Vaglio & Buzio, 2005; Vaglio et al., 2006).

Structural alterations of the aortic wall seen in chronic periaortitis result in part from degradation of the macromolecules, such as collagen and elastin. These changes are associated with excessive production of matrix metalloproteinases (MMPs), which are assumed to orchestrate the widespread matrix destruction (Freestone et al., 1995). The inflammatory infiltrate is thought to play an etiologic role in aneurysm formation by direct local production of matrix-degrading enzymes and production of cytokines that induce resident mesenchymal cell production of MMPs (Newman et al., 1994). Recent findings suggest that both the local mesenchymal cell expression and the macrophage expression of MMPs are required for aneurysm formation (Longo et al., 2002).

Both fibrillar collagen and elastin are highly organized in the lamellar structure of the aortic media. One potential mechanism for the complementary role of MMP-2 and MMP-9 is that MMP-2 primarily acts as a collagenase-initiating cleavage of the triple helix into one- and three-quarter lengths. The single α chains could then be degraded by MMP-9, releasing the coiled elastin and causing it to become fattened and attenuated. Rupture and expansion rates of abdominal aortic aneurysms have been linked to MMP-2 and MMP-9 levels in tissue and plasma (Petersen et al., 2000). Such observations appear consistent with the increased medial atrophy observed within inflammatory abdominal aortic aneurysms, because activated MMPs may weaken the media by causing destruction of elastic and collagen fibers and smooth muscle cells.

As in many other immune-mediated diseases, environmental and infectious agents probably contribute to the pathogenesis of chronic periaortitis. As mentioned above, asbestos exposure and smoking are established risk factors (Uibu et al., 2004). It has been hypothesized that inflammation within the aortic wall may be a response to infection. Both herpes and cytomegalovirus have been described as potential agents (Tanaka et al., 1994). Recent interest has been focused on Chlamydia pneumoniae, which was found to be more prevalent in aneurysmal than in normal aortic tissue (Tang et al., 2005).

5. Clinical features

The clinical presentation of chronic periaortitis is insidious and vague. Lumbar, abdominal or flank pain is present in about 80% of the patients. It has been described as insidious, persistent and dull, poorly localized, unmodified by movement or rest. If the ureters are involved, the pain may be acute and colic-like (Baker et al., 1987; Vaglio et al., 2003; van Bommel et al., 2009). During the initial phases, patients may find relief using non-steroidal anti-inflammatory drugs, but the beneficial effect of these agents is transient (Gilkeson & Allen, 1996; Vaglio et al., 2006).

In addition to pain, the commonest clinical manifestations are systemic symptoms, most likely related to the inflammatory nature of the disease: about 40 to 80% of patients complain of fatigue, anorexia, weight loss and low-grade fever (Baker et al., 1987; Kardar et al., 2002; Vaglio et al., 2003; Scheel et al., 2009). Ureteral obstruction is the most frequent complication of idiopathic retroperitoneal fibrosis. It involves both ureters in a high percentage of cases (50–80%) and may occur simultaneously (Kardar et al., 2002; van Bommel et al., 2007). Ureteric obstruction is commonly due to edema or inflammation rather than fibrosis. This observation is supported by the fact that the obstruction can improve rapidly with corticosteroid therapy (Baker et al., 1987; Nitecki et al., 1996).

In cases of advanced bilateral ureteral obstruction, oliguria and symptoms secondary to uremic syndrome occur (Baker et al., 1987; Sterpetti et al., 1989; Jois et al., 2004). Varicocele and hydrocele, sometimes associated with testicular pain, are not uncommon, and also probably develop because of compression of the gonadal vessels (Baker et al., 1988; Vaglio et al., 2003). Constipation and claudication are less common. Lower limb edema and deep venous thrombosis may occur, probably as a result of inferior vena cava and iliac vein involvement.

Physical examination usually reveals abdominal tenderness and sometimes a palpable, pulsatile and tender abdominal mass. A periumbilical bruit may be heard in patients with inflammatory abdominal aortic aneurysms (Crawford et al., 1985; Nitecki et al., 1996). The combination of abdominal pain, a pulsatile mass with overlying bruit, constitutional symptoms, and high levels of acute-phase reactants usually distinguish inflammatory abdominal aortic aneurysms from noninflammatory abdominal aortic aneurysms.

Laboratory examinations are useful, but not diagnostic for chronic periaortitis. Acute phase reactants such as the erythrocyte sedimentation rate and C-reactive protein are elevated in more than 80% of patients with active disease, in keeping with the presence of a systemic inflammation and are often used to monitor the clinical course of the disease (Kardar et al., 2002; Marcolongo et al., 2004; Vaglio et al., 2006). The erythrocyte sedimentation rate and C-reactive protein dramatically decrease or even normalize after a few weeks of therapy (van Bommel et al., 2007), whereas their sensitivity in heralding relapses is uncertain (Vaglio et al., 2005). A recent retrospective study investigated whether the erythrocyte sedimentation rate and C-reactive protein levels might predict response to glucocorticoid therapy, but found that baseline erythrocyte sedimentation rate and C-reactive protein did not discriminate between chronic periaortitis patients who experienced disease regression and those who showed mass stabilization or progression (Magrey et al., 2009).

Renal dysfunction is related to the severity of ureteral involvement, but only 18-21% of patients actually experiences end-stage renal failure (Baker et al., 1987; Nitecki et al., 1996). Normochromic, normocytic anemia is often present as a result of systemic chronic inflammation. Leukocytosis, eosinophilia, and polyclonal hypergammaglobulinemia may be disclosed in some patients (Gilkeson & Allen, 1996). If polyclonal hypergammaglobulinemia is present, it is worthwhile assessing serum immunoglobulin levels and, if available, IgG subclasses; IgG4 is high in chronic periaortitis patients with features of IgG4-related systemic disease (Vaglio et al, 2011; J.R. Stone, 2011).

Immunologic and autoimmune tests should always be assessed in patients with chronic periaortitis. Antinuclear antibodies have been reported in up to 60% of patients, whereas anti-dsDNA and antiextractable nuclear antigen antibodies are rare (Vaglio et al., 2003). Rheumatoid factor is not uncommon. The presence of these autoantibodies, although non-organ-specific and often positive at low titers, may be a clue to an autoimmune origin of chronic periaortitis. Alternatively, they may be the earliest manifestation of a smoldering disorder that will clinically emerge late in the course of chronic periaortitis.

On the other hand, certain autoantibodies actually indicate the presence of an associated autoimmune disease. When autoimmune thyroiditis coexists, antithyroglobulin and antithyroid microsome antibodies are positive (Vaglio et al., 2003). P-antineutrophil and C-antineutrophil cytoplasmic antibodies have been detected in a few cases of chronic periaortitis associated with small vessel vasculitis, such as Wegener granulomatosis and microscopic polyangiitis (Kaipiainen-Seppanen et al., 1996; Aslangul et al., 2003).

6. Evidence of systemic autoimmunity in chronic periaortitis

Although it has been considered a localized inflammatory disease secondary to atherosclerosis, several genetic, clinical, laboratory and pathologic findings suggest that chronic periaortitis is a systemic autoimmune disease, perhaps involving a vasculitic process of small and medium vessels (Table 1).

Autoimmune Component	Example
Genetics	Association with HLA-DRB1*03, DRB1*0404, DRB1*15 and HLA-B*08 Association with CC chemokine receptor 5 (CCR5) gene delta 32 polymorphism
Autoantibodies	Antinuclear antibody Anti-thyroid microsome and anti-thyroglobulin antibody Anti-neutrophil cytoplasmic antibody Rheumatoid factor Anti-smooth muscle antibody
Association with Autoimmune diseases	Autoimmune thyroiditis Rapidly progressive glomerulonephritis Systemic vasculitis Rheumatoid arthritis Juvenile rheumatoid arthritis Ankylosing spondylitis Systemic lupus erythematosus Antiphospholipid syndrome IgG4-related systemic disease
Histologic finding	Small vessel vasculitis of retroperitoneal vessels and aortic vasa vasorum Ectopic lymphoid follicles with germinal centers in periaortic retroperitoneum and aortic adventitia
Clinical manifestations	Constitutional symptoms, such as fever, fatigue, weight loss, anorexia and sleep disturbances Systemic involvement of large arteries
Laboratory findings	High erythrocyte sedimentation rate High C-reactive protein Anemia
Treatment response	Rapid response to corticosteroids
Prognosis	Chronic-relapsing course

Table 1. Summary of systemic autoimmune components implicated in chronic periaortitis

6.1 Genetics

Genetic association study revealed that patients with chronic periaortitis were associated with certain genetic markers, which is involved in the immune response and commonly associated with autoimmune or inflammatory disease. The HLA system plays a role in conferring susceptibility to chronic periaortitis (Rasmussen et al., 1997; Martorana et al., 2006). The bias in expression of specific HLA alleles are defining features of autoimmune disease.

The HLA-DRB1*03, DRB1*0404, DRB1*15 and HLA-B*08 alleles was significantly higher in patients with chronic periaortitis. These alleles are a well-known marker of autoimmunity, since it is associated with a number of autoimmune diseases such as systemic lupus erythematosus, rheumatoid arthritis, giant cell arteritis, autoimmune thyroiditis, type 1 diabetes mellitus and myasthenia gravis.

The CC chemokine receptor 5 (CCR5) gene delta 32 polymorphism is associated with aneurysmal chronic periaortitis, which creates a truncated, nonfunctional receptor and probably shifts the immune response toward a Th2 pattern (Boiardi L et al., 2011).

6.2 Autoantibodies

Several autoantibodies are positive in varying proportions of patients, which may be a clue to an autoimmune origin of chronic periaortitis. Antinuclear antibodies are positive in up to 50–60% of the cases, although their titer is often low (Vaglio et al., 2003). Anti-thyroid microsome and anti-thyroglobulin antibodies may be positive in 25–30% (Martorana et al., 2006). Other autoantibodies, such as antineutrophil cytoplasmic antibodies, rheumatoid factor, and anti-smooth muscle may also be positive.

6.3 Association with autoimmune disease

Chronic periaortitis are frequently associated with autoimmune diseases involving other organs or structures. Two recent studies have showed a higher incidence of systemic autoimmune diseases. A case-control study comparing inflammatory abdominal aortic aneurysms and noninflammatory abdominal aortic aneurysms showed a higher incidence of systemic autoimmune diseases in the former group (Haug et al., 2003). In another study of 16 consecutive patients with chronic periaortitis, three had antineutrophil cytoplasmic antibody-positive rapid progressive renal disease, three had autoimmune thyroiditis, and one had rheumatoid arthritis (Vaglio et al., 2003).

Another frequently reported association is systemic vasculitides, which in most cases involve small and medium-sized vessel vasculitis, such as Wegener granulomatosis and polyarteritis nodosa (Akman et al., 1983; Hautekeete et al., 1990; De Roux-Serratrice et al., 2002) or unclassifiable systemic vasculitis (Hellstrom & Perez-Stable, 1966; Littlejohn & Keystone, 1981). Antineutrophil cytoplasmic antibody-associated vasculitic syndromes are more and more often reported.

Chronic periaortitis may frequently be associated with fibroinflammatory disorders affecting other organs, IgG4-related systemic disease, which have an autoimmune origin (Matsumoto et al., 2008; Ito et al., 2008; Kasashima et al., 2008; Sakata et al., 2008). Other rheumatic diseases reported in patients with chronic periaortitis include ankylosing spondylitis, juvenile rheumatoid arthritis, systemic lupus erythematosus and antiphospholipid syndrome (Leblanc et al., 2002; Tsai et al., 1996; Okada et al., 1999; Kim et al., 2010).

6.4 Histologic findings

Two peculiar histopathological findings may be interpreted as manifestations of autoimmunity. Firstly, about half of patients with chronic periaortitis had adventitial inflammation with vasa vasoritis in the small retroperitoneal vessels and the aortic vasa vasorum with mononuclear cell infiltration and sometimes fibrinoid necrosis (Mitchinson, 1970; Vaglio et al., 2003; Lindell et al., 1987). Secondly, the inflammatory infiltrate may be organized in lymphoid structures such as lymphoid follicles with germinal centers in both periaortic retroperitoneum and aortic adventitia (Ramshaw & Parums, 1994). Ectopic lymphoid microstructures with germinal centers have been found in autoimmune disorders, such as the synovium in rheumatoid arthritis (Weyand et al., 2001).

6.5 Clinical manifestations

Most patients with chronic periaortitis often complain of constitutional symptoms, such as fever, fatigue, weight loss, anorexia and sleep disturbances, which probably reflect the systemic inflammatory status (Baker et al., 1987; Vaglio et al., 2003). At least in a subgroup of patients, chronic periaortitis is a vasculitis affecting large vessels (Vaglio et al., 2011).

6.6 Laboratory findings

Chronic periaortitis usually present with high concentrations of acute-phase reactants such as erythrocyte sedimentation rate and C-reactive protein, varying degrees of anemia and, in a high percentage of cases, azotemia , which reflect the systemic inflammation (Kardar et al., 2002; Vaglio et al., 2006). The erythrocyte sedimentation rate and C-reactive protein can also be used to monitor the disease course (van Bommel et al., 2007).

6.7 Treatment response

The clinical manifestations of chronic periaortitis promptly subside after the initiation of glucocorticoids therapy, which again is well in agreement with their inflammatory nature. In most patients, they induce remission of the clinical symptoms, normalization of the acute-phase reactant levels, reduction in size of the retroperitoneal mass and also resolution of the obstructive complications (Kardar et al., 2002; Marcolongo et al., 2004; van Bommel et al., 2007; Magrey et al., 2009).

However, glucocorticoids have various significant side effects, which sometimes limit their prolonged use. The combination of glucocorticoids and immunosuppressants such as azathioprine, cyclophosphamide and methotrexate has recently been reported to yield favorable results in patients with chronic periaortitis (Marcolongo et al., 2004; Warnatz et al., 2005).

6.8 Prognosis

As is the case in many inflammatory and autoimmune diseases, chronic periaortitis also has a chronic-relapsing course. The frequency of relapses may depend on the treatment approach, as they occur in 10% to 50% of patients treated with surgery alone and in about 10% when combined immunosuppressive and surgical therapies are used (Baker et al., 1988).

7. IgG4-related systemic disease

In recent years, numerous studies have reported chronic periaortitis in association with IgG4-related systemic disease, a group of autoimmune and fibrosing conditions characterized by high serum levels of IgG4 and tissue infiltration by IgG4-bearing plasma cells (Vaglio et al, 2011; J.R. Stone, 2011). These conditions share common histopathologic characteristics, such as diffuse lymphoplasmacytic infiltration, irregular fibrosis, eosinophilic infiltration, and obliterative phlebitis (Neild et al., 2006; Deshpande et al., 2006; Masaki et al., 2009).

7.1 Idiopathic peritoneal fibrosis with IgG4-related systemic disease

It has become clear that in a subset of patients with idiopathic retroperitoneal fibrosis, the disorder is in fact occurring in the setting of IgG4-related systemic disease. For 10 years, there were several reports that autoimmune pancreatitis could be associated with inflammatory masses within the retroperitoneum, and it was later recognized that both conditions were a manifestation of IgG4-related systemic disease (J.R. Stone, 2011).

In those reports revealed that the retroperitoneal involvement is typically not entirely diffuse, but present primarily as inflammatory masses that often primarily involve the abdominal aorta, the kidneys or the ureters (Hamano et al., 2002; Miyajima et al., 2006; Tanabe et al., 2006). The inflammatory masses are composed of lymphoplasmacytic inflammation and fibrosis with a substantial number of the plasma cells expressing IgG4. The nearly all patients revealed an aortic adventitial involvement, even in the absence of aortic aneurysm formation.

In a recent study of retroperitoneal biopsies of patients with idiopathic retroperitoneal fibrosis, 10 of 17 cases were felt to be due to IgG-related systemic disease (Zen et al., 2009). In these 10 patients, the fraction of plasma cells staining for IgG4 ranged from 35 to 76% compared with 0 to 10% for the other seven patients. Furthermore, for the patients with IgG4-related disease, the mean serum IgG4 concentration was 695 mg/dl (range 154-2330 mg/dl) compared with 30 mg/dl (range 10–53 mg/dl) for the other seven patients.

7.2 Inflammatory abdominal aortic aneurysms with IgG4-related systemic disease

There are several reports which have indicated that a subset of inflammatory abdominal aortic aneurysms cases is in fact a result of IgG4-related systemic disease (Sakata et al., 2008; Kasashima et al., 2008; Qian et al., 2009). A recent study comparing 11 cases of inflammatory abdominal aortic aneurysms to 12 cases of atherosclerotic abdominal aortic aneurysms and demonstrated that the aneurysms defined as inflammatory contained more IgG4+ plasma cells than those defined as atherosclerotic. However, in that study there was no clear delineation as to which inflammatory aneurysms actually represented involvement by IgG4-related systemic disease. In addition, the fraction of plasma cells expressing IgG4 was not reported for either aneurysms group, making it unclear if the enhanced number of IgG4+ plasma cells was simply a manifestation of more plasma cells in general being present in the aneurysms labeled as inflammatory.

There have been several cases reported of inflammatory abdominal aortic aneurysms, which were attributed to IgG4-related systemic disease, and which included pathologic evaluation of the aorta (Kasashima et al., 2008; Ito et al., 2008; Qian et al., 2009). Pathologically, most cases of IgG-4 related inflammatory abdominal aortic aneurysms showed the predominant involvement in adventitia with high fraction of IgG4+ infiltrating plasma cells and high serum IgG levels (J.R. Stone, 2011).

Kasashima et al. reported that four of 10 cases (40%) of inflammatory abdominal aortic aneurysm were due to IgG4-related systemic disease with prominent IgG4+ plasma cell infiltration and high-IgG4 serum levels, whereas the remaining six had a mild (IgG4+ and total) plasma cell infiltration. Inflammation was more evident and tissue eosinophilia predominated in the IgG4-related inflammatory abdominal aortic aneurysms, whereas some degree of neutrophilic infiltration and only rare eosinophils were found in the non-IgG4-related inflammatory abdominal aortic aneurysms. Because inflammatory aneurysms may represent 2–15% of all abdominal aortic aneurysms, this would suggest 1–6% of all abdominal aortic aneurysms could be due to IgG4-related inflammatory abdominal aortic aneurysms (J.R. Stone, 2011).

7.3 Thoracic aortitis with IgG4-related systemic disease

Until now, the six cases of thoracic aortitis due to IgG4-related systemic disease reported, which derived from surgical resections (Khosroshahi et al., 2009; J.H. Stone et al., 2009; Ishida et al., 2009; J.H. Stone et al., 2010; Kasashima et al., 2010). All six patients were men in an old age (65–74 years). The arch was the most commonly involved in five cases, with two cases having involvement of the ascending aorta, and only one case having involvement of the descending aorta. Five of the six patients presented with an aneurysm.

According to histologic assessment, all displayed a prominent lymphoplasmacytic infiltrate, with a high percentage of the plasma cells staining for IgG4 (74–89%). In addition, at least five patients showed an obstructive phlebitis within the adventitia. In three cases, there was a marked predominance for the adventitia compared with the media and intima (J.R. Stone, 2011). Serum IgG4 level was found to be markedly elevated in 2 patients who tested it and both of these patients had documented extra-aortic involvement.

Assessment of all thoracic aortitis cases surgically resected in a 5-year at one institute revealed that IgG4-related systemic disease was responsible for three of four cases of lymphoplasmacytic aortitis and 9% of all cases of thoracic aortitis (J.H. Stone et al., 2010). According to that study, IgG4-related aortitis was present in 0.5% of all thoracic aorta resections. In a subsequent study from Japan, assessment of 125 thoracic aorta resections revealed two cases of IgG4-related aortitis, indicating 1.6% of all resected thoracic aortas contained IgG4-related aortitis (Khosroshahi et al., 2010).

Although much remains to be clarified with regard to the pathogenesis of chronic periaortitis, it is conceivable that IgG4 may represent a link between chronic periaortitis and systemic fibro-inflammatory conditions. The analysis of IgG4-related cases may provide additional clues supporting the possible systemic large-vessel involvement in chronic periaortitis (Vaglio et al., 2011).

8. Conclusion

Chronic periaortitis is a chronic disease characterized by a retroperitoneal fibroinflammatory reaction surrounding the abdominal aorta, which may or may not be dilated. Although it has been considered a localized inflammatory response to advanced atherosclerosis, there is increasing evidence supporting the hypothesis of an underlying systemic autoimmune disease with vasculitic process involving small and medium vessels. Further studies are warranted in order to elucidate the potential triggers of the disease, the pathways leading to the aortic-periaortic inflammation and to the disproportionate fibrogenic reaction.

9. References

Akman N., Avanoglu Y., Karabay K., Erek E., Tokgoz A., Aras E., Girisken G., Tuzuner N. & Avanoglu H. (1983). Henoch-Schoenlein purpura and retroperitoneal fibrosis. *Acta Haematologica*, Vol.70, No.6, (December 1983), pp. 400-401, ISSN 0001-5792

Aslangul E., Ranque B. & Papo T. (2003). Pseudotumoral retroperitoneal fibrosis and localized vasculitis with very high serum levels of anti-PR3 ANCA. *The American Journal of Medicine*, Vol.105, No.3, (August 2003), pp. 250–252, ISSN 0002-9343

Baker LR., Mallinson WJ., Gregory MC., Menzies EA., Cattell WR., Whitfield HN., Hendry WF., Wickham JE. & Joekes AM. (1987). Idiopathic retroperitoneal fibrosis. A retrospective analysis of 60 cases. *British Journal of Urology*, Vol.60, No.6, (December 1987), pp. 497–503, ISSN 0007-1331

Boiardi L., Vaglio A., Nicoli D., Farnetti E., Palmisano A., Pipitone N., Maritati F., Casali B., Martorana D., Moroni G., Buzio C. & Slvarani C. (2011). CC chemokine receptor 5 polymorphism in chronic periaortitis. *Rheumatology (Oxford)*, Vol.50, No.6, (June 2010), pp. 1025-1032 ISSN 1462-0324

Breems DA., Haye H. & van der Meulen J. (2000), The role of advanced atherosclerosis in idiopathic retroperitoneal fibrosis. *The Netherlands Journal of Medicine*, Vol.56, No.2, (February 2000), pp. 38–44, ISSN 0300-2977

Cid MC., Font C., Coll-Vinent B. & Grau M. (1998). Large vessel vasculitides. *Current Opinion in Rheumatology*, Vol.10, No.1, (January 1998), pp. 18–28, ISSN 1040-8711

Corradi D., Maestri R., Palmisano A., Bosio S., Greco P., Mneti L., Ferretti S., Cobelli R., Moroni G., Dei Tos AP., Buzio C. & Vaglio A. (2007). Idiopathic retroperitoneal fibrosis: clinicopathologic features and differential diagnosis. *Kidney International*, Vol.72, No.6 (September2007), pp. 742–753, ISSN 0085-2538

Crawford JL., Stowe CL., Safi HJ., Hallman CH. & Crawford ES. (1985). Inflammatory aneurysms of the aorta. *Journal of Vascular Surgery*, Vol.2, No.1, (January 1985), pp. 113-124, ISSN 0741-5214

Davidson A. & Diamond B. (2001). Autoimmune diseases. *New England Journal of Medicine*, Vol.345, No.5, (August 2001), pp. 340–350, ISSN 0028-4793'

Demko TM., Diamond JR. & Groff J. (1997). Obstructive nephropathy as a result of retroperitoneal fibrosis: a review of its pathogenesis and associations. *Journal of American Society of Nephrology*, Vol.8, No.4, (April 1997), pp. 684–688, ISSN 1046-6673

De Roux-Serratrice C., Serratrice J., Granel B., Dsdier P., Bartoli JM., Pache X., Astoul P., Garbe L., Branchereau A. & Weiller PJ. (2002). Periaortitis heralding Wegener's granulomatosis. *Journal of Rheumatology*, Vol.29, No.2, (February 2002), pp. 392–394, ISSN 0315-162X

Deshpande V., Chicano S., Finkelberg D., Selig MK., Mino-Kenudson M., Brugge WR., Colvin RB. & Lauwers GY. (2006). Autoimmune pancreatitis: a systemic immune complex mediated disease. *The American Journal of Surgical Pathology*, Vol.20, No.12, (December 2006), pp. 1537–1545, ISSN 0147-5185

Doolin EJ., Goldstein H., Kessler B., Vinocur C. & Marchildon MB. (1987). Familial retroperitoneal fibrosis. *Journal of Pediatric Surgery*, Vol.33, No.12 (December 1987), pp. 1092–1094, ISSN 0022-3468

Duffy PG., Johnston SR. & Donaldson RA. (1984). Idiopathic retroperitoneal fibrosis in twins. *Journal of Urology*, Vol.131, No.4, (April 1984), pp. 746, ISSN 0022-5374

Freestone T., Turner RJ., Coady A., Higman DJ., Greenhalgh RM. & Powell JT. (1995). Inflammation and matrix metalloproteinases in the enlarging abdominal aortic aneurysm. *Arteriosclerosis, Thrombosis, and Vascular Biology*, Vol.15, No.8, (August 1995), pp. 1145–1151, ISSN 1079-5642

Haug, ES., Skomsvoll, JF., Jacobsen, G., Halvorson, TB., Saether, OD. & Myhre, HO. (2003). Inflammatory aortic aneurysm is associated with increased incidence of autoimmune disease. *Journal of Vascular Surgery*, Vol.38, No.3, (September 2003), pp. 492-497, ISSN 0741-5214

Hautekeete ML., Babany G., Marcellin P., Gayno S., Palazzo E., Erlinger S. & Benhamou JP. (1990). Retroperitoneal fibrosis after surgery for aortic aneurysm in a patient with periarteritis nodosa: successful treatment with corticosteroids. *Journal of Internal Medicine*, Vol.228, No.5, (November 1990), pp. 533–536, ISSN 0954-6820

Hellstrom HR. & Perezstable EC. (1966). Retroperitoneal fibrosis with disseminated vasculitis and intrahepatic sclerosing cholangitis. (1966). *The American Journal of Medicine*, Vol.40, No.2, (February 1966), pp. 184-187, ISSN 0002-9343

Hellmann DB., Grand DJ. & Freischlag JA. (2007). Inflammatory abdominal aortic aneurysm. *JAMA*, Vol.297, No.4, (January 2007), pp. 395–400, ISSN 1538-3598

Hughes D. & Buckley PJ. (1993). Idiopathic retroperitoneal fibrosis is a macrophage-rich process. Implications for its pathogenesis and treatment. *The American Journal of Surgical Pathology*, Vol.17, No.5, (May 1993), pp. 482–90, ISSN 0147-5185

Gilkeson GS. & Allen NB. (1996). Retroperitoneal fibrosis. A true connective tissue disease. *Rheumatic disease clinics of North America*, Vol.22, No.1, (February 1996), pp. 23-38, ISSN 0889-857X

Ishida M., Hotta M., Kushima R., Asai T. & Okabe H. (2009). IgG4-related inflammatory aneurysm of the aortic arch. *Pathology International*, Vol.59, No.4, (April 2009), pp. 269–273, ISSN 1440-1827

Ito H., Kaizaki Y., Noda Y., Fujii S. & Yamamoto S. (2008). IgG4-related inflammatory abdominal aortic aneurysm associated with autoimmune pancreatitis. *Pathology International*, Vol.58, No.7, (July 2008), pp. 421–6, ISSN 1440-1827

Jagadesham VP., Scott DJ. & Carding SR. (2008). Abdominal aortic aneurysms: an autoimmune disease? *Trends in Moleular Medicine*, Vol.14, No.12, (December 2008), pp. 522-529, ISSN 1471-4914

Jois RN., Gaffney K., Marshall T. & Scott DGI. (2004). Chronic periaortitis. *Rheumatology (Oxford)*, Vol.43, No.11, (November 2004), pp. 1441–1446, ISSN 1462-0324

Kaipiainen-Seppanen O., Jantunen E., Kuusisto J. & Marin S. (1996). Retroperitoneal fibrosis with antineutrophil cytoplasmic antibodies. *Journal of Rheumatology*, Vol.23, No.4, (April 1996), pp. 779–781, ISSN 0315-162X

Kardar AH., Kattan S., Lindstedt E. & Hanash K. (2002). Steroid therapy for idiopathic retroperitoneal fibrosis: dose and duration. *Journal Urology*, Vol.168, No.2, (August 2002), pp. 550–555, ISSN 0022-5347

Kasashima S., Zen Y., Kawashima A., Konishi K., Sasaki H., Endo M., Kawakami K., Zen Y. & Nakanuma Y. (2008). Inflammatory abdominal aortic aneurysm: close relationship to IgG4-related periaortitis. *American Journal of Surgical Pathology*, Vol.32, No.2, (February 2008), pp. 197–204, ISSN 0147-5185

Kasashima S., Zen Y., Kawashima A., Endo M., Matsumoto Y., Kasashima F., Ohtake H. & Nakanuma Y. (2010). A clinicopathologic study of immunoglobulin G4-related sclerosing disease of the thoracic aorta. *Journal of Vascular Surgery*, Vol.52, No.6, (December 2010), pp. 1587-1595, ISSN 1097-6809

Khosroshahi A., Stone JR., Pratt DS., Deshpande V. & Stone JH. (2009). Painless jaundice with serial multiorgan dysfunction. *Lancet*, Vol.373, No.9673, (April 2009), pp. 1494, ISSN 1474-547X

Kim HA., Won JH. & Suh CH. (2010). Chronic periaortitis with antiphospholipid syndrome. *International Journal of Rheumatic Diseases*, Vol.13, No.1, (February 2010), pp. 91-93, ISSN 1756-185X

Leblanc CM., Inman R., Dent P., Smith C., Babyn P. & Laxer RM. (2002). Retroperitoneal fibrosis: an extraarticular manifestation of ankylosing spondylitis. *Arthritis Rheumatism,* Vol.47, No.2, (April 2002), pp. 210–214, ISSN 1474-547X

Lindell OI., Sariola HV. & Lehtonen TA. (1987). The occurrence of vasculitis in perianeurysmal fibrosis. *Journal of Urology,* Vol.138, No.4, (October 1987), pp. 727-729, ISSN 0022-5347

Littlejohn GO. & Keystone EC. (1981). The association of retroperitoneal fibrosis with systemic vasculitis and HLA-B27: a case report and review of the literature. *Journal of Rheumatology,* Vol.8, No.4, (July 1981), pp. 623-629, ISSN 0315-162X

Longo GM., Xiong W., Greiner TC., Zhao Y., Fiotti N. & Baxter BT. (2002). Matrix metalloproteinases 2 and 9 work in concert to produce aortic aneurysms. *The Journal of Clinical Investigation,* Vol.110, No.5, (September 2002), pp. 625–632, ISSN 0021-9783

Magrey MN., Husni ME., Kushner I. & Calabrese LH. (2009). Do acute-phase reactants predict response to glucocorticoid therapy in retroperitoneal fibrosis? *Arthritis Rheumatism,* Vol.61, No.5, (May 2009), pp. 674–679, ISSN 1474-547X

Marcolongo R., Tavolini IM., Laveder F., Busa M., Voventa F., Bassi P. & Semenzato G. (2004). Immunosuppressive therapy for idiopathic retroperitoneal fibrosis: a retrospective analysis of 26 cases. *The American Journal of Medicine,* Vol.116, No.3, (February 2004), pp. 194–197, ISSN 0002-9343

Martorana D., Vaglio A., Greco P., Zanetti A., Moroni G., Salvarani C., Savi M., Buzio C. & Neri TM. (2006). Chronic periaortitis and HLA-DRB1*03: another clue to an autoimmune origin. *Arthritis Rheumatism,* Vol.55, No.1 (February 2006), pp. 126–130, ISSN 0004-3591

Masaki Y., Dong L., Kurose N., Kitagawa K., Morikawa Y., Yamamoto M., Takahashi H., Shinomura Y., Imai K., Saeki T., Azumi A., Nakada S., Sygiyama E., Matsui S., Origuchi T., Nishiyama S., Nishimori I., Nojima T., Yamada K., Kawano M., Kneko M., Miyazaki K., Twubota K. Eguchi K., Tomoda K., Sawaki T., Kawanami T., Tanaka M., Fukushima T., Sugai S. & Umehara H. (2009). Proposal for a new clinical entity, IgG4-positive multiorgan lymphoproliferative syndrome: analysis of 64 cases of IgG4-related disorders. *Annals of the Rheumatic Disease,* Vol.68, No.8, (August 2009), pp. 1310–1315, ISSN 1468-2060

Matsumoto Y., Kasashima S., Kawashima A., Kawashima A., Sasake H., Endo M., Kawakami K., Zen Y. & Nakanuma Y. (2008). A case of multiple immunoglobulin G4-related periarteritis: a timorous lesion of the coronary artery and abdominal aortic aneurysm. *Human Pathology,* Vol.39, No.6, (June 2008), pp. 975–80, ISSN 1532-8392

Meier P., Vogt B. & Blanc E. (2007). Rethinking the Triggering Inflammatory Processes of Chronic Periaortitis. *Nephron Experimental Nephrology,* Vol.105, No.1, (January 2007), pp. e17–e23, ISSN 1660-2129

Miller OF., Snith LJ., Ferrara EX., McAleer IM. & Kaplan GW. (2003). Presentation of idiopathic retroperitoneal fibrosis in the pediatric population. *Journal of Pediatric Surgery,* Vol.38, No.11, (November 2003), pp. 1685-1688, ISSN 1531-5037

Mitchinson MJ. (1970). The pathology of idiopathic retroperitoneal fibrosis. *Journal of Clinical Pathology,* Vol.23, No.8, (November 1970), pp. 681–689, ISSN 0021-9746

Mitchinson MJ. (1984). Chronic periaortitis and periarteritis. *Histopathology*, Vol.8, No.4, (July 1984), pp. 589–600, ISSN 0309-0167

Miyajima N., Koike H., Kawaguchi M., Zen Y., Takahashi K. & Hara N. (2006). Idiopathic retroperitoneal fibrosis associated with IgG4-positive plasmacyte infiltrations and idiopathic chronic pancreatitis. *International Journal of Urology*, Vol.13, No.11, (November 2006), pp. 1442–1444, ISSN 0919-8172

Neild GH., Rodriguez-Justo M., Wall C. & Connolly JO. (2006). Hyper-IgG4 disease: report and characterisation of a new disease. *BMC Medicine*, Vol.4, (October 2006), pp. 23, ISSN 1741-7015

Newman KM., Jean-Claude J., Li H., Ramey WG. & Tilson MD. (1994). Cytokines that activate proteolysis are increased in abdominal aortic aneurysms. *Circulation*, Vol.90, No.5, (November 1994), pp. II224–227, ISSN 0009-7322

Nitecki SS., Hallett JW Jr., Stanson A., Ilstrup DM., Bower TC., Cherry KJ Jr., Gloviczki P. & Pairolero PC. (1996). Inflammatory abdominal aortic aneurysms: a case-control study. *Journal of Vascular Surgery*, Vol.23, No.5, (May 1996), pp. 860–869, ISSN 0741-5214

Okada H., Takahira S., Sugahara S., Nakamoto H. & Suzuki H. (1999). Retroperitoneal fibrosis and systemic lupus erythematosus. *Nephrology, Dialysis, Transplantation*, Vol.14, No.5, (May 1999), pp. 1300–1302, ISSN 0931-0509

Parums DV., Chadwick DR. & Mitchinson MJ. (1986). The localisation of immunoglobulin in chronic periaortitis. *Atherosclerosis*, Vol.61, No.2, (August 1986), pp. 117–125, ISSN 0021-9150

Parums DV. (1990). The spectrum of chronic periaortitis. *Histopathology*, Vol.16, No.6, (December 1990), pp. 423–431, ISSN 0309-0167

Pennell RC., Hollier LH., Lie JT., Bernatz PE., Joyce JW., Pairolero PC., Cherry KJ. & Hallett JW. (1985). Inflammatory abdominal aortic aneurysms: a thirty-year review. *Journal of Vascular Surgery*, Vol.2, No.6, (November 1985), pp. 859-869, ISSN 0741-5214

Petersen E., Gineitis A., Wagberg F. & Angquist KA. (2000). Activity of matrix metalloproteinase-2 and -9 in abdominal aortic aneurysms. Relation to size and rupture. *Eur J Vasc Endovasc Surg*,Vol.20, No.5, (November 2000), pp. 457–461, ISSN 1078-5884

Qian Q., Kashani KB. & Miller DV. Ruptyred abdominal aortic aneurysm related to IgG4 periaortitis. (2009). *New England Journal of Medicine*, Vol.361, No.11, (September 2009), pp. 1121-1123, ISSN 1533-4406

Ramshaw AL. & Parums DV. (1994). The distribution of adhesion molecules in chronic periaortitis. *Histopathology*, Vol.24, No.1, (January 1994), pp. 23–32, ISSN 0309-0167

Ramshaw AL., Roskell DE. & Parums DV. (1994). Cytokine gene expression in aortic adventitial inflammation associated with advanced atherosclerosis (chronic periaortitis). *Journal of Clinical Pathology*, Vol.47, No.8, (August 1994), pp.721–727, ISSN 0021-9746

Rasmussen TE. & Hallett Jr JW. (1997). Inflammatory aortic aneurysms. A clinical review with new perspectives in pathogenesis. *Annals of Surgery*, Vol.225, No.2, (February 1997), pp. 155–164, ISSN 0003-4932

Rasmussen TE., Hallett Jr JW., Metzger RL., Richardson DM., Harmsen WS., Goronzy JJ. & Weyand CM. (1997). Genetic risk factors in inflammatory abdominal aortic aneurysms: polymorphic residue 70 in theHLA-DRB1 gene as a key genetic element. *Journal of Vascular Surgery*, Vol.25, No.2, (February 1997), pp. 356–364, ISSN 0741-5214

Sakata N., Tashiro T., Uesugi N., Kewara T., Furuya K., Hirata Y., Iwasaki H. & Kokima M. (2008). IgG4-positive plasma cells in inflammatory abdominal aortic aneurysm: the possibility of an aortic manifestation of IgG4-related sclerosing disease. *The American Journal of Surgical Pathology*, Vol.32, No.4, (April 2008), pp. 553–559, ISSN 0147-5185

Salvarani C., Pipitone N., Versari A., Vaglio A., Serafini D., Bajocchi G., Slvo D., Buzio C., Greco P. & Boiardi L. (2005). Positron emission tomography (PET): evaluation of chronic periaortitis. *Arthritis Rheumatism*, Vol.53, No.2, (April 2005), pp. 298–303, ISSN 0004-3591

Serra RM., Engle JE., Jones RE. & Schoolwerth AV. (1980). Perianeurysmal retroperitoneal fibrosis. An unusual cause of renal failure. *The American Journal of Medicine*, Vol.68, No.1, (January 1980), pp. 149-153, ISSN 0002-93432

Singh K., Bonaa KH., Jacobsen BK., Bjork L. & Solberg. (2001). Prevalence of and risk factors for abdominal aortic aneurysms in a population-based study: The Tromso Study. *American Journal of Epidemiology*, Vol.154, No.3, (August 2001), pp. 236–244, ISSN 0002-9262

Sterpetti AV., Hunter WJ., Feldhaus RJ., Chansan P., McNamara M., Cisternino S. & Schultz RD. (1989). Inflammatory aneurysms of the abdominal aorta: incidence, pathologic, and etiologic considerations. *Journal of Vascular Surgery*, Vol.9, No.5, (May 1989), pp. 643-650, ISSN 0741-5214

Stone JH., Khosroshahi A., Hilgenberg A., Spooner A., Isselbacher EM. & Stone JR. (2009). IgG4-related systemic disease and lymphoplasmacytic aortitis. *Arthritis Rheumatism*, Vol.60, No.10, (October 2009), pp. 3139–3145, ISSN 1474-547X

Stone JH., Khosroshahi A., Deshpande V. & Stone JR. (2010). IgG4-related systemic disease accounts for a significant proportion of thoracic lymphoplasmacytic aortitis cases. *Arthritis Care Research*, Vol.62, No.3, (March 2010), pp. 316–322, ISSN 2151-4658

Stone JR. (2011). Aortitis, periaortitis, and retroperitoneal fibrosis, as manifestations of IgG4-related systemic disease *Current Opinion in Rheumatology*, Vol.23, No. 1, (January 2011), pp. 88–94, ISSN 1531-6963

Tanaka S., Komori K., Okadome K., Sugimachi K. & Mori R. (1994). Detection of active cytomegalovirus infection in inflammatory aortic aneurysms with RNA polymerase chain reaction. *Journal of Vascular Surgery*, Vol.20, No.2, (August 1994), pp. 235–243, ISSN 0741-5214

Tang T., Boyle JR., Dixon AK. & Varty K. (2005). Inflammatory abdominal aortic aneurysms. *European Journal of Vascular Surgery*, Vol.29, No.4, (April 2005), pp. 353–362, ISSN 1078-5884

Tsai TC., Chang PY., Chen BF., Huang FY. & Shih SL. (1996). Retroperitoneal fibrosis and juvenile rheumatoid arthritis. *Pediatric Nephrology*, Vol.10, No.2, (April 1996), pp. 208-209, ISSN 0931-041X

Uibu T., Oksa P., Auvinen A., Honkanen E., Metsarinne K., Saha H., Uitti J. & Roto P. (2004). Asbestos exposure as a risk factor for retroperitoneal fibrosis. *Lancet*, Vol.363, No.9419, (May 2004), pp. 1422–1426, 1474-547X

Vaglio A., Corradi D., Manenti L., Ferretti L., Garini G. & Buzio C. (2003). Evidence of autoimmunity in chronic periaortitis: a prospective study. *The American Journal of Medicine*, Vol.114, No.6, (April 2003), pp. 454–462, ISSN 0002-9343

Vaglio A. & Buzio C. (2005). Chronic periaortitis: a spectrum of diseases. *Current Opinion in Rheumatology*, Vol.17, No.1, (January 2005), pp. 34–40, ISSN 1531-6963

Vaglio A., Salvarani C. & Buzio C. (2006). Retroperitoneal fibrosis. *Lancet*, Vol.367, No. 9506, (January 2006), pp. 241–251, ISSN 1474-547X

Vaglio A., Greco P., Corradi D., Palmisani A., Martorana D., Ronda N. & Buzio C. (2006). Autoimmune aspects of chronic periaortitis. *Autoimmunity Reviews*, Vol.5, No.7, (August 2006), pp. 458–464, ISSN 1568-9972

Vaglio A., Pipitone N. & Salvarani C. (2011). Chronic periaortitis: a large-vessel vasculitis? *Current Opinion in Rheumatology*, Vol.23, No.1, (January 2011), pp. 1-6, ISSN 1531-6963

van Bommel EF., Siemes C., Hak LE., van der Veer SJ. & Hendriksz TR. (2007). Long-term renal and patient outcome in idiopathic retroperitoneal fibrosis treated with prednisone. *American Journal of Kidney Disease*, Vol.49, No.5, (May 2007), pp. 615–625, ISSN 1523-6838

van Bommel EF., van Tits LJ., van den Berg EA., Prins J. & Stalenhoef AF. (2011). Autoantibodies against oxidized low-density lipoprotein and lipid profile in patients with chronic periaortitis: case–control study. *Rheumatol International*, Vol 31, No.2, (February 2011), pp. 201-208, ISSN 1437-160X

Vanoli M., Daina E., Salvarani C., Sabbadini MG., Rossi C., Bacchiani G., Schieppati A., Baldissera E., Bertolini G. & Itaka Study Group. (2005). Takayasu's arteritis: A study of 104 Italian patients. *Arthritis Rheumatism*, Vol.53, No.1, (February 2005), pp. 100–107, ISSN 0004-3591

von Fritschen U., Malzfeld E., Clasen A. & Kortmann H. (1999). Inflammatory abdominal aortic aneurysm: A postoperative course of retroperitoneal fibrosis. *Journal of Vascular Surgery*, Vol.30, No.6, (December 1999), pp. 1090–1098, ISSN 0741-5214

Warnatz K., Keskin AG., Uhl C., Scholz C., Katzenwadel A., Vaith P., Peter HH. & Walker UA. (2005). Immunosuppressive therapy of chronic periaortitis: a retrospective study of 20 patients with chronic periaortitis and a review of the literature. *Annals of the Rheumatic Disease*, Vol.64, No.6, (June 2005), pp. 828–833, ISSN 0003-4967

Weyand CM., Kurtin PJ. & Goronzy JJ. (2001). Ectopic lymphoid organogenesis: a fast track for autoimmunity. The *American Journal of Pathology*, Vol.159, No.3, (September 2001), pp. 787-793, ISSN 0002-9440

Yusuf K., Murat B., Unal A., Ulku K., Taylan K., Ozerdem O., Erdal Y. & Tahsin Y. (2007). Inflammatory abdominal aortic aneurysm: predictors of long-term outcome in a casecontrol study. *Surgery*, Vol.141, No.1, (January 2007), pp. 83–89, ISSN 0886-0440

Zen Y., Onodera M., Inoue D., Kitao A., Matsui O., Nohara T., Namiki M., Kasashima S., Kawashima A., Matsumoto Y., Katayanagi K., Murata T., Ishizawa S., Hosaka N., Hosaks N., Kuriki K. & Kakanuma Y. (2009). Retroperitoneal fibrosis: a clinicopathologic study with respect to immunoglobulin G4. *The American Journal of Surgical Pathology*, Vol.33, No.12, (December 2009), pp. 1833–1839, ISSN 1532-0979

17

Endothelial Progenitor Cells: New Targets to Control Autoimmune Disorders

Sarah L. Brice, Andrew J. Sakko, Pravin Hissaria and Claudine S. Bonder
Human Immunology, Centre for Cancer Biology, SA Pathology, Co-operative Research Centre for Biomarker Translation, LaTrobe University, Australia

1. Introduction

The formation of blood vessels is essential for preparing a closed circulatory system in the body, and for supply of oxygen and nutrients to all tissues and organs. One of the key mechanisms behind many autoimmune diseases is abnormal blood vessel structure and function. This dysfunction is reflected in some of the serious manifestations of rheumatoid arthritis (RA), type 1 diabetes mellitus (T1DM) and systemic sclerosis (SSc) that are currently difficult to treat, such as loss of fingers due to reduced blood flow, kidney failure due to renal hypertensive crisis and heart failure due to pulmonary arterial hypertension. The cells that line blood vessels (endothelial cells) not only confine blood to the vessels but actively participate in the recruitment of circulating cell subsets to sites of inflammation and vascular permeability for the exchange of solutes and gases. Collectively, endothelial cells play many roles in the development and maintenance of blood vessels. Blood vessel development occurs primarily via one of two mechanisms, angiogenesis (the generation of blood vessels from pre-existing vasculature) and vasculogenesis (the recruitment of endothelial progenitor cells from the bone marrow to sites of vascularisation). In recent decades, extensive studies have revealed that a variety of factors and their receptors regulate angiogenesis in vertebrates, including vascular endothelial growth factor (VEGF)-VEGFRs, angiopoietin-Tie, Ephrins-EphRs and Delta-Notch (reviewed by Karamysheva (Karamysheva, 2008)). Indeed, targeting these molecules has resulted in significant advances in the treatment of cancer and cardiovascular disease. However, the burden of diseases that involve vascular dysfunction is immense and continues to rise with drug resistance, intolerance and ineffectiveness being significant contributors. Less is known about the mechanisms underpinning vasculogenesis and despite an explosion of research in this area over the past decade we are yet to fully exploit these cells for therapeutic benefit (Sen et al., 2011, Sieveking and Ng, 2009). This chapter discusses whether the endothelial progenitor cells (EPCs) from patients with autoimmune diseases, such as RA, T1DM and SSc, behave differently from normal EPCs and whether there are factors in the serum of these patients that may be responsible for this abnormal behaviour. The altered behaviour of EPCs in patients with autoimmune disease is poorly understood, based on limited studies to date. This chapter addresses whether EPCs would be a prime target for therapeutic intervention in the serious complications of autoimmune disease.

2. Vascular dysfunction in autoimmune disease

2.1 Rheumatoid arthritis

RA is a chronic and debilitating autoimmune disease that affects the joints. The disease is characterised by inflammation of the synovial tissue, which lines the joints and tendons. In healthy tissue, the synovium is made up of synovial cells, a network of capillaries and lymphatic vessels, and a well-organized matrix containing proteoglycan aggregates. Between the cartilage and synovium is the synovial fluid, which nourishes and lubricates the joint. In RA, cells of lympho-haematopoietic origin, e.g. T-helper cells, B cells and macrophages, infiltrate the synovium. The synovium also becomes thickened, from a layer of 1–2 cells to approximately 6–8 cells, and becomes locally invasive at the interface with the cartilage and the bone or tendon. The volume of the synovial fluid eventually increases in volume as a result of oedema, which causes swelling of the joints and pain.

Several lines of evidence indicate that RA is associated with aberrant and severe vasculogenesis (i.e. the de novo formation of blood vessels) within the inflamed joints (Paleolog, 2009, Grisar et al., 2007, Grisar et al., 2005, Herbrig et al., 2006, Hirohata et al., 2004, Jodon de Villeroche et al., 2010, Ruger et al., 2004, Silverman et al., 2007). One of the first observations of vasculogenesis in RA was the discovery that the synovial fluids from patients with RA contained a low molecular weight vasculogenesis factor apparently identical to that derived from tumours (Brown et al., 1980). Subsequent studies revealed that synovial fluid from patients with RA stimulated proliferation of human endothelial cells (Kumar et al., 1985) and the formation of tubular networks (Semble et al., 1985). A study of synovial tissue histology from patients with RA revealed that there is a significant correlation between the number of synovial blood vessels and vessel proliferation, mononuclear cell infiltration, fibrosis and clinical measurements of joint tenderness (Rooney et al., 1988). Capillaries are distributed more deeply in the synovium from patients with RA (Stevens et al., 1991). The different stages of rheumatoid arthritis are shown in Figure 1 (upper panel). Although perivascular mononuclear cell infiltration and increased thickness of the synovial lining layer are observed in tissue from both inflamed and non-inflamed joints of RA patients, vascular proliferation is seen only in tissues from inflamed joints (FitzGerald et al., 1991). In addition, endothelial cells lining blood vessels within RA synovium have been shown to express cell cycle-associated antigens such as proliferating cell nuclear antigen and Ki67, and integrin alpha 5 beta 3, which is associated with vascular proliferation (Ceponis et al., 1998). Hypoxia, which can activate vasculogenesis factors and cause further invasion of the synovium, is another common event that occurs within the synovial joints in RA (FitzGerald et al., 1991, Muz et al., 2009). Taken together, these studies indicate that vascular dysfunction in synovial tissue is a likely therapeutic target in RA.

2.2 Type 1 diabetes mellitus

T1DM is a life-long autoimmune disease characterised by hyperglycaemia. Hyperglycaemia in T1DM occurs when the number of insulin-producing ß-cells in the pancreatic Islets of Langerhans drops below the number required to control glycaemia. Hyperglycaemia leads to macrovascular complications, such as coronary artery disease, peripheral arterial disease, and stroke, and microvascular complications, such as diabetic nephropathy, neuropathy, and retinopathy. Onset is early in life and patients exhibit increased risks of renal failure, blindness, amputation, stroke and heart attack (Shapiro et al., 2006). Best available practice with insulin therapy is not a cure as it does not protect the remaining islets from inflammatory attack or the patient from long-term complications.

Insulin-producing ß-cells, which comprise 60-80% of islet mass, are crucial for the maintenance of normal blood sugar. Pancreatic islets are highly metabolically active and densely vascularised with specialized endothelium - they receive 10% of pancreatic blood flow despite comprising only 1% of tissue mass. Pancreatic islets come under a myriad of cellular assaults during isolation including ischemia, enzymatic damage and physical stress. Dysfunction of the endothelium plays a critical role in the development of vascular complications in T1DM (Stehouwer et al., 1997, Flyvbjerg, 2000). Clinical trials have shown that hyperglycaemia leads to changes in the proliferation of endothelial cells, barrier function and the adhesion of other circulating cells to endothelial cells (Schalkwijk and Stehouwer, 2005). This vascular dysfunction may be mediated by several distinct mechanisms and different stages of diabetic retinopathy are shown in Figure 1 (middle panel). Hyperglycaemia results in an increase in intracellular glucose, which leads to an increase in the conversion of glucose to sorbitol via the polyol pathway. This increase in sorbitol can cause osmotic stress, tissue hypoxia and oxidative stress (Williamson et al., 1993, Schalkwijk and Stehouwer, 2005). Hyperglycaemia also results in activation of protein kinase C, which can cause dysregulation of vascular permeability and blood flow, basement membrane thickening and impaired fibrinolysis (Williamson et al., 1993, Chen et al., 2000). In addition, hyperglycaemia causes increased glucosamine-6-phosphate and consequently increased transcription of cytokines such as transforming growth factor beta, which can regulate the proliferation and apoptosis of endothelial cells (Nerlich et al., 1998, Ziyadeh, 2004). Greater insight into the mechanisms underlying endothelial dysfunction may lead to important treatment strategies which can reduce the morbidity and mortality rate caused by endothelial dysfunction in patients with T1DM.

2.3 Systemic sclerosis

SSc is a heterogeneous disease in which vascular dysfunction, extensive fibrosis and autoimmunity are the hallmark characteristics. The aetiology of SSc is unknown as there are many unresolved questions as to both cause and initiating factors (Geyer and Muller-Ladner, 2011). Multiple genetic and environmental factors, combined with other specific factors (e.g. alterations to the immune system, vasculature and extracellular matrix) are the most likely causes of this insidious disorder. The pathophysiology of SSc is diverse and includes abnormal immunologic processes such as cytokine and chemokine dysregulation, abnormal T cell signalling, B cell dysfunction, endothelial injury, aberrant wound healing due to dysregulation of matrix homeostasis, abnormalities in the fibrinolytic system, polymorphisms in critical molecules of the immune system and matrix homeostasis, and microchimerism due to foetal/maternal placental exchange of HLA compatible cells (Gabrielli et al., 2009).

Vascular dysfunction is an early event in SSc (Kahaleh, 2008) and the different stages of SSc are shown in Figure 1 (lower panel). The preferred site of early lesions in SSc is the perivascular space. Progressive wall thickening and perivascular infiltrates are features of the vascular lesions in this compartment, indicating the involvement of vascular smooth-muscle cells and pericytes. Endothelial cells are the only type of mesodermal cell that

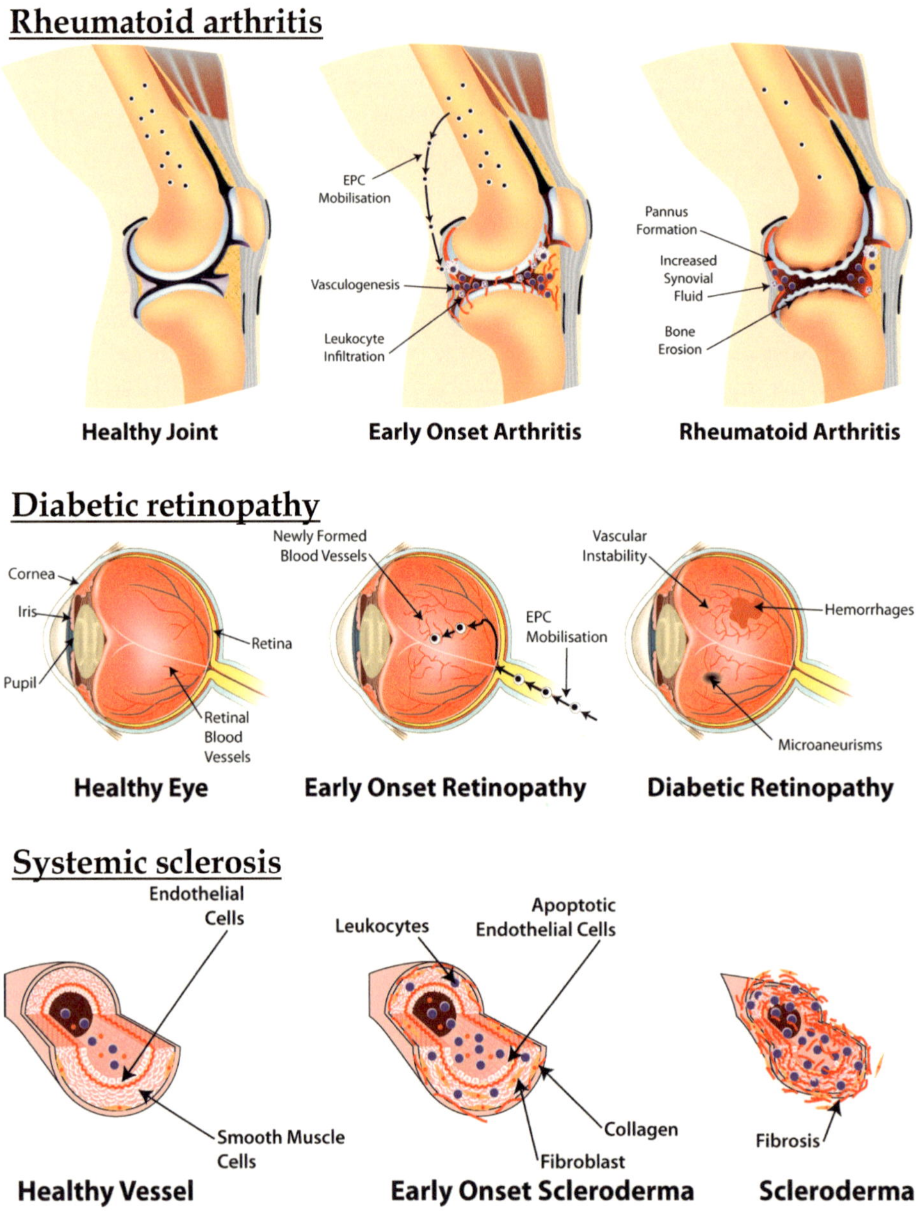

In rheumatoid arthritis (upper panel), circulating endothelial progenitor cells (EPCs) and vasculogenesis are causally linked to the influx of pro-inflammatory **leukocytes** and increased capillary beds contribute to thickening of the synovial lining and joint pain. In diabetic patients with proliferative retinopathy (middle panel), infiltrating EPCs contribute to the dense vascularisation in the eye and reduced vascular stability associated with blindness. Vascular injury is one of the early events in the pathogenesis of systemic sclerosis (lower panel) and is characterized by endothelial-cell damage and apoptosis, the proliferation of fibroblasts, production of collagen and **infiltration** of circulating leukocytes. Despite the increased number of circulating EPCs in these patients, the endothelial layer of the vasculature remains denuded and is ultimately obliterated.

Fig. 1. Vascular dysfunction in autoimmune disease.

undergo apoptosis in early SSc, whereas vascular smooth-muscle cells and pericytes proliferate vigorously. This vascular damage, which eventually occurs in almost all organs (Harrison et al., 1993), presents as large gaps between endothelial cells, loss of integrity of the endothelial lining, and the formation of vacuoles in the endothelial cell cytoplasm. In addition, several basal lamina-like layers build up, mononuclear immune cells infiltrate the vessel walls, obliterative microvascular lesions occur, and the capillaries rarefy (Prescott et al., 1992, Fleming et al., 2008). In the later stages of SSc, relatively few small blood vessels remain. Serum levels of VEGF are high in SSc despite the progressive loss of blood vessels (Distler et al., 2004, Davies et al., 2006), possibly as a result of an adaptive response to hypoxia (Fleming et al., 2008, Kuwana et al., 2004, Cipriani et al., 2007). The molecular mechanisms underlying this defect in vasculogenesis are unknown and both vasculogenic (Davies et al., 2006, Distler et al., 2004) and anti-vasculogenic (Fleming et al., 2008, Hebbar et al., 2000, Scheja et al., 2000) factors have been detected in early SSc. Inflammatory cytokines, such as tumour necrosis factor (TNF), can stimulate or inhibit angiogenesis depending on the duration of the stimulus (Sainson et al., 2008). Collectively, these data indicate that vascular dysfunction is a common event in SSc and an important therapeutic target.

3. Endothelial progenitor cells

EPCs were first discovered in peripheral blood by Asahara and colleagues in 1997 (Asahara et al., 1997). This discovery revealed that vasculogenesis occurs after post-natal development. Vascular insult or disease causes the upregulation of cytokines such as VEGF, stromal cell-derived factor-1 (SDF-1) matrix metalloproteinase 9 (MMP9), hypoxia inducible factor 1α (HIF-1α) and erythropoietin (EPO) at the site of injury and this stimulates the release of EPCs from the stem cell niche in the bone marrow into the circulation (Aicher et al., 2005). EPCs then follow the cytokine gradient to the site of vascular trauma where they contribute to vasculogenesis either by (1) paracrine assistance (via production of VEGF and endothelial nitric oxide synthase (eNOS)) (2) integration or (3) new vessel formation (Figure 2).

There are currently two distinct ways in which EPCs are identified, i.e. (1) they are directly identified in the peripheral blood by the surface antigen expression of any combination of CD133, CD34 and VEGR2 or (2) they are isolated from either peripheral blood (Asahara et al., 1997), umbilical cord blood (Asahara et al., 1997, Shi et al., 1998) or bone marrow (Shi et al., 1998) and cultured ex vivo. The complication associated with using the cell surface markers CD133, CD34 and VEGFR2 to identify EPCs is that these markers are not exclusively expressed on EPCs and can be found on many other cell types including the closely related haematopoietic progenitors and mature endothelial cells as well as fibroblasts, epithelial cells and cancer stem cells (Hirschi et al., 2008, Kumar and Caplice, 2010). Further evidence of a need to standardise the isolation technique, culture conditions and phenotyping strategy is exemplified by Case et al., who suggest that it is not possible to culture EPCs from a CD133+ CD34+ VEGFR2+-sorted population (Case et al., 2007).

Currently, the term 'EPC' is used to describe two populations of cells cultured in vitro, both of which show vascular potential, but differ in both phenotype and function. The first EPC population to be characterised in vitro were the early-outgrowth EPCs, or colony forming unit-endothelial cells (CFU-ECs). Early-outgrowth EPCs form colonies after 3-5 days in culture on fibronectin-coated wells, consist of multiple thin, flat cells emanating from a

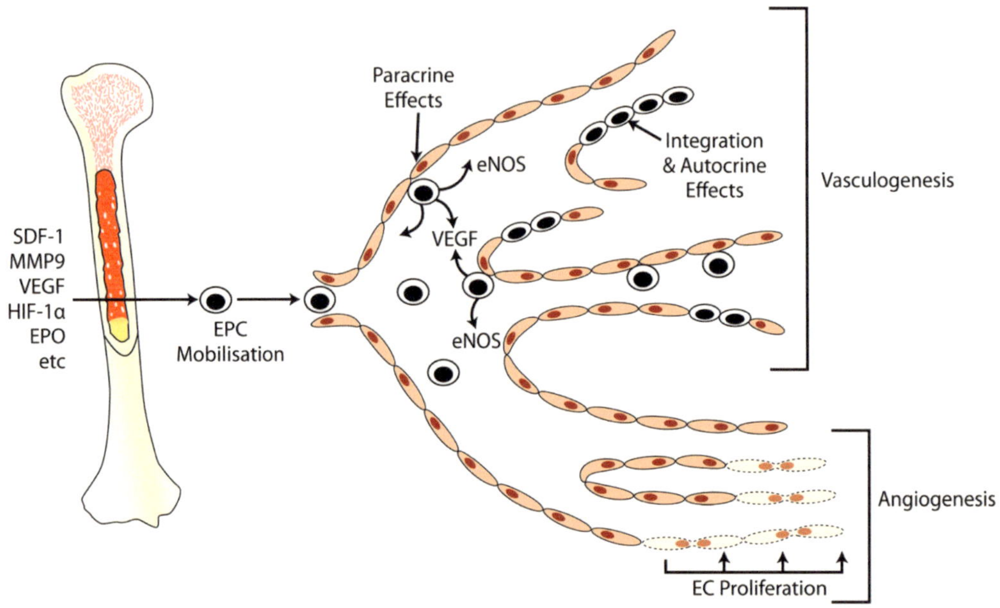

Recruitment of endothelial cells from pre-existing vessel walls or circulating endothelial progenitor cells (EPCs) play a critical role in blood vessel development and repair during disease states. Mobilised bone-marrow derived EPCs with high proliferative capacity may have the potential to home to a site for vascularisation and act in a paracrine or autocrine way to promote vessel wall development. Abbreviations: SDF-1, stromal derived factor -1; MMP9, matrix metalloproteinase 9; VEGF, vascular endothelial growth factor; HIF-1α, hypoxia inducible factor 1α; EPO, erythropoietin; eNOS, endothelial nitric oxide.

Fig. 2. Model of postnatal angiogenesis and vasculogenesis.

central cluster of round cells and express CD133, VEGFR2 and CD34 (Hur et al., 2004). Early-outgrowth EPCs secrete pro-angiogenic factors (Hur et al., 2004, Rehman et al., 2003, Yoon et al., 2005), but are not able to form tubes when seeded alone in Matrigel (Rehman et al., 2003, Timmermans et al., 2007, Yoder et al., 2007, Yoon et al., 2005). When transplanted into mice, they are able to increase capillary density in a model of limb ischemia (Hur et al., 2004, Yoon et al., 2005), suggesting that they contribute to tube formation through paracrine mechanisms. Early-outgrowth EPCs express the pan-leukocyte marker CD45 and the myeloid marker CD14 and have been shown to be of monocyte origin (Medina et al., 2010) and are thus not considered true endothelial cell progeny.

The second EPC population to be characterised are the late-outgrowth EPCs, which as also referred to as outgrowth endothelial cells (OECs) and endothelial colony forming cells (ECFCs). Late-outgrowth EPCs can be isolated from bone marrow, cord blood and peripheral blood and form colonies with distinct cobblestone morphology, similar to that of endothelial cells within 2-4 weeks when cultured on either collagen or gelatin (Lin et al., 2000, Shi et al., 1998). Late-outgrowth EPCs have 10 times the proliferative capacity of mature ECs, they express mature endothelial cell markers including von Willebrand factor (vWF), CD31 and VEGFR2, but not the progenitor marker CD133 and they are able to form tubes in Matrigel (Bompais et al., 2004, Ingram et al., 2004, Lin et al., 2000, Rehman et al., 2003, Timmermans et al., 2007, Yoder et al., 2007, Yoon et al., 2005). Late-outgrowth EPCs have been shown to increase neovascularisation in a mouse limb ischemic model (Hur et al., 2004, Yoon et al., 2005) and are haemangioblastic in origin (Medina et al., 2010) and are thus considered to be true endothelial cell progeny.

Whilst the monocytic early-outgrowth EPCs and the haemangioblastic late-outgrowth EPCs are distinct EPC populations, the combined therapeutic potential of these two EPC populations is greater than either of the EPC populations when delivered individually in a mouse model of limb ischemia (Yoon et al., 2005), suggesting that these EPC populations may function synergistically during vasculogenesis.

4. Endothelial progenitor cells in autoimmune disease

4.1 Endothelial progenitor cells in rheumatoid arthritis

The association between EPC numbers and RA has brought about conflicting results (Table 1). Some studies have reported a lower circulating EPC number in RA patients compared with controls (Grisar et al., 2005, Herbrig et al., 2006), whilst others report higher numbers (Jodon de Villeroche et al., 2010) and a few report no differences (Egan et al., 2008, Kuwana et al., 2004). A schematic of a potential role for EPCs in RA is depicted in Figure 1 (upper panel).

In the studies that reported lower circulating EPC numbers in patients with active RA compared to healthy controls (Grisar et al., 2005, Herbrig et al., 2006), the circulating EPCs were identified through the expression of CD133, CD34 and VEGFR2 and the formation of early-outgrowth EPC colonies. It is highly likely that these studies were not specifically identifying a pure EPC population, but rather a mixed population consisting of both early-outgrowth EPCs, late-outgrowth EPCs and haematopoietic progenitors, as the biomarkers used to identify EPCs are not specific for any one cell type.

In contrast, Jodan de Villeroche et al used a method to exclusively identify haemangioblastic late-outgrowth EPCs distinct from monocytic early-outgrowth EPCs (Jodon de Villeroche et al., 2010). Jodan de Villeroche et al exclusively monitored the number of late-outgrowth EPCs by detecting Lin-/7-aminoactinomycin (7-AAD)-/CD34+/CD133+/VEGFR2+ cells from CD14 depleted peripheral blood. This detection panel eliminated apoptotic cells (using 7-AAD) and early-outgrowth EPCs (through CD14 depletion). Using these methods this study revealed that RA patients with active RA had significantly higher levels of circulating late-outgrowth EPCs compared with controls. To complement these findings, this study also investigated the formation of late-outgrowth EPC colonies and found that RA patients had a higher number of late-outgrowth colonies compared to controls. This study was the first to implement a method that made a distinction between the two EPC populations.

4.2 Endothelial progenitor cells in type 1 diabetes mellitus

A decrease in EPC number and function has been associated with T1DM and has been reported by several groups (Table 2). However before comparisons can be made between studies, it is important to consider the methods used to quantify EPC numbers in these studies. Circulating EPC numbers were quantified either by surface antigen expression on peripheral blood mononuclear cells (PBMNCs) (Brunner et al., 2009, Sibal et al., 2009), through the culture of early-outgrowth EPC colonies (Asnaghi et al., 2006) or through the uptake of acetylated LDL and binding of UEA-l to cultured PBMNCs (Loomans et al., 2004). To the best of our knowledge, there are currently no reports on the correlation between T1DM and the growth of late-outgrowth EPCs.

Reference	Method of EPC identification	Comments
Grisar et al., 2005	Expression of CD133/CD34/VEGFR2 from PBMNC using flow cytometry.	EPCs were lower in active RA patients compared to healthy controls when assessing surface antigen expression.
	In vitro culture of PBMNCs and detection of early-outgrowth EPCs colonies.	Reduced number of early-outgrowth EPC colonies in active RA patients compared to healthy controls.
Grisar et al., 2007	Expression of CD133/CD34/VEGFR2 from PBMNC using flow cytometry.	TNF may be partly responsible for the reduction of circulating EPCs seen in RA patients.
Egan et al., 2008	Expression of CD133/CD117/CD34/CD31 from PBMNCs using flow cytometry.	No difference in the number of EPCs in RA patients and healthy controls when assessing surface antigen expression.
	In vitro culture of PBMNCs and detection of early-outgrowth EPCs colonies.	Reduced number of early-outgrowth EPCs in active RA patients compared to healthy controls.
		Early-outgrowth EPC colony numbers were associated with cardiovascular risk.
Jodon de Villeroche et al., 2010	Surface antigen profile Lin-/7AAD-/CD34+/CD133+/VEGFR2+ from CD14-depleted PBMNCs using flow cytometry.	RA patients had higher numbers of circulating EPCs than healthy controls.
	In vitro culture PBMNCs and detection of late-outgrowth colonies.	Circulating EPCs correlated with disease activity.
Herbrig et al., 2006	In vitro culture of PMNCs and assessment of Ac-LDL uptake, UEA-1 lectin binding and the surface antigen profile VE-cadherin+/CD31+/VEGFR2+/CD146-.	EPCs from RA patients showed reduced migratory activity in response to VEGF.

Abbreviations: RA, rheumatoid arthritis; PBMNCs, peripheral blood mononuclear cells; EPCs, endothelial progenitor cells; Ac-LDL, acetylated-low density lipoprotein; UEA-1 lectin, *Ulex Europaeus* Lectin; TNF, tumour necrosis factor; VEGF, vascular endothelial growth factor.

Table 1. Studies that have reported aberrant EPC numbers in patients with RA.

EPC dysfunction has been seen in patients with T1DM, as shown by Loomans et al. when conditioned media from EPCs isolated from T1DM patients impaired in vitro tube formation of HUVEC (Loomans et al., 2004). An inverse relationship between the number of

EPCs and HbA1C in patients has also been identified (Loomans et al., 2004). Moreover, there appears to be an association between the progression of diabetic retinopathy and the level of circulating EPCs. In patients with T1DM and proliferative retinopathy a marked increase in circulating EPCs has been reported (Asnaghi et al., 2006, Brunner et al., 2009). Conversely, circulating EPC numbers have been identified as being lower in patients with T1DM and non-proliferative retinopathy (Brunner et al., 2009). These studies highlight how atypical EPC numbers and function are associated with T1DM pathology and a schematic of a potential role for EPCs in diabetic retinopathy is depicted in Figure 1 (middle panel).

Reference	**Method of EPC identification**	**Comments**
Loomans et al., 2004	In vitro culture of PMNCs and assessment of Ac-LDL uptake, UEA-1 lectin binding and CD31 expression.	T1DM patients had lower EPC levels compared to healthy controls.
Sibal et al., 2009	Expression of CD133/CD34/VEGFR2/VE-cadherin from PBMNC using flow cytometry.	EPC counts were lower in patients with T1DM compared to healthy controls.
Asnaghi et al., 2006	Immunostaining with CD133 and CD31	Patients with T1DM and retinopathy had higher EPC levels than healthy controls and patients with T1DM and no retinopathy.
	In vitro culture of PBMNCs and detection of early-outgrowth EPCs colonies.	Patients with T1DM and no retinopathy had lower EPC levels than healthy controls and patients with T1DM and retinopathy.
Brunner et al., 2008	CPC surface antigen profile CD133+/CD34+	Patients with T1DM and proliferative retinopathy had increased levels of mature EPCs.
	EPCs surface antigen profile CD133+/CD34+/VEGFR2+	Patients with T1DM and nonproliferative retinopathy had decreased levels of EPCs.
	Mature surface antigen profile CD133+/CD34+/VEGFR2+/CD31+	
	Nonmature surface antigen profile CD133+/CD34+/VEGFR2+/CD31-	

Abbreviations: T1DM, type 1 diabetes mellitus; PBMNCs, peripheral blood mononuclear cells; EPCs, endothelial progenitor cells; CPC, circulating progenitor cells; Ac-LDL, acetylated-low density lipoprotein; UEA-1 lectin, *Ulex Europaeus* Lectin

Table 2. Studies that have reported aberrant EPC numbers in patients with T1DM.

4.3 Endothelial progenitor cells in systemic sclerosis

Aberrant EPC numbers within the circulation of patients with SSc has been described extensively (Table 3). The majority of these studies used flow cytometry to assess EPC numbers using various combinations of the markers CD133, CD34 and VEGFR2. As mentioned previously, the use of these markers does not unambiguously identify circulating EPCs as they are expressed by other progenitor cells and mature endothelial cells. Avouac et al describe the most stringent method of EPC identification, which involved culturing the PBMNCs from both SSc patients and healthy controls and assessing late-outgrowth EPC colony formation. This study showed that the number of late-outgrowth EPC colonies correlated with the number of circulating EPCs detected using the surface antigen profile Lin-/7AAD-/CD34+/CD133+/VEGFR2+ (Avouac et al., 2008).

Reference	Method of EPC identification	Comments
Allanore et al., 2007	Expression of CD133/CD34 from PBMNC using flow cytometry.	SSc patients had higher numbers of EPCs than osteoarthritis patients, but lower than RA patients.
Yamaguchi et al., 2010	In vitro culture of PBMNCs depleted for platelets. Expression of CD34/VEGFR1/CD1a/CD83/CD80 using flow cytometry and CD31/CD144 by immunohistochemistry.	The number of early-outgrowth EPCs was higher in SSc patients compared to RA patients and healthy controls. Early-outgrowth EPCs derived from SSc patients showed greater vascular potential in vitro and in vivo than early-outgrowth EPCs derived from healthy controls.
Kuwana et al., 2004	Expression of CD133/CD34/VEGR2 from CD34-enriched PBMNC using flow cytometry.	EPCs were lower in SSc patients compared to RA patients and healthy controls. Levels of angiogenic factors within the circulation were higher in SSc patients than in health controls.
Kuwana et al., 2006	Expression of CD133/CD34/VEGR2 from CD34-enriched PBMNC using flow cytometry.	Atorvastatin treatment resulted in an increase in circulating EPCs from baseline, however levels did not reach those of healthy controls.
Del Papa et al., 2004	Surface antigen profile CD133+/CD34+ from PBMNC using flow cytometry.	High levels of EPCs in patients with SSc and counts were higher in early stages of disease.
Del Papa et al., 2006	Surface antigen profile CD133+/CD45- from PBMNC and BM using flow cytometry.	Circulating EPCs were higher in patients with early stage disease, but not in those with late stage disease. BM EPCs were reduced and functionally impaired.
Avouac et al., 2008	Surface antigen profile Lin-/7AAD-/CD34+/CD133+/VEGFR2+ from PBMNCs detected using flow cytometry. In vitro culture of PBMNCs and detection of late-outgrowth colonies.	Circulating EPC levels were higher in SSc patients than in healthy controls. Positive correlation between the number of late-outgrowth EPC colonies and the level of circulating EPCs detected by flow cytometry in patients with SSc.

Abbreviations: SSc, systemic sclerosis; PBMNCs, peripheral blood mononuclear cells; EPCs, endothelial progenitor cells; BM, bone marrow.

Table 3. Studies that have reported aberrant EPC numbers in patients with SSc.

It has been well documented that circulating EPC numbers are elevated in patients with SSc (Allanore et al., 2007, Avouac et al., 2008, Del Papa et al., 2004, Del Papa et al., 2006, Yamaguchi et al., 2010). However, two studies by Kuwana and colleagues have reported reduced EPC numbers in SSc patients (Kuwana et al., 2006, Kuwana et al., 2004). Del Papa et al showed that in early stage SSc (3-5 years) there appears to be an increase in circulating EPCs and post 5 years, there appears to be either a normal or decreased number of circulating EPCs (Del Papa et al., 2006). A schematic of a potential role for EPCs in SSc is depicted in Figure 1 (lower panel). There is also evidence to suggest that the vascular function of EPCs from SSc patients is actually higher than that of healthy controls as early-outgrowth EPCs from SSc patients are able to promote tube formation of HUVEC in vitro as well as enhance tumour growth and blood vessel formation in vivo (Yamaguchi et al., 2010).

5. Therapeutic intervention targeting EPCs in autoimmune diseases

There have been rapid advances in the field of therapeutic angiogenesis since the original description of bone marrow derived EPCs in 1997 (Asahara et al., 1997). Most of these bench-to-bed-side studies have been done in models of atherosclerosis and acute ischemic events such as myocardial infarction (MI) and critical limb ischemia. The first pre-clinical studies in these diseases were executed (within four years of their initial discovery) in a MI model in mice (Kocher et al., 2001) and demonstrated improvement in angiogenesis and cardiac function. This was followed by a series of publications showing the effectiveness of EPCs in preventing the extent of damage (Orlic et al., 2001) after MI as well as effectiveness in the large vessel occlusive damage (Griese et al., 2003) and prevention of atherosclerosis in a highly prone mouse model (Rausher et al, 2003). However, the exact mechanism of action of these interventions, in particular whether the benefit was due to neo-angiogenesis modulated by EPCs or due to paracrine mechanisms that improved the survival of resident endothelial cells, is not entirely clear.

There was a rapid transition of these studies to humans as autologous marrow transplantation became a relatively safe and well established procedure in haematological malignancies and non-invasive methods to mobilise bone marrow progenitors became well established. In 2002, there were two studies published reporting the benefit of locally injecting ex-vivo expanded autologous bone marrow derived mononuclear cells in MI critical lower limb ischemia (Strauer et al., 2002, Tateishi-Yuyama et al., 2002). Furthermore, there have been multiple randomised controlled trials looking at the effectiveness of bone marrow derived cell therapies, which have been reviewed in a recent meta-analysis (Martin-Rendon et al., 2008).

The therapeutic use of EPCs in inflammatory diseases is more complicated as they have been implicated in pathogenesis of the inflammatory process as well as being an important cause of long term morbidity. There have been no studies of direct intervention with EPCs in autoimmune diseases. This is mainly due to their differential effects on the immunopathogenesis of these diseases. Attempts to understand this field are further bedevilled by observations of patients with systemic lupus erythematosus (SLE) who exhibit a significant decrease in circulating EPCs as well as a striking increase in premature atherosclerosis of unclear aetiology (de Leeuw et al., 2005, Westerweel et al., 2007) demonstrating no significant difference in EPC number between SLE patients without and with advanced coronary artery calcification (Baker et al., 2011). As detailed above, the inflammatory milieu in autoimmune diseases is characterized by neo-angiogenesis and as such it would seem that increased EPCs might contribute to inflammation. On the other hand, the most common cause of long term morbidity and mortality in these diseases is attributed to atherosclerosis and its complications where EPCs might have beneficial effect. There have been numerous studies looking at the effect of various disease modifying therapies in patients with autoimmune diseases on the circulating EPCs (both monocytic and haemangioblastic) reviewed in a recent article (Westerweel and Verhaar, 2009). These studies show an increase in the levels of circulating haemangioblastic EPCs after various immunosuppressive therapies including anti-TNF drugs, corticosteroids and hydroxychloroquine in these patients. However, the association of these changes with long term clinically useful outcome, such as incidence of atherosclerosis and coronary artery disease, has not been demonstrated. This finding is intriguing as it is well known from long term clinical studies that corticosteroids are known to promote atherosclerosis and anti-TNF medications reduce long term morbidity and mortality due to this complication (Kaplan, 2010). Moreover, methotrexate, a commonly used disease modifying agent in various autoimmune diseases is known to induce EPC apoptosis in vitro (Herbrig et al., 2006) but has beneficial effects in patients.

There needs to be better understanding of the role of EPCs in the different stages of the disease, i.e. early active versus long standing, and its pathophysiological implications relating to long term outcome of patients to be able to design studies with intervention directed at EPCs. The knowledge of various paracrine mechanisms involved in the beneficial effects of EPCs in atherosclerosis models might help to dissect the pathways involved in neo-angiogenesis versus survival of resident endothelial cells. This knowledge can then be exploited to design intervention at various stages of autoimmune diseases.

6. Conclusions

Faced with an ever-increasing burden of autoimmune diseases such as RA, T1DM and SSc, modern medicine is confronted with the need to provide new therapies that not only mitigate the symptoms of these diseases but may also facilitate regeneration of organ function. Given their role in development and in maintaining and repairing injured vessels, stem and progenitor cells represent an exciting alternative for regenerative medicine. Since their first identification over a decade ago, the use of EPCs as a diagnostic tool or therapeutic was greeted with great enthusiasm. However, progress in their clinical application remains limited by identification and *ex vivo* expansion factors, and as a result, variable functional attributes. It can be seen from the aforementioned examples that the timing and methods used to detect EPCs can greatly affect the outcome of studies. The major issues associated with EPC identification within the circulation are (1) identifying the bone marrow progenitors from the circulating mature endothelial cells and (2) defining the distinction between haemangioblastic late-outgrowth EPCs and monocytic early-outgrowth EPCs. These matters are the focus of ongoing research, especially the search for a unique EPC marker. Nevertheless, EPCs are a robust biomarker of vascular dysfunction (based on their direct interaction and influence on endothelial function), and the unique ability to monitor their peripheral number or function as a marker of response to therapy. Notwithstanding the current knowledge regarding EPC cell signalling, activation and migration, the precise mechanisms of activation of these cells and their functional significance is not known. In the research setting, continued understanding of EPC function improves insight into vasculogenesis, and the pathology of vascular dysfunction in autoimmune disease.

7. Acknowledgements

This work was supported by the Co-operative Research Centre for Biomarker Translation (Transbio Ltd) and Arthritis Australia. CSB is a Heart Foundation Research Fellow and we thank P. Dunne for preparation of the figures.

8. References

Aicher, A., Zeiher, A. M. & Dimmeler, S. 2005. Mobilizing endothelial progenitor cells. *Hypertension,* 45, 321-5.

Allanore, Y., Batteux, F., Avouac, J., Assous, N., Weill, B. & Kahan, A. 2007. Levels of circulating endothelial progenitor cells in systemic sclerosis. *Clin Exp Rheumatol,* 25, 60-6.

Asahara, T., Murohara, T., Sullivan, A., Silver, M., Van Der Zee, R., Li, T., Witzenbichler, B., Schatteman, G. & Isner, J. M. 1997. Isolation of putative progenitor endothelial cells for angiogenesis. *Science,* 275, 964-7.

Asnaghi, V., Lattanzio, R., Mazzolari, G., Pastore, M. R., Ramoni, A., Maestroni, A., Ruggieri, D., Luzi, L., Brancato, R. & Zerbini, G. 2006. Increased clonogenic potential of circulating endothelial progenitor cells in patients with type 1 diabetes and proliferative retinopathy. *Diabetologia,* 49, 1109-11.

Avouac, J., Juin, F., Wipff, J., Couraud, P. O., Chiocchia, G., Kahan, A., Boileau, C., Uzan, G. & Allanore, Y. 2008. Circulating endothelial progenitor cells in systemic sclerosis: association with disease severity. *Ann Rheum Dis,* 67, 1455-60.

Baker, J. F., Zhang, L., Imadojemu, S., Sharpe, A., Patil, S., Moore, J. S., Mohler, E. R., 3rd & Von Feldt, J. 2011. Circulating endothelial progenitor cells are reduced in SLE in the absence of coronary artery calcification. *Rheumatol Int.*

Bompais, H., Chagraoui, J., Canron, X., Crisan, M., Liu, X. H., Anjo, A., Tolla-Le Port, C., Leboeuf, M., Charbord, P., Bikfalvi, A. & Uzan, G. 2004. Human endothelial cells derived from circulating progenitors display specific functional properties compared with mature vessel wall endothelial cells. *Blood,* 103, 2577-84.

Brown, R. A., Weiss, J. B., Tomlinson, I. W., Phillips, P. & Kumar, S. 1980. Angiogenic factor from synovial fluid resembling that from tumours. *Lancet,* 1, 682-5.

Brunner, S., Schernthaner, G. H., Satler, M., Elhenicky, M., Hoellerl, F., Schmid-Kubista, K. E., Zeiler, F., Binder, S. & Schernthaner, G. 2009. Correlation of different circulating endothelial progenitor cells to stages of diabetic retinopathy: first in vivo data. *Invest Ophthalmol Vis Sci,* 50, 392-8.

Case, J., Mead, L. E., Bessler, W. K., Prater, D., White, H. A., Saadatzadeh, M. R., Bhavsar, J. R., Yoder, M. C., Haneline, L. S. & Ingram, D. A. 2007. Human CD34+AC133+VEGFR-2+ cells are not endothelial progenitor cells but distinct, primitive hematopoietic progenitors. *Exp Hematol,* 35, 1109-18.

Ceponis, A., Konttinen, Y. T., Imai, S., Tamulaitiene, M., Li, T. F., Xu, J. W., Hietanen, J., Santavirta, S. & Fassbender, H. G. 1998. Synovial lining, endothelial and inflammatory mononuclear cell proliferation in synovial membranes in psoriatic and reactive arthritis: a comparative quantitative morphometric study. *Br J Rheumatol,* 37, 170-8.

Chen, S., Apostolova, M. D., Cherian, M. G. & Chakrabarti, S. 2000. Interaction of endothelin-1 with vasoactive factors in mediating glucose-induced increased permeability in endothelial cells. *Lab Invest,* 80, 1311-21.

Cipriani, P., Guiducci, S., Miniati, I., Cinelli, M., Urbani, S., Marrelli, A., Dolo, V., Pavan, A., Saccardi, R., Tyndall, A., Giacomelli, R. & Cerinic, M. M. 2007. Impairment of endothelial cell differentiation from bone marrow-derived mesenchymal stem cells: new insight into the pathogenesis of systemic sclerosis. *Arthritis Rheum,* 56, 1994-2004.

Davies, C. A., Jeziorska, M., Freemont, A. J. & Herrick, A. L. 2006. The differential expression of VEGF, VEGFR-2, and GLUT-1 proteins in disease subtypes of systemic sclerosis. *Hum Pathol,* 37, 190-7.

De Leeuw, K., Kallenberg, C. & Bijl, M. 2005. Accelerated atherosclerosis in patients with systemic autoimmune diseases. *Ann N Y Acad Sci,* 1051, 362-71.

Del Papa, N., Colombo, G., Fracchiolla, N., Moronetti, L. M., Ingegnoli, F., Maglione, W., Comina, D. P., Vitali, C., Fantini, F. & Cortelezzi, A. 2004. Circulating endothelial cells as a marker of ongoing vascular disease in systemic sclerosis. *Arthritis Rheum,* 50, 1296-304.

Del Papa, N., Quirici, N., Soligo, D., Scavullo, C., Cortiana, M., Borsotti, C., Maglione, W., Comina, D. P., Vitali, C., Fraticelli, P., Gabrielli, A., Cortelezzi, A. & Lambertenghi-Deliliers, G. 2006. Bone marrow endothelial progenitors are defective in systemic sclerosis. *Arthritis Rheum,* 54, 2605-15.

Distler, O., Distler, J. H., Scheid, A., Acker, T., Hirth, A., Rethage, J., Michel, B. A., Gay, R. E., Muller-Ladner, U., Matucci-Cerinic, M., Plate, K. H., Gassmann, M. & Gay, S. 2004. Uncontrolled expression of vascular endothelial growth factor and its receptors leads to insufficient skin angiogenesis in patients with systemic sclerosis. *Circ Res,* 95, 109-16.

Egan, C. G., Caporali, F., Garcia-Gonzalez, E., Galeazzi, M. & Sorrentino, V. 2008. Endothelial progenitor cells and colony-forming units in rheumatoid arthritis: association with clinical characteristics. *Rheumatology (Oxford),* 47, 1484-8.

Fitzgerald, O., Soden, M., Yanni, G., Robinson, R. & Bresnihan, B. 1991. Morphometric analysis of blood vessels in synovial membranes obtained from clinically affected and unaffected knee joints of patients with rheumatoid arthritis. *Ann Rheum Dis,* 50, 792-6.

Fleming, J. N., Nash, R. A., Mcleod, D. O., Fiorentino, D. F., Shulman, H. M., Connolly, M. K., Molitor, J. A., Henstorf, G., Lafyatis, R., Pritchard, D. K., Adams, L. D., Furst, D. E. & Schwartz, S. M. 2008. Capillary regeneration in scleroderma: stem cell therapy reverses phenotype? *PLoS One,* 3, e1452.

Flyvbjerg, A. 2000. Putative pathophysiological role of growth factors and cytokines in experimental diabetic kidney disease. *Diabetologia,* 43, 1205-23.

Gabrielli, A., Avvedimento, E. V. & Krieg, T. 2009. Scleroderma. *N Engl J Med,* 360, 1989-2003.

Geyer, M. & Muller-Ladner, U. 2011. The pathogenesis of systemic sclerosis revisited. *Clin Rev Allergy Immunol,* 40, 92-103.

Griese, D. P., Ehsan, A., Melo, L. G., Kong, D., Zhang, L., Mann, M. J., Pratt, R. E., Mulligan, R. C. & Dzau, V. J. 2003. Isolation and transplantation of autologous circulating endothelial cells into denuded vessels and prosthetic grafts: implications for cell-based vascular therapy. *Circulation,* 108, 2710-5.

Grisar, J., Aletaha, D., Steiner, C. W., Kapral, T., Steiner, S., Saemann, M., Schwarzinger, I., Buranyi, B., Steiner, G. & Smolen, J. S. 2007. Endothelial progenitor cells in active rheumatoid arthritis: effects of tumour necrosis factor and glucocorticoid therapy. *Ann Rheum Dis,* 66, 1284-8.

Grisar, J., Aletaha, D., Steiner, C. W., Kapral, T., Steiner, S., Seidinger, D., Weigel, G., Schwarzinger, I., Wolozcszuk, W., Steiner, G. & Smolen, J. S. 2005. Depletion of endothelial progenitor cells in the peripheral blood of patients with rheumatoid arthritis. *Circulation,* 111, 204-11.

Harrison, A., Lusk, J. & Corkill, M. 1993. Reliability of skin score in scleroderma. *Br J Rheumatol,* 32, 170.

Hebbar, M., Peyrat, J. P., Hornez, L., Hatron, P. Y., Hachulla, E. & Devulder, B. 2000. Increased concentrations of the circulating angiogenesis inhibitor endostatin in patients with systemic sclerosis. *Arthritis Rheum,* 43, 889-93.

Herbrig, K., Haensel, S., Oelschlaegel, U., Pistrosch, F., Foerster, S. & Passauer, J. 2006. Endothelial dysfunction in patients with rheumatoid arthritis is associated with a reduced number and impaired function of endothelial progenitor cells. *Ann Rheum Dis,* 65, 157-63.

Hirohata, S., Yanagida, T., Nampei, A., Kunugiza, Y., Hashimoto, H., Tomita, T., Yoshikawa, H. & Ochi, T. 2004. Enhanced generation of endothelial cells from CD34+ cells of the bone marrow in rheumatoid arthritis: possible role in synovial neovascularization. *Arthritis Rheum,* 50, 3888-96.

Hirschi, K. K., Ingram, D. A. & Yoder, M. C. 2008. Assessing identity, phenotype, and fate of endothelial progenitor cells. *Arterioscler Thromb Vasc Biol,* 28, 1584-95.

Hur, J., Yoon, C. H., Kim, H. S., Choi, J. H., Kang, H. J., Hwang, K. K., Oh, B. H., Lee, M. M. & Park, Y. B. 2004. Characterization of two types of endothelial progenitor cells and their different contributions to neovasculogenesis. *Arterioscler Thromb Vasc Biol,* 24, 288-93.

Ingram, D. A., Mead, L. E., Tanaka, H., Meade, V., Fenoglio, A., Mortell, K., Pollok, K., Ferkowicz, M. J., Gilley, D. & Yoder, M. C. 2004. Identification of a novel hierarchy of endothelial progenitor cells using human peripheral and umbilical cord blood. *Blood,* 104, 2752-60.

Jodon De Villeroche, V., Avouac, J., Ponceau, A., Ruiz, B., Kahan, A., Boileau, C., Uzan, G. & Allanore, Y. 2010. Enhanced late-outgrowth circulating endothelial progenitor cell levels in rheumatoid arthritis and correlation with disease activity. *Arthritis Res Ther,* 12, R27.

Kahaleh, B. 2008. Vascular disease in scleroderma: mechanisms of vascular injury. *Rheum Dis Clin North Am,* 34, 57-71; vi.

Kaplan, M. J. 2010. Cardiovascular complications of rheumatoid arthritis: assessment, prevention, and treatment. *Rheum Dis Clin North Am,* 36, 405-26.

Karamysheva, A. F. 2008. Mechanisms of angiogenesis. *Biochemistry (Mosc),* 73, 751-62.

Kocher, A. A., Schuster, M. D., Szabolcs, M. J., Takuma, S., Burkhoff, D., Wang, J., Homma, S., Edwards, N. M. & Itescu, S. 2001. Neovascularization of ischemic myocardium by human bone-marrow-derived angioblasts prevents cardiomyocyte apoptosis, reduces remodeling and improves cardiac function. *Nat Med,* 7, 430-6.

Kumar, A. H. & Caplice, N. M. 2010. Clinical potential of adult vascular progenitor cells. *Arterioscler Thromb Vasc Biol,* 30, 1080-7.

Kumar, P., Erroi, A., Sattar, A. & Kumar, S. 1985. Weibel-Palade bodies as a marker for neovascularization induced by tumor and rheumatoid angiogenesis factors. *Cancer Res,* 45, 4339-48.

Kuwana, M., Kaburaki, J., Okazaki, Y., Yasuoka, H., Kawakami, Y. & Ikeda, Y. 2006. Increase in circulating endothelial precursors by atorvastatin in patients with systemic sclerosis. *Arthritis Rheum,* 54, 1946-51.

Kuwana, M., Okazaki, Y., Yasuoka, H., Kawakami, Y. & Ikeda, Y. 2004. Defective vasculogenesis in systemic sclerosis. *Lancet,* 364, 603-10.

Lin, Y., Weisdorf, D. J., Solovey, A. & Hebbel, R. P. 2000. Origins of circulating endothelial cells and endothelial outgrowth from blood. *J Clin Invest,* 105, 71-7.

Loomans, C. J., De Koning, E. J., Staal, F. J., Rookmaaker, M. B., Verseyden, C., De Boer, H. C., Verhaar, M. C., Braam, B., Rabelink, T. J. & Van Zonneveld, A. J. 2004. Endothelial progenitor cell dysfunction: a novel concept in the pathogenesis of vascular complications of type 1 diabetes. *Diabetes,* 53, 195-9.

Martin-Rendon, E., Brunskill, S. J., Hyde, C. J., Stanworth, S. J., Mathur, A. & Watt, S. M. 2008. Autologous bone marrow stem cells to treat acute myocardial infarction: a systematic review. *Eur Heart J,* 29, 1807-18.

Medina, R. J., O'neill, C. L., Sweeney, M., Guduric-Fuchs, J., Gardiner, T. A., Simpson, D. A. & Stitt, A. W. 2010. Molecular analysis of endothelial progenitor cell (EPC) subtypes reveals two distinct cell populations with different identities. *BMC Med Genomics,* 3, 18.

Muz, B., Khan, M. N., Kiriakidis, S. & Paleolog, E. M. 2009. Hypoxia. The role of hypoxia and HIF-dependent signalling events in rheumatoid arthritis. *Arthritis Res Ther,* 11, 201.

Nerlich, A. G., Sauer, U., Kolm-Litty, V., Wagner, E., Koch, M. & Schleicher, E. D. 1998. Expression of glutamine:fructose-6-phosphate amidotransferase in human tissues: evidence for high variability and distinct regulation in diabetes. *Diabetes,* 47, 170-8.

Orlic, D., Kajstura, J., Chimenti, S., Limana, F., Jakoniuk, I., Quaini, F., Nadal-Ginard, B., Bodine, D. M., Leri, A. & Anversa, P. 2001. Mobilized bone marrow cells repair the infarcted heart, improving function and survival. *Proc Natl Acad Sci U S A,* 98, 10344-9.

Paleolog, E. M. 2009. The vasculature in rheumatoid arthritis: cause or consequence? *Int J Exp Pathol,* 90, 249-61.

Prescott, R. J., Freemont, A. J., Jones, C. J., Hoyland, J. & Fielding, P. 1992. Sequential dermal microvascular and perivascular changes in the development of scleroderma. *J Pathol,* 166, 255-63.

Rehman, J., Li, J., Orschell, C. M. & March, K. L. 2003. Peripheral blood "endothelial progenitor cells" are derived from monocyte/macrophages and secrete angiogenic growth factors. *Circulation,* 107, 1164-9.

Rooney, M., Condell, D., Quinlan, W., Daly, L., Whelan, A., Feighery, C. & Bresnihan, B. 1988. Analysis of the histologic variation of synovitis in rheumatoid arthritis. *Arthritis Rheum,* 31, 956-63.

Ruger, B., Giurea, A., Wanivenhaus, A. H., Zehetgruber, H., Hollemann, D., Yanagida, G., Groger, M., Petzelbauer, P., Smolen, J. S., Hoecker, P. & Fischer, M. B. 2004.

Endothelial precursor cells in the synovial tissue of patients with rheumatoid arthritis and osteoarthritis. *Arthritis Rheum,* 50, 2157-66.
Sainson, R. C., Johnston, D. A., Chu, H. C., Holderfield, M. T., Nakatsu, M. N., Crampton, S. P., Davis, J., Conn, E. & Hughes, C. C. 2008. TNF primes endothelial cells for angiogenic sprouting by inducing a tip cell phenotype. *Blood,* 111, 4997-5007.
Schalkwijk, C. G. & Stehouwer, C. D. 2005. Vascular complications in diabetes mellitus: the role of endothelial dysfunction. *Clin Sci (Lond),* 109, 143-59.
Scheja, A., Wildt, M., Wollheim, F. A., Akesson, A. & Saxne, T. 2000. Circulating collagen metabolites in systemic sclerosis. Differences between limited and diffuse form and relationship with pulmonary involvement. *Rheumatology (Oxford),* 39, 1110-3.
Semble, E. L., Turner, R. A. & Mccrickard, E. L. 1985. Rheumatoid arthritis and osteoarthritis synovial fluid effects on primary human endothelial cell cultures. *J Rheumatol,* 12, 237-41.
Sen, S., Mcdonald, S. P., Coates, P. T. & Bonder, C. S. 2011. Endothelial progenitor cells: novel biomarker and promising cell therapy for cardiovascular disease. *Clin Sci (Lond),* 120, 263-83.
Shapiro, A. M., Ricordi, C., Hering, B. J., Auchincloss, H., Lindblad, R., Robertson, R. P., Secchi, A., Brendel, M. D., Berney, T., Brennan, D. C., Cagliero, E., Alejandro, R., Ryan, E. A., Dimercurio, B., Morel, P., Polonsky, K. S., Reems, J. A., Bretzel, R. G., Bertuzzi, F., Froud, T., Kandaswamy, R., Sutherland, D. E., Eisenbarth, G., Segal, M., Preiksaitis, J., Korbutt, G. S., Barton, F. B., Viviano, L., Seyfert-Margolis, V., Bluestone, J. & Lakey, J. R. 2006. International trial of the Edmonton protocol for islet transplantation. *N Engl J Med,* 355, 1318-30.
Shi, Q., Rafii, S., Wu, M. H., Wijelath, E. S., Yu, C., Ishida, A., Fujita, Y., Kothari, S., Mohle, R., Sauvage, L. R., Moore, M. A., Storb, R. F. & Hammond, W. P. 1998. Evidence for circulating bone marrow-derived endothelial cells. *Blood,* 92, 362-7.
Sibal, L., Aldibbiat, A., Agarwal, S. C., Mitchell, G., Oates, C., Razvi, S., Weaver, J. U., Shaw, J. A. & Home, P. D. 2009. Circulating endothelial progenitor cells, endothelial function, carotid intima-media thickness and circulating markers of endothelial dysfunction in people with type 1 diabetes without macrovascular disease or microalbuminuria. *Diabetologia,* 52, 1464-73.
Sieveking, D. P. & Ng, M. K. 2009. Cell therapies for therapeutic angiogenesis: back to the bench. *Vasc Med,* 14, 153-66.
Silverman, M. D., Haas, C. S., Rad, A. M., Arbab, A. S. & Koch, A. E. 2007. The role of vascular cell adhesion molecule 1/ very late activation antigen 4 in endothelial progenitor cell recruitment to rheumatoid arthritis synovium. *Arthritis Rheum,* 56, 1817-26.
Stehouwer, C. D., Lambert, J., Donker, A. J. & Van Hinsbergh, V. W. 1997. Endothelial dysfunction and pathogenesis of diabetic angiopathy. *Cardiovasc Res,* 34, 55-68.
Stevens, C. R., Blake, D. R., Merry, P., Revell, P. A. & Levick, J. R. 1991. A comparative study by morphometry of the microvasculature in normal and rheumatoid synovium. *Arthritis Rheum,* 34, 1508-13.
Strauer, B. E., Brehm, M., Zeus, T., Kostering, M., Hernandez, A., Sorg, R. V., Kogler, G. & Wernet, P. 2002. Repair of infarcted myocardium by autologous intracoronary mononuclear bone marrow cell transplantation in humans. *Circulation,* 106, 1913-8.

Tateishi-Yuyama, E., Matsubara, H., Murohara, T., Ikeda, U., Shintani, S., Masaki, H., Amano, K., Kishimoto, Y., Yoshimoto, K., Akashi, H., Shimada, K., Iwasaka, T. & Imaizumi, T. 2002. Therapeutic angiogenesis for patients with limb ischaemia by autologous transplantation of bone-marrow cells: a pilot study and a randomised controlled trial. *Lancet,* 360, 427-35.

Timmermans, F., Van Hauwermeiren, F., De Smedt, M., Raedt, R., Plasschaert, F., De Buyzere, M. L., Gillebert, T. C., Plum, J. & Vandekerckhove, B. 2007. Endothelial outgrowth cells are not derived from CD133+ cells or CD45+ hematopoietic precursors. *Arterioscler Thromb Vasc Biol,* 27, 1572-9.

Westerweel, P. E., Luijten, R. K., Hoefer, I. E., Koomans, H. A., Derksen, R. H. & Verhaar, M. C. 2007. Haematopoietic and endothelial progenitor cells are deficient in quiescent systemic lupus erythematosus. *Ann Rheum Dis,* 66, 865-70.

Westerweel, P. E. & Verhaar, M. C. 2009. Endothelial progenitor cell dysfunction in rheumatic disease. *Nat Rev Rheumatol,* 5, 332-40.

Williamson, J. R., Chang, K., Frangos, M., Hasan, K. S., Ido, Y., Kawamura, T., Nyengaard, J. R., Van Den Enden, M., Kilo, C. & Tilton, R. G. 1993. Hyperglycemic pseudohypoxia and diabetic complications. *Diabetes,* 42, 801-13.

Yamaguchi, Y., Okazaki, Y., Seta, N., Satoh, T., Takahashi, K., Ikezawa, Z. & Kuwana, M. 2010. Enhanced angiogenic potency of monocytic endothelial progenitor cells in patients with systemic sclerosis. *Arthritis Res Ther,* 12, R205.

Yoder, M. C., Mead, L. E., Prater, D., Krier, T. R., Mroueh, K. N., Li, F., Krasich, R., Temm, C. J., Prchal, J. T. & Ingram, D. A. 2007. Redefining endothelial progenitor cells via clonal analysis and hematopoietic stem/progenitor cell principals. *Blood,* 109, 1801-9.

Yoon, C. H., Hur, J., Park, K. W., Kim, J. H., Lee, C. S., Oh, I. Y., Kim, T. Y., Cho, H. J., Kang, H. J., Chae, I. H., Yang, H. K., Oh, B. H., Park, Y. B. & Kim, H. S. 2005. Synergistic neovascularization by mixed transplantation of early endothelial progenitor cells and late outgrowth endothelial cells: the role of angiogenic cytokines and matrix metalloproteinases. *Circulation,* 112, 1618-27.

Ziyadeh, F. N. 2004. Mediators of diabetic renal disease: the case for tgf-Beta as the major mediator. *J Am Soc Nephrol,* 15 Suppl 1, S55-7.

18

Autoimmune Disorders and Lymphomas

Dolcetti R.[1], Ponzoni M.[2,3], Mappa S.[2,4] and Ferreri A.J.M.[2]
[1]*Cancer Bioimmunotherapy Unit, Dept of Oncology, National Cancer Institute CRO-IRCCS,*
[2]*Unit of Lymphoid Malignancies, Dept of Onco-Hematology,*
[3]*Pathology Unit,* [4]*Internal Medicine Unit; San Raffaele Scientific Institute*
Italy

1. Introduction

Patients affected by autoimmune diseases have demonstrated an increased risk of developing lymphoid malignancies. Non-Hodgkin lymphomas (NHL) have consistently been associated with several autoimmune conditions, such as, by way of example, rheumatoid arthritis (RA), Sjögren syndrome (SS) and systemic lupus erythematosus (SLE). Similarly, even if based on fewer studies, an increased risk of malignant lymphomas has also been associated with celiac disease, dermatitis herpetiformis, Hashimoto's thyroiditis, and autoimmune haemolytic anemia. An association between other autoimmune conditions, such as inflammatory bowel diseases (Crohn's disease and ulcerative colitis), psoriasis and systemic sclerosis, and a higher risk of lymphoproliferative disorders has not been consistently proven (Askling *et al*, 2005, von Roon *et al*, 2007, Boffetta *et al*, 2001, Gelfand *et al*, 2006, Chatterjee *et al*, 2005). The magnitude of these associations varies widely among different studies. Reported relative risk is about two-fold in RA, 9-18 fold in SS, 3-6 fold in SLE, celiac disease and Hashimoto thyroiditis, and 2-10 fold in dermatitis herpetiformis. Epidemiologic analysis by NHL subtype have shown that diffuse large B-cell lymphoma (DLBCL) is more frequently associated with RA and SS, while extranodal marginal zone lymphoma, in the respective target organs, is strongly associated with SS (Theander *et al*, 2004) and Hashimoto's thyroiditis. Celiac disease is associated with a 520-fold increased risk of enteropathy-associated T-cell lymphoma of the small intestine (EATL). Autoimmune conditions of the skin including psoriasis, pemphigus and discoid lupus erythematosus have an increased risk of T-cell cutaneous lymphoma (Anderson *et al*, 2009). Hodgkin lymphoma has also been associated with some autoimmune conditions, such as RA, SLE and sclerodermia. On the other hand, it is still unclear why other autoimmune conditions, such as type 1 mellitus diabetes, multiple sclerosis, and sarcoidosis do not present an increased risk of lymphoma development. The exact mechanism of lymphomagenesis in the contest of autoimmunity remains largely unexplained, but it may be related to chronic antigenic stimulation, chronic inflammatory response and deficiency in immunesurveillance, promoting a multistep process of genetic instability resulting in accumulation of genetic alterations. In addition, immunosuppressive medications (e.g., methotrexate) may concur to alter patient's immune status. In this chapter, we review the mainstream of epidemiologic studies, discuss the pathways underlying autoimmunity and lymphomas as well as mechanisms of lymphomagenesis, and summarize the characteristics of the various autoimmune diseases that may be associated with lymphoma. Therapeutic options for these clinically intriguing conditions are also discussed.

2. Epidemiologic studies

The first report of an association between autoimmunity and lymphomas was made in 1966 (Mellors, 1966). Notwithstanding the low incidence of autoimmune and lymphoproliferative disorders in the general population, large patients groups and long observation periods are needed to establish an association between these two conditions. In the past, many population-based case-control and cohort studies were carried out to confirm the consistence of an association between these two diseases. Registry-based cohort studies, which are generally based on hospital discharge diagnosis records, are able to evaluate large cohort of patients affected by different autoimmune disorders following them for the occurrence of cancer, usually using cancer registries. This method allows studying large number of patients with autoimmune diseases although lymphoma occurrence is a rare event. Despite the adequate statistical power of these studies, they may over select patients with severe disease, missing patients who are treated only as outpatients. On the other hand, case-control studies of lymphoma patients allows the evaluation of large numbers of well-characterized cancer cases, providing for a wider range of information about lymphoma subtype and covariate exposure of interest, with the disadvantage of rarity of some autoimmune disorders, the low statistical power and control selection bias. Therefore, both study designs have limitations in evaluating the consistence of this peculiar association. Another important limitation of these studies is the potential bias due to reverse causality (i.e., undiagnosed lymphoma causing paraneoplastic inflammation misclassified as rheumatic disease). Many studies have reported in fact a major risk of lymphoma development during the first year after diagnosis of autoimmune disease or have excluded from analysis this time interval. A meta-analysis of all previous available cohort studies relating SLE, RA and SS to the risk of NHL development showed that NHL is more frequent in patients affected by autoimmune diseases than in the general population, especially for SS and SLE (Zintzaras *et al*, 2005). Importantly, a reason for the inconsistent associations between many autoimmune conditions and NHL overall risk may lie in the molecular, morphologic and etiologic heterogeneity of the different NHL subtypes. One of the largest epidemiologic study published has performed a pooled analysis of self-reported autoimmune conditions and NHL different subtypes, including 29.423 participants in 12 case-control studies over Europe, North America and Australia (Ekstrom Smedby *et al*, 2008). The study concluded that an increased risk of NHL is associated only with few autoimmune disorders and that these associations are stronger for some lymphoma subtypes than others. In fact, a 6.5-fold increased risk of NHL was associated with SS, which is lower than in previous reports including only cohorts of hospitalized patients that may present a more severe form of disease. It has been observed a 250-fold increased risk of parotid gland NHL and a 1.000-fold increased risk of marginal zone B-cell lymphoma of mucosa-associated lymphoid tissue (MALT)-type of the parotid gland and an association with DLBCL. SLE has been associated with a 2.7-fold increased risk of NHL, in particular, DLBCL and MALT lymphomas. Haemolytic anaemia has been associated with DLBCL. In patients with celiac disease, an increased overall risk for NHL was not observed; only associations with entheropathy-associated T-cell lymphoma of small intestine and anaplastic large T-cell lymphoma have been detected. Regarding RA, an overall increased risk of NHL was not observed, but only a moderately increased risk in patients treated with corticosteroids or immunosuppressant. Finally, inflammatory bowel disorders, type I diabetes, sarcoidosis, pernicious anaemia, and multiple sclerosis were not associated with increased risk of NHL. Importantly, this analysis demonstrated a persistent risk of lymphoma development also after ten year of autoimmune disease duration, excluding the risk of autoimmune phenomena triggered by yet undiagnosed lymphomas. Another large population-based case-control study form the U.S. Surveillance Epidemiology and End Results-Medicare database has been conducted on 44.350 lymphoid malignancy cases (> 67 years) and 122.531 population-based controls (Anderson *et al*, 2009). Association between specific lymphoid malignancy subtypes and various autoimmune conditions has been also investigated. Although the study was limited to subjects over age 65, the strongest association by NHL subtype was observed between DLBCL and RA and SS; T-cell lymphoma and haemolytic anaemia, psoriasis, discoid lupus erythematosus, and celiac

Studies	**Disease**	**NHL**	**95% CI**	**HL**	**95% CI**	***p***
Zintzaras, 2005	Reumatoid arthritis	3.9 (SIR)	2.5-5.9	-	-	-
	Systemic lupus erythematosus	7.4	3.3-17	-	-	-
	Primary Sjögren syndrome	18.8	9.5-37.3	-	-	-
Engels, 2005	Reumatoid arthritis	1.3 (OR)	0.8-2.1	-	-	0.24
	Systemic lupus erythematosus	1.3	0.3-5.6	-	-	0.72
	Primary Sjögren syndrome	4.9	0.6-43	-	-	0.11
Landgren, 2006	Reumatoid arthritis	-	-	2.7 (OR)	1.9-4.0	-
	Systemic lupus erythematosus	-	-	5.8	2.2-15.1	-
	Systemic scleroderma	-	-	0.6	0.1-6.2	-
	Hashimoto thyroiditis	-	-	2.0	0.3-14	-
Ekstrom Smedby, 2008	Reumatoid arthritis	1.06 (OR)	0.87-1.29	-	-	< 0.1
	Systemic lupus erythematosus	2.69	1.68-4.3	-	-	0.39
	Primary Sjögren syndrome	4.75	1.79-12.6	-	-	0.93
	Secondary Sjögren syndrome	9.57	2.9-31.6	-	-	-
	Celiac disease	1.5	0.89-2.54	-	-	0.72
Anderson, 2009	Rheumatoid arthritis (OR)	1.2	1.1-1.3	1.5 (OR)	1.1-2.0	-
	Systemic lupus erythematosus	1.5	1.2-1.9	3.5	1.9-6.7	-
	Sjögren syndrome	1.9	1.5-2.3	1.6	0.6-4.4	-
	Systemic scleroderma	1.4	0.9-2.2	2.5	0.6-10	-
	Hashimoto thyroiditis	1.1	0.8-1.4	2.1	1.0-4.8	-
	Celiac disease	1.5	0.9-2.5	-	-	-

Table 1. Epidemiologic studies

disease; marginal zone lymphoma and SLE and haemolytic anaemia; Hodgkin lymphoma (HL) and SLE. Additional analysis excluding data for up to 5 years before the diagnosis of malignancy have been also performed to exclude reverse causality, i.e., lymphoma causing autoimmune disorder. Another population based case-control study disclosed a solid association between NHL and SS and a small increase in NHL risk associated with SLE (Engels *et al*, 2005). While most epidemiologic studies demonstrated a consistent association between autoimmunity and NHL, there are only limited data on the risk of developing HL in these settings. A population-based case-control study during a 40-year period analyzed the association between 32 autoimmune disorders and risk of developing HL (Landgren *et al*, 2006), reporting a statistically significant increased risk to develop HL in patients with personal history of RA, SLE, sarcoidosis, or ITP. In addition, personal or family history of sarcoidosis and ulcerative colitis was associated with significantly increased risk of HL.

3. Pathogenesis

The aetiology of NHL remains largely unexplained, but some well-established risk factors have been identified. Under normal conditions, B and T lymphocytes respond to antigenic stimulation in a regulated manner and proliferative responses are self-limited. Immune dysregulation, leading to a continue lymphocyte proliferation, is considered to play a major role in lymphomagenesis, as demonstrated by an increased risk of lymphoma development in states of immunosuppression (i.e. following organ transplant or hereditary and acquired immunodeficiency syndromes). In addition, the occurrence of specific subtypes of NHL in

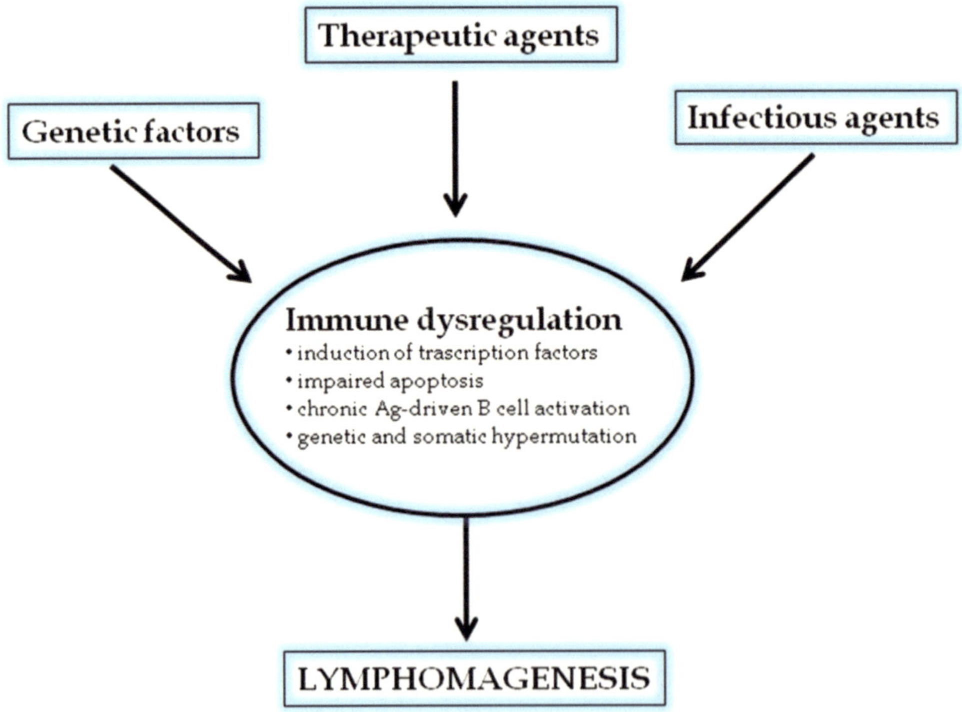

Fig. 1. Proposed pathogenetic factors of lymphomagenesis in the context of autoimmunity

the context of infectious conditions suggests a pathogenic role also for inflammation and chronic immune stimulation. Autoimmune diseases have been considered a possible predisposing factor for lymphoma development as they are characterized by impairment of immune responses leading to a loss of tolerance to self-antigens, a deregulated lymphocyte reactivity with production of autoantibodies against specific tissues and organs. It is conceivable that a sustained antigen-driven B proliferation may increase the risk of adverse genetic events that may finally result in the emergence of a neoplastic clone.

3.1 Immune dysregulation

In the development of lymphoma at primary sites, such as MALT lymphomas arising in the parotid gland during the course of SS or in the thyroid gland in the case of chronic thyroiditis, and as T-cell lymphoma in small intestine of patients with celiac disease, a critical role is played by local chronic antigen-driven stimulation leading to the genesis of organized lymphoid tissue, the so called "tertiary" lymphoid tissue, characterized by organ-specific T- or B-cell proliferation, polyclonality and, eventually, oligo-monoclonality.

3.1.1 Tertiary lymphoid tissue

Chronic inflammatory infiltrates resembling the secondary lymphoid organs have been previously described as "tertiary lymphoid organs" (Picker, 1992) and can be induced by the same mediators of lymphoid ontogenesis, such as tumor necrosis factor (TNF)-beta and other members of the TNF family (Kratz *et al*, 1996), through induction of transcription factors, adhesion molecules, lymphoid-tissue-homing chemokines, and other cytokines (Hjelmstrom, 2001). The transcription factor named nuclear factor kappa-B (NF-κB) is induced by TNF proteins and is involved in lymphoid tissue development through chemokines, adhesion molecules and members of the TNF family themselves. TNF proteins are also required for the normal expression of CXCL13 and CCL21, two homing chemokines crucial for lymphoid neogenesis (Ngo *et al*, 1999). CXCR13 is normally produced by stromal cells in lymphoid tissues and attracts naive B cells and activated and memory T cells *in vitro* (Legler et al, 1998). CCL21 is a ligand for the CCR7 receptor that directs the migration of naive T cells and dendritic cells. Expression of CXCL13 and CCL21 has been found in disease models of chronic inflammation characterized by lymphoid neogenesis (Hjelmstrom, 2001). Chronic autoimmune diseases are characterized by a chronic inflammatory infiltrate in the target organs, with mononuclear cells and lymphoid follicles. The thyroid gland in patients affected by Hashimoto's thyroiditis is organized in a structure that resembles a lymph node, including germinal centres, plasma cells and high endothelial venules (Knecht *et al*, 1981, Kabel *et al*, 1989). Also the thymus of patients affected by autoimmune myasthenia gravis is characterized by the presence of ectopic lymphoid follicles with germinal centres containing activated B lymphocytes and plasma cells that produce autoantibodies (Soderstrom *et al*, 1970, Leprince *et al*, 1990). SS is characterized by the presence of antigen-driven proliferation of B cells and lymphoid follicles with clonally expanded lymphocytes (Freimark *et al*, 1989, Stott *et al*, 1998). Similarly, there is an evidence for lymphoid neogenesis in the chronic synovial inflammation of patients with RA (Watson *et al*, 1994, Randen *et al*, 1995); B cell diversification, somatic hypermutation and plasma cells development occur in the synovial germinal centres (Schroder *et al*, 1996, Kim *et al*, 1999) and the homing chemokine CXCL13 seems to be present in the synovial follicles of patients with RA (Hjelmstrom, 2001).

Expansion of B self-reactive lymphocytes is normally limited by several checkpoint mechanisms able to prevent the development of both autoimmunity and lymphoma. Both such diseases may be the result of a multistep process which ends up with the elimination of such aforementioned checkpoints. This multistep process regards both inherited and somatic mutations of genes involved in these pathways. For example, germinal and somatic mutations of *Fas* are associated with both autoimmune diseases and lymphoproliferative disorders, probably by inhibition of apoptosis. Somatic mutations occur physiologically in lymphocytes, during the course of somatic hypermutation of immunoglobulin genes in the germinal centre of lymphoid follicles of lymph nodes and spleen. VDJ recombination, isotype switching and somatic hypermutation, requiring double strand break and DNA rejoining, are susceptible to error and are known to activate oncogenes and inactivate tumour suppression mechanisms. Secondly, the epidemiological evidence of overlapping pathogenesis between autoimmunity and lymphoma may be explained by an enhanced lymphocyte proliferation resulting in increased rates of somatic mutations (Goodnow, 2007). Acquisition of distinct chromosomal translocations among reactive B cells, such as the t(11;18) in the course of *Helicobacter pylori*-positive chronic gastritis, is known to promote lymphomagenesis. Conversely, a similar risk was not found in other settings characterized by chronic immune responses, such as allergic diseases (Soderberg *et al*, 2006) or inflammatory bowel disease (Smedby *et al*, 2006).

3.1.2 Triad autoimmunity-lymphoproliferation-lymphoma in Sjögren's Syndrome

Among all autoimmune diseases, SS better reflects the mechanism of the triad autoimmunity-lymphoproliferation-lymphoma. The underlying chronic inflammation, in fact, promotes the formation of organized lymphoid tissue, with a crucial role played by TNF-beta, characterized by the presence of high endothelial venules, dendritic cells and follicular dendritic cells, antigen-driven clonal proliferation of B cells, and lymphoid follicles with clonally expanded lymphocytes (Stott *et al*, 1998, Harris, 1999). The SS-associated chronic lymphoproliferation varies from benign to MALT-type lesions, MALT lymphomas, and even aggressive lymphomas (Burke, 1999). In fact, chronic antigen-driven polyclonal B-cell activation in SS seems to support selection and expansion of auto-reactive B-cell clones through the processes of class switch recombination and somatic hypermutation (Stott *et al*, 1998). Subsequent studies confirmed the selective accumulation of a B cell population characterized by a high rate of mutations in productively rearranged VL chain genes (Jacobi *et al*, 2002, Gellrich *et al*, 1999). The genetic instability associated with DNA hypermutation can favour the escape of malignant B cell clones with the consequent development of an overt B-cell lymphoma (Royer *et al*, 1997). The processes of class switch recombination and somatic hypermutation seem to critically depend on the enzyme activation-induced cytidine deaminase (AID). It has been shown (Bombardieri *et al*, 2007) that AID deaminase is expressed within follicular dendritic cell networks of the salivary gland of patients with SS, in a comparable way to that of secondary lymphoid organs, supporting the hypothesis that ectopic lymphoid tissue recapitulates the molecular setting necessary for local autoantibody production and B-cell expansion. The evolution of a non-malignant B-cell clone present in the parotid gland of a single patient with SS followed at multiple time points over a 7-year period to overt B-cell lymphoma has been documented (Gasparotto *et al*, 2003). In this case, lymphoma evolution occurred in a different site (lung) from that of the primary localization of B-cell proliferation (parotid gland), providing evidence that the pulmonary neoplastic clone derived from the salivary gland clone, possibly through the acquisition of oncogenic alterations in cell regulatory genes able to confer a more aggressive phenotype.

3.1.3 *BAFF* deregulation and apoptotic resistance

Whether local antigen-driven stimulation and chronic inflammatory processes are important for the development of distant (typically nodal) NHL such as DLBCL is not yet known. Disease severity and inflammatory load are important determinants of NHL development in SS and RA (Theander *et al*, 2006, Baecklund *et al*, 2006a), with an increased risk of occurrence of DLBCL in these autoimmune disorders (Smedby *et al*, 2008), including factors related to cytokine profile, T cell subset balance and apoptotic resistance (Theander *et al*, 2006, Eguchi, 2001). In RA and SLE, apoptotic resistance is increased and mediated by *Bcl-2* expression, activation of NF-κB by inflammatory cytokines and growth factors, and abnormalities in the expression of B-cell activating factor (*BAFF*) (Eguchi, 2001, Mackay *et al*, 2005). *BAFF* is a critical regulator of B-cell homeostasis, and its excessive production causes multiple autoimmune symptoms in mice models and compromises apoptosis of autoreactive B cells. Deregulated BAFF expression has been described to lead to disease progression and perpetuation of humoral autoimmunity. Patients affected by systemic autoimmune diseases, such as SS, RA and SLE, have increased levels of BAFF in serum and synovial fluid with respect to healthy people. Moreover, serum levels of BAFF in SS correlate with the level of autoantibodies, and with rheumatoid factor in patients with RA. *BAFF* has been therefore proposed to play a major role in the development of SS and to contribute in the development of B-cell malignancies. In SS patients, the overexpression of *BAFF* can cause an excessive immunoglobulin production. In salivary glands of patients with SS, the reduced level of apoptosis among BAFF-expressing cells might lead to maintain signalling for tissue-infiltrating B cells to proliferate and to become autoantibody-producing plasma cells, contributing to germinal centres formation and lymphoma development. Finally, mice carrying a BAFF transgene become highly susceptible to lymphoproliferation, autoimmunity and lymphoma development (Mackay *et al*, 1999). The possible pathogenetic role of BAFF in SS and lymphomagenesis has led to the development of agents neutralizing BAFF as a new therapeutic option for such patients (Szodoray & Jonsson, 2005). Belimumab, the fully human recombinant IgG monoclonal antibody to soluble B-lymphocyte stimulator human antibody (anti-Blys; LymphoStat-B) binds soluble BAFF and prevents interaction with its receptor (Baker *et al*, 2003). Encouraging results have been reported by two large phase III randomized controlled trials of belimumab versus placebo in seropositive SLE patients with stable disease receiving standard of care treatment. The study showed that belimumab improved several markers of disease activity (in the central nervous system, vascular, musculoskeletal, immunologic and cutaneous) and promoted reduction of average steroid dose compared to placebo. Belimumab also determined significative changes in immunologic parameters, such as reduction of IgG and IgM and autoantibodies, increase in C3 and C4 levels, reduction of circulating CD20+ B cells (Thanou-Stavraki & Sawalha, 2011). In summary, a continuous antigen-driven stimulation in a microenvironment where normal regulatory mechanisms are absent may promote both autoimmunity and lymphoma development.

3.2 Genetic factors

Several studies explored the relationship between genetic factors and development of lymphoid malignancies in the different settings of autoimmunity. It has been suggested that some inherited mutations could be involved in pathogenesis of both diseases. For example, inherited mutations of the *TNFSRF6* gene, which encodes the transmembrane protein *Fas* (CD59), a major mediator of lymphocyte apoptosis, lead to a genetic defect in apoptosis responsible of a familial syndrome called "autoimmune lymphoproliferative syndrome of childhood" (ALPS or Canale-Smith syndrome) characterized by chronic, non-malignant diffuse lymphadenopathy and hepatosplenomegaly together with hypergammaglobulinemia, autoantibodies and/or overt autoimmune diseases. These patients are at high risk of developing lymphomas, almost exclusively of the B-cell immunophenotype (HL, follicular, Burkitt and T-cell rich B-cell lymphoma) (Jackson & Puck, 1999) with an incidence of 13% (6 out 46) among cases studied at the US National Institute of Health, with intervals from the onset of ALPS of 6-48 years (Mackay & Rose, 2001). However, previous population-based case control studies have failed to demonstrate that a family history of autoimmune disease is a risk factor for lymphoma development. A multicenter US study on 759 patients observed that a family history of dermatomyositis was associated with NHL, but not family history of 14 other autoimmune diseases (Engels *et al*, 2005). A statistically significant increase in risk of HL among patients with a family history of sarcoidosis or ulcerative colitis has been reported, but no association with a family history of other autoimmune conditions has been demonstrated (Landgren *et al*, 2006). Finally, an association between the risk of lymphoma development and a family history of a wide range of autoimmune diseases has not been detected in a population-based case-control study on 24,728 NHL patients (Mellemkjaer *et al*, 2008). Likewise, an increased risk of lymphoma occurrence among the first-degree relatives of RA patients has not been proven (Ekstrom *et al*, 2003). Therefore, studies evaluating whether genetic factors play a major role in lymphoma development have failed to prove a consistent association in the context of most autoimmune diseases and available data about inherited mutations are still inconsistent.

3.3 Therapeutic agents

The role played by autoimmune disease therapy in the subsequent lymphoma development was extensively analyzed, although with inconclusive results. This seems to be due to a selection bias related to the fact that patients requiring therapy usually show a more aggressive disease. Thus, the comparison between treated and untreated patients may result in a falsely increased treatment-associated risk. Disease modifying anti-rheumatic drugs (DMARDs) such as methotrexate and azathioprine have been suggested to increase the relative risk of malignant lymphoma (Baecklund *et al*, 2006b, Bernatsky *et al*, 2008, Askling *et al*, 2009, Wolfe & Michaud, 2007). However, several large population-based studies failed to demonstrate an increased risk linked to methotrexate *per se* (Baecklund et al, 2006b, Mariette et al, 2002, Wolfe & Michaud, 2004). Corticosteroids, a mainstream of treatment of inflammatory diseases, have never been consistently associated with lymphoma development (Baecklund *et al*, 2006b). Studies about the relationship between nonsteroidal anti-inflammatory drugs (NSAID) and lymphoma are also inconsistent (Baecklund *et al*, 2006b, Sorensen *et al*, 2003). The only exception is constituted by 8 cases of hepatosplenic γδ T-cell lymphoma diagnosed among young patients treated with infliximab or adalimumab for inflammatory bowel disease. All patients were receiving concomitant immunosuppressive therapy with azathioprine or prednisone and it was not possible to ascertain if anti-TNF medication had an exclusive role in the pathogenesis of these lymphomas (Mackey *et al*, 2007). Conversely, although it has not been definitively demonstrated, postponing therapy could contribute to lymphoma development; this could be due to a chronic worsening of the inflammatory microenvironment promoted by uncontrolled disease. In a population-based case-control study (Smedby *et al*, 2006), an increased risk of lymphoma occurrence was detected in patients with RA treated with NSAIDs, corticosteroids and other immunosuppressants but it was not confirmed in untreated patients. This may be related to the fact that the first cohort of patients had a more severe disease with higher levels of chronic inflammation that contributed to lymphoma development.

3.3.1 NSAIDs and steroids

Regular use of aspirin and NSAIDs has been hypothesized to be associated with reduced risk of development of colorectal cancer (RR= 0.5-0.8), and possibly of other cancers as stomach, breast, lung, pancreas, and ovary. Decreased cancer risk may be related to inhibition of prostaglandin synthesis, enhancement of cellular immune response or induction of apoptosis. RA patients, who frequently use long-lasting high doses of both aspirin and other NSAIDs, have a decreased risk of colorectal cancer and possibly female breast cancer (Beauparlant *et al*, 1999). Some prospective cohort and case-control studies analyzed the association between aspirin and non-aspirin NSAID use and risk of NHL with contradictory results. An inverse association was documented in a population-based case-control study (OR=0.72; 95% CI= 0.56-0.91) (Holly *et al*, 1999) and a near significant association between regular use of aspirin and moderate decrease of NHL has also been reported in another hospital-based case-control study in men (OR= 0.82; 95% CI= 0.65-1.04), while women who used acetaminophen regularly experienced a 71% elevation in the risk of B-cell NHL (OR= 1.71; 95% CI 1.18-2.50) (Baker *et al*, 2005). A potential protective effect of analgesic use on NHL risk in women but not in men has also been reported (Beiderbeck *et al*, 2003). Conversely, a positive association between use of aspirin or acetaminophen and NHL has been observed among women, but not among men (RR=1.96; 95% CI=0.56-3.08) in a population-based study (Bernstein & Ross, 1992) and a suggestive positive association has also been reported in a prospective study cohort (RR=1.40; 95% CI= 0.99-1.97). This association was lost when aspirin was evaluated alone (Cerhan *et al*, 2003). Finally, no association between aspirin and other analgesics and lymphoma or leukaemia was observed in two other hospital-based case-control studies (Rosenberg *et al*, 1995, Cartwright *et al*, 1988) and in a large study cohort (Sorensen *et al*, 2003). Although the exact reason of this gender discrepancies is unclear, a different response to pharmacologic agents could be referred to women's lower body weight and high percentage of body fat or to endocrine milieu (Meibohm *et al*, 2002). In fact, clearance of both aspirin and acetaminophen positively correlates with body size and is faster in man rather than women (Miners *et al*, 1986) and some metabolizing enzymes are induced by hormones. Treatment with corticosteroids is one of the mainstreams of the management of systemic inflammatory diseases, because of their strong and fast anti-inflammatory effects. A linkage between corticosteroids and lymphoma risk was suspected in some studies (Bernstein & Ross, 1992, Kato *et al*, 2002, Zhang *et al*, 2004), whereas this association was excluded by others (Engels *et al*, 2005, Smedby *et al*, 2006, Beiderbeck *et al*, 2003, Chang *et al*, 2005). For example, a markedly reduced risk of lymphoma associated with steroid treatment has been observed in RA patients, also after adjustment for disease severity (Baecklund *et al*, 2006a). Also a case-control study of 378 patients with RA-associated lymphoma demonstrated that treatment with oral steroids was associated with a 30% reduced risk of lymphoma (OR=0.69; 95%

CI=0.51-0.94); this feature remained also after adjustment for DMARDs treatment, disease activity and use of intra-articular steroids. Moreover, treatment up to 2 years showed no protective effect, while a treatment of more than 2 years was associated with a markedly reduced risk. Analysis by lymphoma subtype showed the strongest association between oral steroids and DLBCL (Hellgren *et al*, 2010b). The reduced lymphoma risk associated with steroid therapy might be explained by a reduced inflammatory activity induced by these drugs. Conversely, a meta-analysis of case-control and cohort studies reported between 1992 and 2006 failed to prove an increased risk of lymphoma development over the last decades during which there has been an increased use of immunomodulatory drugs such as corticosteroids and NSAID, disproving thus any possible link between therapy and cancer (Bernatsky *et al*, 2007).

3.3.2 Anti-TNF agents

The use of biologic drugs as antagonists of TNF has been extensively evaluated for safety profile both in randomized (Bongartz *et al*, 2006, Leombruno *et al*, 2009) and observational studies (Wolfe & Michaud, 2007, Setoguchi *et al*, 2006, Askling *et al*, 2005). TNF plays an important role in tumour growth control and host defence, and biologic therapy targeting TNF determines an important immunomodulation, raising thus the concern of a possible increased risk of malignancies in patients treated with anti-TNF antibodies. Regarding short-term cancer risk, meta-analysis of clinical trials suggested an increased risk of cancer development (Bongartz *et al*, 2006, Leombruno *et al*, 2009, Bongartz *et al*, 2009), but observational studies did not confirm these results. Randomized controlled trials provide balanced groups for analysis and a well-selected study population but, on the other hand, considering that the time interval from the onset of cancer until its clinical manifestation is counted in years and not in months, any long-term effect of therapy cannot be correctly estimated using data from clinical trials. In addition, the overall number of cancers in these trials is modest, particularly in the control arm. In a review of data from the MedWatch post-market adverse event surveillance system of FDA, 26 cases of spontaneous lymphoproliferative disorders following treatment with etanercept or infliximab have been reported, with an estimated incidence of 19.9 per 10.000 person-year for etanercept and 6.6 per 100.000 person-year for infliximab (Brown *et al*, 2002). These concerns were confirmed also by a meta-analysis of cancer risk in patients affected by RA treated with infliximab or adalimumab in randomized controlled trials, excluding patients treated with etanercept (Bongartz *et al*, 2006), which reported a pooled odds ratio for malignancy in the TNF treated vs. untreated patients of 3.3 (95% CI 1.2-9.1) in a dose-dependent manner. However, included trials were heterogeneous in terms of disease activity, disease duration and previous or concomitant DMARD treatment and usually lasted between 3 months and 1 year, a relatively short interval for estimating cancer incidence. A subsequent update of this meta-analysis with additional data reported an odds ratio of 2.02 (Costenbader *et al*, 2006). Conversely, these results were not confirmed by another meta-analysis assessing 18 randomized controlled trials for a total of 8.808 RA patients (Leombruno *et al*, 2009). Observational studies provide a major number of patients and longer follow-up, but they have also some limitations. The first one is the non-random assignment to treatment, patients with more severe arthritis being more likely treated, and so that outcome could be related to severity of disease rather than treatment. Other limitations may be due to less selected study subjects and introduced bias such as age, sex, smoking history, disease activity and baseline use of corticosteroids. Another bias could be introduced by physician's decision not to prescribe anti-TNF treatment to a patient with a history of malignancies. Finally, last reason for the divergence between data from trials and from observational studies is the control chosen in the latter. In fact, patients newly starting therapy with anti-TNF should be compared with patients newly starting therapy with other agents for the same disease (Ray, 2003). In Sweden, patients treated with anti-TNF drugs were included in a regional register since the introduction of etanercept and infliximab in 1999 (Geborek *et al,* 2002). A study comparing 757 patients treated with etanercept or infliximab from 1999 to 2002 with 800 patients who received conventional therapy showed no increased risk in solid tumors in anti-TNF treated patients, but, interestingly, five cases of lymphoma were identified among these patients (1.603 person-year), and, compared with conventional-therapy cohort, the relative risk of lymphoma in patients treated with anti-TNF agents was 4.9 (95% CI 0.9-26.2) (Geborek *et al,* 2005). Lymphoma incidence from follow-up of 18.572 American RA patients compared with general population allowed to detect 29 cases of lymphoma, with an overall relative risk for lymphoma of 1.9 in patients with RA not treated with TNF antagonists and tripled (2.9) in patients receiving treatment with TNF antagonists; 2.6 in those receiving infliximab with or without etanercept; and 3.8 in those receiving etanercept with or without infliximab (Wolfe & Michaud, 2004). The increased risk in the TNF antagonist treated group might be due to the fact that patients with the highest risk of lymphoma received TNF antagonists. Consequently, the authors were unable to conclude whether the increased standardized rate ratios were related to RA or truly associated with the drugs. Additionally, this study was not adjusted for patient characteristics other than age and sex. Analysis of cancer risk in TNF antagonists users using a Swedish registry of anti-TNF treated patients and community-based RA patients detected five cases of lymphoma per 1.603 person-year in the treated group and two cases per 3.948 person-year in the comparison group (Franklin *et al,* 2005). The adjusted hazard ratio for lymphoma was 4.9 in anti-TNF treated group, suggesting a large increase in risk. Again, RA severity in patients never treated with anti-TNF agents may be minor. The comparison between a cohort of 4.160 RA patients treated with anti-TNF agents with 53.067 patients with untreated RA, showed that patients with RA are at increased risk of lymphomas in line with previous estimations, and using these expected RA rates as reference, that patients treated with TNF antagonists were not at any additional increased lymphoma risk compared with untreated patients (Askling *et al,* 2005). A cohort study using patients with RA treated with methotrexate (MTX) as a control group did not show any significant increase in the risk of cancer in biologic DMARDS users. This particular control group has been chosen because of similar disease severity between patients treated with these two strategies, and investigators have concluded that it is unlikely that RA patients who have received biologic agents have a greater risk of lymphoproliferative disorders compared with those treated with MTX (Setoguchi *et al,* 2006). A single observational study has reported relative risk for cancer occurrence per single anti-TNF agent (infliximab, etanercept, adalimumab), finding a positive association between biologic therapy and skin cancers, but not with other malignancies, with a median time of exposure of 3.0 years, for any of the three agents separately. However, patients were not followed-up from the start of anti-TNF therapy and so any assessment of risk per time since treatment start was not carried out (Wolfe & Michaud, 2007). Finally, the largest population-based study with the longest observation period investigating cancer risks associated with anti-TNF therapy in RA patients has failed to prove an overall increase of risk during the first 6 years after treatment start and during follow-up time. In fact patients treated with anti-TNF drugs had the same cancer risk of naïve patients and of those starting MTX or DMARDs combination therapy. Incidence or relative risk of cancer does not increase with time nor with duration of active therapy (Askling *et al*, 2009).

Studies	Overall	95% CI	Infliximab	95% CI	Etanercept	95% CI	Adalimumab	95% CI
Wolfe, 2004	1.9 (SIR)	1.3-2.7	2.6	1.4-4.5	3.8	1.9-7.5	-	-
Geborek, 2005	11.5 (SIR)	3.7-26.9	-	-	-	-	-	-
Askling, 2005	1.9 (SIR)	1.7-2.1	-	-	-	-	-	-
Setoguchi, 2006	1.11 (HR)	0.51-2.37	-	-	-	-	-	-
Wolfe, 2007	1.7 (SIR)	1.3-2.2	0.9	0.4-2.1	1.3	0.6-2.8	1.3	0.2-10
Leombruno, 2008	1.26 (OR)	0.52-3.06	-	-	-	-	-	-

Table 2. Lymphoma risk and anti-TNF agents

3.3.3 Methotrexate

Methotrexate (MTX) is a widely used DMARD in the context of autoimmune diseases. RA patients treated with MTX may develop a lymphoproliferative disorder (LPD) resembling lymphomas occurring in immunosuppressed patients (Ellman *et al*, 1991, Kingsmore *et al*, 1992, Liote *et al*, 1995). LPD develops in RA patients at a frequency 2.0-5-fold higher than in general population. MTX-LPD is classified along with other iatrogenic immunodeficiency-related LPDs by WHO classification (Swerdlow *et al*, 2008) and, among these, DLBCL accounts for about 50% of cases, with frequent extranodal involvement and HL for 10-20% of cases. MTX-LPD and non-MTX-LPD seem to share similar clinical findings in RA patients, such as sex, age, primary site, stage and outcome (5-year OS: 59% vs. 53%) (Hoshida *et al*, 2007). Conversely, other papers did not confirm increased incidence of lymphoma in MTX-treated RA patients, even after long-term follow-up (Moder *et al*, 1995, Bologna *et al*, 1997, Kremer, 1997, Weinblatt *et al*, 1998). In a prospective series of 18.572 RA patients, treatment with MTX alone has not been associated with an increased standardized incidence ratio for lymphoma with respect to untreated patients (1.7 vs 1.0) (Wolfe & Michaud, 2004). These results confirmed those reported in a 3-year national prospective study on French RA patients treated with MTX. Investigators have found no increase in lymphoma risk among treated patients compared with French general population. However, in the latter study, authors did not even find an increased lymphoma risk in RA patients overall compared to general population (Mariette *et al*, 2002). There are some case reports of lymphoma regression after MTX discontinuation in patients treated for autoimmune diseases (Liote *et al*, 1995, Kamel *et al*, 1993, Salloum *et al*, 1996). Complete remission occurred generally within 4 weeks after discontinuation of MTX and appeared to persist over a median follow-up of 15 months (4-60). On the other hand, partial remission occurred in a time interval longer than four weeks, often about 2-3 months later (Rizzi *et al*, 2009). Regression of LPD after MTX discontinuation can be considered an evidence of the carcinogenic potential of MTX. This drug in fact is capable to directly induce reactivation of Epstein-Barr virus (EBV) infection with release of virions (Feng *et al*, 2004). An immunodeficient state provides the conditions for the development of lymphoma possibly through the activation of the oncogenic EBV. The EBV positive rate among patients affected by autoimmune disease and lymphoma is about 30% (Hoshida *et al*, 2007, Kamel *et al*, 1993). Moreover, patients affected by RA have an elevated number of EBV-infected circulating B lymphocytes and a major T-cell defect in EBV-specific suppression (Tosato *et al*, 1984). Taken together, the oncogenic role of EBV, the impaired immune response of RA patients to EBV and the additional immunosuppressive effect of MTX may account for EBV-positive lymphoma development in a small number of RA patients treated with MTX (Baecklund *et al*, 1998). The monoclonal antibody rituximab is currently used for the treatment of LPD after allogeneic transplantation. There are still few reports about its use for MTX-LPDs and more studies are warranted to elucidate its potential therapeutic role in this context.

4. Autoimmune entities

	Most frequent subtype	**Risk factors**
Rheumatoid arthritis	Diffuse large B- cell lymphoma	High inflammatory activity Male gender
Sjögren syndrome	MALT lymphoma	Low serum immunoglobulins levels High serum β2 microglobulin level Disappearance of a positive rheumatoid factor Hypocomplementemia Low CD4 levels Palpable purpura, parotid gland enlargement
Systemic lupus erythematosus	Diffuse large B- cell lymphoma	Autoimmune haemolytic anaemia Leukopenia Chronic thrombocytopenia Salivary gland swellings Pulmonary infiltrates and/or recurrent pneumonia
Hashimoto's thyroiditis	MALT lymphoma and diffuse large B-cell lymphoma	-
Systemic sclerosis	B-cell lymphomas	-
Celiac disease	Entheropathy-type T-cell lymphoma	Inadequate gluten-free diet
Dermatitis herpetiformis	Entheropathy-type T-cell lymphoma	Inadequate gluten-free diet

Table 3. Most frequent histologic subtypes associated with singular autoimmune entities and known risk factors

4.1 Rheumatoid arthritis

RA is a multisystem chronic autoimmune disorder affecting joint and almost any organ system, with inflammatory nodules formation, interstitial lung disease and leukocytoclastic vasculitis (Turesson & Matteson, 2004). Several studies have demonstrated that patients with RA have a 2-fold increased risk of developing lymphoma (Ekstrom *et al*, 2003, Franklin *et al*, 2006) and a link between disease severity and lymphoma risk exist (Smedby *et al*, 2006, Baecklund *et al*, 2006a). A nested case-control study performed to determine factors predisposing to lymphoma development in RA patients demonstrated that a high inflammatory activity is the greater risk factor with a an odds ratio of 25.8 compared with low inflammatory activity (Baecklund *et al*, 1998). Furthermore, a study on Felty syndrome, a complication of severe RA, reported a 13-fold relative risk for lymphoma compared with that of general population (Gridley *et al*, 1994). Men affected by RA display a higher standardized incidence ratio for the development of NHL and HL than female (Gridley *et al*, 1993). Finally, a personal history of lymphoma in the years preceding diagnosis of autoimmune disease is not more common in patients affected by RA than expected in general population, while the increased risk of lymphoma development occurs in the first 10 years from RA diagnosis. This proves that shared susceptibility or common risk factors are not the major explanation for this increased risk, but it indicates a critical link between the RA disease or its therapy and the subsequent lymphoma development (Hellgren *et al*, 2010a). Interestingly, the reported relative risk rates remained relatively constant over time despite therapeutic changes occurred in RA.

4.1.1 Pathogenesis

The increased risk of lymphoma development in RA patients may arise from the interaction of multiple factors: activation of autoimmune B lymphocytes, chronic inflammation, poor EBV control and immunosuppressive therapy (Balandraud *et al*, 2005). It has been hypothesized that a constant immune stimulation of B cells by auto-antigens may result in both synovitis and lymphocyte activation, finally leading to malignant transformation (Symmons, 1985). Evidence of a B-cell activation is derived from the finding of increased levels of B cell activating factors in RA patients, such as BLy and APRIL, which are produced in the synovial lesions and can drive B cell expansion (Mackay *et al*, 2005, Seyler *et al*, 2005). Moreover, several studies have also reported oligoclonal B cell expansion both in the synovium and in the peripheral blood of RA patients (Berek & Kim, 1997). Whether the increased risk is entirely a consequence of the disease and/or of its treatment is not yet fully ascertained. Patients with RA may lack immunocompetence, being more susceptible to lymphoma development, or immunosuppressive treatment may concur to weaken the patient's immune response. Therefore, lymphoma in RA could be due to a too strong or insufficient immunosuppressive therapy (Weyand *et al*, 2006). A matched case-control study on 378 consecutive Swedish RA patients in whom lymphoma occurred between 1964 and 1995 and 378 healthy controls showed that 48% of lymphoma cases were DLBCLs, and, within those, EBV infection was detected in 12% of lymphomas. Approximately half of the patients had received corticosteroids; 44% had received intra-articular injection of steroids; over 70% of patients had been treated with DMARDs, most frequently antimalarial agents; a few patients had received azathioprine (6%) or MTX (6%) and none had received anti-TNF therapy. An increased lymphoma risk was found only in the azathioprine-treated group, while oral steroids proved to reduce this risk (OR 0.6), especially the intra-articular steroid treatment (OR 0.2). Patients affected both by RA and lymphoma had received similar treatment than those without lymphoma (Baecklund *et al*, 2006a). In a Japanese cohort of RA patients not treated with immunosuppressive drugs, DLBCL was again the most frequently detected histotype and EBV was present in 30% of cases. Four cases were HL, all of them EBV positive (Hoshida *et al*, 2004). The increased risk of NHL development could be referred to the impaired capacity of RA patients to control infection of EBV (Balandraud *et al*, 2005). EBV is an oncogenic herpes virus involved in the pathogenesis of several lymphomas in the context of states of immunodeficiency (Young & Rickinson, 2004, Ambinder, 2003). EBV is not usually found in DLBCL of immunocompetent patients (Ambinder, 2003). EBV-related lymphomagenesis is characteristic in the setting of organ or bone marrow transplantation and congenital or acquired immunodeficiency disorders (Loren *et al*, 2003). Patients affected by RA have an impaired immune response to EBV. High serum titre of anti-EBV specific antibodies have been detected in some RA patients (Alspaugh *et al*, 1981), EBV-specific CD8+ T cells have been found in synovial fluid (Tan *et al*, 2000) and EBV DNA was isolated from the joints of RA patients (Edinger *et al*, 1999). An impaired control of the outgrowth of EBV infected cells in vitro was also observed (Tosato *et al*, 1981). This hypothesis is also supported by studies of EBV load in RA patients. In fact an increase in shedding of EBV in saliva and in the proportion of EBV-infected circulating B cells in RA patients has been shown (Tosato *et al*, 1984, Yao *et al*, 1986). The mean EBV load in peripheral blood of RA patients is more than 8-fold greater than in normal healthy control, similarly to what occurs in transplant recipients (Balandraud *et al*, 2003). Nonetheless, the overall incidence of EBV positivity in NHL reported in previous cohorts is 24% (Baecklund *et al*, 2006a, Mariette *et al*, 2002), too low to entirely justify the increased incidence of lymphomas among these patients.

4.1.2 Lymphoma subtypes

DLBCL is the most common lymphoma subtype in RA patients, with a prevalence of 48%-67% among all NHL (Mariette *et al*, 2002, Baecklund *et al*, 2003), a slightly higher incidence with respect to the general population of western countries, where DLCBL represents the 30-40% of all NHL. DLBCLs can be further subdivided into germinal centre-like (GC) and activated B cell-like subtypes by gene expression profiling, characterized by a different cellular origin and a different prognosis. The majority of RA patients develops a DLBCL of non GC subtype, particular those with a severe and longstanding disease. These lymphomas are characterized by advanced stage at diagnosis, rapid progression and a worse prognosis (5-year OS: 16% vs. 33% for the GC subtypes). In those patients presenting a severe disease and a continuous immune stimulation, the proliferative drive might determine an increased risk of genetic aberrations, particularly in the peripheral activated B cells, the expansion of an uncontrolled peripheral B cell clone and therefore the development of a non-GC DLBCL. Otherwise, alternative pathways are also probably involved in lymphomagenesis, since only a minor proportion of DLBCL are of GC subtype (30%) and other lymphoma subtypes have also been reported in RA patients (Baecklund *et al*, 2006a). The human germinal-centre associated lymphoma protein (HGAL) is a marker of GC B cell derivation, expressed in the cytoplasm of GC lymphocytes and in lymphomas of GC derivation (Lossos *et al*, 2003, Natkunam *et al*, 2005), which inhibits cell migration in normal GC cells and lymphoma cells (Lu *et al*, 2007). HGAL immunoreactivity has been found in 38 (34%) of 111 RA-DLBCLs (Baecklund *et al*, 2006b), a lower proportion than that reported in DLBCL in general (68%)

(Natkunam *et al*, 2005), but not surprising giving the fact that the majority of RA-DLBCLs are of the non-GC type. HGAL expression has been associated with a limited-stage disease and better survival. The expression of HGAL as a GC marker may thus been associated with a better clinical course in RA-DLBCLs.

4.2 Sjögren Syndrome

SS is a chronic systemic autoimmune disease clinically characterized by dry mouth (xerostomia) and dry eyes (keratoconjunctivite sicca) (Kassan & Moutsopoulos, 2004). It is distinguished by a lymphoproliferative sialadenitis (LESA) with lymphocyte infiltration of salivary ducts, ductal epithelial cell proliferation and apoptosis (Daniels, 1984). This disorder can occur either alone, known as primary SS, or in the context of other systemic autoimmune disorders, such as RA, systemic sclerosis, SLE, which is known as secondary SS. Compared with the general population, an increased risk of developing NHL during the course of such disease was reported (Kassan *et al*, 1978, Ioannidis *et al*, 2002). Patients affected by SS, in fact, have an increased relative risk of 28 fold to develop extranodal MALT lymphoma (MZL) of the salivary gland and a 11-fold increased risk of developing a DLBCL arising *de novo* or by transformation of a previous indolent lymphoma (Smedby *et al*, 2006). Relative risk to develop a lymphoma is 8.7 for patients with primary SS form and 4.5 for patients with a secondary SS (Kauppi *et al*, 1997). NHL is the major complication during the course of the disease, with a prevalence of 4.3% (Voulgarelis *et al*, 1999). The high risk of lymphoma development suggests that it originates locally as a consequence of chronic lymphocyte activation due to the autoimmune setting.

4.2.1 Pathogenesis

Lymphocytes have a central role in the pathogenesis of both SS and lymphoma, but whether T or B lymphocytes play the leading role is controversial. From one side, biopsies of salivary and lachrymal glands are characterized by a mixed infiltrate of predominant CD4 and CD8 T cells, showing restriction of TCR usage (Adamson *et al*, 1983). On the other side, primary SS is characterized by increased monoclonal Ig and by the development of lymphomas of B-cell type. A B-cell mediated autoimmune response occurs in the salivary glands. A wide variety of nuclear auto-antigens are immune targets in SS patients. Anti-nuclear antibody as anti-SSA/Ro and anti-SSB/La are detectable in 70-85% of patients (Jonsson *et al*, 2003). The cause of B-cell hyperactivity in primary SS is not known. Exocrine glands of SS patients show an accumulation of B cells clustering in benign polyclonal aggregates (Brandtzaeg & Johansen, 2005), harbouring mutated IgVH genes and therefore being GC, marginal zone or memory B cells. Successively, an evolution from benign to malignant B lymphoproliferation has been described in the course of primary SS, but not of secondary (Anderson & Talal, 1972). Initial benign polyclonal clusters of B-cells enlarge to organize lymphoid follicle-like structures with germinal centres (GCs), in which plasma cells differentiate. The role of local antigens is crucial for the development of these extralymphoid GCs (Youinou *et al*, 2010). The evolution from a benign B-cell aggregate to a malignant lymphoma may be therefore the consequence of the autoimmune response through the selection and expansion of a monoclonal B-cell clone (Friedman *et al*, 1991). Mutations of *p53* are also involved in lymphoma development in these patients (Tapinos *et al*, 1999). Approximately 20% of SS patients exhibits monoclonal Igs in the serum and urine and mixed monoclonal cryoglobulinemia (MMC) with an IgMk monoclonal rheumatoid factor (RF) component (Youinou *et al*, 1988, Tzioufas *et al*, 1986). Monoclonality therefore correlates with the transition from the autoimmune state to NHL. Various studies on clonality have demonstrated that SS patients with the same and persistent monoclonal B-cell expansion in follow-up biopsies are at higher risk of lymphoma developing. MALT lymphoma cells are found only in glands for years and a subsequent spread outside the salivary may involve the lymph nodes and other extranodal organs (Royer *et al*, 1997).

4.2.2 Clinical characteristics

The development of a malignant lymphoproliferation occurs only in a subset of SS patients and is characterized by the emergence of clinical and serologic parameters in the initial phases of disease, the monitoring of which is important for early detection of malignancy and timely therapeutic intervention (Tzioufas *et al*, 1986, Moutsopoulos *et al*, 1983). Usually, median age at lymphoma diagnosis is 58 years, and the median time from SS diagnosis is 7.5 years (Voulgarelis *et al*, 1999). MZL is the most common histologic subtype, but also follicular lymphoma, lymphoplasmacytoid lymphoma and DLBCL have been reported (Kassan *et al*, 1978, Valesini *et al*, 1997, Mariette, 1999). MZL in SS patients is generally localized at diagnosis (stage I and II) and is characterized by a small tumour burden, good performance status and normal lactate dehydrogenase serum levels. The salivary glands are the most commonly involved organs, with parotid gland enlargement being the main presenting symptom, but near 20% of these lymphomas involve other extra-nodal sites, such as stomach, nasopharynx, skin, liver, kidney, and lung, justifying indeed the importance of a complete staging at diagnosis. Bone marrow involvement is rare (10% of cases) and B symptoms are uncommon. Other clinical manifestations are skin vasculitis, peripheral nerve and renal involvement, anemia, lymphopenia, monoclonal immunoglobulins and mixed monoclonal cryoglobulinemia (MMC) (Voulgarelis *et al*, 1999). Indolent lymphomas arisen in SS patients experience high-grade transformation, mostly in DLBCLs, in about 10% of cases. This evolution is characterized by nodal and extra-nodal dissemination and a unfavourable prognosis, with a median overall survival shorter than two years (Voulgarelis *et al*, 1999). It has been proven by immunohistochemical and genotypic studies that such DLBCLs arise from the same clone as indolent lymphomas, as a consequence of genetic alterations such as p53 allelic loss or mutation, hypermethylation of p15 and p16 genes, deletion of p16 gene (Du *et al*, 1996, Neumeister *et al*, 1997).

4.2.3 Risk factors

Some risk factors for lymphoma development have been identified in SS patients. Lymphoma risk seems to increase with disease severity, expressed by decreased levels of serum immunoglobulins, high serum β2-microglobulin levels and disappearance of a previous positive rheumatoid factor (FR) (Anderson & Talal, 1972, Anaya *et al*, 1996); parotid gland enlargement, splenomegaly, lymphadenopathy (Kassan *et al*, 1978); low C4 levels and palpable purpura (Ioannidis *et al*, 2002, Skopouli *et al*, 2000); MMC (Tzioufas *et al*, 1996). A higher relative risk of developing lymphoproliferative disorders in patients with an early onset of disease has been suggested, with a significant and independent association between lymphoma development and low C4 levels (Ramos-Casals *et al*, 2005). An adverse prognostic value of low levels of C3 (Theander *et al*, 2004), vasculitis, severe involvement in parotid scintigraphy, hypocomplementaemia and/or cryoglobulins at diagnosis (Brito-

Zeron *et al*, 2007) have been proposed in patients with primary SS. Patients with such risk factors should be closely monitored.

4.2.4 Lymphoma treatment

Many patients with localized MALT lymphoma may be managed with a "wait and watch" policy, with a median overall survival of 6.4 years (Voulgarelis *et al*, 1999). In a retrospective study (Ambrosetti *et al*, 2004), no difference in outcome between patients treated with surgery, radiotherapy or chemotherapy and those who were not treated has been reported. Single-agent chemotherapy is indicated (alkylating agents; purine analogues; monoclonal antibody rituximab) for multiple extra-nodal disease. The purine analogue cladribine has been associated with a 75% complete remission rate in patients with SS-associated MALT lymphoma (Voulgarelis *et al*, 2002); while the efficacy of the anti-CD20 monoclonal antibody rituximab is controversial (Pijpe *et al*, 2005, Quartuccio *et al*, 2009). Combined chemotherapy (CHOP-like regimens) should be reserved to patients with high tumour burden or aggressive lymphoma. R-CHOP regimen has been associated with complete remission (duration 10-23 months) in four patients with SS-aggressive NHL. Importantly, certain signs and symptoms of MC type II (purpura, peripheral neuropathy and arthralgias) significantly improved with treatment, the levels of circulating cryoglobulins and RF decreased, and C4 levels returned to normal (Voulgarelis *et al*, 2006).

4.3 Systemic Lupus Erythematosus

SLE is a systemic autoimmune disease characterized by variable severity and a multisystem involvement, including cardiovascular, musculoskeletal, excretory, respiratory, and neurological involvement. Prognosis of SLE patients has considerably improved during the last decades, with an increase in 5-year survival from <50% before 1955 to >90% nowadays (Moss *et al*, 2002), due to the use of novel therapeutic options. Nevertheless, the incidence of late complications seems to be increased and mortality due to malignancies remains higher than that of general population (Nossent *et al*, 2007). This could be referred to the common pathogenic pathways in lupus and cancer. Lupus and various malignancies share some risk factors, such as genetic predisposition, viral infections (EBV), hormones (insulin-like growth factor, prolactin, oestrogen, and growth hormone) (Bernatsky *et al*, 2002, Poole *et al*, 2009). Another shared characteristic is represented by antiphospholipid antibodies, frequently present in both diseases and recently associated with cancer development (Tincani *et al*, 2010). SLE has been associated with a 2.7 - 4.1 fold increased risk of NHL development (Ekstrom Smedby *et al*, 2008, Abu-Shakra *et al*, 1993, Ekstrom *et al*, 2003), and some studies have also suggested a link between SLE and HL (Landgren *et al*, 2006, Bernatsky *et al*, 2007). A multi-site international cohort study calculated a standardized incidence ratio (SIR) for all hematologic malignancies of 2.75 and for NHL of 3.64 (Bernatsky *et al*, 2005b). As far as HL, same authors observed a SIR of 2.4 in another large multi-site international cohort (Bernatsky *et al*, 2007). The pooled analysis combining these data with those of other large cohort studies provided a SIR estimate for HL in SLE of 3.16. Generally, aggressive lymphomas, such as DLBCL are more common in SLE patients (Smedby *et al*, 2006, Simon *et al*, 2007, Bernatsky *et al*, 2005a, Lofstrom *et al*, 2007). In general population, DLBCL accounts for 30% of all lymphomas, but in SLE patients this percentage is between 38% and 64% (Smedby *et al*, 2006, Bernatsky *et al*, 2005a, King & Costenbader, 2007). No subtyping into germinal-centre like or activated B-cell like subtype has been reported.

4.3.1 Pathogenesis

Concerning genetic predisposition, a possible reason for the increased risk of NHL in SLE is that distinct major histocompatibility complex (MHC)-haplotypes may predispose to both disorders (Okada *et al*, 1991). The role of immunosuppressive therapy is controversial; it may impair immune defence resulting in an increased risk of lymphomagenesis. However, SLE patients who have never been treated with immunosuppressive agents have the highest rate of NHL incidence during the first year from diagnosis, suggesting that the increased risk is not related to cumulative doses of therapy (Kiss *et al*, 2010). A nested case-cohort study performed to assess the HR for cancer within a multi-site international SLE cohort after exposure to immunosuppressive drugs (anti-malarial drugs, systemic glucocorticoids, NSAIDs, aspirin) showed an adjusted HR for overall cancer risk of 0.82. This risk seems to be higher when only haematological malignancies are considered (Bernatsky *et al*, 2008). In addition to extrinsic risk factors, there are also defects in the immune system contributing to the development of both SLE and lymphomas, as the abnormal B-cell activation due to the chronic and persistent antigen-stimulation, cell-cycle deregulation and impaired apoptosis, which leads to uncontrolled cell proliferation, an exaggerated humoral autoimmune response and the increased risk of oncogene translocation (Illes *et al*, 2009). The impaired immune response in SLE is thus characterized by the accumulation of activated self-reactive B and T cells (Xu & Wiernik, 2001). Many studies have underlined the role of impaired apoptosis in this process. For example, the MRL/lpr mouse, a murine SLE model, has defects in the *Fas* gene, leading to defects in apoptosis and subsequent development of SLE (Watanabe-Fukunaga *et al*, 1992). Mice with mutations of *PTEN*, a tumor suppressor gene, which impairs the *Fas*-mediated elimination of activated lymphocytes, develop SLE characterized by ANA antibodies, glomerulonephritis and lymphadenopathies (Di Cristofano *et al*, 1999). Also *bcl-2*, a proto-oncogene involved in the majority of B NHL, is highly expressed in SLE (Aringer *et al*, 1994), causing prolonged survival of auto-reactive B cells and thus favouring malignant transformation (Xu & Wiernik, 2001). The persistent clonal expansion of benign hyperactive B and T cells retained in lymph node of SLE patients in response to self-antigens exposes these cells to DNA damage, ultimately leading to neoplastic transformation (Xu & Wiernik, 2001). Increased serum levels of type-I Interferons (IFNs a/b) is also associated with active SLE disease (Theofilopoulos *et al*, 2005). The IFNs are cytokines that inhibit cell proliferation and modulate cell survival (Banchereau & Pascual, 2006), and also inhibit apoptosis induced by signalling through B-cell receptor (Su & David, 1999). The p202a murine protein is a member of the interferon-inducible p200-protein family (Choubey & Kotzin, 2002). Increased levels of the p202 protein in splenic B cells of B6.Nba2 SLE susceptible mice determine defects of apoptosis and accumulation of B cells in the spleen (Xin *et al*, 2006) probably by inhibiting p53-mediated transcriptional activation of genes that encode pro-apoptotic proteins as well as transcriptional repression of genes that encode anti-apoptotic proteins. It is therefore possible that increased levels of p202 in B cells also contribute to enhance the risk of developing B-cell malignancies (Veeranki & Choubey, 2010). The murine p202 protein does not have any human homologue, but the human IFI16 protein, a member of the p200-protein family, is functionally similar. An increased expression of IFI16 protein in normal human cells determines cellular growth arrest and up to 29% of SLE patients present high auto-antibodies titres to the IFI16 protein (Choubey *et al*, 2008). IFI16 protein binds p53, so basal and IFN-induced increased levels of IFI16 in SLE patients may inhibit the p53 mediated transcription of target genes (Choubey *et al*, 2008). Finally, SLE patients have high plasma levels of BAFF (Do & Chen-Kiang, 2002), which activates NF-kB (Laabi & Strasser, 2000). Mice overexpressing BAFF develop a SLE-like disease and exhibit B-cell activation (Mackay *et al*, 1999). Also the increased level of IFI16 protein in B cells is capable to activate the NF-kB transcription factor, which persistent activation has been related to the development of B cell malignancies (Vallabhapurapu & Karin, 2009). In addition, NF-kB induces IL-6 expression (Choubey & Panchanathan, 2008). Overall, these results suggest that the triad IFI16/NF-kB/IL-6 could be involved in the development of B-cell malignancies in SLE patients. Recently, it was also shown that antiribosomal-P-protein (anti-P) antibodies, present in nearly 15-20% of patients with SLE active disease, cross react with phospholipids (Caponi *et al*, 2007), enhancing the production of TNF-alfa and IL-6 by monocytes (Toubi & Shoenfeld, 2007), which increases proliferation of normal and clonal B cells. The role of EBV in the pathogenesis of lymphoma in SLE patients has not been fully investigated. An increased prevalence of EBV infection in young patients with SLE has been reported (James *et al*, 1997) and there are some observations that, in some cases, EBV may be a trigger of lymphomagenesis in SLE (Verdolini *et al*, 2002). In contrast, in a retrospective study analyzing lymphoma development in a large cohort of SLE patients, EBV positivity was found only in 17% of cases (King & Costenbader, 2007). Whether EBV infection causes SLE and/or lymphoma independently has not yet been ascertained.

4.3.2 Clinical characteristics

The emerge of NHL in a SLE patient is clinically difficult to recognize in the current practice, due to the fact that many lymphoma characteristics are already part of the autoimmune disease (lymphadenopathy, fever, weight loss, hepato-splenomegaly, cytopenias, autoantibodies), raising the possibility that SLE might be a paraneoplastic syndrome appearing in the context of the lymphoid malignancy. Some clinical SLE characteristics as haematological manifestations (autoimmune haemolytic anaemia, leukopenia, hyperglobulinemia, chronic thrombocytopenia) (King & Costenbader, 2007), sicca symptoms/salivary gland swellings, pulmonary infiltrates, and/or recurrent pneumonia (Lofstrom *et al*, 2007) have been associated with increased risk of developing lymphoma. The common involvement of mucosal membranes, salivary glands and lung parenchyma in patients developing a lymphoma could be due to the fact that, in an immune-deficient patient, an impaired barrier for exogenous agents, as viruses, favour recurrent infections, which may be involved in lymphomagenesis. Median age at lymphoma diagnosis is 50 years, with a median time interval from SLE diagnosis of 17.8 years (King & Costenbader, 2007). Diffuse large B cell lymphoma is the most common subtype (King & Costenbader, 2007). After diagnosis of NHL a 5-year survival probability of 47%-50% has been estimated (Bernatsky *et al*, 2005b, Lofstrom *et al*, 2007), and mortality in patients with both diseases is usually due to progressive B-cell malignancy (Xu & Wiernik, 2001).

4.4 Hashimoto's thyroiditis

Hashimoto's thyroiditis (HT) is an autoimmune chronic inflammatory disease of the thyroid, histologically characterized by a severe and progressive lymphocytic infiltration causing destruction of the glandular parenchyma and consequent goitre development and hypothyroidism. It commonly affects middle-aged women (Aozasa, 1990). The activation of CD4+ T lymphocytes specific for thyroid antigens is considered the trigger of the autoimmune process in HT (Weetman & McGregor, 1994, Dayan & Daniels, 1996). Autoantibodies produced in HT are specific for thyreoglobulin, thyroperoxidase and the thyroid stimulating hormone receptor (TSH-R). The first two antibodies are not detected in all patients. Antibodies against TSH-R block the activation of this receptor, causing the functional impairment of the thyroid. On the other side, activated CD4+ T cells recruit cytotoxic CD8+ T cells and B cells into the thyroid causing the direct killing of thyroid cells. Patients affected by HT are at increased risk of developing primary thyroid lymphoma (PTL) with a relative risk of 67 fold for marginal zone B-cell lymphoma of MALT-type (Holm *et al*, 1985). Lymphoma typically occurs 20-30 years after the diagnosis of thyroiditis (Pedersen & Pedersen, 1996). HT is not only associated with thyroidal MALT lymphoma, but also with other extranodal lymphomas. In a retrospective study on 80 patients affected by MALT lymphoma, 13 (16%) had a concomitant diagnosis of HT; four of these patients had thyroidal lymphoma and nine had extra-thyroidal lymphomas (gastric, orbital, small intestinal, and salivary gland lymphomas) (Troch *et al*, 2008). PTL represents 5% of all thyroid malignancies (Staunton & Greening, 1973) and MALT lymphoma represent 25% of all PTLs (Thieblemont *et al*, 2002, Derringer *et al*, 2000). About 50% of patients diagnosed with PTL have a clinical history of HT (Niitsu *et al*, 2007, Rossi, 2009), even if only 0.5% of patients with HT develop PTL.

4.4.1 Pathogenesis

It has been hypothesized that the chronic antigenic stimulation caused by the autoimmune and inflammatory process in HT leads to the proliferation of newly formed lymphoid tissue and ultimately to malignant transformation. The thyroid gland does not contain native lymphoid tissue (Holm *et al*, 1985, Isaacson, 1997). The lymphoid tissue present in HT thyroid gland share many features with MALT (Hyjek & Isaacson, 1988). The presence of clonal B-cell populations has been demonstrated in HT thyroid specimens also in patients without evidence of lymphoma development (Saxena *et al*, 2004). The clonal IgH gene rearrangements carried by thyroid lymphomas may already be evident in the oligoclonal rearrangements characterizing HT, and a fraction of thyroid lymphomas use the same IgH utilized by anti-thyroid auto-antibodies (Rossi, 2009, Moshynska & Saxena, 2008). IGVH genes are extensively targeted by aberrant somatic hypermutation in thyroid DLBCL, MALT and follicular lymphoma, and also in 2 of 14 (14.3%) patients affected by HT, suggesting that these genetic alterations represent an early step in the process of B-cell lymphomagenesis. This aberrant activity of somatic hypermutation may introduce activating mutations and may cause genetic instability, favouring chromosomal translocation (Takakuwa *et al*, 2009).

4.4.2 Clinical characteristics

Patients developing a PTL clinically present a rapid growth of a thyroid mass, associated with hoarseness, stridor or, less commonly, with dysphagia or dyspnoea. The presence of B symptoms is uncommon in indolent subtypes (Ansell *et al*, 1999). Up to 90% of patients usually presents with early stage I or II lymphoma (Graff-Baker *et al*, 2010). The most common histologic subtypes are B cell-type, in particular MALT lymphomas and DLBCL. The other histological subtypes are exceptional (Thieblemont *et al*, 2002). MALT lymphoma is an indolent lymphoma, with a 5-year disease-free survival of over 95% (Graff-Baker *et al*, 2010) and the disease tends to remain localized for a long time. Conversely, aggressive DLBCL usually arise from a pre-existing MALT lymphoma and a component of residual MALT lymphoma can be still found (Niitsu *et al*, 2007). DLBCL has a dismal prognosis despite polychemotherapic regimens, with a 5 year probability of survival of 44% (Thieblemont *et al*, 2002). Only rare cases of HL of the thyroid have been reported in the literature, but any association with underlying thyroiditis cannot be ascertained because of the small number of cases (Wang *et al*, 2005). Older age at diagnosis is associated with decreased disease-free survival (Graff-Baker *et al*, 2010). Tissue biopsies should be considered the gold standard for histological diagnosis (Thieblemont *et al*, 2002).

4.4.3 Therapy

Local treatment, such as surgical excision and radiotherapy, could represent a valid treatment strategy for patients with stage I or II MALT lymphoma of the thyroid gland (Tsang *et al*, 2003). Complete surgical resection improves prognosis over incomplete resection, with a 5-year OS of 100% (Thieblemont *et al*, 2002), although most authors currently believe that total thyroidectomy is unnecessary, exposing patients to the risks of surgery (recurrent laryngeal nerve damage and hypoparathyroidism) without conferring any survival advantage (Tupchong *et al*, 1986, Ruggiero *et al*, 2005, Klyachkin *et al*, 1998). Involved field radiotherapy is associated with a 5-year OS of 90% (Laing *et al*, 1994). Nonetheless, patients with thyroid malignant lymphoma treated with radiotherapy seem to have a higher incidence of hypothyroidism than those treated with chemotherapy (Tamura *et al*, 1981). Localized treatment plays a minor role in DLBCL, which requires aggressive anthracycline-based chemotherapy regimens (CHOP or CHOP-like), associated with rituximab, a monoclonal antibody directed against B-cell specific antigen CD20, and followed by involved-field radiotherapy. Chemotherapy alone may be considered in selected patients younger than 60 years and with no adverse prognostic factors (Reyes *et al*, 2005). Rituximab is effective for autoimmune thyroid diseases such as Grave's disease (El Fassi *et al*, 2007a, El Fassi *et al*, 2007b). The use of rituximab monotherapy in three cases of HT-related thyroid MALT lymphoma has also been reported. Rituximab monotherapy determined a significant decrease of anti-thyroid autoantibody levels, but it is still unknown whether thyroid dysfunction can be restored, and its use remains still controversial in HT (Kahara *et al*, 2011).

4.5 Systemic sclerosis

Systemic sclerosis (SSc) is a multisystem inflammatory disease with autoimmune features. It is characterized by vascular abnormalities and fibrosis of the skin and internal organs. Some retrospective studies have reported an increased risk of malignancies in SSc patients (Abu-Shakra *et al*, 1993, Rosenthal *et al*, 1993, Derk *et al*, 2006), but data on the link between SSc and lymphoproliferative disorders are still controversial. This association was first proposed in 1953 (ZATUCHNI *et al*, 1953) and successively several epidemiological studies have been performed to explore this risk (Chatterjee *et al*, 2005, Hill *et al*, 2003, Duncan & Winkelmann, 1979). A number of sporadic case reports have underlined the association between SSc and NHL, particularly with aggressive B-cell subtypes (Arnaud *et al*, 2006, Derk *et al*, 2004, Haviv *et al*, 1997) and some authors observed an increased risk of NHL among SSc patients, primarily within the first year after the onset of disease, but not beyond 4 years of follow up (Landgren *et al*, 2006, Mellemkjaer *et al*, 2008, Rosenthal *et al*, 1993). Conversely, other studies failed to demonstrate a consistent association between SSc and lymphomas (Chatterjee *et al*, 2005, Rosenthal *et al*, 1995, Roumm & Medsger, 1985). In some cases, systemic sclerosis could even represent a paraneoplastic syndrome (Vettori *et al*, 2010). In a population-based cohort study from south-west England to determine if patients with scleroderma have an increased risk of malignancy compared with general population, the highest risk among patients affected by scleroderma was found for haematological malignancies, especially for NHL (RR=25.8) (Siau *et al,* 2010). Another retrospective analysis of 218 Hungarian patients with SSc followed during a period of 12 years showed lymphoma development in three of them (1.38%), all of B cell phenotype, within 2 years after the onset of SSc. The incidence of lymphoma in this cohort was 38.3 cases per 100.000 patients per year (Szekanecz *et al,* 2008). Considering 24 studies analyzed in a review, characteristics associated to NHL development are old age, female sex, diffuse cutaneous subset and early disease. B-cell lymphoma represents the most frequent histotype and the interval between diagnosis of SSc and lymphoma onset is usually short (Vettori *et al,* 2010). Some sporadic cases have also reported an association with HL (Rosenthal *et al,* 1993, Duggal *et al,* 2002, Kedar *et al,* 1979, Hall *et al,* 1978).

4.5.1 Pathogenesis

The pathophysiological relationship between scleroderma and malignancy remains poorly understood. There might be multiple pathways leading to cancer in general, and lymphoproliferative disorders in particular. B cells have many pathogenic roles in SSc (Sato *et al,* 2004). SSc patients are indeed characterized by alterations of the B-cell homeostasis, such as expansion of naïve cells, decreased number of circulating but activated memory cells and defective natural killer cells activity (Sato *et al,* 2004, Horikawa *et al,* 2005). Therefore, altered B cell functions may be responsible of the higher incidence of B NHL. Also TGF-β, a cytokine involved in the regulation of connective tissue proteins, which is highly expressed in SSc tissues, might play an important role since dysregulated signalling of the TGF-β is capable to induce tumorigenesis (Grady, 2005). Moreover, the malignant transformation might be a consequence of chronic tissue damage. Finally, EBV-encoded small RNAs have been detected in the majority of DLBCLs associated with systemic rheumatic diseases, including SSc (Kojima *et al,* 2006). In conclusion, a clear relationship between SSc and NHL has not yet been ascertained and further studies with higher number of patients are required to clarify the coexistence of these two entities.

4.6 Celiac disease

Celiac disease (CD) is a chronic autoimmune enteropathy affecting small-intestine, triggered by gluten proteins from wheat, barley and rye. The small-intestinal mucosal injury caused by the autoimmune response determines malabsorption which results in gastrointestinal symptoms (diarrhoea, weight loss, abdominal pain, anorexia, lactose intolerance, abdominal distension and irritability) and/or non-gastrointestinal features (iron-deficiency anaemia, dermatitis herpetiformis, chronic fatigue, joint pain/inflammation, migraines, depression, attention-deficit disorder, epilepsy, osteoporosis/osteopenia, infertility and/or recurrent fetal loss, vitamin deficiencies, short stature, failure to thrive, delayed puberty, dental defects and autoimmune disorders). The diagnosis of CD is based on histologic characteristics of small-bowel biopsy and on clinical and histological remission after a strict gluten-free diet. The presence of circulating CD-associated antibodies, such as IgA against the endomysium of connective tissue and against tissue transglutaminase, at time of diagnosis and their normalization after a gluten-free diet support the diagnosis of CD. Most CD patients display specific pairs of allelic variants in two HLA genes, HLA-DQA1 and

HLA-DQB1. Adhering to a strict gluten-free diet usually results in healing of the damaged small-intestinal mucosa and improvement of intestinal absorption. A gluten-free diet is sufficient to treat the majority of patients. Two–5% of patients with adult-onset CD, especially those diagnosed above the age of 50, does not respond to a gluten-free diet (Tack *et al*, 2010a). Refractory celiac disease (RCD) is defined when clinical and histological symptoms recur after a good response to a gluten-free diet or persist after more than 12 months of strict diet. Patients affected by CD are at increased risk of lymphoma development, not only primary gastrointestinal, but at any site. The occurrence of an EATL is the main cause of death in RCD patient. About 50-60% of patients with RCD type II develop an EATL within 5 years (Al-Toma *et al*, 2007, Di Sabatino & Corazza, 2009, Daum *et al*, 2003). Despite the strong association between CD and EATL, the majority of lymphomas associated with CD are of different histologies, such as DLBCL and peripheral T cell lymphomas (Catassi *et al*, 2002, Mearin *et al*, 2006, Smedby *et al*, 2005, Halfdanarson *et al*, 2010).

4.6.1 Epidemiology

Earlier estimates of risk of NHL in CD amply varies, from no increased risk (Collin *et al*, 1994) to a 42-fold (Holmes *et al*, 1989) or a 69-fold increased risk of NHL (Corrao *et al*, 2001). A significant increased risk of NHL among CD patients has been reported, with a SIR of 2.2 (95% CI 1.3-3.6) for B-cell NHL and 3.6 (95% CI 2.3-5.2) for lymphomas of non-intestinal origin (Smedby *et al*, 2005), most common subtype being DLBCL. The RR for T cell NHL was 50-fold increased. Patients with B-cell lymphomas have been demonstrated to have a better prognosis that those with T cell NHL (Halfdanarson *et al*, 2010). To investigate the frequency of CD among patients with NHL a prospective, multi-centre case-control study was conducted in 10 European countries between 1998 and 2002, showing that patients with CD have a significantly increased risk of developing NHL (OR=2.6 95%CI=1.4-4.9) in comparison with the general population. Importantly, the increased frequency of CD in NHL occurred in those celiac patients diagnosed clinically before screening and not in undiagnosed CD (Mearin *et al*, 2006). Another large nationwide population-based study assessed and compared risk of developing a lymphoproliferative disease among three different classes of subjects: patients affected by CD, patients with small bowel intestinal inflammation and patients with latent CD. It was showed an increased risk of lymphoproliferative malignancy (HR=2.82 95% CI 2.36-3.37) associated with the presence of a biopsy-proven CD, even after 5 years of follow up, but not with latent CD. The increased risk regarded NHL of the T cell and the B cell type as well as HL (Elfstrom *et al*, 2011). The risk of developing a lymphoma in CD patients is related to the age of diagnosis of CD. As a matter of fact, mean age at diagnosis of patients who develops a cancer is higher than that of patients who did not (Silano *et al*, 2007). This could be due to the diagnostic delay causing a prolonged period of dietary exposure to gluten (Holmes *et al*, 1989, Corrao *et al*, 2001). The risk of developing a malignancy in patients with CD who adhere to a gluten-free diet for five consecutive years or more is not increased compared with that of general population (Holmes *et al*, 1989, Lewis *et al*, 1996, Silano *et al*, 2008).

4.6.2 EATL

EATL is an intestinal tumour of intraepithelial T lymphocytes, usually presenting as a neoplasm composed of large lymphoid cells and often associated with necrosis and an inflammatory background, including large number of histiocytes and eosinophils. The adjacent intestinal mucosa frequently shows enteropathy with villous atrophy, crypt hyperplasia, increased *lamina propria* lymphocytes and plasma cells and intraepithelial lymphocytosis (Chott *et al*, 1998). In 10-20% of cases, lymphoma is composed of monomorphic medium-sized cells with no inflammatory background and rare necrosis (type II EATL) and may occur sporadically, not associated with CD. EATL more often occurs in the jejunum or ileum as one or more ulcerating mucosal lesions that invade the wall of intestine and frequently cause perforation. The time interval between diagnosis of CD and development of lymphoma varies from 2 months to more than 5 years (Ilyas *et al*, 1995). HLA genotyping shows that patients with EATL have the CD-associated DQA1*0501, DQB1*0201 phenotype, and additional HLA-DR/DQ alleles may increase the risk of lymphoma (Wright, 1995).

4.6.2.1 Pathogenesis

RCD patients can be classified as RCD type I and type II. Type-II RCD patients have >20% phenotypically aberrant intraepithelial lymphocytes (IEL), expressing cytoplasmatic CD3, but lacking surface expression of CD3, CD4 and CD8, while type-I RCD patients have normal IEL (Cellier *et al*, 2000, Patey-Mariaud De Serre *et al*, 2000). IEL with aberrant phenotype also show monoclonal T-cell receptor (TCR)-gamma rearrangement (Bagdi *et al*, 1999), suggesting that these cells constitute a neoplastic population. Moreover, in those patients with type II RCD who subsequently develop EATL, the IEL share the same monoclonal TCR-gamma as the subsequent T-cell lymphoma (Cellier *et al*, 2000, Cellier *et al*, 1998, Daum *et al*, 2005, Ashton-Key *et al*, 1997) and carry gain of chromosome 1q in common with 16% of EATL (Verkarre *et al*, 2003). Therefore, type II RCD may be considered an example of cryptic intraepithelial T-cell lymphoma (Daum *et al*, 2001). CD30+ IEL in RCD II seem to indicate a worse prognosis, including risk of developing lymphoma (Farstad *et al*, 2002). Also interleukin 15 (IL15) might play a role in lymphomagenesis. Uncontrolled overexpression of IL15 by enterocytes in patients with type-II RCD promotes and maintain activation of IEL, favouring the emergence of T-cell clonal proliferations and the subsequent transformation into EATL (Mention *et al*, 2003).

4.6.2.2 Clinical characteristics and prognosis

EATL often present at older age (mean > 60 years) and in patients with a reduced performance status. In most cases disease is disseminated at diagnosis. Patients generally present with abdominal pain, often associated with jejunal perforation, weight loss, diarrhoea or bowel obstruction. Since obstruction and perforation are frequent, many cases are diagnosed at laparotomy. EATL is characterized by multifocal presentation in 10-25% of cases. Neurologic symptoms are reported in approximately 6% of adults with CD, of which cerebellar ataxia is the most frequent one. EATL is an aggressive malignancy that, if untreated, leads to death due to multifocal intestinal perforation caused by refractory malignant ulcers. The prognosis of EATL is very poor compared with that of intestinal B cell lymphomas (Domizio *et al*, 1993). It shows low chemosensitivity, rapid tumour growth and a tendency to dissemination with about 80% of patients experiencing relapse, even after 5 years of follow up, and a 1- and 5-year survival rates of 31-39% and 8-20% respectively (Al-Toma *et al*, 2007, Daum *et al*, 2003). Overall, the dismal prognosis of these patients reflects in part late diagnosis and in part the poor performance status due to the compromised immunological and nutritional status (Gale *et al*, 2000). Stage is the main prognostic factor, with a 5-year cause-specific survival higher than 60% for patients with limited disease and 25% for those with advanced stage (d'Amore *et al*, 1994, Chott *et al*, 1992).

4.6.2.3 Therapy

A standard treatment for patients with EATL has not been established, and reported results are overall unsatisfactory. Most patients with EATL are managed with a surgical approach as the primary strategy. Even if surgery is not a curative approach, debulking and resection of masses at high risk of perforation following chemotherapy or occlusion are frequently indicated in these patients. Involved-field radiotherapy 35 Gy was indicated in some patients with bulky disease or incomplete resection (Novakovic *et al*, 2006), but it is used almost exclusively with palliative purposes. Combined treatment modality with debulking surgery followed by systemic anthracycline-containing polichemotherapy, with or without consolidation radiotherapy, showed an ORR of 58%, a 5-year FFS of 3% and a 5-year OS of 20-25% (Domizio *et al*, 1993, Gale *et al*, 2000, d'Amore *et al*, 1994, Morton *et al*, 1993). Many patients are unable to complete the chemotherapy program and do not receive radiotherapy due to rapid disease progression, poor nutritional and performance status, associated with local and systemic complications (Daum *et al*, 2003, Gale *et al*, 2000). Given the dismal prognosis of patients treated with conventional chemotherapy, some authors assessed feasibility and activity of high-dose chemotherapy supported by autologous stem cell transplantation as upfront treatment of EATL, with conflicting results. Most of these studies are based on small retrospective series of patients with disomogeneous characteristics, and utilizing different conditioning regimens (Al-Toma *et al*, 2007, Bishton & Haynes, 2007). High-dose chemotherapy with IVE/MTX (ifosfamide, vincristine, etoposide, methotrexate) followed by ASCT has been associated with significantly better outcome in comparison with historical controls treated with conventional anthracycline-based chemotherapy. In fact, patients treated with IVE/MTX-ASCT had an improved remission rate (69% vs. 42%); lower death rates and higher 5-year PFS and OS (52% vs. 22% and 60% vs. 22%, respectively) (Sieniawski *et al*, 2010). Interestingly, chemotherapy supported by ASCT may also prevent EATL development in patients with RCD (Meijer *et al*, 2004). In fact, in a retrospective series of 18 patients with RCD type II, 13 patients successfully underwent conditioning with fludarabine and melphalan supported by ASCT, with a significant reduction of the aberrant T-cells in duodenal biopsies associated with improvement in clinical well-being and normalization of hematologic and biochemical markers. After a follow up > 2 years EATL developed only in one transplanted patients, with a 4-year survival rate of 66% (Tack *et al*, 2010b). Alemtuzumab, a humanized anti-CD52 monoclonal antibody has been rarely used in EATL. The combination of gemcitabine and alemtuzumab has been successfully used in an elderly patients with poor performance status and extra-intestinal dissemination of EATL both at diagnosis and relapse (Soldini *et al*, 2008). Another patient with EATL was treated with alemtuzumab-CHOP combination at diagnosis in a prospective phase II trial on T-cell lymphomas achieving a short-lasting complete remission (Gallamini *et al*, 2007). Moreover, alemtuzumab was successfully used in the treatment of a patient with RCD at high risk of developing EATL, obtaining a total recovery of duodenal biopsy (Vivas *et al*, 2006). Patients with refractory or relapsed EATL and without formal contraindications should be therefore managed with high-dose chemotherapy supported by ASCT. Two patients in CR were treated with allogeneic SCT with reduced intensity conditioning regimen, with a HLA identical sibling donor. Both patients relapsed within few months after transplantation (van de Water *et al*, 2010).

4.7 Dermatitis herpetiformis

Dermatitis herpetiformis (DH) is a gluten-sensitive skin disease characterized by an itchy, blistering rash which diagnosis is based on the presence of granular IgA deposits in the epidermal-dermal junction observed by direct immunofluorescence. About 75-80% of patients have an associated gluten-sensitive enteropathy with villous atrophy identical to that found in CD, even if gastrointestinal symptoms are rare, and the remaining show increased amount of $\gamma\delta$ receptor bearing T lymphocytes in the jejunal mucosa (Savilahti *et al*, 1992, Reunala, 1998). Both enteropathy and cutaneous rash recover with a gluten-free diet and relapse when diet is withdrawn (Fry *et al*, 1973, Reunala *et al*, 1977), suggesting that DH might be a cutaneous manifestation of CD. Moreover, almost all patients affected by DH carry the HLA alleles DQA1*0501 and DQB1*0201 typical of CD (Fronek *et al*, 1991). Since 1970, it is thought that patients with DH but without clinical sign of CD have an increased risk of developing cancer (Gjone & Nordoy, 1970), and some cases of patients with DH and lymphoma were reported (Jenkins *et al*, 1983, Reunala *et al*, 1982). The first large population-based cohort study assessing lymphoma risk in DH included 976 patients affected by DH without concomitant CD diagnosed from 1964 to 1983 in Sweden (Sigurgeirsson *et al*, 1994). The RR of developing cancer resulted 1.4 (95% CI= 1.1-1.7) in male patients and 1.2 (95% CI= 0.8-1.7) in female patients. This increased risk lost significance if lymphomas were excluded from analysis. In fact, analyzing cancer by subtype, it was found only a significant association with NHL (RR 5.4 95% CI= 2.2-11.1 in male patients and 4.5 95% CI=0.9-13.2 in female patients). The median time between the first admission to hospital and diagnosis of lymphoma was 4 years and the median age at diagnosis was 64 years. Most lymphomas were localized outside the gastrointestinal tract and were of the B cell phenotype. Only one case was classified as EATL. DH indeed is not only associated with EATL, but also with B-cell lymphomas, which may occur both within and outside the gastrointestinal tract as nodal or extranodal disease (Hervonen *et al*, 2005, Viljamaa *et al*, 2006). One possible reason for this discrepancy may be the less severe small bowel damage in DH with respect to that in CD. Occurrence of malignancy was assessed in another DH-patient cohort mainly treated with dapsone and gluten-free diet compared with patients affected by CD and general population (Collin *et al*, 1996). This study cohort included 305 consecutive Finnish patients diagnosed with DH from 1970 to 1992 and 383 patients diagnosed with CD. The only significantly increased SIR was that for NHL among patients with DH (10.3; 95% CI 2.8-26.3), while the overall incidence of other malignancies was not increased. Of four patients who developed NHL, three were adhering to a gluten-free diet, but two for less than five years, which is probably a too short period to exhibit a protective effect against malignancy (Holmes *et al*, 1989). Extension of the follow up period for a further 12 years confirmed that patients who have adhered to a strict gluten-free diet for more than 5 years have no increased risk of developing lymphoma compared to the general population (Lewis *et al*, 1996), supporting the protective role of a gluten-free diet against lymphoma development in DH (Hervonen *et al*, 2005). Moreover, three patients had abnormal small bowel villous architecture, while one patient had normal mucosa, implying that a normal small bowel mucosa in DH does not protect from lymphoma. Another retrospective cohort study has reported a 2-fold increased risk for malignant lymphoma (SIR=1.9; 95% CI 0.8-3.9) (Askling *et al*, 2002). Importantly, NHL occurrence seems to be reduced in DH patients whose diagnosis was made over the recent years (Viljamaa *et al*, 2006) maybe due to a less adherence of patients to a gluten-free diet in the past, not considered as essential as nowadays in DH. First-degree relatives of patients with DH or CD have an higher risk of developing a gluten-sensitive enteropathy (Hervonen *et al*, 2002). This is not true for lymphoma risk, as demonstrated in a large series of patients with DH and their first-degree relatives, where three lymphoma cases (0.2%) were diagnosed among 1.825 first-degree relatives, compared with the prevalence in the general population of 0.1%. The aetiopathology of lymphoma development in patients with DH is unknown, but several mechanisms may be involved, such as the polyclonal stimulation of B or T lymphocytes by gluten in the gastrointestinal tract, leading to the transformation in a malignant clone.

5. Conclusions

The relationship existing between autoimmunity and cancer continues to fascinate clinicians and physicians. Many pathogenic and therapeutic overlaps have been demonstrated so far in these two intriguing and closely interrelated fields but several challenges remain open to future development. The exact pathogenic mechanism connecting both diseases remain still poorly understood and additional studies will explore genetic, biologic and inflammatory mechanisms underlying lymphoma development. Further epidemiologic studies are needed to ascertain which host factors may predispose in the setting of an autoimmune disease to develop a malignancy in general, and a lymphoproliferative disorder in particular, in order to define more accurately the pre-treatment risk. Finally, more surveillance studies will clarify if novel immunomodulatory treatments increase or decrease lymphoma risk. A more clear elucidation of these critical issues will lead to the development of novel therapeutic options able to improve the prevention and/or treatment of lymphomas in the setting of autoimmunity.

6. References

Abu-Shakra, M., Guillemin, F. & Lee, P. (1993) Cancer in systemic sclerosis. *Arthritis and Rheumatism*, 36, 460-464.

Adamson, T.C.,3rd, Fox, R.I., Frisman, D.M. & Howell, F.V. (1983) Immunohistologic analysis of lymphoid infiltrates in primary sjogren's syndrome using monoclonal antibodies. *Journal of Immunology (Baltimore, Md.: 1950)*, 130, 203-208.

Alspaugh, M.A., Henle, G., Lennette, E.T. & Henle, W. (1981) Elevated levels of antibodies to epstein-barr virus antigens in sera and synovial fluids of patients with rheumatoid arthritis. *The Journal of Clinical Investigation*, 67, 1134-1140.

Al-Toma, A., Verbeek, W.H., Hadithi, M., von Blomberg, B.M. & Mulder, C.J. (2007) Survival in refractory coeliac disease and enteropathy-associated T-cell lymphoma: Retrospective evaluation of single-centre experience. *Gut*, 56, 1373-1378.

Ambinder, R.F. (2003) Epstein-barr virus-associated lymphoproliferative disorders. *Reviews in Clinical and Experimental Hematology*, 7, 362-374.

Ambrosetti, A., Zanotti, R., Pattaro, C., Lenzi, L., Chilosi, M., Caramaschi, P., Arcaini, L., Pasini, F., Biasi, D., Orlandi, E., D'Adda, M., Lucioni, M. & Pizzolo, G. (2004) Most cases of primary salivary mucosa-associated lymphoid tissue lymphoma are associated either with sjoegren syndrome or hepatitis C virus infection. *British Journal of Haematology*, 126, 43-49.

Anaya, J.M., McGuff, H.S., Banks, P.M. & Talal, N. (1996) Clinicopathological factors relating malignant lymphoma with sjogren's syndrome. *Seminars in Arthritis and Rheumatism*, 25, 337-346.

Anderson, L.A., Gadalla, S., Morton, L.M., Landgren, O., Pfeiffer, R., Warren, J.L., Berndt, S.I., Ricker, W., Parsons, R. & Engels, E.A. (2009) Population-based study of autoimmune conditions and the risk of specific lymphoid malignancies. *International Journal of Cancer.Journal International Du Cancer*, 125, 398-405.

Anderson, L.G. & Talal, N. (1972) The spectrum of benign to malignant lymphoproliferation in sjogren's syndrome. *Clinical and Experimental Immunology*, 10, 199-221.

Ansell, S.M., Grant, C.S. & Habermann, T.M. (1999) Primary thyroid lymphoma. *Seminars in Oncology*, 26, 316-323.

Aozasa, K. (1990) Hashimoto's thyroiditis as a risk factor of thyroid lymphoma. *Acta Pathologica Japonica*, 40, 459-468.

Aringer, M., Wintersberger, W., Steiner, C.W., Kiener, H., Presterl, E., Jaeger, U., Smolen, J.S. & Graninger, W.B. (1994) High levels of bcl-2 protein in circulating T lymphocytes, but not B lymphocytes, of patients with systemic lupus erythematosus. *Arthritis and Rheumatism*, 37, 1423-1430.

Arnaud, L., Chryssostalis, A., Terris, B., Pavy, S., Chaussade, S., Kahan, A. & Allanore, Y. (2006) Systemic sclerosis and gastric MALT lymphoma. *Joint, Bone, Spine : Revue Du Rhumatisme*, 73, 105-108.

Ashton-Key, M., Diss, T.C., Pan, L., Du, M.Q. & Isaacson, P.G. (1997) Molecular analysis of T-cell clonality in ulcerative jejunitis and enteropathy-associated T-cell lymphoma. *The American Journal of Pathology*, 151, 493-498.

Askling, J., Linet, M., Gridley, G., Halstensen, T.S., Ekstrom, K. & Ekbom, A. (2002) Cancer incidence in a population-based cohort of individuals hospitalized with celiac disease or dermatitis herpetiformis. *Gastroenterology*, 123, 1428-1435.

Askling, J., Brandt, L., Lapidus, A., Karlen, P., Bjorkholm, M., Lofberg, R. & Ekbom, A. (2005) Risk of haematopoietic cancer in patients with inflammatory bowel disease. *Gut*, 54, 617-622.

Askling, J., van Vollenhoven, R.F., Granath, F., Raaschou, P., Fored, C.M., Baecklund, E., Dackhammar, C., Feltelius, N., Coster, L., Geborek, P., Jacobsson, L.T., Lindblad, S., Rantapaa-Dahlqvist, S., Saxne, T. & Klareskog, L. (2009) Cancer risk in patients with rheumatoid arthritis treated with anti-tumor necrosis factor alpha therapies: Does the risk change with the time since start of treatment? *Arthritis and Rheumatism*, 60, 3180-3189.

Askling, J., Fored, C.M., Baecklund, E., Brandt, L., Backlin, C., Ekbom, A., Sundstrom, C., Bertilsson, L., Coster, L., Geborek, P., Jacobsson, L.T., Lindblad, S., Lysholm, J., Rantapaa-Dahlqvist, S., Saxne, T., Klareskog, L. & Feltelius, N. (2005) Haematopoietic malignancies in rheumatoid arthritis: Lymphoma risk and characteristics after exposure to tumour necrosis factor antagonists. *Annals of the Rheumatic Diseases*, 64, 1414-1420.

Baecklund, E., Ekbom, A., Sparen, P., Feltelius, N. & Klareskog, L. (1998) Disease activity and risk of lymphoma in patients with rheumatoid arthritis: Nested case-control study. *BMJ (Clinical Research Ed.)*, 317, 180-181.

Baecklund, E., Sundstrom, C., Ekbom, A., Catrina, A.I., Biberfeld, P., Feltelius, N. & Klareskog, L. (2003) Lymphoma subtypes in patients with rheumatoid arthritis: Increased proportion of diffuse large B cell lymphoma. *Arthritis and Rheumatism*, 48, 1543-1550.

Baecklund, E., Iliadou, A., Askling, J., Ekbom, A., Backlin, C., Granath, F., Catrina, A.I., Rosenquist, R., Feltelius, N., Sundstrom, C. & Klareskog, L. (2006a) Association of chronic inflammation, not its treatment, with increased lymphoma risk in rheumatoid arthritis. *Arthritis and Rheumatism,* 54, 692-701.

Baecklund, E., Backlin, C., Iliadou, A., Granath, F., Ekbom, A., Amini, R.M., Feltelius, N., Enblad, G., Sundstrom, C., Klareskog, L., Askling, J. & Rosenquist, R. (2006b) Characteristics of diffuse large B cell lymphomas in rheumatoid arthritis. *Arthritis and Rheumatism,* 54, 3774-3781.

Bagdi, E., Diss, T.C., Munson, P. & Isaacson, P.G. (1999) Mucosal intra-epithelial lymphocytes in enteropathy-associated T-cell lymphoma, ulcerative jejunitis, and refractory celiac disease constitute a neoplastic population. *Blood,* 94, 260-264.

Baker, J.A., Weiss, J.R., Czuczman, M.S., Menezes, R.J., Ambrosone, C.B. & Moysich, K.B. (2005) Regular use of aspirin or acetaminophen and risk of non-hodgkin lymphoma. *Cancer Causes & Control : CCC,* 16, 301-308.

Baker, K.P., Edwards, B.M., Main, S.H., Choi, G.H., Wager, R.E., Halpern, W.G., Lappin, P.B., Riccobene, T., Abramian, D., Sekut, L., Sturm, B., Poortman, C., Minter, R.R., Dobson, C.L., Williams, E., Carmen, S., Smith, R., Roschke, V., Hilbert, D.M., Vaughan, T.J. & Albert, V.R. (2003) Generation and characterization of LymphoStat-B, a human monoclonal antibody that antagonizes the bioactivities of B lymphocyte stimulator. *Arthritis and Rheumatism,* 48, 3253-3265.

Balandraud, N., Roudier, J. & Roudier, C. (2005) What are the links between epstein-barr virus, lymphoma, and tumor necrosis factor antagonism in rheumatoid arthritis? *Seminars in Arthritis and Rheumatism,* 34, 31-33.

Balandraud, N., Meynard, J.B., Auger, I., Sovran, H., Mugnier, B., Reviron, D., Roudier, J. & Roudier, C. (2003) Epstein-barr virus load in the peripheral blood of patients with rheumatoid arthritis: Accurate quantification using real-time polymerase chain reaction. *Arthritis and Rheumatism,* 48, 1223-1228.

Banchereau, J. & Pascual, V. (2006) Type I interferon in systemic lupus erythematosus and other autoimmune diseases. *Immunity,* 25, 383-392.

Beauparlant, P., Papp, K. & Haraoui, B. (1999) The incidence of cancer associated with the treatment of rheumatoid arthritis. *Seminars in Arthritis and Rheumatism,* 29, 148-158.

Beiderbeck, A.B., Holly, E.A., Sturkenboom, M.C., Coebergh, J.W., Stricker, B.H. & Leufkens, H.G. (2003) No increased risk of non-hodgkin's lymphoma with steroids, estrogens and psychotropics (netherlands). *Cancer Causes & Control : CCC,* 14, 639-644.

Berek, C. & Kim, H.J. (1997) B-cell activation and development within chronically inflamed synovium in rheumatoid and reactive arthritis. *Seminars in Immunology,* 9, 261-268.

Bernatsky, S., Lee, J.L. & Rahme, E. (2007) Non-hodgkin's lymphoma--meta-analyses of the effects of corticosteroids and non-steroidal anti-inflammatories. *Rheumatology (Oxford, England),* 46, 690-694.

Bernatsky, S., Clarke, A. & Ramsey-Goldman, R. (2002) Malignancy and systemic lupus erythematosus. *Current Rheumatology Reports,* 4, 351-358.

Bernatsky, S., Ramsey-Goldman, R., Isenberg, D., Rahman, A., Dooley, M.A., Sibley, J., Boivin, J.F., Joseph, L., Armitage, J., Zoma, A. & Clarke, A. (2007) Hodgkin's lymphoma in systemic lupus erythematosus. *Rheumatology (Oxford, England),* 46, 830-832.

Bernatsky, S., Joseph, L., Boivin, J.F., Gordon, C., Urowitz, M., Gladman, D., Fortin, P.R., Ginzler, E., Bae, S.C., Barr, S., Edworthy, S., Isenberg, D., Rahman, A., Petri, M., Alarcon, G.S., Aranow, C., Dooley, M.A., Rajan, R., Senecal, J.L., Zummer, M., Manzi, S., Ramsey-Goldman, R. & Clarke, A.E. (2008) The relationship between cancer and medication exposures in systemic lupus erythaematosus: A case-cohort study. *Annals of the Rheumatic Diseases,* 67, 74-79.

Bernatsky, S., Ramsey-Goldman, R., Rajan, R., Boivin, J.F., Joseph, L., Lachance, S., Cournoyer, D., Zoma, A., Manzi, S., Ginzler, E., Urowitz, M., Gladman, D., Fortin, P.R., Edworthy, S., Barr, S., Gordon, C., Bae, S.C., Sibley, J., Steinsson, K., Nived, O., Sturfelt, G., St Pierre, Y. & Clarke, A. (2005a) Non-hodgkin's lymphoma in systemic lupus erythematosus. *Annals of the Rheumatic Diseases,* 64, 1507-1509.

Bernatsky, S., Boivin, J.F., Joseph, L., Rajan, R., Zoma, A., Manzi, S., Ginzler, E., Urowitz, M., Gladman, D., Fortin, P.R., Petri, M., Edworthy, S., Barr, S., Gordon, C., Bae, S.C., Sibley, J., Isenberg, D., Rahman, A., Aranow, C., Dooley, M.A., Steinsson, K., Nived, O., Sturfelt, G., Alarcon, G., Senecal, J.L., Zummer, M., Hanly, J., Ensworth, S., Pope, J., El-Gabalawy, H., McCarthy, T., St Pierre, Y., Ramsey-Goldman, R. & Clarke, A. (2005b) An international cohort study of cancer in systemic lupus erythematosus. *Arthritis and Rheumatism,* 52, 1481-1490.

Bernstein, L. & Ross, R.K. (1992) Prior medication use and health history as risk factors for non-hodgkin's lymphoma: Preliminary results from a case-control study in los angeles county. *Cancer Research,* 52, 5510s-5515s.

Bishton, M.J. & Haynes, A.P. (2007) Combination chemotherapy followed by autologous stem cell transplant for enteropathy-associated T cell lymphoma. *British Journal of Haematology,* 136, 111-113.

Boffetta, P., Gridley, G. & Lindelof, B. (2001) Cancer risk in a population-based cohort of patients hospitalized for psoriasis in sweden. *The Journal of Investigative Dermatology,* 117, 1531-1537.

Bologna, C., Picot, M.C., Jorgensen, C., Viu, P., Verdier, R. & Sany, J. (1997) Study of eight cases of cancer in 426 rheumatoid arthritis patients treated with methotrexate. *Annals of the Rheumatic Diseases,* 56, 97-102.

Bombardieri, M., Barone, F., Humby, F., Kelly, S., McGurk, M., Morgan, P., Challacombe, S., De Vita, S., Valesini, G., Spencer, J. & Pitzalis, C. (2007) Activation-induced cytidine deaminase expression in follicular dendritic cell networks and interfollicular large B cells supports functionality of ectopic lymphoid neogenesis in autoimmune sialoadenitis and MALT lymphoma in sjogren's syndrome. *Journal of Immunology (Baltimore, Md.: 1950),* 179, 4929-4938.

Bongartz, T., Warren, F.C., Mines, D., Matteson, E.L., Abrams, K.R. & Sutton, A.J. (2009) Etanercept therapy in rheumatoid arthritis and the risk of malignancies: A systematic review and individual patient data meta-analysis of randomised controlled trials. *Annals of the Rheumatic Diseases,* 68, 1177-1183.

Bongartz, T., Sutton, A.J., Sweeting, M.J., Buchan, I., Matteson, E.L. & Montori, V. (2006) Anti-TNF antibody therapy in rheumatoid arthritis and the risk of serious infections and malignancies: Systematic review and meta-analysis of rare harmful effects in randomized controlled trials. *JAMA : The Journal of the American Medical Association,* 295, 2275-2285.

Brandtzaeg, P. & Johansen, F.E. (2005) Mucosal B cells: Phenotypic characteristics, transcriptional regulation, and homing properties. *Immunological Reviews,* 206, 32-63.

Brito-Zeron, P., Ramos-Casals, M., Bove, A., Sentis, J. & Font, J. (2007) Predicting adverse outcomes in primary sjogren's syndrome: Identification of prognostic factors. *Rheumatology (Oxford, England),* 46, 1359-1362.

Brown, S.L., Greene, M.H., Gershon, S.K., Edwards, E.T. & Braun, M.M. (2002) Tumor necrosis factor antagonist therapy and lymphoma development: Twenty-six cases reported to the food and drug administration. *Arthritis and Rheumatism,* 46, 3151-3158.

Burke, J.S. (1999) Are there site-specific differences among the MALT lymphomas--morphologic, clinical? *American Journal of Clinical Pathology,* 111, S133-43.

Caponi, L., Anzilotti, C., Longombardo, G. & Migliorini, P. (2007) Antibodies directed against ribosomal P proteins cross-react with phospholipids. *Clinical and Experimental Immunology,* 150, 140-143.

Cartwright, R.A., McKinney, P.A., O'Brien, C., Richards, I.D., Roberts, B., Lauder, I., Darwin, C.M., Bernard, S.M. & Bird, C.C. (1988) Non-hodgkin's lymphoma: Case control epidemiological study in yorkshire. *Leukemia Research,* 12, 81-88.

Catassi, C., Fabiani, E., Corrao, G., Barbato, M., De Renzo, A., Carella, A.M., Gabrielli, A., Leoni, P., Carroccio, A., Baldassarre, M., Bertolani, P., Caramaschi, P., Sozzi, M., Guariso, G., Volta, U., Corazza, G.R. & Italian Working Group on Coeliac Disease and Non-Hodgkin's-Lymphoma. (2002) Risk of non-hodgkin lymphoma in celiac disease. *JAMA : The Journal of the American Medical Association,* 287, 1413-1419.

Cellier, C., Delabesse, E., Helmer, C., Patey, N., Matuchansky, C., Jabri, B., Macintyre, E., Cerf-Bensussan, N. & Brousse, N. (2000) Refractory sprue, coeliac disease, and enteropathy-associated T-cell lymphoma. french coeliac disease study group. *Lancet,* 356, 203-208.

Cellier, C., Patey, N., Mauvieux, L., Jabri, B., Delabesse, E., Cervoni, J.P., Burtin, M.L., Guy-Grand, D., Bouhnik, Y., Modigliani, R., Barbier, J.P., Macintyre, E., Brousse, N. & Cerf-Bensussan, N. (1998) Abnormal intestinal intraepithelial lymphocytes in refractory sprue. *Gastroenterology,* 114, 471-481.

Cerhan, J.R., Anderson, K.E., Janney, C.A., Vachon, C.M., Witzig, T.E. & Habermann, T.M. (2003) Association of aspirin and other non-steroidal anti-inflammatory drug use with incidence of non-hodgkin lymphoma. *International Journal of Cancer.Journal International Du Cancer,* 106, 784-788.

Chang, E.T., Smedby, K.E., Hjalgrim, H., Schollkopf, C., Porwit-MacDonald, A., Sundstrom, C., Tani, E., d'Amore, F., Melbye, M., Adami, H.O. & Glimelius, B. (2005) Medication use and risk of non-hodgkin's lymphoma. *American Journal of Epidemiology,* 162, 965-974.

Chatterjee, S., Dombi, G.W., Severson, R.K. & Mayes, M.D. (2005) Risk of malignancy in scleroderma: A population-based cohort study. *Arthritis and Rheumatism,* 52, 2415-2424.

Chott, A., Dragosics, B. & Radaszkiewicz, T. (1992) Peripheral T-cell lymphomas of the intestine. *The American Journal of Pathology,* 141, 1361-1371.

Chott, A., Haedicke, W., Mosberger, I., Fodinger, M., Winkler, K., Mannhalter, C. & Muller-Hermelink, H.K. (1998) Most CD56+ intestinal lymphomas are CD8+CD5-T-cell lymphomas of monomorphic small to medium size histology. *The American Journal of Pathology*, 153, 1483-1490.

Choubey, D. & Panchanathan, R. (2008) Interferon-inducible Ifi200-family genes in systemic lupus erythematosus. *Immunology Letters*, 119, 32-41.

Choubey, D. & Kotzin, B.L. (2002) Interferon-inducible p202 in the susceptibility to systemic lupus. *Frontiers in Bioscience : A Journal and Virtual Library*, 7, e252-62.

Choubey, D., Deka, R. & Ho, S.M. (2008) Interferon-inducible IFI16 protein in human cancers and autoimmune diseases. *Frontiers in Bioscience : A Journal and Virtual Library*, 13, 598-608.

Collin, P., Pukkala, E. & Reunala, T. (1996) Malignancy and survival in dermatitis herpetiformis: A comparison with coeliac disease. *Gut*, 38, 528-530.

Collin, P., Reunala, T., Pukkala, E., Laippala, P., Keyrilainen, O. & Pasternack, A. (1994) Coeliac disease--associated disorders and survival. *Gut*, 35, 1215-1218.

Corrao, G., Corazza, G.R., Bagnardi, V., Brusco, G., Ciacci, C., Cottone, M., Sategna Guidetti, C., Usai, P., Cesari, P., Pelli, M.A., Loperfido, S., Volta, U., Calabro, A., Certo, M. & Club del Tenue Study Group. (2001) Mortality in patients with coeliac disease and their relatives: A cohort study. *Lancet*, 358, 356-361.

Costenbader, K.H., Glass, R., Cui, J. & Shadick, N. (2006) Risk of serious infections and malignancies with anti-TNF antibody therapy in rheumatoid arthritis. *JAMA : The Journal of the American Medical Association*, 296, 2201; author reply 2203-4.

d'Amore, F., Brincker, H., Gronbaek, K., Thorling, K., Pedersen, M., Jensen, M.K., Andersen, E., Pedersen, N.T. & Mortensen, L.S. (1994) Non-hodgkin's lymphoma of the gastrointestinal tract: A population-based analysis of incidence, geographic distribution, clinicopathologic presentation features, and prognosis. danish lymphoma study group. *Journal of Clinical Oncology : Official Journal of the American Society of Clinical Oncology*, 12, 1673-1684.

Daniels, T.E. (1984) Labial salivary gland biopsy in sjogren's syndrome. assessment as a diagnostic criterion in 362 suspected cases. *Arthritis and Rheumatism*, 27, 147-156.

Daum, S., Cellier, C. & Mulder, C.J. (2005) Refractory coeliac disease. *Best Practice & Research.Clinical Gastroenterology*, 19, 413-424.

Daum, S., Ullrich, R., Heise, W., Dederke, B., Foss, H.D., Stein, H., Thiel, E., Zeitz, M. & Riecken, E.O. (2003) Intestinal non-hodgkin's lymphoma: A multicenter prospective clinical study from the german study group on intestinal non-hodgkin's lymphoma. *Journal of Clinical Oncology : Official Journal of the American Society of Clinical Oncology*, 21, 2740-2746.

Daum, S., Weiss, D., Hummel, M., Ullrich, R., Heise, W., Stein, H., Riecken, E.O., Foss, H.D. & Intestinal Lymphoma Study Group. (2001) Frequency of clonal intraepithelial T lymphocyte proliferations in enteropathy-type intestinal T cell lymphoma, coeliac disease, and refractory sprue. *Gut*, 49, 804-812.

Dayan, C.M. & Daniels, G.H. (1996) Chronic autoimmune thyroiditis. *The New England Journal of Medicine*, 335, 99-107.

Derk, C.T., Conway, R.T. & Jimenez, S.A. (2004) Primary B-cell lymphoma of the tongue in a patient with systemic sclerosis. *Oral Oncology*, 40, 103-106.

Derk, C.T., Rasheed, M., Artlett, C.M. & Jimenez, S.A. (2006) A cohort study of cancer incidence in systemic sclerosis. *The Journal of Rheumatology*, 33, 1113-1116.

Derringer, G.A., Thompson, L.D., Frommelt, R.A., Bijwaard, K.E., Heffess, C.S. & Abbondanzo, S.L. (2000) Malignant lymphoma of the thyroid gland: A clinicopathologic study of 108 cases. *The American Journal of Surgical Pathology,* 24, 623-639.

Di Cristofano, A., Kotsi, P., Peng, Y.F., Cordon-Cardo, C., Elkon, K.B. & Pandolfi, P.P. (1999) Impaired fas response and autoimmunity in pten+/- mice. *Science (New York, N.Y.),* 285, 2122-2125.

Di Sabatino, A. & Corazza, G.R. (2009) Coeliac disease. *Lancet,* 373, 1480-1493.

Do, R.K. & Chen-Kiang, S. (2002) Mechanism of BLyS action in B cell immunity. *Cytokine & Growth Factor Reviews,* 13, 19-25.

Domizio, P., Owen, R.A., Shepherd, N.A., Talbot, I.C. & Norton, A.J. (1993) Primary lymphoma of the small intestine. A clinicopathological study of 119 cases. *The American Journal of Surgical Pathology,* 17, 429-442.

Du, M.Q., Xu, C.F., Diss, T.C., Peng, H.Z., Wotherspoon, A.C., Isaacson, P.G. & Pan, L.X. (1996) Intestinal dissemination of gastric mucosa-associated lymphoid tissue lymphoma. *Blood,* 88, 4445-4451.

Duggal, L., Gupta, S., Aggarwal, P.K., Sachar, V.P. & Bhalla, S. (2002) Hodgkin's disease and scleroderma. *The Journal of the Association of Physicians of India,* 50, 1186-1188.

Duncan, S.C. & Winkelmann, R.K. (1979) Cancer and scleroderma. *Archives of Dermatology,* 115, 950-955.

Edinger, J.W., Bonneville, M., Scotet, E., Houssaint, E., Schumacher, H.R. & Posnett, D.N. (1999) EBV gene expression not altered in rheumatoid synovia despite the presence of EBV antigen-specific T cell clones. *Journal of Immunology (Baltimore, Md.: 1950),* 162, 3694-3701.

Eguchi, K. (2001) Apoptosis in autoimmune diseases. *Internal Medicine (Tokyo, Japan),* 40, 275-284.

Ekstrom Smedby, K., Vajdic, C.M., Falster, M., Engels, E.A., Martinez-Maza, O., Turner, J., Hjalgrim, H., Vineis, P., Seniori Costantini, A., Bracci, P.M., Holly, E.A., Willett, E., Spinelli, J.J., La Vecchia, C., Zheng, T., Becker, N., De Sanjose, S., Chiu, B.C., Dal Maso, L., Cocco, P., Maynadie, M., Foretova, L., Staines, A., Brennan, P., Davis, S., Severson, R., Cerhan, J.R., Breen, E.C., Birmann, B., Grulich, A.E. & Cozen, W. (2008) Autoimmune disorders and risk of non-hodgkin lymphoma subtypes: A pooled analysis within the InterLymph consortium. *Blood,* 111, 4029-4038.

Ekstrom, K., Hjalgrim, H., Brandt, L., Baecklund, E., Klareskog, L., Ekbom, A. & Askling, J. (2003) Risk of malignant lymphomas in patients with rheumatoid arthritis and in their first-degree relatives. *Arthritis and Rheumatism,* 48, 963-970.

El Fassi, D., Clemmensen, O., Nielsen, C.H., Silkiss, R.Z. & Hegedus, L. (2007a) Evidence of intrathyroidal B-lymphocyte depletion after rituximab therapy in a patient with graves' disease. *The Journal of Clinical Endocrinology and Metabolism,* 92, 3762-3763.

El Fassi, D., Nielsen, C.H., Bonnema, S.J., Hasselbalch, H.C. & Hegedus, L. (2007b) B lymphocyte depletion with the monoclonal antibody rituximab in graves' disease: A controlled pilot study. *The Journal of Clinical Endocrinology and Metabolism,* 92, 1769-1772.

Elfstrom, P., Granath, F., Ekstrom Smedby, K., Montgomery, S.M., Askling, J., Ekbom, A. & Ludvigsson, J.F. (2011) Risk of lymphoproliferative malignancy in relation to small intestinal histopathology among patients with celiac disease. *Journal of the National Cancer Institute,* 103, 436-444.

Ellman, M.H., Hurwitz, H., Thomas, C. & Kozloff, M. (1991) Lymphoma developing in a patient with rheumatoid arthritis taking low dose weekly methotrexate. *The Journal of Rheumatology,* 18, 1741-1743.
Engels, E.A., Cerhan, J.R., Linet, M.S., Cozen, W., Colt, J.S., Davis, S., Gridley, G., Severson, R.K. & Hartge, P. (2005) Immune-related conditions and immune-modulating medications as risk factors for non-hodgkin's lymphoma: A case-control study. *American Journal of Epidemiology,* 162, 1153-1161.
Farstad, I.N., Johansen, F.E., Vlatkovic, L., Jahnsen, J., Scott, H., Fausa, O., Bjorneklett, A., Brandtzaeg, P. & Halstensen, T.S. (2002) Heterogeneity of intraepithelial lymphocytes in refractory sprue: Potential implications of CD30 expression. *Gut,* 51, 372-378.
Feng, W.H., Cohen, J.I., Fischer, S., Li, L., Sneller, M., Goldbach-Mansky, R., Raab-Traub, N., Delecluse, H.J. & Kenney, S.C. (2004) Reactivation of latent epstein-barr virus by methotrexate: A potential contributor to methotrexate-associated lymphomas. *Journal of the National Cancer Institute,* 96, 1691-1702.
Franklin, J., Lunt, M., Bunn, D., Symmons, D. & Silman, A. (2006) Incidence of lymphoma in a large primary care derived cohort of cases of inflammatory polyarthritis. *Annals of the Rheumatic Diseases,* 65, 617-622.
Franklin, J.P., Symmons, D.P. & Silman, A.J. (2005) Risk of lymphoma in patients with RA treated with anti-TNFalpha agents. *Annals of the Rheumatic Diseases,* 64, 657-658.
Freimark, B., Fantozzi, R., Bone, R., Bordin, G. & Fox, R. (1989) Detection of clonally expanded salivary gland lymphocytes in sjogren's syndrome. *Arthritis and Rheumatism,* 32, 859-869.
Friedman, D.F., Cho, E.A., Goldman, J., Carmack, C.E., Besa, E.C., Hardy, R.R. & Silberstein, L.E. (1991) The role of clonal selection in the pathogenesis of an autoreactive human B cell lymphoma. *The Journal of Experimental Medicine,* 174, 525-537.
Fronek, Z., Cheung, M.M., Hanbury, A.M. & Kagnoff, M.F. (1991) Molecular analysis of HLA DP and DQ genes associated with dermatitis herpetiformis. *The Journal of Investigative Dermatology,* 97, 799-802.
Fry, L., Seah, P.P., Riches, D.J. & Hoffbrand, A.V. (1973) Clearance of skin lesions in dermatitis herpetiformis after gluten withdrawal. *Lancet,* 1, 288-291.
Gale, J., Simmonds, P.D., Mead, G.M., Sweetenham, J.W. & Wright, D.H. (2000) Enteropathy-type intestinal T-cell lymphoma: Clinical features and treatment of 31 patients in a single center. *Journal of Clinical Oncology : Official Journal of the American Society of Clinical Oncology,* 18, 795-803.
Gallamini, A., Zaja, F., Patti, C., Billio, A., Specchia, M.R., Tucci, A., Levis, A., Manna, A., Secondo, V., Rigacci, L., Pinto, A., Iannitto, E., Zoli, V., Torchio, P., Pileri, S. & Tarella, C. (2007) Alemtuzumab (campath-1H) and CHOP chemotherapy as first-line treatment of peripheral T-cell lymphoma: Results of a GITIL (gruppo italiano terapie innovative nei linfomi) prospective multicenter trial. *Blood,* 110, 2316-2323.
Gasparotto, D., De Vita, S., De Re, V., Marzotto, A., De Marchi, G., Scott, C.A., Gloghini, A., Ferraccioli, G. & Boiocchi, M. (2003) Extrasalivary lymphoma development in sjogren's syndrome: Clonal evolution from parotid gland lymphoproliferation and role of local triggering. *Arthritis and Rheumatism,* 48, 3181-3186.
Geborek, P., Crnkic, M., Petersson, I.F., Saxne, T. & South Swedish Arthritis Treatment Group. (2002) Etanercept, infliximab, and leflunomide in established rheumatoid

arthritis: Clinical experience using a structured follow up programme in southern sweden. *Annals of the Rheumatic Diseases,* 61, 793-798.

Geborek, P., Bladstrom, A., Turesson, C., Gulfe, A., Petersson, I.F., Saxne, T., Olsson, H. & Jacobsson, L.T. (2005) Tumour necrosis factor blockers do not increase overall tumour risk in patients with rheumatoid arthritis, but may be associated with an increased risk of lymphomas. *Annals of the Rheumatic Diseases,* 64, 699-703.

Gelfand, J.M., Shin, D.B., Neimann, A.L., Wang, X., Margolis, D.J. & Troxel, A.B. (2006) The risk of lymphoma in patients with psoriasis. *The Journal of Investigative Dermatology,* 126, 2194-2201.

Gellrich, S., Rutz, S., Borkowski, A., Golembowski, S., Gromnica-Ihle, E., Sterry, W. & Jahn, S. (1999) Analysis of V(H)-D-J(H) gene transcripts in B cells infiltrating the salivary glands and lymph node tissues of patients with sjogren's syndrome. *Arthritis and Rheumatism,* 42, 240-247.

Gjone, E. & Nordoy, A. (1970) Dermatitis herpetiformis, steatorrhoea, and malignancy. *British Medical Journal,* 1, 610.

Goodnow, C.C. (2007) Multistep pathogenesis of autoimmune disease. *Cell,* 130, 25-35.

Grady, W.M. (2005) Transforming growth factor-beta, smads, and cancer. *Clinical Cancer Research: An Official Journal of the American Association for Cancer Research,* 11, 3151-3154.

Graff-Baker, A., Sosa, J.A. & Roman, S.A. (2010) Primary thyroid lymphoma: A review of recent developments in diagnosis and histology-driven treatment. *Current Opinion in Oncology,* 22, 17-22.

Gridley, G., Klippel, J.H., Hoover, R.N. & Fraumeni, J.F.,Jr. (1994) Incidence of cancer among men with the felty syndrome. *Annals of Internal Medicine,* 120, 35-39.

Gridley, G., McLaughlin, J.K., Ekbom, A., Klareskog, L., Adami, H.O., Hacker, D.G., Hoover, R. & Fraumeni, J.F.,Jr. (1993) Incidence of cancer among patients with rheumatoid arthritis. *Journal of the National Cancer Institute,* 85, 307-311.

Halfdanarson, T.R., Rubio-Tapia, A., Ristow, K.M., Habermann, T.M., Murray, J.A. & Inwards, D.J. (2010) Patients with celiac disease and B-cell lymphoma have a better prognosis than those with T-cell lymphoma. *Clinical Gastroenterology and Hepatology: The Official Clinical Practice Journal of the American Gastroenterological Association,* 8, 1042-1047.

Hall, S.W., Gillespie, J.J. & Tenczynski, T.F. (1978) Generalized lipodystrophy, scleroderma, and hodgkin's disease. *Archives of Internal Medicine,* 138, 1303-1304.

Harris, N.L. (1999) Lymphoid proliferations of the salivary glands. *American Journal of Clinical Pathology,* 111, S94-103.

Haviv, Y.S., Ben-Yehuda, A., Polliack, A. & Safadi, R. (1997) Lymphoma and systemic sclerosis--an uncommon association or possible coincidence of two disorders with a fatal outcome. *European Journal of Haematology,* 59, 194-196.

Hellgren, K., Smedby, K.E., Feltelius, N., Baecklund, E. & Askling, J. (2010a) Do rheumatoid arthritis and lymphoma share risk factors?: A comparison of lymphoma and cancer risks before and after diagnosis of rheumatoid arthritis. *Arthritis and Rheumatism,* 62, 1252-1258.

Hellgren, K., Iliadou, A., Rosenquist, R., Feltelius, N., Backlin, C., Enblad, G., Askling, J. & Baecklund, E. (2010b) Rheumatoid arthritis, treatment with corticosteroids and risk of malignant lymphomas: Results from a case-control study. *Annals of the Rheumatic Diseases,* 69, 654-659.

Hervonen, K., Vornanen, M., Kautiainen, H., Collin, P. & Reunala, T. (2005) Lymphoma in patients with dermatitis herpetiformis and their first-degree relatives. *The British Journal of Dermatology*, 152, 82-86.

Hervonen, K., Hakanen, M., Kaukinen, K., Collin, P. & Reunala, T. (2002) First-degree relatives are frequently affected in coeliac disease and dermatitis herpetiformis. *Scandinavian Journal of Gastroenterology*, 37, 51-55.

Hill, C.L., Nguyen, A.M., Roder, D. & Roberts-Thomson, P. (2003) Risk of cancer in patients with scleroderma: A population based cohort study. *Annals of the Rheumatic Diseases*, 62, 728-731.

Hjelmstrom, P. (2001) Lymphoid neogenesis: De novo formation of lymphoid tissue in chronic inflammation through expression of homing chemokines. *Journal of Leukocyte Biology*, 69, 331-339.

Holly, E.A., Lele, C., Bracci, P.M. & McGrath, M.S. (1999) Case-control study of non-hodgkin's lymphoma among women and heterosexual men in the san francisco bay area, california. *American Journal of Epidemiology*, 150, 375-389.

Holm, L.E., Blomgren, H. & Lowhagen, T. (1985) Cancer risks in patients with chronic lymphocytic thyroiditis. *The New England Journal of Medicine*, 312, 601-604.

Holmes, G.K., Prior, P., Lane, M.R., Pope, D. & Allan, R.N. (1989) Malignancy in coeliac disease--effect of a gluten free diet. *Gut*, 30, 333-338.

Horikawa, M., Hasegawa, M., Komura, K., Hayakawa, I., Yanaba, K., Matsushita, T., Takehara, K. & Sato, S. (2005) Abnormal natural killer cell function in systemic sclerosis: Altered cytokine production and defective killing activity. *The Journal of Investigative Dermatology*, 125, 731-737.

Hoshida, Y., Tomita, Y., Zhiming, D., Yamauchi, A., Nakatsuka, S., Kurasono, Y., Arima, Y., Tsudo, M., Shintaku, M. & Aozasa, K. (2004) Lymphoproliferative disorders in autoimmune diseases in japan: Analysis of clinicopathological features and epstein-barr virus infection. *International Journal of Cancer.Journal International Du Cancer*, 108, 443-449.

Hoshida, Y., Xu, J.X., Fujita, S., Nakamichi, I., Ikeda, J., Tomita, Y., Nakatsuka, S., Tamaru, J., Iizuka, A., Takeuchi, T. & Aozasa, K. (2007) Lymphoproliferative disorders in rheumatoid arthritis: Clinicopathological analysis of 76 cases in relation to methotrexate medication. *The Journal of Rheumatology*, 34, 322-331.

Hyjek, E. & Isaacson, P.G. (1988) Primary B cell lymphoma of the thyroid and its relationship to hashimoto's thyroiditis. *Human Pathology*, 19, 1315-1326.

Illes, A., Varoczy, L., Papp, G., Wilson, P.C., Alex, P., Jonsson, R., Kovacs, T., Konttinen, Y.T., Zeher, M., Nakken, B. & Szodoray, P. (2009) Aspects of B-cell non-hodgkin's lymphoma development: A transition from immune-reactivity to malignancy. *Scandinavian Journal of Immunology*, 69, 387-400.

Ilyas, M., Niedobitek, G., Agathanggelou, A., Barry, R.E., Read, A.E., Tierney, R., Young, L.S. & Rooney, N. (1995) Non-hodgkin's lymphoma, coeliac disease, and epstein-barr virus: A study of 13 cases of enteropathy-associated T- and B-cell lymphoma. *The Journal of Pathology*, 177, 115-122.

Ioannidis, J.P., Vassiliou, V.A. & Moutsopoulos, H.M. (2002) Long-term risk of mortality and lymphoproliferative disease and predictive classification of primary sjogren's syndrome. *Arthritis and Rheumatism*, 46, 741-747.

Isaacson, P.G. (1997) Lymphoma of the thyroid gland. *Current Topics in Pathology.Ergebnisse Der Pathologie,* 91, 1-14.

Jackson, C.E. & Puck, J.M. (1999) Autoimmune lymphoproliferative syndrome, a disorder of apoptosis. *Current Opinion in Pediatrics,* 11, 521-527.

Jacobi, A.M., Hansen, A., Kaufmann, O., Pruss, A., Burmester, G.R., Lipsky, P.E. & Dorner, T. (2002) Analysis of immunoglobulin light chain rearrangements in the salivary gland and blood of a patient with sjogren's syndrome. *Arthritis Research,* 4, R4.

James, J.A., Kaufman, K.M., Farris, A.D., Taylor-Albert, E., Lehman, T.J. & Harley, J.B. (1997) An increased prevalence of epstein-barr virus infection in young patients suggests a possible etiology for systemic lupus erythematosus. *The Journal of Clinical Investigation,* 100, 3019-3026.

Jenkins, D., Lynde, C.W. & Stewart, W.D. (1983) Histiocytic lymphoma occurring in a patient with dermatitis herpetiformis. *Journal of the American Academy of Dermatology,* 9, 252-256.

Jonsson, R., Gordon, T.P. & Konttinen, Y.T. (2003) Recent advances in understanding molecular mechanisms in the pathogenesis and antibody profile of sjogren's syndrome. *Current Rheumatology Reports,* 5, 311-316.

Kabel, P.J., Voorbij, H.A., de Haan-Meulman, M., Pals, S.T. & Drexhage, H.A. (1989) High endothelial venules present in lymphoid cell accumulations in thyroids affected by autoimmune disease: A study in men and BB rats of functional activity and development. *The Journal of Clinical Endocrinology and Metabolism,* 68, 744-751.

Kahara, T., Iwaki, N., Kaya, H., Kurokawa, T., Yoshida, T., Ishikura, K. & Usuda, R. (2011) Transition of thyroid autoantibodies by rituximab treatment for thyroid MALT lymphoma. *Endocrine Journal,* 58, 7-12.

Kamel, O.W., van de Rijn, M., Weiss, L.M., Del Zoppo, G.J., Hench, P.K., Robbins, B.A., Montgomery, P.G., Warnke, R.A. & Dorfman, R.F. (1993) Brief report: Reversible lymphomas associated with epstein-barr virus occurring during methotrexate therapy for rheumatoid arthritis and dermatomyositis. *The New England Journal of Medicine,* 328, 1317-1321.

Kassan, S.S. & Moutsopoulos, H.M. (2004) Clinical manifestations and early diagnosis of sjogren syndrome. *Archives of Internal Medicine,* 164, 1275-1284.

Kassan, S.S., Thomas, T.L., Moutsopoulos, H.M., Hoover, R., Kimberly, R.P., Budman, D.R., Costa, J., Decker, J.L. & Chused, T.M. (1978) Increased risk of lymphoma in sicca syndrome. *Annals of Internal Medicine,* 89, 888-892.

Kato, I., Koenig, K.L., Shore, R.E., Baptiste, M.S., Lillquist, P.P., Frizzera, G., Burke, J.S. & Watanabe, H. (2002) Use of anti-inflammatory and non-narcotic analgesic drugs and risk of non-hodgkin's lymphoma (NHL) (united states). *Cancer Causes & Control : CCC,* 13, 965-974.

Kauppi, M., Pukkala, E. & Isomaki, H. (1997) Elevated incidence of hematologic malignancies in patients with sjogren's syndrome compared with patients with rheumatoid arthritis (finland). *Cancer Causes & Control : CCC,* 8, 201-204.

Kedar, A., Khan, A.B., Mattern, J.Q., Fisher, J., Thomas, P.R. & Freeman, A.I. (1979) Autoimmune disorders complicating adolescent hodgkin's disease. *Cancer,* 44, 112-116.

Kim, H.J., Krenn, V., Steinhauser, G. & Berek, C. (1999) Plasma cell development in synovial germinal centers in patients with rheumatoid and reactive arthritis. *Journal of Immunology (Baltimore, Md.: 1950),* 162, 3053-3062.

King, J.K. & Costenbader, K.H. (2007) Characteristics of patients with systemic lupus erythematosus (SLE) and non-hodgkin's lymphoma (NHL). *Clinical Rheumatology,* 26, 1491-1494.

Kingsmore, S.F., Hall, B.D., Allen, N.B., Rice, J.R. & Caldwell, D.S. (1992) Association of methotrexate, rheumatoid arthritis and lymphoma: Report of 2 cases and literature review. *The Journal of Rheumatology,* 19, 1462-1465.

Kiss, E., Kovacs, L. & Szodoray, P. (2010) Malignancies in systemic lupus erythematosus. *Autoimmunity Reviews,* 9, 195-199.

Klyachkin, M.L., Schwartz, R.W., Cibull, M., Munn, R.K., Regine, W.F., Kenady, D.E., McGrath, P.C. & Sloan, D.A. (1998) Thyroid lymphoma: Is there a role for surgery? *The American Surgeon,* 64, 234-238.

Knecht, H., Saremaslani, P. & Hedinger, C. (1981) Immunohistological findings in hashimoto's thyroiditis, focal lymphocytic thyroiditis and thyroiditis de quervain. comparative study. *Virchows Archiv.A, Pathological Anatomy and Histology,* 393, 215-231.

Kojima, M., Itoh, H., Shimizu, K., Saruki, N., Murayama, K., Higuchi, K., Tamaki, Y., Matsumoto, M., Hirabayashi, K., Igarishi, S., Masawa, N. & Nakamura, S. (2006) Malignant lymphoma in patients with systemic rheumatic disease (rheumatoid arthritis, systemic lupus erythematosus, systemic sclerosis, and dermatomyositis): A clinicopathologic study of 24 japanese cases. *International Journal of Surgical Pathology,* 14, 43-48.

Kratz, A., Campos-Neto, A., Hanson, M.S. & Ruddle, N.H. (1996) Chronic inflammation caused by lymphotoxin is lymphoid neogenesis. *The Journal of Experimental Medicine,* 183, 1461-1472.

Kremer, J.M. (1997) Is methotrexate oncogenic in patients with rheumatoid arthritis? *Seminars in Arthritis and Rheumatism,* 26, 785-787.

Laabi, Y. & Strasser, A. (2000) Immunology. lymphocyte survival--ignorance is BLys. *Science (New York, N.Y.),* 289, 883-884.

Laing, R.W., Hoskin, P., Hudson, B.V., Hudson, G.V., Harmer, C., Bennett, M.H. & MacLennan, K.A. (1994) The significance of MALT histology in thyroid lymphoma: A review of patients from the BNLI and royal marsden hospital. *Clinical Oncology (Royal College of Radiologists (Great Britain)),* 6, 300-304.

Landgren, O., Engels, E.A., Pfeiffer, R.M., Gridley, G., Mellemkjaer, L., Olsen, J.H., Kerstann, K.F., Wheeler, W., Hemminki, K., Linet, M.S. & Goldin, L.R. (2006) Autoimmunity and susceptibility to hodgkin lymphoma: A population-based case-control study in scandinavia. *Journal of the National Cancer Institute,* 98, 1321-1330.

Legler, D.F., Loetscher, M., Roos, R.S., Clark-Lewis, I., Baggiolini, M. & Moser, B. (1998) B cell-attracting chemokine 1, a human CXC chemokine expressed in lymphoid tissues, selectively attracts B lymphocytes via BLR1/CXCR5. *The Journal of Experimental Medicine,* 187, 655-660.

Leombruno, J.P., Einarson, T.R. & Keystone, E.C. (2009) The safety of anti-tumour necrosis factor treatments in rheumatoid arthritis: Meta and exposure-adjusted pooled analyses of serious adverse events. *Annals of the Rheumatic Diseases,* 68, 1136-1145.

Leprince, C., Cohen-Kaminsky, S., Berrih-Aknin, S., Vernet-Der Garabedian, B., Treton, D., Galanaud, P. & Richard, Y. (1990) Thymic B cells from myasthenia gravis patients are activated B cells. phenotypic and functional analysis. *Journal of Immunology (Baltimore, Md.: 1950),* 145, 2115-2122.

Lewis, H.M., Renaula, T.L., Garioch, J.J., Leonard, J.N., Fry, J.S., Collin, P., Evans, D. & Fry, L. (1996) Protective effect of gluten-free diet against development of lymphoma in dermatitis herpetiformis. *The British Journal of Dermatology,* 135, 363-367.

Liote, F., Pertuiset, E., Cochand-Priollet, B., D'Agay, M.F., Dombret, H., Numeric, P., D'Anglejan, G. & Kuntz, D. (1995) Methotrexate related B lymphoproliferative disease in a patient with rheumatoid arthritis. role of epstein-barr virus infection. *The Journal of Rheumatology,* 22, 1174-1178.

Lofstrom, B., Backlin, C., Sundstrom, C., Ekbom, A. & Lundberg, I.E. (2007) A closer look at non-hodgkin's lymphoma cases in a national swedish systemic lupus erythematosus cohort: A nested case-control study. *Annals of the Rheumatic Diseases,* 66, 1627-1632.

Loren, A.W., Porter, D.L., Stadtmauer, E.A. & Tsai, D.E. (2003) Post-transplant lymphoproliferative disorder: A review. *Bone Marrow Transplantation,* 31, 145-155.

Lossos, I.S., Alizadeh, A.A., Rajapaksa, R., Tibshirani, R. & Levy, R. (2003) HGAL is a novel interleukin-4-inducible gene that strongly predicts survival in diffuse large B-cell lymphoma. *Blood,* 101, 433-440.

Lu, X., Chen, J., Malumbres, R., Cubedo Gil, E., Helfman, D.M. & Lossos, I.S. (2007) HGAL, a lymphoma prognostic biomarker, interacts with the cytoskeleton and mediates the effects of IL-6 on cell migration. *Blood,* 110, 4268-4277.

Mackay, F., Sierro, F., Grey, S.T. & Gordon, T.P. (2005) The BAFF/APRIL system: An important player in systemic rheumatic diseases. *Current Directions in Autoimmunity,* 8, 243-265.

Mackay, F., Woodcock, S.A., Lawton, P., Ambrose, C., Baetscher, M., Schneider, P., Tschopp, J. & Browning, J.L. (1999) Mice transgenic for BAFF develop lymphocytic disorders along with autoimmune manifestations. *The Journal of Experimental Medicine,* 190, 1697-1710.

Mackay, I.R. & Rose, N.R. (2001) Autoimmunity and lymphoma: Tribulations of B cells. *Nature Immunology,* 2, 793-795.

Mackey, A.C., Green, L., Liang, L.C., Dinndorf, P. & Avigan, M. (2007) Hepatosplenic T cell lymphoma associated with infliximab use in young patients treated for inflammatory bowel disease. *Journal of Pediatric Gastroenterology and Nutrition,* 44, 265-267.

Mariette, X. (1999) Lymphomas in patients with sjogren's syndrome: Review of the literature and physiopathologic hypothesis. *Leukemia & Lymphoma,* 33, 93-99.

Mariette, X., Cazals-Hatem, D., Warszawki, J., Liote, F., Balandraud, N., Sibilia, J. & Investigators of the Club Rhumatismes et Inflammation. (2002) Lymphomas in rheumatoid arthritis patients treated with methotrexate: A 3-year prospective study in france. *Blood,* 99, 3909-3915.

Mearin, M.L., Catassi, C., Brousse, N., Brand, R., Collin, P., Fabiani, E., Schweizer, J.J., Abuzakouk, M., Szajewska, H., Hallert, C., Farre Masip, C., Holmes, G.K. & Biomed Study Group on Coeliac Disease and Non-Hodgkin Lymphoma. (2006) European multi-centre study on coeliac disease and non-hodgkin lymphoma. *European Journal of Gastroenterology & Hepatology,* 18, 187-194.

Meibohm, B., Beierle, I. & Derendorf, H. (2002) How important are gender differences in pharmacokinetics? *Clinical Pharmacokinetics,* 41, 329-342.

Meijer, J.W., Mulder, C.J., Goerres, M.G., Boot, H. & Schweizer, J.J. (2004) Coeliac disease and (extra)intestinal T-cell lymphomas: Definition, diagnosis and treatment. *Scandinavian Journal of Gastroenterology.Supplement,* (241), 78-84.

Mellemkjaer, L., Pfeiffer, R.M., Engels, E.A., Gridley, G., Wheeler, W., Hemminki, K., Olsen, J.H., Dreyer, L., Linet, M.S., Goldin, L.R. & Landgren, O. (2008) Autoimmune disease in individuals and close family members and susceptibility to non-hodgkin's lymphoma. *Arthritis and Rheumatism,* 58, 657-666.

Mellors, R.C. (1966) Autoimmune disease in NZB-bl mice. II. autoimmunity and malignant lymphoma. *Blood,* 27, 435-448.

Mention, J.J., Ben Ahmed, M., Begue, B., Barbe, U., Verkarre, V., Asnafi, V., Colombel, J.F., Cugnenc, P.H., Ruemmele, F.M., McIntyre, E., Brousse, N., Cellier, C. & Cerf-Bensussan, N. (2003) Interleukin 15: A key to disrupted intraepithelial lymphocyte homeostasis and lymphomagenesis in celiac disease. *Gastroenterology,* 125, 730-745.

Miners, J.O., Grgurinovich, N., Whitehead, A.G., Robson, R.A. & Birkett, D.J. (1986) Influence of gender and oral contraceptive steroids on the metabolism of salicylic acid and acetylsalicylic acid. *British Journal of Clinical Pharmacology,* 22, 135-142.

Moder, K.G., Tefferi, A., Cohen, M.D., Menke, D.M. & Luthra, H.S. (1995) Hematologic malignancies and the use of methotrexate in rheumatoid arthritis: A retrospective study. *The American Journal of Medicine,* 99, 276-281.

Morton, J.E., Leyland, M.J., Vaughan Hudson, G., Vaughan Hudson, B., Anderson, L., Bennett, M.H. & MacLennan, K.A. (1993) Primary gastrointestinal non-hodgkin's lymphoma: A review of 175 british national lymphoma investigation cases. *British Journal of Cancer,* 67, 776-782.

Moshynska, O.V. & Saxena, A. (2008) Clonal relationship between hashimoto thyroiditis and thyroid lymphoma. *Journal of Clinical Pathology,* 61, 438-444.

Moss, K.E., Ioannou, Y., Sultan, S.M., Haq, I. & Isenberg, D.A. (2002) Outcome of a cohort of 300 patients with systemic lupus erythematosus attending a dedicated clinic for over two decades. *Annals of the Rheumatic Diseases,* 61, 409-413.

Moutsopoulos, H.M., Steinberg, A.D., Fauci, A.S., Lane, H.C. & Papadopoulos, N.M. (1983) High incidence of free monoclonal lambda light chains in the sera of patients with sjogren's syndrome. *Journal of Immunology (Baltimore, Md.: 1950),* 130, 2663-2665.

Natkunam, Y., Lossos, I.S., Taidi, B., Zhao, S., Lu, X., Ding, F., Hammer, A.S., Marafioti, T., Byrne, G.E.,Jr, Levy, S., Warnke, R.A. & Levy, R. (2005) Expression of the human germinal center-associated lymphoma (HGAL) protein, a new marker of germinal center B-cell derivation. *Blood,* 105, 3979-3986.

Neumeister, P., Hoefler, G., Beham-Schmid, C., Schmidt, H., Apfelbeck, U., Schaider, H., Linkesch, W. & Sill, H. (1997) Deletion analysis of the p16 tumor suppressor gene in gastrointestinal mucosa-associated lymphoid tissue lymphomas. *Gastroenterology,* 112, 1871-1875.

Ngo, V.N., Korner, H., Gunn, M.D., Schmidt, K.N., Riminton, D.S., Cooper, M.D., Browning, J.L., Sedgwick, J.D. & Cyster, J.G. (1999) Lymphotoxin alpha/beta and tumor necrosis factor are required for stromal cell expression of homing chemokines in B and T cell areas of the spleen. *The Journal of Experimental Medicine,* 189, 403-412.

Niitsu, N., Okamoto, M., Nakamura, N., Nakamine, H., Bessho, M. & Hirano, M. (2007) Clinicopathologic correlations of stage IE/IIE primary thyroid diffuse large B-cell lymphoma. *Annals of Oncology : Official Journal of the European Society for Medical Oncology / ESMO,* 18, 1203-1208.

Nossent, J., Cikes, N., Kiss, E., Marchesoni, A., Nassonova, V., Mosca, M., Olesinska, M., Pokorny, G., Rozman, B., Schneider, M., Vlachoyiannopoulos, P.G. & Swaak, A.

(2007) Current causes of death in systemic lupus erythematosus in europe, 2000--2004: Relation to disease activity and damage accrual. *Lupus,* 16, 309-317.

Novakovic, B.J., Novakovic, S. & Frkovic-Grazio, S. (2006) A single-center report on clinical features and treatment response in patients with intestinal T cell non-hodgkin's lymphomas. *Oncology Reports,* 16, 191-195.

Okada, T., Takiura, F., Tokushige, K., Nozawa, S., Kiyosawa, T., Nakauchi, H., Hirose, S. & Shirai, T. (1991) Major histocompatibility complex controls clonal proliferation of CD5+ B cells in H-2-congenic new zealand mice: A model for B cell chronic lymphocytic leukemia and autoimmune disease. *European Journal of Immunology,* 21, 2743-2748.

Patey-Mariaud De Serre, N., Cellier, C., Jabri, B., Delabesse, E., Verkarre, V., Roche, B., Lavergne, A., Briere, J., Mauvieux, L., Leborgne, M., Barbier, J.P., Modigliani, R., Matuchansky, C., MacIntyre, E., Cerf-Bensussan, N. & Brousse, N. (2000) Distinction between coeliac disease and refractory sprue: A simple immunohistochemical method. *Histopathology,* 37, 70-77.

Pedersen, R.K. & Pedersen, N.T. (1996) Primary non-hodgkin's lymphoma of the thyroid gland: A population based study. *Histopathology,* 28, 25-32.

Picker, L.J. (1992) Mechanisms of lymphocyte homing. *Current Opinion in Immunology,* 4, 277-286.

Pijpe, J., van Imhoff, G.W., Spijkervet, F.K., Roodenburg, J.L., Wolbink, G.J., Mansour, K., Vissink, A., Kallenberg, C.G. & Bootsma, H. (2005) Rituximab treatment in patients with primary sjogren's syndrome: An open-label phase II study. *Arthritis and Rheumatism,* 52, 2740-2750.

Poole, B.D., Templeton, A.K., Guthridge, J.M., Brown, E.J., Harley, J.B. & James, J.A. (2009) Aberrant epstein-barr viral infection in systemic lupus erythematosus. *Autoimmunity Reviews,* 8, 337-342.

Quartuccio, L., Fabris, M., Salvin, S., Maset, M., De Marchi, G. & De Vita, S. (2009) Controversies on rituximab therapy in sjogren syndrome-associated lymphoproliferation. *International Journal of Rheumatology,* 2009, 424935.

Ramos-Casals, M., Brito-Zeron, P., Yague, J., Akasbi, M., Bautista, R., Ruano, M., Claver, G., Gil, V. & Font, J. (2005) Hypocomplementaemia as an immunological marker of morbidity and mortality in patients with primary sjogren's syndrome. *Rheumatology (Oxford, England),* 44, 89-94.

Randen, I., Mellbye, O.J., Forre, O. & Natvig, J.B. (1995) The identification of germinal centres and follicular dendritic cell networks in rheumatoid synovial tissue. *Scandinavian Journal of Immunology,* 41, 481-486.

Ray, W.A. (2003) Population-based studies of adverse drug effects. *The New England Journal of Medicine,* 349, 1592-1594.

Reunala, T. (1998) Dermatitis herpetiformis: Coeliac disease of the skin. *Annals of Medicine,* 30, 416-418.

Reunala, T., Helin, H., Kuokkanen, K. & Hakala, T. (1982) Lymphoma in dermatitis herpetiformis: Report on four cases. *Acta Dermato-Venereologica,* 62, 343-346.

Reunala, T., Blomqvist, K., Tarpila, S., Halme, H. & Kangas, K. (1977) Gluten-free diet in dermatitis herpetiformis. I. clinical response of skin lesions in 81 patients. *The British Journal of Dermatology,* 97, 473-480.

Reyes, F., Lepage, E., Ganem, G., Molina, T.J., Brice, P., Coiffier, B., Morel, P., Ferme, C., Bosly, A., Lederlin, P., Laurent, G., Tilly, H. & Groupe d'Etude des Lymphomes de l'Adulte (GELA). (2005) ACVBP versus CHOP plus radiotherapy for localized aggressive lymphoma. *The New England Journal of Medicine,* 352, 1197-1205.

Rizzi, R., Curci, P., Delia, M., Rinaldi, E., Chiefa, A., Specchia, G. & Liso, V. (2009) Spontaneous remission of "methotrexate-associated lymphoproliferative disorders" after discontinuation of immunosuppressive treatment for autoimmune disease. review of the literature. *Medical Oncology (Northwood, London, England),* 26, 1-9.

Rosenberg, L., Palmer, J.R., Zauber, A.G., Warshauer, M.E., Strom, B.L., Harlap, S. & Shapiro, S. (1995) Relation of benzodiazepine use to the risk of selected cancers: Breast, large bowel, malignant melanoma, lung, endometrium, ovary, non-hodgkin's lymphoma, testis, hodgkin's disease, thyroid, and liver. *American Journal of Epidemiology,* 141, 1153-1160.

Rosenthal, A.K., McLaughlin, J.K., Gridley, G. & Nyren, O. (1995) Incidence of cancer among patients with systemic sclerosis. *Cancer,* 76, 910-914.

Rosenthal, A.K., McLaughlin, J.K., Linet, M.S. & Persson, I. (1993) Scleroderma and malignancy: An epidemiological study. *Annals of the Rheumatic Diseases,* 52, 531-533.

Rossi, D. (2009) Thyroid lymphoma: Beyond antigen stimulation. *Leukemia Research,* 33, 607-609.

Roumm, A.D. & Medsger, T.A.,Jr. (1985) Cancer and systemic sclerosis. an epidemiologic study. *Arthritis and Rheumatism,* 28, 1336-1340.

Royer, B., Cazals-Hatem, D., Sibilia, J., Agbalika, F., Cayuela, J.M., Soussi, T., Maloisel, F., Clauvel, J.P., Brouet, J.C. & Mariette, X. (1997) Lymphomas in patients with sjogren's syndrome are marginal zone B-cell neoplasms, arise in diverse extranodal and nodal sites, and are not associated with viruses. *Blood,* 90, 766-775.

Ruggiero, F.P., Frauenhoffer, E. & Stack, B.C.,Jr. (2005) Thyroid lymphoma: A single institution's experience. *Otolaryngology--Head and Neck Surgery : Official Journal of American Academy of Otolaryngology-Head and Neck Surgery,* 133, 888-896.

Salloum, E., Cooper, D.L., Howe, G., Lacy, J., Tallini, G., Crouch, J., Schultz, M. & Murren, J. (1996) Spontaneous regression of lymphoproliferative disorders in patients treated with methotrexate for rheumatoid arthritis and other rheumatic diseases. *Journal of Clinical Oncology : Official Journal of the American Society of Clinical Oncology,* 14, 1943-1949.

Sato, S., Fujimoto, M., Hasegawa, M. & Takehara, K. (2004) Altered blood B lymphocyte homeostasis in systemic sclerosis: Expanded naive B cells and diminished but activated memory B cells. *Arthritis and Rheumatism,* 50, 1918-1927.

Savilahti, E., Reunala, T. & Maki, M. (1992) Increase of lymphocytes bearing the gamma/delta T cell receptor in the jejunum of patients with dermatitis herpetiformis. *Gut,* 33, 206-211.

Saxena, A., Alport, E.C., Moshynska, O., Kanthan, R. & Boctor, M.A. (2004) Clonal B cell populations in a minority of patients with hashimoto's thyroiditis. *Journal of Clinical Pathology,* 57, 1258-1263.

Schroder, A.E., Greiner, A., Seyfert, C. & Berek, C. (1996) Differentiation of B cells in the nonlymphoid tissue of the synovial membrane of patients with rheumatoid arthritis. *Proceedings of the National Academy of Sciences of the United States of America,* 93, 221-225.

Setoguchi, S., Solomon, D.H., Weinblatt, M.E., Katz, J.N., Avorn, J., Glynn, R.J., Cook, E.F., Carney, G. & Schneeweiss, S. (2006) Tumor necrosis factor alpha antagonist use and cancer in patients with rheumatoid arthritis. *Arthritis and Rheumatism,* 54, 2757-2764.

Seyler, T.M., Park, Y.W., Takemura, S., Bram, R.J., Kurtin, P.J., Goronzy, J.J. & Weyand, C.M. (2005) BLyS and APRIL in rheumatoid arthritis. *The Journal of Clinical Investigation,* 115, 3083-3092.

Siau, K., Laversuch, C.J., Creamer, P. & O'Rourke, K.P. (2010) Malignancy in scleroderma patients from south west england: A population-based cohort study. *Rheumatology International.*

Sieniawski, M., Angamuthu, N., Boyd, K., Chasty, R., Davies, J., Forsyth, P., Jack, F., Lyons, S., Mounter, P., Revell, P., Proctor, S.J. & Lennard, A.L. (2010) Evaluation of enteropathy-associated T-cell lymphoma comparing standard therapies with a novel regimen including autologous stem cell transplantation. *Blood,* 115, 3664-3670.

Sigurgeirsson, B., Agnarsson, B.A. & Lindelof, B. (1994) Risk of lymphoma in patients with dermatitis herpetiformis. *BMJ (Clinical Research Ed.),* 308, 13-15.

Silano, M., Volta, U., Vincenzi, A.D., Dessi, M., Vincenzi, M.D. & Collaborating Centers of the Italian Registry of the Complications of Coeliac Disease. (2008) Effect of a gluten-free diet on the risk of enteropathy-associated T-cell lymphoma in celiac disease. *Digestive Diseases and Sciences,* 53, 972-976.

Silano, M., Volta, U., Mecchia, A.M., Dessi, M., Di Benedetto, R., De Vincenzi, M. & Collaborating centers of the Italian registry of the complications of coeliac disease. (2007) Delayed diagnosis of coeliac disease increases cancer risk. *BMC Gastroenterology,* 7, 8.

Simon, Z., Tarr, T., Ress, Z., Gergely, L., Kiss, E. & Illes, A. (2007) Successful rituximab-CHOP treatment of systemic lupus erythematosus associated with diffuse large B-cell non-hodgkin lymphoma. *Rheumatology International,* 28, 179-183.

Skopouli, F.N., Dafni, U., Ioannidis, J.P. & Moutsopoulos, H.M. (2000) Clinical evolution, and morbidity and mortality of primary sjogren's syndrome. *Seminars in Arthritis and Rheumatism,* 29, 296-304.

Smedby, K.E., Baecklund, E. & Askling, J. (2006) Malignant lymphomas in autoimmunity and inflammation: A review of risks, risk factors, and lymphoma characteristics. *Cancer Epidemiology, Biomarkers & Prevention : A Publication of the American Association for Cancer Research, Cosponsored by the American Society of Preventive Oncology,* 15, 2069-2077.

Smedby, K.E., Askling, J., Mariette, X. & Baecklund, E. (2008) Autoimmune and inflammatory disorders and risk of malignant lymphomas--an update. *Journal of Internal Medicine,* 264, 514-527.

Smedby, K.E., Akerman, M., Hildebrand, H., Glimelius, B., Ekbom, A. & Askling, J. (2005) Malignant lymphomas in coeliac disease: Evidence of increased risks for lymphoma types other than enteropathy-type T cell lymphoma. *Gut,* 54, 54-59.

Smedby, K.E., Hjalgrim, H., Askling, J., Chang, E.T., Gregersen, H., Porwit-MacDonald, A., Sundstrom, C., Akerman, M., Melbye, M., Glimelius, B. & Adami, H.O. (2006) Autoimmune and chronic inflammatory disorders and risk of non-hodgkin lymphoma by subtype. *Journal of the National Cancer Institute,* 98, 51-60.

Soderberg, K.C., Jonsson, F., Winqvist, O., Hagmar, L. & Feychting, M. (2006) Autoimmune diseases, asthma and risk of haematological malignancies: A nationwide case-control study in sweden. *European Journal of Cancer (Oxford, England : 1990),* 42, 3028-3033.

Soderstrom, N., Axelsson, J.A. & Hagelqvist, E. (1970) Postcapillary venules of the lymph node type in the thymus in myasthenia. *Laboratory Investigation; a Journal of Technical Methods and Pathology,* 23, 451-458.

Soldini, D., Mora, O., Cavalli, F., Zucca, E. & Mazzucchelli, L. (2008) Efficacy of alemtuzumab and gemcitabine in a patient with enteropathy-type T-cell lymphoma. *British Journal of Haematology,* 142, 484-486.

Sorensen, H.T., Friis, S., Norgard, B., Mellemkjaer, L., Blot, W.J., McLaughlin, J.K., Ekbom, A. & Baron, J.A. (2003) Risk of cancer in a large cohort of nonaspirin NSAID users: A population-based study. *British Journal of Cancer,* 88, 1687-1692.

Staunton, M.D. & Greening, W.P. (1973) Clinical diagnosis of thyroid cancer. *British Medical Journal,* 4, 532-535.

Stott, D.I., Hiepe, F., Hummel, M., Steinhauser, G. & Berek, C. (1998) Antigen-driven clonal proliferation of B cells within the target tissue of an autoimmune disease. the salivary glands of patients with sjogren's syndrome. *The Journal of Clinical Investigation,* 102, 938-946.

Su, L. & David, M. (1999) Inhibition of B cell receptor-mediated apoptosis by IFN. *Journal of Immunology (Baltimore, Md.: 1950),* 162, 6317-6321.

Swerdlow, S.H., Campo, E., Harris, N.L., Jaffe, E.S., Pileri, S., Stein, H., Thiele, J. & Vardiman J.W. (2008) WHO classification of tumours of haematopoietic and lymphoid tissues.

Symmons, D.P. (1985) Neoplasms of the immune system in rheumatoid arthritis. *The American Journal of Medicine,* 78, 22-28.

Szekanecz, E., Szamosi, S., Gergely, L., Keszthelyi, P., Szekanecz, Z. & Szucs, G. (2008) Incidence of lymphoma in systemic sclerosis: A retrospective analysis of 218 hungarian patients with systemic sclerosis. *Clinical Rheumatology,* 27, 1163-1166.

Szodoray, P. & Jonsson, R. (2005) The BAFF/APRIL system in systemic autoimmune diseases with a special emphasis on sjogren's syndrome. *Scandinavian Journal of Immunology,* 62, 421-428.

Tack, G.J., Verbeek, W.H., Schreurs, M.W. & Mulder, C.J. (2010a) The spectrum of celiac disease: Epidemiology, clinical aspects and treatment. *Nature Reviews. Gastroenterology & Hepatology,* 7, 204-213.

Tack, G.J., Wondergem, M.J., Al-Toma, A., Verbeek, W.H., Schmittel, A., Machado, M.V., Perri, F., Ossenkoppele, G.J., Huijgens, P.C., Schreurs, M.W., Mulder, C.J. & Visser, O.J. (2010b) Auto-SCT in refractory celiac disease type II patients unresponsive to cladribine therapy. *Bone Marrow Transplantation,* .

Takakuwa, T., Miyauchi, A. & Aozasa, K. (2009) Aberrant somatic hypermutations in thyroid lymphomas. *Leukemia Research,* 33, 649-654.

Tamura, K., Shimaoka, K. & Friedman, M. (1981) Thyroid abnormalities associated with treatment of malignant lymphoma. *Cancer,* 47, 2704-2711.

Tan, L.C., Mowat, A.G., Fazou, C., Rostron, T., Roskell, H., Dunbar, P.R., Tournay, C., Romagne, F., Peyrat, M.A., Houssaint, E., Bonneville, M., Rickinson, A.B., McMichael, A.J. & Callan, M.F. (2000) Specificity of T cells in synovial fluid: High frequencies of CD8(+) T cells that are specific for certain viral epitopes. *Arthritis Research,* 2, 154-164.

Tapinos, N.I., Polihronis, M. & Moutsopoulos, H.M. (1999) Lymphoma development in sjogren's syndrome: Novel p53 mutations. *Arthritis and Rheumatism,* 42, 1466-1472.

Thanou-Stavraki, A. & Sawalha, A.H. (2011) An update on belimumab for the treatment of lupus. *Biologics : Targets & Therapy,* 5, 33-43.

Theander, E., Manthorpe, R. & Jacobsson, L.T. (2004) Mortality and causes of death in primary sjogren's syndrome: A prospective cohort study. *Arthritis and Rheumatism,* 50, 1262-1269.

Theander, E., Henriksson, G., Ljungberg, O., Mandl, T., Manthorpe, R. & Jacobsson, L.T. (2006) Lymphoma and other malignancies in primary sjogren's syndrome: A cohort study on cancer incidence and lymphoma predictors. *Annals of the Rheumatic Diseases,* 65, 796-803.

Theofilopoulos, A.N., Baccala, R., Beutler, B. & Kono, D.H. (2005) Type I interferons (alpha/beta) in immunity and autoimmunity. *Annual Review of Immunology,* 23, 307-336.

Thieblemont, C., Mayer, A., Dumontet, C., Barbier, Y., Callet-Bauchu, E., Felman, P., Berger, F., Ducottet, X., Martin, C., Salles, G., Orgiazzi, J. & Coiffier, B. (2002) Primary thyroid lymphoma is a heterogeneous disease. *The Journal of Clinical Endocrinology and Metabolism,* 87, 105-111.

Tincani, A., Taraborelli, M. & Cattaneo, R. (2010) Antiphospholipid antibodies and malignancies. *Autoimmunity Reviews,* 9, 200-202.

Tosato, G., Steinberg, A.D. & Blaese, R.M. (1981) Defective EBV-specific suppressor T-cell function in rheumatoid arthritis. *The New England Journal of Medicine,* 305, 1238-1243.

Tosato, G., Steinberg, A.D., Yarchoan, R., Heilman, C.A., Pike, S.E., De Seau, V. & Blaese, R.M. (1984) Abnormally elevated frequency of epstein-barr virus-infected B cells in the blood of patients with rheumatoid arthritis. *The Journal of Clinical Investigation,* 73, 1789-1795.

Toubi, E. & Shoenfeld, Y. (2007) Clinical and biological aspects of anti-P-ribosomal protein autoantibodies. *Autoimmunity Reviews,* 6, 119-125.

Troch, M., Woehrer, S., Streubel, B., Weissel, M., Hoffmann, M., Mullauer, L., Chott, A. & Raderer, M. (2008) Chronic autoimmune thyroiditis (hashimoto's thyroiditis) in patients with MALT lymphoma. *Annals of Oncology : Official Journal of the European Society for Medical Oncology / ESMO,* 19, 1336-1339.

Tsang, R.W., Gospodarowicz, M.K., Pintilie, M., Wells, W., Hodgson, D.C., Sun, A., Crump, M. & Patterson, B.J. (2003) Localized mucosa-associated lymphoid tissue lymphoma treated with radiation therapy has excellent clinical outcome. *Journal of Clinical Oncology : Official Journal of the American Society of Clinical Oncology,* 21, 4157-4164.

Tupchong, L., Hughes, F. & Harmer, C.L. (1986) Primary lymphoma of the thyroid: Clinical features, prognostic factors, and results of treatment. *International Journal of Radiation Oncology, Biology, Physics,* 12, 1813-1821.

Turesson, C. & Matteson, E.L. (2004) Management of extra-articular disease manifestations in rheumatoid arthritis. *Current Opinion in Rheumatology,* 16, 206-211.

Tzioufas, A.G., Boumba, D.S., Skopouli, F.N. & Moutsopoulos, H.M. (1996) Mixed monoclonal cryoglobulinemia and monoclonal rheumatoid factor cross-reactive idiotypes as predictive factors for the development of lymphoma in primary sjogren's syndrome. *Arthritis and Rheumatism,* 39, 767-772.

Tzioufas, A.G., Manoussakis, M.N., Costello, R., Silis, M., Papadopoulos, N.M. & Moutsopoulos, H.M. (1986) Cryoglobulinemia in autoimmune rheumatic diseases. evidence of circulating monoclonal cryoglobulins in patients with primary sjogren's syndrome. *Arthritis and Rheumatism,* 29, 1098-1104.

Valesini, G., Priori, R., Bavoillot, D., Osborn, J., Danieli, M.G., Del Papa, N., Gerli, R., Pietrogrande, M., Sabbadini, M.G., Silvestris, F. & Valsecchi, L. (1997) Differential risk of non-hodgkin's lymphoma in italian patients with primary sjogren's syndrome. *The Journal of Rheumatology,* 24, 2376-2380.

Vallabhapurapu, S. & Karin, M. (2009) Regulation and function of NF-kappaB transcription factors in the immune system. *Annual Review of Immunology,* 27, 693-733.

van de Water, J.M., Cillessen, S.A., Visser, O.J., Verbeek, W.H., Meijer, C.J. & Mulder, C.J. (2010) Enteropathy associated T-cell lymphoma and its precursor lesions. *Best Practice & Research.Clinical Gastroenterology,* 24, 43-56.

Veeranki, S. & Choubey, D. (2010) Systemic lupus erythematosus and increased risk to develop B cell malignancies: Role of the p200-family proteins. *Immunology Letters,* 133, 1-5.

Verdolini, R., Bugatti, L., Giangiacomi, M., Nicolini, M., Filosa, G. & Cerio, R. (2002) Systemic lupus erythematosus induced by epstein-barr virus infection. *The British Journal of Dermatology,* 146, 877-881.

Verkarre, V., Romana, S.P., Cellier, C., Asnafi, V., Mention, J.J., Barbe, U., Nusbaum, S., Hermine, O., Macintyre, E., Brousse, N., Cerf-Bensussan, N. & Radford-Weiss, I. (2003) Recurrent partial trisomy 1q22-q44 in clonal intraepithelial lymphocytes in refractory celiac sprue. *Gastroenterology,* 125, 40-46.

Vettori, S., Staibano, S., Mascolo, M., Ilardi, G. & Valentini, G. (2010) Non-hodgkin's lymphoma in systemic sclerosis: Case and literature review. *Clinical Rheumatology,* 29, 1-6.

Viljamaa, M., Kaukinen, K., Pukkala, E., Hervonen, K., Reunala, T. & Collin, P. (2006) Malignancies and mortality in patients with coeliac disease and dermatitis herpetiformis: 30-year population-based study. *Digestive and Liver Disease : Official Journal of the Italian Society of Gastroenterology and the Italian Association for the Study of the Liver,* 38, 374-380.

Vivas, S., Ruiz de Morales, J.M., Ramos, F. & Suarez-Vilela, D. (2006) Alemtuzumab for refractory celiac disease in a patient at risk for enteropathy-associated T-cell lymphoma. *The New England Journal of Medicine,* 354, 2514-2515.

von Roon, A.C., Reese, G., Teare, J., Constantinides, V., Darzi, A.W. & Tekkis, P.P. (2007) The risk of cancer in patients with crohn's disease. *Diseases of the Colon and Rectum,* 50, 839-855.

Voulgarelis, M., Giannouli, S., Tzioufas, A.G. & Moutsopoulos, H.M. (2006) Long term remission of sjogren's syndrome associated aggressive B cell non-hodgkin's lymphomas following combined B cell depletion therapy and CHOP (cyclophosphamide, doxorubicin, vincristine, prednisone). *Annals of the Rheumatic Diseases,* 65, 1033-1037.

Voulgarelis, M., Petroutsos, G., Moutsopoulos, H.M. & Skopouli, F.N. (2002) 2-chloro-2'-deoxyadenosine in the treatment of sjogren's syndrome-associated B cell lymphoproliferation. *Arthritis and Rheumatism,* 46, 2248-2249.

Voulgarelis, M., Dafni, U.G., Isenberg, D.A. & Moutsopoulos, H.M. (1999) Malignant lymphoma in primary sjogren's syndrome: A multicenter, retrospective, clinical study by the european concerted action on sjogren's syndrome. *Arthritis and Rheumatism,* 42, 1765-1772.

Wang, S.A., Rahemtullah, A., Faquin, W.C., Roepke, J., Harris, N.L. & Hasserjian, R.P. (2005) Hodgkin's lymphoma of the thyroid: A clinicopathologic study of five cases and review of the literature. *Modern Pathology : An Official Journal of the United States and Canadian Academy of Pathology, Inc,* 18, 1577-1584.

Watanabe-Fukunaga, R., Brannan, C.I., Copeland, N.G., Jenkins, N.A. & Nagata, S. (1992) Lymphoproliferation disorder in mice explained by defects in fas antigen that mediates apoptosis. *Nature,* 356, 314-317.

Watson, W.C., Tooms, R.E., Carnesale, P.G. & Dutkowsky, J.P. (1994) A case of germinal center formation by CD45RO T and CD20 B lymphocytes in rheumatoid arthritic subchondral bone: Proposal for a two-compartment model of immune-mediated disease with implications for immunotherapeutic strategies. *Clinical Immunology and Immunopathology,* 73, 27-37.

Weetman, A.P. & McGregor, A.M. (1994) Autoimmune thyroid disease: Further developments in our understanding. *Endocrine Reviews,* 15, 788-830.

Weinblatt, M.E., Maier, A.L., Fraser, P.A. & Coblyn, J.S. (1998) Longterm prospective study of methotrexate in rheumatoid arthritis: Conclusion after 132 months of therapy. *The Journal of Rheumatology,* 25, 238-242.

Weyand, C.M., Goronzy, J.J. & Kurtin, P.J. (2006) Lymphoma in rheumatoid arthritis: An immune system set up for failure. *Arthritis and Rheumatism,* 54, 685-689.

Wolfe, F. & Michaud, K. (2007) The effect of methotrexate and anti-tumor necrosis factor therapy on the risk of lymphoma in rheumatoid arthritis in 19,562 patients during 89,710 person-years of observation. *Arthritis and Rheumatism,* 56, 1433-1439.

Wolfe, F. & Michaud, K. (2004) Lymphoma in rheumatoid arthritis: The effect of methotrexate and anti-tumor necrosis factor therapy in 18,572 patients. *Arthritis and Rheumatism,* 50, 1740-1751.

Wright, D.H. (1995) The major complications of coeliac disease. *Bailliere's Clinical Gastroenterology,* 9, 351-369.

Xin, H., D'Souza, S., Jorgensen, T.N., Vaughan, A.T., Lengyel, P., Kotzin, B.L. & Choubey, D. (2006) Increased expression of Ifi202, an IFN-activatable gene, in B6.Nba2 lupus susceptible mice inhibits p53-mediated apoptosis. *Journal of Immunology (Baltimore, Md.: 1950),* 176, 5863-5870.

Xu, Y. & Wiernik, P.H. (2001) Systemic lupus erythematosus and B-cell hematologic neoplasm. *Lupus,* 10, 841-850.

Yao, Q.Y., Rickinson, A.B., Gaston, J.S. & Epstein, M.A. (1986) Disturbance of the epstein-barr virus-host balance in rheumatoid arthritis patients: A quantitative study. *Clinical and Experimental Immunology,* 64, 302-310.

Youinou, P., Devauchelle-Pensec, V. & Pers, J.O. (2010) Significance of B cells and B cell clonality in sjogren's syndrome. *Arthritis and Rheumatism,* 62, 2605-2610.

Youinou, P., Papadopoulos, N.M., Katsikis, P., Pennec, Y.L., Jouquan, J., Lelong, A. & Moutsopoulos, H.M. (1988) Monoclonal immunoglobulins in the serum of patients with primary sjogren's syndrome. *Clinical and Experimental Rheumatology,* 6, 247-252.

Young, L.S. & Rickinson, A.B. (2004) Epstein-barr virus: 40 years on. *Nature Reviews.Cancer,* 4, 757-768.

Zatuchni, J., Campbell, W.N. & Zarafonetis, C.J. (1953) Pulmonary fibrosis and terminal bronchiolar (alveolar-cell) carcinoma in scleroderma. *Cancer,* 6, 1147-1158.

Zhang, Y., Holford, T.R., Leaderer, B., Zahm, S.H., Boyle, P., Morton, L.M., Zhang, B., Zou, K., Flynn, S., Tallini, G., Owens, P.H. & Zheng, T. (2004) Prior medical conditions and medication use and risk of non-hodgkin lymphoma in connecticut united states women. *Cancer Causes & Control : CCC,* 15, 419-428.

Zintzaras, E., Voulgarelis, M. & Moutsopoulos, H.M. (2005) The risk of lymphoma development in autoimmune diseases: A meta-analysis. *Archives of Internal Medicine,* 165, 2337-2344.

19

A Possible Link Between Autoimmunity and Cancer

Erika Cristaldi, Giulia Malaguarnera,
Alessandra Rando and Mariano Malaguarnera
University of Catania
Italy

1. Introduction

The most important cause of mortality after cardiovascular diseases is due to cancer, that affects both young and elderly people. The increasing incidence of tumour discovery is a consequence of improving diagnosis techniques and sensitization acts, thus facilitating a precocious identification and consequently an immediate therapeutic approach (Malaguarnera et al., 2010).

Autoimmune diseases represent one of the main growing health problem worldwide with wide variations in incidence and severity (Silink, 2002). Autoimmune diseases arise from an overactive immune response of the body against substances and tissues normally present in the body and they are due to the breakdown of immune tolerance to specific self-antigens.

Cancers and autoimmunity are often coincident—more coincident than is generally appreciated; thereby it has been raised more interest the relationship and the possible temporal consequence between autoimmune disease and cancer onset. Particularly, since a high level of autoimmunity is unhealthy, a low level of autoimmunity may actually be beneficial, thereby autoimmune reactions may be considered as a defence processes played by the host against tumour, or it may be possible that the anti-tumour immune response may result in elicitation of auto-antibodies against various auto-antigens, including self antigens expressed in tumour cells.

Some autoimmune diseases, such as Sjögren's syndrome, rheumatoid arthritis and systemic lupus erythematosus have been associated with the development of lymphoproliferative malignancies (Kiss et al., 2010), and a pleyade of autoantibodies have been found in patients with solid tumours (Bei et al., 2009). In addition, patients with dermatomyositis have a greater risk of developing solid-organ malignancies than the general population. In these patients, cancer can precede, parallel or follow myositis diagnosis (Zampieri et al., 2010).

The mechanism behind disease etiology remains unknown for most autoimmune diseases. This situation is distinct from cancer where our understanding of how genetic mutations lead to disease, is increasing. These advancements in cancer biology may have provided a very important piece to the autoimmunity puzzle. However, the relationship between cancer and autoimmunity is not well known. Despite minimal supporting evidence, the standard model for explaining this coincidence is that autoimmunity leads to cancer due to the rapid cell division associated with the regeneration of damaged tissues at the site of inflammation (Coussens & Werb, 2002). The relationship between autoimmunity and cancer was investigated, focusing on implication of immune system, apoptosis and new therapeutic agents for autoimmune diseases.

2. Break tolerance mechanisms in autoimmune diseases

The clinical signs and symptoms of different autoimmune diseases overlap, and individual patients often present with syndromes that combine features of more than one disease. Different autoimmune diseases share some genetic predisposing factors, including human leukocyte antigen (HLA) alleles (SLEGEN et al., 2008) or the T-cell regulatory gene CTLA-4 (Ueda et al., 2003). Our current knowledge suggests that multiple mutation might be needed before a self-reactive clone bypasses sequential tolerance-checkpoints and gives rise to an autoimmune disease (Baechler et al., 2003). The development of autoantibodies reflects a loss of B- and T- cell tolerance, which might result from a combination of genetic predisposition, persistent inflammatory responses, abnormal handling of apoptotic material and immune complexes, abnormal presentation of self-antigens and other events. As a high level of autoimmunity is unhealthy, a low level of autoimmunity may actually be beneficial. First, low-level autoimmunity might aid in the recognition of neoplastic cells by $CD8^+$ T cells, and thus reducing the incidence of cancer. Second, autoimmunity may have an important role, allowing a rapid immune response in the early stages of an infection when the availability of foreign antigens limits the response (i.e., when there are few pathogens present).

Diseases such as rheumatoid arthritis and tireotoxicosis are associated with the loss of immunological tolerance, which is the ability of an individual to ignore self, while reacting to non-self. This breakage leads to the immune system mounting an effective and specific immune response against self determinants. The exact genesis of immunological tolerance is still unclear, but several theories have been proposed to explain its origin. Two hypotheses have gained widespread attention among immunologists:

- Clonal Deletion theory, proposed by Burnet (1988), according to which self-reactive lymphoid cells are destroyed during their development. The extent to which the thymus can mediate tolerance to tissue-specific proteins and how organ specific tolerance is mediated remains an open question. While some tissue-specific proteins might reach the thymus through the circulation, this mechanism may be unnecessary due to expression within the thymus of the autoimmune regulator protein AIRE, which acts as a promiscuous ubiquitin ligase with the potential function of controlling transcription of a broad array of tissue-specific target genes in thymic epithelial cells (Nagamine et al., 1997).
- Clonal Anergy theory, proposed by Nossal et al. (1982), in which self-reactive T- or B-cells become inactivated in the normal individual and cannot amplify the immune response. This process is based upon the requirement of two signals for T-cell activation. The first is provided by the recognition of MHC-complexes and the second is due to the interaction between CD28 on T cells and B7 on activated antigen presenting cell (APC), that are induced by pro-inflammatory factors, such as bacterial products, pro-inflammatory cytokines, and other signals.

Previously, conditions such as cancer could not stimulate immune responses due to lack of co-stimulatory signals. However, this notion was based on cancers at late or advanced stages of disease, when tumour-induced immunosuppression may be at its highest degree (e.g. through production of the regulatory cytokines, transforming growth factor (TGF)-β and IL-10); in fact there is a considerable potential for newly transformed cells to evoke danger signals through the engagement of pro-inflammatory signaling pathways (Eisenlohr & Rothstein, 2006).

3. Autoimmune diseases and cancer - pathogenetic aspects

Positive associations have been reported between certain lymphomas and inflammation, autoimmune disease and infectious agents (Rosenquist, 2008).
Normally, tolerance checkpoints silence self-reactive T and B cells by preventing uncontrolled stimulation through self-antigens exposure. Several observations suggest that lymphocyte clones having bypassed tolerance mechanisms may be involved both in autoimmunity and malignancy (Goodnow, 2007). There are epidemiological observations of autoimmunity and lymphoma occurring simultaneously in diseases like systemic lupus erythematosus, rheumatoid arthritis and Sjögren's syndrome regardless of the use of immunosuppressive therapy (Bernatsky et al., 2007).
Infectious agents causing lymphomas can be classified according to several mechanisms. First, some viruses can directly transform lymphocytes as for Burkitt's lymphomas that may occur following infection with HIV; as well as T-cell lymphomas may occur following chronic antigen challenge with wheat in celiac disease (Cellier et al., 2000). Second, some infections increase lymphoma risk through chronic immune stimulation (Engels, 2007), which is also present in autoimmune diseases. Since uncontrolled stimulation of antigen receptors and lymphocyte proliferation triggered by chronic infection (e.g. Helicobacter pylori) may result in mucosa-associated lymphoid- tissue B-cell lymphomas (Suarez et al.,2006), it may be supposed that chronic stimulation of autoreactive cells paired with somatic hypermutation and recombinase activator gene (RAG) activity directed at non-antigen receptor loci may underlie lymphoma in systemic lupus erythematosus, rheumatoid arthritis and Sjögren's syndrome (Schuetz et al., 2010).
Treatments for autoimmune and chronic inflammatory disorders could also affect the risk of lymphoproliferative malignancies. Another reason for the association could be shared environmental risk factors (Landgren et al., 2006), and in some autoimmune diseases genetic mutations are discovered, leading to lymphoproliferation (Turbyville & Rao, 2010). Somatic mutations in lymphocytes may additionally contribute to the pathogenesis of autoimmunity and lymphoid malignancies as observed in patients with autoimmune lymphoproliferative syndrome carrying a mutated FAS gene in a single hematopoietic stem cell that contributes to a small fraction of blood cells. These patients may present with autoimmune symptoms and lymphoma formation just like patients with inherited FAS mutations (Holzelova et al., 2004).

4. The role of adaptive immunity

4.1 Treg cells

Regulatory T (Treg) cells are currently considered as key players in the mechanisms of peripheral immune tolerance. They are classified in natural and inducible $CD4^+CD25^+$ $FOXP3^+$ Treg cells. The transcription regulator FOXP3 (Forkhead box P3) appears to be required for the development, maintenance, and suppressor function of Treg cells (Hori et al., 2003), and the loss of FOXP3 in Treg cells - or its reduced expression - leads to the acquisition of effector T-cell properties including the production of non-Treg cell specific cytokines (Wan & Flavell, 2007). Treg cells are engaged in the control of immune self-tolerance, allograft rejection, allergy, and are also important for inhibiting the effector functions during infection and tumours development. In addition, the removal or a functional defect of Treg cells from normal rodents leads to the development of various autoimmune diseases (Weiner, 2001), because these cells actively suppress the activation and expansion of autoreactive immune cells.

Sometimes the studies investigating the role of Treg cells in SLE, have given controversial results (Khun et al., 2009). Most studies have found a reduced or normal frequency of Treg cells in SLE (La Cava, 2008), although other studies may have shown increased number. It has been observed a decreased number of Treg cells, during active disease flares (Miyara et al., 2005) and active SLE pediatric patients, thereby showing a poor suppressive capacity and an inverse correlation between Treg cells and disease activity as well as autoantibody levels (Lee et al., 2006). However, treatment with corticosteroids and/or immunosuppressive agents has been found to promote an increase in the number of Treg cells, particularly of peripheral Treg cells. Also, increased mRNA levels of CD25, FOXP3, and GITR have been found in B-cell depleted patients treated with rituximab at the time of B cell repopulation (Cepika et al., 2007).

In the collagen-induced arthritis model of systemic joint inflammation, the adoptive transfer of Treg cells protects from disease, whereas a depletion of Treg cells accelerates it (Morgan et al., 2005). Furthermore, in patients with early rheumatoid arthritis (RA), a reduced number of peripheral Treg cells is observed (Lawson et al., 2006), although the synovial fluid can often contain increased numbers of Treg cells (Cao et al., 2003).

Furthermore, increased frequency of $Foxp3^+$ Treg cells has been documented in tumour tissues and peripheral blood of patients with several types of cancer consistent with a role in tumour escape from immunological control. And also, not only the quantitative aspect of Treg cells, but also their functions are different between tumour patients and healthy control. Treg cells are considered inhibitors of anti-tumour immunity and $CD4^+CD25^+Foxp3^+$ regulatory T cells have been considered as a candidate for cancer immunotherapy for over a decade. Attempts to block or eliminate Treg cells have been made by the use of chemotherapy; these strategies, aimed at block Treg cells induction and migration, may be clinically useful, as suggested by experimental evidences in tumour models (Langier et al., 2010).

Data concerning the role of $CD4^+CD25^+$ regulatory T cells in human cancer derived from a work, which showed that the presence of such Treg cells in advanced ovarian cancer correlated with reduced survival (Curiel et al., 2004). In addition, TGF-β is a cytokine produced by Treg and Type 1 T regulatory cells, that is involved in the suppression of T cell proliferation and function (M.L. Chen et al., 2005). The experimental results supplied by other researchs indicate that TGF-β, secreted by ovarian carcinoma cells, owns vital function in the process of converting peripheral $CD4^+CD25^-$ T cells into $CD4^+CD25^+$ regulatory T cells, likely providing a possible immunotherapeutic target for ovarian cancer (Zheng et al., 2004).

One of the new therapeutic approach to cancer is based on the adoptive transfer of tumour-specific cytotoxic T cells and anti-CD25 antibodies. A combination of Treg cell-depletion, using anti-CD25 monoclonal antibodies, and cytotoxic T lymphocytes administration is a possible approach for treatment of cancers which enable further exploration in the clinical setting (Ohmura et al., 2008), though these future approaches suggest a possible development of autoimmune diseases, due to decreased Treg cells occurrence.

4.2 Dendritic cells

Dendritic cells have been recognized as the most efficient antigen presenting cells that have the capacity to initiate naïve T-cell response *in vitro* and *in vivo*. During their differentiation and maturation pathways, DCs can efficiently capture, process and present antigens for T-cell activation. The functional activities of DCs mainly depend on their state of activation and differentiation: iDC are involved in the maintenance of peripheral tolerance whereas mature DC can efficiently induce the development of effector T cells. Thereby, accumulated iDCs, which are educated at the tumour site, act as functional inhibitors of a tumour-specific immune response in cancer, immature pDCs are activated by Toll-like receptors, which lead to B- and T-cell immune responses in autoimmune disease (Lang et al., 2005). The immunological tolerance is produced by tumour-derived soluble factors (TDSFs) and immature dendritic cells (iDCs), which inhibit DC and T-cell activation, and exclusively inhibit the DNA–IgG immune complex, inducing pro-inflammatory responses needed for an immune response. Immunological ignorance is produced by reduced levels of tumour antigens. Dendritic cells not only initiate T-cell responses, but are also involved in silencing T-cell immune response. DC can play a central role in the development of T-cell tolerance, and its maintenance in the periphery is critical for the prevention of autoimmunity.

4.3 T helper 17 cells (Th17)

T helper 17 cells constitute a third subset of T helper cells that are important in the development of autoimmune diseases and in the immune response against infections. These cells are characterized as preferential producers of IL-17A, IL-17F, IL-21, IL-22 and IL-26 in humans. The IL-17 production is required to differentiate Th17 cells, from IFN-γ producing Th1 cells, or IL-4 producing Th2 cells. IL-17 (A and F) induces production of a broad range of pro-inflammatory cytokines and chemokines, including IL-6, colony-stimulating factors, chemokines (CCL2, CCL7, CXCL1, and CCL20), human β-defensin-2 and matrix metalloproteinases (MMP-3 and MMP-13), by a variety of cells (Weaver et al., 2007). Conversely, inhibition of IL-17 signaling leads to impaired host defence against bacterial infection (Ye et al., 2001) and resistance to autoimmune diseases (Yang et al., 2008). IL-17 regulates host defence against infectious organisms through promoting granulopoiesis and neutrophil trafficking (Linden et al., 2005).

Although FOXP3^{+} Treg cells are critical for control of autoimmunity and inflammation (Sakaguchi, 2004), Th17 cells have been implicated in mediating inflammation and autoimmune diseases (Weaver et al., 2007). It has been shown that the balance between Treg and Th17 cells is a key factor which regulates T-helper cell function relating to the Th1/Th2 shift in autoimmune disease and graft versus host disease (GVHD) (Afzali et al., 2007). In fact, elevated levels of IL-17 have been associated with inflammatory diseases in humans, including rheumatoid arthritis, scleritis, uveitis, asthma, systemic lupus erythematosus, and allograft rejection (Kolls & Linden, 2004).

However, there are limited information on the balance between Treg and Th17 cells in cancer patients and on the active role played by Th 17 in anti-tumour immunity (Kryczek et al., 2009). The function of IL-17 in tumour immunity is a controversial subject. The effects of IL-17 on tumour development are directly influenced by the existence of an adaptive immune system. In the presence of lymphocytes, IL-17 promotes tumour rejection, whereas in the absence of those, IL-17 favours tumour growth and angiogenesis (Martin-Orozco & Chen Dong, 2009a). By using IL-17-deficient mice in a model of lung melanoma, it has been provided direct evidence for a protective role of IL-17 in anti tumour responses (Martin-

Orozco et al., 2009b). It has also found that Th17 cells provided better protection to tumours than Th1 cells, and this difference was largely due to their unique ability to promote CD8+ T cell priming. In Th17- but not Th1-treated tumour-bearing mice, it has been observed increased numbers of CD8+ T cells in the lung, suggesting that Th17 cells may promote the activation or recruitment of tumour antigen-specific CD8+ T cells (Martin-Orozco et al., 2009 b). There are data supporting the existence of IL17-producing effector CD8+ T cells (Tc17) which are also induced by IL23 and may play a role in cancer development as well as in autoimmunity (Ciric et al., 2009). Thereby, the protective role of Th 17 cells, inhibiting tumour growth, may influence the onset of autoimmune diseases.

5. Apoptosis mechanism

Apoptosis is an active, genetically controlled process of cell death required to ensure that the rate of cell division were balanced by the rate of cell death in multicellular organisms. The control of apoptosis is critical for the homeostasis of the immune system as it happens during infections, where antigen specific lymphocytes need to rapidly proliferate. After clearance of the infectious microbe lymphocytes need to die in order to prevent dysregulated proliferation with the consequence of leukemia or lymphoma (Lorenz et al., 2000). Importantly, as explained below, during apoptotic breakdown many nuclear constituents are post-translation modified, possibly altering antigenicity. Therefore it is not surprising that failure to achieve programmed cell death and to clear apoptotic cell fragments may be discussed as a key pathogenetic factor leading to autoimmunity. This could be explained by a failure to kill an autoreactive cell or by inducing autoantibodies against apoptotically modified cellular constituents. If the preload is excessive, as in massive cell death (e.g. upon infection), regulatory clearance mechanisms cannot effectively remove apoptotic residuals and thereby allowing the persistence of antigens for stimulation of the immune system. During apoptosis, the cellular contents of the nucleus, cytosol and membrane are brought together in close proximity, a mechanism that could lead to epitope spreading (Vidalino et al., 2009). Altered structures of intracellular proteins produced during cleavage events in apoptosis could also be a source of immunogenic antigens. Altered apoptosis mechanism is associated with the pathogenesis of a wide array of diseases: cancer, neurodegeneration, autoimmunity, heart disease and others.

5.1 Phases of apoptotic death

Apoptotic cell death can be divided into a "triggering phase" (e.g., ligation of "dedicated death receptor" such as Fas, or withdrawal of growth/survival factors), a "signaling phase" (e.g., protein kinase cascades that include MAPK family, JNK and p38), an "execution phase" (e.g., activation of caspases and nucleases), and a "burial phase" (e.g. phagocytosis of dying cells by neighboring cells) *(*Utz & Anderson, 1998*)*.

5.1.1 Triggering phase

Fas ligand (FasL) and tumor necrosis factor α (TNF-α) are the prototypical inducers of apoptosis. These ligands induce clustering of their respective receptors (Fas, TNFR-I or TNFR-II), which leads to recruitment of the early signal-transducing molecules. The Fas/FasL system is the most studied receptor mediated apoptotic pathway. Fas/Apo-1/CD95 is a type I trans membrane protein with a cysteine-rich extracellular domain and is a member of the tumor necrosis factor receptor (TNFR) superfamily (Itoh & Nagata, 1993*)*. A variety of cell types express Fas, but differing between tissues for the expression levels. Its ligand, FasL, is a type II transmembrane protein that can also exist as a soluble factor in a stable trimer configuration (Mountz et al.,1994). On ligation of FasL, Fas trimerizes and recruits an adaptor protein known as Fas-associated protein with death domain (FADD, also called MORT-1) through its intracellular death domain (Chinnaiyan et al., 1995). The cytotoxic signal is further propagated as FADD recruits and interacts with another adapter protein as FADD-like interleukin-1β converting enzyme (FLICE), also known as caspase-8 (Muzio et al., 1997). Formation of the Fas-FADD-FLICE/ caspase-8 complex, known as death-inducing signal complex (DISC), facilitates the autocleavage and activation of caspase- 8 (Kischkel et al., 1995). A protein known as inhibitor of FLICE (I-FLICE) and FLICE-inhibitory protein (FLIP) can prevent the formation of DISC required for further apoptotic signaling (Irmler et al., 1997).

5.1.2 Signaling phase

Apoptosis is a multistep process and protein kinases have been implicated both in the upstream induction phase of apoptosis and in the downstream execution stage, as the direct targets for caspases. The serine/threonine protein kinases that have been suggested to play a role in apoptosis are the mitogen- activated protein kinase (MAPK) family, specifically, p42/ 44 ERK, p38 MAPK and c-Jun N-terminal kinase (JNK), cyclic AMP-dependent protein kinase A (PKA), protein kinase B (PKB), or Akt and protein kinase C (PKC). The activation of JNK/SAPK and p38 MAP kinases is generally associated with the promotion of apoptosis, while p42/44 ERK activity inhibits apoptosis (Mc Cubrey et al., 2000).

5.1.3 Execution phase

In mammalian cells, activation of caspases is achieved through at least two independent mechanisms which are initiated by distinct caspases, but results in activation of common executioner caspases. Once activated, caspase-8 can induce either directly or indirectly the activation of a number of distal caspases such as caspase-3, -6 and -7 (CD95 type I cells) (Muzio et al., 1997). Another pathway for caspase activation involves cytochrome c, which in mammalian cells is often released from the mitochondria into the cytosol during apoptosis (CD95 type II cells) (Scaffidi et al., 1999) (fig.1).

5.2 The cell death regulator: Bcl-2 and TNF-R

The B cell leukemia-2 (Bcl-2) was the first mammalian cell death regulator identified. Bcl-2 and the tumor necrosis factor receptor (TNF-R) family contribute to the regulation of apoptosis with their corresponding ligands. The proto-oncogene Bcl-2 has been cloned from the t(14:18) chromosomal translocation breakpoint in human follicular centre B lymphoma (Korsmeyer, 1995) and its function was first discovered when it was over-expressed in cytokine-dependent haematopoietic cell lines. Upon removal of the growth factor, Bcl-2 promoted survival of these cells in the quiescent state (Gerl & Vaux, 2005). An important discovery from the studies in lymphocytes was that Bcl-2 did not only promote survival of growth factor-deprived cells but could inhibit apoptosis triggered by a broad range of physiological or experimentally applied cytotoxic stimuli (Sentman et al., 1991). Bcl-2 family can be divided into two groups according to their function: those which are structurally most similar to Bcl-2 and inhibit apoptosis, on the other side there are the members of the Bcl-2 family that enhance cell death. The mitochondrial pathway, is triggered by

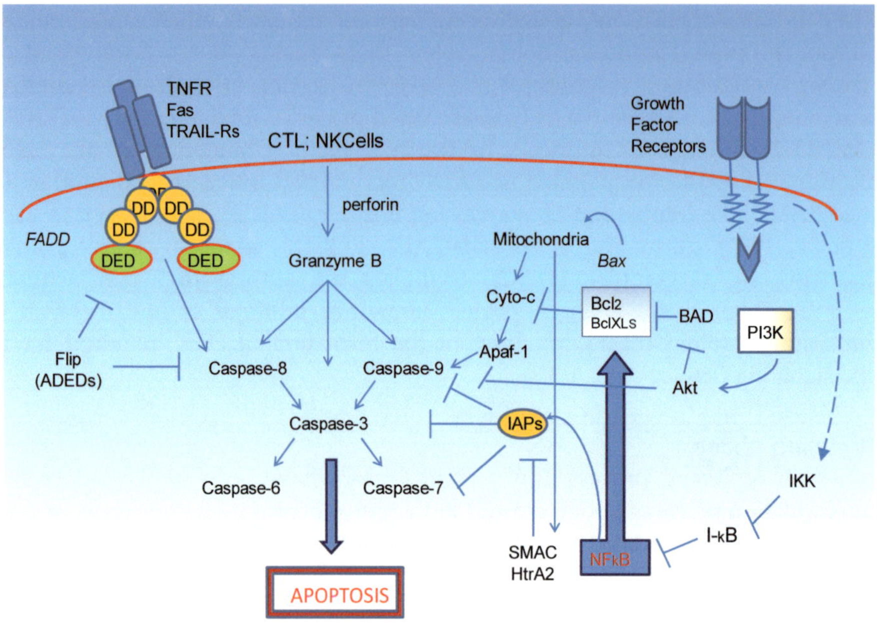

Fig. 1. ADEDs: Anti-apoptotic Death Effector Domain proteins; Akt: serine/threonine protein kinase ; Apaf-1: Apoptotic protease activating factors-1; BAD: Bcl-2-associated death promoter protein; Bax: Bcl-2–associated X protein; Bcl-2: B-cell lymphoma 2; Bcl-xl: B-cell lymphoma-extra large; CTL: Cytolytic T-cells; Cyto-c: Cytochrome-c; DED: Death Effector Domains; FADD: Fas-associated death domain; Flip: FLICE (Fadd-Like Interleukin-1β Converting Enzyme) inhibitory protein; HTRA2/Omi: mammalian homolog of the bacterial high temperature requirement protein (HTRA); IAPs: Inhibitor of apoptosis protein; IKK: IκB kinase ; IκB: Inhibitor of κB ; NFkB: nuclear factor kappa-B; NK: Natural Killer; PI3K: phosphatidylinositol 3-kinase ; SMAC: Second Mitocondrial-derived Activator of Caspase ; TNFR: Tumor Necrosis Factor Receptors; TRAIL-Rs: TNF-related apoptosis inducing ligand-Receptors.

proapoptotic members of the Bcl-2 family. In response to environmental cues these proteins engage another set of proapoptotic Bcl-2 members, the Bax sub family residing on the mitochondrial outer membranes or in the cytosol. The interaction induces the latter to oligomerize and insert into the mitochondrial membrane (Eskes et al., 2000). Here the complex acts to trigger the sudden and complete release of cytochrome c and other proteins from all of the mitochondria in the cell. Bcl-2 block death by preventing the mitochondrial release of the intermembrane proteins, including cytochrome c (Moriishi et al., 1999). A protein with the dual name of Smac/DIABLO is released from the mitochondria along with cytochrome c during apoptosis, and this protein functions to promote caspase activation by associating with the Apaf- 1 apoptosome and inhibiting inhibitor of apoptosis proteins.

Members of the tumour necrosis factor (TNF) receptor family and their corresponding ligands are critical regulators of apoptosis, and also control other cellular processes (Wallach, 1997). CD95 (also called Fas or APO-1) and p55 TNF-RI receptors, and a few other members of the family, contain a cytoplasmic region, called "death domain" (DD), which is essential for inducing apoptosis (Tartaglia et al., 1993). Upon receptor activation, the death domain undergoes interaction with a death domain in the adaptor proteins FADD (Fas-Associated protein with Death Domain)/Mort-1 or TRADD (Tumor necrosis factor receptor type 1-associated DEATH domain protein) (Hsu et al., 1996). FADD/MORT 1 binds directly to CD95 and indirectly to p55 TNF-R I via TRADD, and it is essential for cell death signaling from both receptors. This complex binds caspase-8, therefore inducing its self-processing (Boldin et al., 1996). The members of the TNF receptor family (death receptors) bearing death domain can also activate signaling pathways that promote survival, proliferation, and differentiation of cells. Signaling via TRADD is essential for TNF-induced activation of Jun kinase and its absence renders cells less susceptible to the pro-apoptotic activity of TNF (Yeh et al., 1997). Death domain RIP (receptor-interacting protein) kinase is required for TNF-receptor transduced activation of NF-kB and its absence also sensitizes cells to TNF-induced apoptosis (Kelliher 1998). This indicates that Jun kinase and NF-kB elicit signals that protect cells against death receptor-induced apoptosis. Moreover, FADD/MORT1, which was originally thought to transducing only a death signal (Hsu et al., 1996), it is now known to be also essential for mitogen-induced proliferation of T lymphocytes (Zhang et al., 1998).

5.3 The role of apoptosis in development, function and homeostasis of lymphocytes

Apoptosis plays a critical role in the immune system, both during the development of B and T cells in primary lymphoid organs as well as during immune responses of mature lymphocytes (Strasser et al., 1995). Programmed cell death is thought to be responsible for the elimination of immature B and T cells that failed to receive a survival signal due to both the lack of growth factors, and either to the failure to productively rearrange antigen receptor genes, or failure of the T cell antigen receptor on thymocytes to bind to MHC molecules on stromal cells (lack of positive selection) (Lu & Osmond, 1997). The effector functions of activated lymphocytes (i.e. secretion of antibodies, production of cytokines or cytotoxicity) are potentially hazardous and it is therefore beneficial to delete these cells when an infection has been overcome (Strasser et al., 1995). The survival of T lymphoblasts is controlled by two distinct mechanisms, both availability of growth factors (e.g. IL-2) and exposure to death ligands (e.g. Fas ligand), which are produced by T cells themselves as a consequence of repeated TCR stimulation (Brunner et al., 1995). The lack of IL-2 triggers a death pathway that can be inhibited by Bcl-2, instead the pathway triggered by Fas ligand is insensitive to Bcl-2 and its homologues (Newton et al., 1998). The death pathway controlled by growth factors and Bcl-2 is thought to be responsible for removing T cells activated by foreign, non-persisting antigens, while death receptor-signaling is critical for removal of activated T cells specific to self-antigens or persistent foreign antigens (Van Parijs et al., 1998).

6. Apoptosis in autoimmune disease

The association between autoimmunity and apoptotic cell death is under extensive investigation. The process of apoptosis defines a series of biochemical and morphologic events that contribute to the normal homeostasis and regulation of immune autoreactivity (Mevorach et al., 1998). During apoptosis, the cellular components as the nucleus, cytosol and, membrane are brought together in close proximity, a mechanism that could lead to epitopes spreading. Altered structures of intracellular proteins produced during cleavage events in apoptosis could also be a source of immunogenic antigens, as cleavage by granzyme B is a common phenomenon for the release of autoantigens. If cell death is excessive, regulatory clearance mechanisms may not effectively remove apoptotic debris, thereby leading to the persistence of antigens for immune system stimulation. Also, the resistance to clearance by defective proteins may lead to autoimmune phenomenon. Furthermore, the rapid clearance of apoptotic cells by macrophages is important to inhibit inflammation and autoimmune responses against intracellular antigens. Mice deficient in receptor tyrosine kinases, such as Tyro 3, Axl, and Mer, have defective clearance of apoptotic cells, lymphadenopathy, and features of autoimmunity (Scott et al., 2001). A common feature of autoimmune diseases such as systemic lupus erythematosus, systemic sclerosis, Sjogren's syndrome, and mixed connective tissue disease is the breakdown of tolerance to self antigens, which induces the production of antibodies reactive with multiple self proteins (Von Muhlen & Tan, 1995). Accumulating evidences show that modifications of autoantigens during apoptosis lead to the development of autoantibodies, thus bypassing normal mechanisms of tolerance (Amoura et al., 1999). Furthermore, direct evidence exists associating faulty apoptotic machinery with the development of autoimmune disease in experimental models and in human disease. Genetic evidences have shown that defects in individual cell-death genes can lead to autoimmune disease. In humans, direct evidence was found in deficient Fas patients, leading to the development of the autoimmune lymphoproliferative syndrome, manifested by lymphadenopathy, renal disease and hemolytic anemia. This syndrome parallels the autoimmune phenomena found in mrl/lpr mice that lack the Fas protein (Straus et al., 1999). In addition, expression of a bcl-2 transgene in mouse B lymphocytes causes extended survival of B lineage cells, sustained humoral immune responses and consequently accumulation of non-transformed B cells and plasma cells and increased levels of serum Ig (O'Reilly et al.,1997). Auto-antibody-secreting plasma cells have been found in normal individuals, but they had no detrimental effect since they were relatively infrequent and short-lived. Expression of a bcl-2 transgene prolongs the survival of such cells and consequently auto-antibodies reach pathogenic levels.

6.1 Apoptosis and systemic lupus erythematosus

Systemic lupus erythematosus (SLE) is an autoimmune disease clinically characterized by a broad variety of symptoms, mostly affecting the joints. In Europe the incidence of this disease is about 1/10,000. Based on new therapeutic approaches, most of the patients will experience a remission and about 90% of SLE patients are still alive after a five year follow-up (Pons-Estel, et al., 2010). The etiopathogenesis of SLE, although partially understood, is due to multifactorial process. Genetic predisposition in association with environmental factors, including infectious agents, drugs, occupational factors, and food may lead to profound alterations in immune system (Love,1994). These changes include the appearance of autoantibodies with different specificity, altered T cell function, as well as a defective phagocytosis and changes in oncogenes (Kalden et al., 1991). In the pathogenesis of systemic lupus erythematosus an important role is due to a dysregulated apoptosis, which may contribute to development of the disease, regulating the induction of nuclear antibodies frequently found in SLE. This hypothesis is partly based on experiments with an animal model used for SLE (i.e. MRL/lpr mice). Mutational inactivation of the genes encoding CD95 (lpr) or its ligand, Fas ligand (gld), cause lymphadenopathy and SLE-like autoimmune disease in mice (Adachi et al., 1995). Two spontaneous mutations found in the CD95 gene have been considered the cause of deficient expression of a membrane molecule Fas/Apo-1 (CD95). Animals with a deficient expression of Fas/Apo 1 molecule showed an insufficient elimination of lymphocytes, leading to the assumption that autoreactive lymphocytes could survive and consequently cause autoimmune phenomena (Watson et al., 1992). However, in all humans with SLE the Fas/Apo-1 dependent apoptosis pathway was unaffected (Mysler et al., 1994), and patients with a defect in the Fas/Apo-1 molecule develop a non malignant lymphoproliferation (Rieux-Laucat, 1995). Although this, it has been reported in patients with SLE increased numbers of apoptotic lymphocytes and macrophages (Emlen et al., 1994). Likely, this could be the result of both a fail during the apoptosis phase and an increased triggering of apoptosis, thus delaying the end of programmed cell death process. A sustained apoptotic activity, due to continuous stimuli, is responsible of producing autoantigens, which may lead to the development of autoantibodies directed against macromolecular complex, thereby acting some pathologic effects. In summary, SLE is a complex disorder in which defects in apoptosis and impaired clearance are strong contributing factors for susceptibility, onset and severity of the disease.

6.2 Apoptosis in rheumatoid arthritis

Rheumatoid arthritis (RA) is a chronic inflammatory disease, characterized by chronic synovial inflammation and synovial cell proliferation, both responsible of "pannus" production. Its development is related to mononuclear cell infiltration, neoangiogenesis, and abnormal proliferation of fibroblast-like synoviocytes (FLS). The pathogenesis of the rheumatoid pannus, has been partly explained by a study on FLS biology (Pap et al., 2000). Two general mechanisms contribute to synovial hyperplasia: increased FLS proliferation and decreased synoviocyte apoptosis. However, apoptotis of synovial cells has been also identified in histologic sections, suggesting that the relative rate of apoptotic cells to proliferating cells is suppressed in proliferating tissues such as in the synovium of RA patients (Sekine et al., 1996). Several studies have examined the mechanisms that could contribute to the resistance against Fas-mediated apoptosis in RA, demonstrating that though Fas is normally expressed by the cells of the pannus both *in vivo* and *in vitro*, the persistence of synovial proliferation in RA patients may lead to bone damage and cartilage erosion (Kawakami et al., 1999). The function of the Fas/FasL system seems to be inadequate to eliminate the cells in the proliferating RA synovium suggesting a strong anti-apoptotic effect in the RA joint.

FLICE inhibitory protein (Flip) is highly expressed at sites of erosion, in the pannus, in the lining, and in the areas of the synovial tissue where apoptosis has not been observed (Perlman et al., 2001). This prospect was supported by the fact that, when synovial tissues were examined by immunohistochemistry, high levels of Flip were associated with low levels of apoptosis in early RA. In contrast, decreased Flip was detected later in the disease course, and this was related with increased apoptosis and decreased numbers of macrophages (Catrina et al., 2002). In addition, it has been supposed that the potential beneficial effects of TNF-α antagonist therapy might be related to the reduction of Flip, which would permit Fas/FasL-mediated apoptosis and result in subsequent clinical improvement.

In the antigen-induced arthritis model of RA, Bcl-2 was present at sites of early erosion and correlated with levels for erosion and inflammation, thus supporting the importance of this factor. Since either the presence of Bcl-2 or anti-apoptotic Bcl-2 family members (Bcl-2, Bcl-xL, A1 and myeloid-cell leukaemia sequence 1) at sites of early erosion in antigen-induced model of arthritis was greatly expressed on synovial fibroblasts, in the synovial lining and in the sublining region from RA patients, it has been largely examined the potential mechanisms that may contribute to the augmented expression of Bcl-2 (Perlman et al., 2001). Activated NF-kB, has been implicated in the regulation of gene transcription that contributes to cytokine generation, expression of cell surface adhesion epitopes, lymphocyte maturation, protection from TNF-α induced apoptosis, and antigen processing and presentation by MHC class I molecules. NF-kB is expressed in almost all cell types, and plays a significant role in regulating the production of inflammatory cytokines, such as TNF-α, IL-1 and IL-6, as well as anti-apoptotic molecules such as Flip (Pope & Perlman, 2000). Different cytokines such as IL-lβ, platelet-derived growth factor (PDGF), basic fibroblast growth factor (bFGF), transforming growth factor β (TGF-β) and TNF-α are present in synovial tissues of RA patients, promoting the proliferation of human synovial cells. Fas antigen expression on synovial cells is inhibited by the addition of TGF-βl with up-regulation of Bcl-2, Bcl-xL and XIAP. The expression of FLIP, is increased in bFGF-treated synovial cells. These results show that bFGF treatment augmented the expression of FLIP, resulting in resistance toward Fas-mediated apoptosis. The tumour suppressor gene p53 regulates cell cycle, DNA repair, and inhibits angiogenesis. Although, early study reported an upregulation of p53 expression in RA joints (Firestein et al., 1996), a more recent interesting study about the role of several genes, involved in apoptosis mechanisms, reported that p53 gene was deeply reduced in peripheral blood mononuclear cells from patients with RA, SLE, insulin-dependent diabetes mellitus and multiple sclerosis compared with that in normal controls; thus suggesting, that the decreased expression of p53, might contribute to the development of autoimmune disease, possibly by failing to eliminate potentially pathogenetic cells (Maas et al., 2002). Its increase is due to DNA damage, thus permitting DNA repair through cell cycle prolongation, or leading to apoptosis in more severe cases. Deletions, mutations or other mechanisms leading to its lost are often associated with tumour growth.

Although Fas and FasL are greatly expressed on synovial lining macrophages, paucity of apoptosis within the joint might be the result of a variety of mechanisms. An improved understanding of the mechanisms regulating apoptosis will provide insights to aid with a more effective therapy patients with RA.

6.3 Apoptosis and Sjögren's syndrome

Sjögren's syndrome (SS) is a chronic autoimmune disorder, occurring primarily in women, affecting the salivary and lacrimal glands. The histopathological changes in the minor salivary gland biopsy are characterized by the infiltration of these glands by mononuclear cells with secondary destruction of the parenchymal tissue, resulting in oral and ocular dryness (Moutsopoulos et al., 1980). The pathogenesis of glandular damage in Sjögren's syndrome is currently poorly understood; however, the predominance among the infiltrating mononuclear cells of activated $CD4^{+}$ T cells suggests that cell-mediated immunity plays an important role in tissue destruction (Skopouli et al., 1991). In recent years, it has been reported that the expression of the apoptosis regulating-proteins in salivary glands of Sjögren's syndrome patients suggests a role for apoptotic cell death in the pathogenesis of glandular damage (Patel & McHugh, 2000). The resistance of infiltrating mononuclear cells to apoptosis may result in longer survival that might also increase the production of pro-inflammatory cytokines and autoantibodies, or predispose to the late development of lymphoma in some Sjögren's syndrome patients. T lymphocytes induce apoptotic cell death through either the release of proteases, such as perforin and granzymes, or the interaction of FasL, expressed by activated $CD4^+$ T cells, with Fas on target cells (Russell & Ley, 2002). In murine models, defective signaling and blocked apoptosis caused by mutations in Fas or FasL resulted in autoimmune disease as well as lymphadenopathy (Skarstein et al., 1997). Corresponding mutations were not found in genes encoding Fas and FasL in primary Sjögren's syndrome patients (Bolstad et al., 2000). However, it has been suggested that increased levels of Fas induced apoptosis among epithelial cells explaining the damage of the glands. On the other hand, increased expression of intracellular anti-apoptotic molecules could lead to dysregulation of apoptosis and the formation of large foci of infiltrating mononuclear cells. In the field of autoimmune disease, a common feature is the lack of specific serum markers of disease. Among the most widely used serological markers in confirming the diagnosis of Sjögren's syndrome (SS), there are anti-SSB/La and SSA / Ro antibodies, with a prevalence between 70 and 80% . Although this prevalence is high, they are not specific for Sjögren's syndrome, but also found patients with other autoimmune diseases: anti-SSA / Ro in 35% of patients with systemic lupus erythematosus and 85% of patients with congenital heart block (BCC), and anti-SSB / La in 15% of patients with systemic lupus erythematosus. SSA and SSB are two ribonucleoproteins, located mainly in the nucleus and in the cytoplasm. In patients with Sjögren's syndrome it has been recently studied a new autoantibody that recognizes a structural protein, bound to actin, and that is part of the cytoplasmic skeleton: the α-fodrin (Ulbricht et al., 2003). The fodrin has a localization predominantly near the inner surface of the cell membrane and physiologically it participates in the process of cellular secretion. When antibodies directed against the α-fodrin are present, the cellular mechanism of secretion is impaired. Since the salivary glands are rich in α-fodrin, their secretory mechanism is inhibited, resulting in xerostomia and keratoconjunctivitis sicca. Therefore α-fodrin antibodies would more precocious than those commonly used in the diagnosis of SS (anti-Ro and anti-La), especially in the early stages of the disease. The cleaved α-fodrin fragment has been shown to be a marker of apoptosis (Janicke et al., 1998). Furthermore, a monospecific antibody recognizing the cleaved α-fodrin is available. In Sjögren's syndrome, cleaved α-fodrin autoantigen is greatly expressed on ductal epithelium, on sporadic acinar cells and strongly associated with infiltrating mononuclear cells, however it is rarely detected in normal salivary glands. Further studies are required to verify the specific association of cleaved α-fodrin with primary and secondary Sjögren's syndrome. Therefore based on results of studies of SS-like disease in mice, there may be 2 distinct phases in the pathogenesis of SS (Humphreys-Beher et al., 1999). The first, a lymphocyte-independent step may be characterized by a genetically determined anomaly responsible for epithelial cell apoptosis, resulting in either the production of nucleosomes or the exposure on the cell membrane of autoantigens, such as α-fodrin, SS-A (Ro), and SS-B (La) ribonucleoproteins. In fact, apoptosis allows the translocation either of the ribonucleoproteins SS-A (Ro) and SS-B (La) or the cytoplasmic protein α-fodrin on epithelial cell membranes, where they may be exposed to antigen-presenting cells such as macrophages, and thus generate an autoimmune response (McArthur et al., 2002). After this phase, an elevated expression of proinflammatory cytokines and metalloproteases also may occur, with consequent degradation of epithelial basal membranes (Pérez et al., 2000). The second phase is characterized by mononuclear cells (MNC) infiltration, lymphocyte mediated apoptosis through Fas/FasL interaction, perforin and granzyme B release and production of cytokines

(IFN-γ, TNF-α, and TGF-β1) leading to glandular damage and secretory flow injury (Perez et al., 2000). Improved understanding of the primary cellular events responsible for the glandular damage occurring in SS may allow the discovery of new therapeutic strategies able to interfere with the mediators of apoptosis and thus prevent epithelial cell death and consequent impairment of secretory function.

7. Apoptosis and malignancies

Altered function of apoptosis mechanism occurs frequently in cancers and has been implicated in many events relevant for the pathogenesis and progression of tumours, including cell accumulation caused by failure of programmed cell death (Reed, 1999). Thereby, it may be induce a permissive environment for genetic instability and oncogene activation, promote resistance to immune cell attack, and contribute to resist to the cytotoxic effects of chemotherapy and radiation, allowing tumour cell survival. In the same way, defects in DNA repair and chromosome segregation normally trigger cell suicide as a defence mechanism for eradicating genetically unstable cells. Apoptosis defects permit the survival of the genetically unstable cells, and thus provide opportunities of selection of progressively aggressive clones (Anthoney et al., 1996). In addition, apoptosis defects play a role in tumour resistance to hypoxia, growth factor deprivation, immune surveillance mechanisms, chemotherapy, and radiation (Medh & Thompson, 2000). Tumour immunosuppression that favours tumour progression and metastasis is the consequence of the activation of an immunosuppressive network, mediated by several tumour-derived soluble factors, such as interleukin- 10 (IL-10), transforming growth factor (TGF)- β and vascular endothelial growth factor (VEGF), and which involves the primary tumour site, secondary lymphoid organs and peripheral vessels (Zou, 2005). There are different pathways leading to dysregulated immune responses in cancer and autoimmune disease, such as the impaired clearance of apoptotic cells, played by macrophages. Although the fact that tumour cells generate pro-inflammatory conditions, the immune cells induce an anti-inflammatory environment , due to impaired clearance of apoptotic cells by macrophages during the turnover of tumour cells. The impaired clearance of apoptotic cells induces anti-DNA antibodies to self-antigens that lead to a pseudo-autoimmune status, which, provoking a pro-inflammatory response, allows tumour progression (Kim et al., 2005). The increased concentration of autoantibodies and dendritic cells can induce the production of $CD4^+$ $CD25^+$ regulatory T cells (Tregs) that inhibit T-cell function, causing immunological tolerance (Ward et al., 2004). Thus, it is likely that cancer immunosuppression is produced by tumour-derived soluble factors, due to an anti-inflammatory response to immune cells triggered by a defective apoptotic cell clearance, and increased concentration of Treg cells.

There are significant differences in immunological dysregulation between cancer and autoimmune disease. In the first case, the impaired clearance of apoptotic cells causes accumulation of autoantibodies, which is attributed to the inhibition of T-cell function through increased Treg cells, which play a crucial role in immunological tolerance in cancer cells. In autoimmune diseases, defective apoptotic cell clearance causes accumulation of DNA–IgG immune complexes, which provokes an immune response through Toll-like receptor 9 (TLR9), leading to tissue injury. Unfortunately, the Treg cells are decreased and dysregulated, in this case (Lang et al., 2005).

7.1 Apoptosis and the genes that control it - effect on the malignant phenotype

Elucidation of the genetic alterations of molecules with a central role in apoptosis pathway has provided new insights into tumour biology, revealing novel strategies for combating cancer. More weight has been placed on core apoptosis components such as, Bcl-2 family proteins, death receptor signaling, endogenous inhibitors of caspases, transcriptional control of apoptosis, apoptosis regulation by oncogenes and tumour suppressor genes. The proteins of Bcl-2 family play a key role in the normal regulation of apoptosis and aberrant expression of members of this family has been associated with several tumours. The anti-apoptotic members include Bcl-2 and Bcl-xl and the pro-apoptotic members include Bax, Bad, Bim, Bid (Chang et al., 2003). Experiments involving knockout mice have contributed to our understanding of the role of Bcl-2 family members in tumourigenesis. Bad-knockout mice develop B-cell lymphomas and are less able to hold-out with sub-lethal doses of γ-irradiation (Ranger et al., 2003), while Bid-knockout mice develop myelomonocytic leukemia (Zinkel et al., 2005). Interesting results, involving tumours and Bcl-2, derive from studies undergone on human beings. Over-expression of Bcl-2 has been observed in both B-cell lymphomas (where it was originally discovered) as well as in non-Hodgkin's lymphomas. Furthermore, over-expression of Bcl-2 has been observed in solid tumours such as lung, renal, stomach, and brain cancer. Instead, lower levels of Bcl-2 have been observed in breast cancers. However, either over-expression of Bcl-2 in some subtypes of lymphoma or low levels in breast cancer correlate with poor prognosis (Gascoyne et al., 1997; Chang et al.,2003). It seems that the prognostic value of Bcl-2 expression differs between tumour types and in some cases there may be no correlation with disease progression. The importance of p53 in maintaining genome stability is exemplified by the finding that approximately half of all human tumours carry mutant p53. At present, there are > 10 million people with tumours that contain inactivated p53, while a similar number have tumours in which the p53 pathway is in part blocked by inactivation of other signaling components (Brown et al., 2009). It is well confirmed that the p53 response is defective in most cancers, either by mutations or deletions in the p53 gene, or by alterations in the p53 pathway caused by other oncogenic events. These observations have raised a wide range of clinical possibilities both for diagnosis and treatment, rendering p53 an ideal target for anti-cancer drug design. p53 mutations, the first tumour suppressor gene linked to apoptosis, occur in the most of human tumours and are often associated with advanced tumour stage and poor patient prognosis. Studies using p53 knockout mice demonstrated that endogenous p53 could play a part in apoptosis, in fact p53 has been required for radiation-induced cell death in the thymus, but not cell death induced by glucocorticoids or other apoptotic stimuli (Lowe et al., 1993). p53 can exhibits different and global functions (e.g. promote apoptosis, cell-cycle arrest and senescence). Evidences indicate that p53 apoptotic activity is important in tumour suppression. Therefore, the occurrence of p53 mutations correlates with a decreased apoptosis in some transgenic mice (Attardi & Jacks, 1999) and in clonal progression of tumour cells (Bardeesy et al., 1995). Furthermore alterations of several p53 effectors in apoptosis (e.g. Bax, apaf-1 and casp-9) can promote oncogenic transformation and tumour development in mouse model systems (Soengas et al., 1999). Activation of p53 is sufficient to directly or indirectly trigger apoptosis by inducing pro-apoptotic Bcl-2 family members (Schuler et al., 2000). In addition, alterations in genes encoding various modulators of NF-kB can occur in several types of B-cell malignancies, including non-Hodgkin lymphomas, B-chronic lymphocytic leukemia, and multiple myeloma (Rayet & Gelinas, 1999).

8. The role of TNF-α antagonist therapy in cancer onset

As biologic therapy becomes more common in treating a spectrum of conditions, awareness of side-effects is becoming more important. Mouse models and in vitro experiences indicate that TNF-α plays an important role in tumour growth control. Thus, anti- TNF-α agents might influence the risk of malignancy.

TNF-α is one of main regulator of chronic inflammation and contributes to tumour development, therefore suggesting a role in the progression of solid tumours. However, therapy with TNF-blockers, such as infliximab or etanercept, in patients with advanced cancer was well tolerated, with no evidence of disease acceleration (E.R. Brown et al., 2008). Nevertheless, a systematic review and metanalysis of data from randomized controlled trials of monoclonal antibodies against TNF-α in patients with rheumatoid arthritis showed that there were 29 case of cancers in patients with infliximab group compared to 3 in the control group (Bongartz et al., 2006). In a study of 404 patients with Crohn's disease and 404 matched controls, there were 3 cases of breast cancer in the infliximab-exposed group compared to 1 case in the other group (Biancone et al., 2006). In the Swedish nationwide cancer registry, 4160 patients exposed to TNF-α antagonists (etanercept, infliximab, or adalimumab) were identified (Askling et al., 2005a). Although it has been reported 67 solid cancers, including 8 cases of breast cancer, it has not been found excess risk of solid cancer in this cohort.

TNF-α generates a variety of cellular responses that may either promote or inhibit tumourigenesis. This variability may explain the discrepancies in study results. Some studies on experimental models suggest increased tumour progression with TNF-α blockade. Clinical trials, in contrast, suggest that TNF-α blockade may decrease the activity of solid cancers (kidney and breast). These discordant data generate uncertainty about the potential effects of TNF-α antagonists on the risk of human malignancies in general and on male breast cancer in particular (Williams, 2008). Infliximab is a chimeric mouse-human monoclonal antibody targeting TNF-α. Blocking the actions of tumour necrosis factor-alpha is highly effective in treating several inflammatory disorders. Although safety data have been encouraging, there are reports of immunosuppressive sequelae resulting from the use of the drug.

The soluble dimeric form of p75 TNF receptor, etanercept, binds free TNF in the circulation and cell-bound TNF, thus acting as a competitive inhibitor, blocking TNF interaction with TNF receptors on cell surface (Tsimberidou & Giles, 2002). It inhibits binding of both TNF and lymphotoxin (LT)-a (also known as TNF-β) to cell surface TNF receptors, rendering TNF biologically inactive. It has been postulated that etanercept acts both as a cytokine carrier and TNF antagonist, and can modulate biological responses that are induced or regulated by TNF, such as expression of adhesion molecules responsible for leukocyte migration (Tsimberidou & Giles, 2002). Etanercept has shown activity and is currently indicated in patients with moderately to severely active rheumatoid arthritis; moderately to severely active polyarticular-course juvenile rheumatoid arthritis with inadequate response to disease-modifying antirheumatic drugs; or psoriatic arthritis (Lovell et al., 2000; Mease et al., 2000). In a pilot study, it was given Etanercept to 13 patients affected by cutaneous T-cell lymphoma (CTCL), because of the role played by TNF in tumour progression. An improvement was observed in patients with early disease, and a larger cohort of patients with early disease merits investigation, while it is unlikely that it will be effective in patients with advanced CTCL (Tsimberidou et al., 2004).

Adalimumab is a fully human recombinant IgG1 monoclonal antibody with specificity for human TNF-α. Bongartz et al. (2006) conducted a systematic review and meta-analysis that included 9 trials employing either infliximab or adalimumab in 3493 patients with RA versus 1512 patients taking placebo to further elucidate the carcinogenic potential of TNF-α blockers. The odds ratio for malignancy was found to be 3.3, and the incidence of cancer was associated with higher doses of the biologic. For patients treated with anti-TNF-α antibodies included in these trials, the number needed to harm was 154 within the 6- to 12-month follow-up period. But the study failed to give some adjustments.

The relationship between lymphoma and TNF-α blockers has been documented in a few case reports focusing on psoriasis patients. One report reviewed relevant data in the MedWatch postmarketing adverse event surveillance system run by the Food and Drug Administration and discovered 26 cases of lymphoma following treatment with either etanercept (18 cases) or infliximab (8 cases) (S.L. Brown, 2002). Frequently, those receiving etanercept were reported to be taking MTX concurrently (5 of 18) or had a history of prior exposure to MTX (4 of 18), or a history of exposure to another immunosuppressive agent (4 of 18). Another noteworthy clinical feature of the lymphomas observed was the very short latent period of only few weeks between the initiation of anti-TNF therapy and the development of malignancy.

In two instances (one etanercept, one infliximab), lymphoma regression was observed following discontinuation of the TNF-α -blocker in the absence of specific cytotoxic therapy directed toward the lymphoma.

The association between lymphoma and biologic therapy was weakened by data reported by Askling et al. (2005b) who epidemiologically studied cohorts of RA patients with either long-standing disease, incident disease, or TNF-α -antagonist treated disease linked with the Swedish Cancer Registry. The lymphoma risk in those treated with TNF-blockers was no higher versus the other RA cohorts, given that the standardized incidence ratio (SIR) for RA patients on TNF blockers was 2.9 and not statistically significant after adjustment for sex, age, and disease duration from the SIR of 2.0 in control subjects with RA.

A study reviewed 1440 patients having psoriasis treated with etanercept for more than 5 years, without founding any increase of malignancies (Burge, 2003). However, a multitude of recent case reports have begun to strengthen the link between anti-TNF-α therapy and induction or rapid reactivation of latent malignancies.

In the literature many case-reports were found about the cancer onset after anti-TNF-α therapy, such as anorectal carcinoma (Melichar et al.,_2006) and non-Hodgkin Lymphoma (Bickston et al., 1999) after infliximab therapy in Crohn's disease, cutaneous and systemic T-cell lymphoma after treatment with infliximab and also with etanercept (Adams et al., 2004).

One reason for the safety concerns surrounding anti-TNF-α therapy is the role of the members of the TNF family in normal immune system development and function (Bazzoni & Beutler, 1996). However, "knock-out" mutations of the TNF gene complex in mouse models of disease cause an increased susceptibility to certain infections, but not autoimmunity or malignancy (Erickson et al., 1994). In addition, it is noteworthy the absence of a clear immunosuppressive effects of TNF antagonism in preclinical and human studies. Thus, in contrast to the pleiotropic effects of TNF with the immune system, blockade of TNF with infliximab does not suppress global immune function in the manner of drugs such as azathioprine (Meenan et al., 1997). Therapy with infliximab has not been associated with decreases in absolute lymphocyte counts (Meenan et al., 1997), development of anergy (Feldmann et al., 1997), or emergence of opportunistic viral and fungal infections. Together,

these data suggest that blockade of TNF with a drug such as infliximab may lead to limited and selective rather than broad-spectrum immune suppression.
Also for adalimumab therapy carried on patients affected by rheumatoid arthritis it was observed the incidence of cancer, especially the onset of melanoma in two patients, after two years from the start of therapy with adalimumab (Dewan et al., 2009).
However, it is not easy to establish clearly the real risk associated with anti- TNF-α therapies because of various confounding factors including possible increased predisposition to cancer due to the underlying disorder and the concomitant or prior use of other potentially cancer-promoting therapies.

9. Possible link between autoimmune diseases and cancer

In many systemic autoimmune diseases, where disproportional humoral autoimmune responses are pivotal in the pathogenesis (e.g. systemic lupus erythematosus and Sjögren's syndrome), exaggerated B-cell processes exist, resembling B-cell malignancies (Illes et al., 2009). Both conditions are characterized by cell-cycle regulation abnormalities, which affect lymphocyte survival, proliferation and differentiation, as well.

9.1 Systemic lupus erythematosus

Systemic lupus erythematosus (SLE) is a systemic autoimmune disease, characterized by a wide array of symptoms and organ involvements, leading to varying disease courses and outcome. In patients with SLE, the incidence and risk of malignancy development is increased. The malignancies occurred frequently in SLE patients are Non-Hodgkin's Lymphoma, Hodgkin's Lymphoma, as well as solid tumours, as lung, cervical and breast cancer (Kiss et al., 2010).
The frequent occurrence of malignancies can be associated with the common pathogenetic pathways for cancer and autoimmune disease development. This phenomenon is reinforced by the following notions: generally, in autoimmune diseases malignancies occur with high frequency; in neoplastic disorders, autoimmune diseases can develop, as part of the paraneoplastic syndrome; also, immunosuppressive treatment in autoimmune diseases increases the development of malignancies (Zintzaras et al., 2005).
The long-term, in many instances aggressive immunosuppressive treatment in lupus is evidently related to the development of malignant transformations and manifest tumours. Besides these common extrinsic etiological factors, the intrinsic errors of the immune system contribute to the development of both disease entities (Bernatsky et al., 2002).

9.1.1 Cancer before systemic lupus erythematosus

Since the clinical appearance of Non-Hodgkin's Lymphoma and systemic lupus erythematosus is similar, and it is sometimes difficult to distinguish the two disease entities in the initial phases, these raise the possibility that SLE might be a paraneoplastic syndrome and appears on the grounds of the lymphoid malignancy (Kiss et al., 2010).

9.1.2 Cancer after systemic lupus erythematosus

The pathogenic background behind the more frequent presence of NHL in SLE can be due to the chronic, persistent antigen-stimulus, chronic inflammation, uncontrolled B cell proliferation, defected apoptosis, and the increased risk of oncogene translocation. Common environmental and genetic factors, linked with major histocompatibility complex (MHC)-associated genes, further contribute to lymphomagenesis in lupus. Also, treatment with immunomodulating and immunosuppressive drugs, commonly used in SLE can contribute to the development of lymphomagenesis, either by directly causing mutagenesis, or by weakening the immune surveillance, which can lead to uncontrolled B cell proliferation (Kiss et al., 2010).

In 9% of SLE patients may occur some inflammatory diseases, such as pneumonitis-fibrosis or bronchiolitis obliterans organizing pneumonia, that may lead to a chronic stimulation and extensive DNA damage which underlie lung cancer.

Moreover, in female affected by SLE it has been reported a higher risk of breast cancer, without any family history or exogenous hormonal exposure (Ramsey-Goldman et al., 1998). Thereby, likely the pathological immune responses triggered by the autoimmune disease can lead to uncontrolled cell proliferation and decreased apoptosis, and breast cancer development, indeed (Kiss et al.,2010).

9.1.3 Antiphospholipid antibodies

Another link between lupus and malignant diseases can be served by antiphospholipid antibodies (aPL), frequently present in SLE and cancer as well.

Patients with cancer are at higher risk of thromboembolic complications than healthy people for many reasons. It is known that an important thrombogenic mechanism is mediated by antiphospholipid antibodies (aPL). Although the evidence on their association, the relationship between aPL presence and cancer is contradictory. It is unclear whether aPL antibody positivity has a pathogenetic role in the development of thromboses or whether, in contrast, these antibodies are an epiphenomenon in cancer patients (Reinstein & Shoenfeld, 2007).

In the last years a higher prevalence of aPL antibodies was observed in patients with solid tumours compared to controls (Zuckerman et al., 1995) and in patients with haematological malignancies (Pusterla et al., 2004). The reasons of this increased antibody production are only partially clarified: their production may be induced by particular immunotherapy of cancer such as interferon α (Becker et al., 1994) or started by immune system response to new tumour antigens (Sawamura et al., 1994).

In particular it is possible that autoantibodies to malignant cells arise secondary to changes in the cell membrane that induce exposure of certain antigens that are normally facing the intracellular compartment (Reinstein & Shoenfeld, 2007), then activating pathogenetic autoreactive human T cells (Yamaguchi et al., 2007). In this context, it has been reported that viable tumour cells (Fernandes et al., 2006) as well as tumour blood vessels (Ran et al., 2002) showed increased exposure of anionic phospholipids on the outer layer of their membranes, directly triggering coagulation cascade by providing a procoagulatory surface (Vogt et al., 1997). Therefore, tumour microenvironment may be a source of anionic lipid surfaces that facilitate aPL antibodies production. It is also possible that tumoural cells directly synthetize antibodies as in the case of multiple myeloma or Waldenstrom's macroglobulinemia (Tincani et al., 2010).

Moreover, an interesting study carried on aPL antibodies healthy carriers, reported that the major cause of morbidity and mortality was the occurrence of malignancies, in particular non-Hodgkin's lymphoma seemed to affect this group with an higher incidence than the general population (Finazzi, 1997).

9.2 Rheumatic arthritis

The link between autoimmune phenomena, particularly rheumatic arthritis, and cancers has been suggested in several studies. It may be due to the generation of autoantibodies against self and non-self antigens, paraneoplastic syndromes or by chemotherapy.

As the presence of autoantibodies has been identified in the sera of patients both with solid tumours and haematological malignancies, it may be considered as the consequence of the immune response against the tumour (Conrad, 2000).

The natural autoantibodies (NAA), frequently occurring in high titres in the sera of patients with multiple myeloma, Waldenstrom's macroglobulinemia, chronic lymphocytic leukaemia, and B cell lymphoma, are generated by CD5+ B cells. They are mainly IgM, which bind with low affinity self and non-self antigens, and they also have rheumatoid factor activity (Abu-Shakra et al., 2001). This autoantibody activity is the result of malignant transformation of B cells, that produce autoantibodies (Dighiero, 1998).

9.2.1 Cancer after rheumatic arthritis

An increased occurrence of malignancies in patients with established rheumatoid arthritis (RA) has been found by several studies (Bernatsky et al., 2006). In most cases, the higher rate of cancer is linked to the use of immunosuppressive therapy, and the tumour generally takes several years to develop.

9.2.2 Cancer before rheumatic arthritis

However, the early manifestation of an occult malignancy may be a rapid-onset arthritis mimicking rheumatoid arthritis. More often, the rheumatoid arthritis-like syndrome precedes the development of cancer by 6–12 months. (Racanelli et al., 2008)

Rheumatoid arthritis-like syndromes have been associated with malignancies of the lung, colon, breast, ovary, stomach and oropharynx cancer and with haematopoietic malignancies. (Andrai et al., 2006)

Patients with paraneoplastic rheumatic disease generally exhibit a form of asymmetric polyarthritis that may be confused with seronegative rheumatoid arthritis or spondyloarthropathy.

The paraneoplastic disorders disappear after surgical removal or pharmacological treatment of the cancer, otherwise these treatments have any influence on rheumatic symptoms that are tumour-associated (Naschitz, 2001).

9.3 Polymyositis and dermatomyositis

The association between malignancy and autoimmune myositis, in particular polymyositis (PM) and dermatomyositis (DM), has been largely described (Briani et al., 2006). The diagnosis of tumour can precede, parallel or follow myositis diagnosis. Most commonly cancer is diagnosed after the onset of myositis, but in many cases the course of the myopathy paralleled the course of the tumour (Zampieri et al., 2010). The incidence of cancer in patients with an established autoimmune myopathies was estimated ranging from 6% to 60% (Hill et al., 2001). In contrast, the incidence of myopathies as an early manifestation of an occult malignancies is undefined.

9.3.1 Cancer before autoimmune myositis

The malignancies more frequently associated with PM and DM are ovarian, colorectal, breast, and lung cancer (Wakata et al., 2002). The so called "paraneoplastic" inflammatory myopathies are autoimmune myositis, that develop in patients with primary cancer as the consequence of its presence. In the paraneoplastic syndromes the surgical removal or pharmacological treatment of cancer results in the disappearance of the clinical symptoms of the paraneoplastic disease (Raccanelli et al., 2008). Some myopathies can develop also in response to chemotherapeutic agents used to treat cancer (Chakravarty & Genovese, 2003). The paraneoplastic myositis show different clinical features and laboratory data, as well as a later onset and a lower or absent response to immunosuppressive drugs (Buchbinder et al., 2001).

9.3.2 Cancer after autoimmune myositis

Patients with DM have a greater risk of developing malignancy than the general population, while PM patients seem to be associated to a lesser extent to an increased risk. Also the drugs used to treat autoimmune myositis can be responsible for cancer onset in these patients. These drugs are administered in order to modulate the response of immune system and therefore their use can induce an altered state of immune surveillance which can be responsible for the consequent development of tumour (Szekanecz et al., 2006).
The pathogenetic molecular mechanisms underlying the association between cancer and myositis are still unknown, even though some hypotheses have been purposed (Eisenlohr & Rothstein, 2006). It is possible that an immune response directed against cancer cells in both breast and lung adenocarcinoma, as well as hepatocellular carcinoma, cross-reacts with regenerating muscle cells (Casciola-Rosen et al., 2005). These regenerating muscle fibers and tumour cells expressing myositis specific autoantigens, may be responsible for the induction of autoimmune response in those patients with a predisposing genetic background to autoimmunity. Casciola-Rosen et al. (2005) have been demonstrated that some tumours (e.g. breast, lung adenocarcinoma, and hepatocellular carcinoma), but not the corresponding normal tissues, express high levels of myositis autoantigens. It has been also demonstrated that in affected muscles from myositis patients, regenerating myoblasts overexpress myositis specific autoantigens and notably the expression of these autoantigens by tumour cells as well as by regenerating myoblasts, indicates a possible antigenic similarity between the two cell populations (Casciola-Rosen et al., 2005).

9.4 Sjögren's syndrome

The link between Sjögren's syndrome (SS) and non-Hodgkin's lymphoma (NHL) is one of the strongest among all the known associations between systemic autoimmune diseases and malignancies. The occurrence of NHL has been reported to be as much as 44-fold greater in Sjögren's syndrome than in the general population (Kovács et al., 2010). In the majority of patients, the histopathologic type of lymphoma is mucosa-associated lymphoid tissue (MALT) type B cell lymphoma, i.e. extranodal marginal zone B cell lymphoma, and in about 30% of SS patients, other types of NHL can be observed. In SS, the predominant cellular components of the focal lymphocytic infiltration in the salivary glands are CD4+T lymphocytes. The evolution of a malignant proliferation of B-lymphocytes from this inflammatory infiltration is due to a complex process. The ultimate step in this process is the transition from benign B cell proliferation to malignant expansion. The uncontrolled expansion of B-lymphocytes is a result of various genetic alterations, typically translocations involving immunoglobulin gene loci and proto-oncogenes or other genes involved in cell-cycle regulation (Kovács et al., 2010).

10. Conclusion

The relationship between autoimmunity and cancer has been investigated, focusing on implication of immune system, apoptosis and new therapeutic agents for autoimmune diseases. Autoimmune diseases, characterized by chronic inflammatory state, with continuous antigenic stimulation, may contribute to haematological malignancies and solid tumours development. However , the role of new therapeutic agents, as biologic drugs used more frequently in autoimmune diseases treatment, is controversial and need further studies in depth, since they may be involved in cancer onset, as well. The autoimmune diseases, as rheumatoid disorders, systemic lupus erythematosus or myositis may occur before or concomitant with a tumour, as paraneoplastic syndromes, which regress after cancer removal.

Apoptosis is a critical regulator of cellular and humoral immune responses, appearing to play a critical role in the deletion of lymphocytes after an inflammatory state, as well as in the control of tumour cell survival, leading to unchecked tumour growing, if the genes of apoptosis show some mutations. Therefore, understanding normal apoptosis mechanisms is critical for developing a better know-how from which to undertake strategies for improving autoimmune diseases and cancer therapy.

In addition, it is an interesting task the different immune responses against autoantigen occurring during autoimmunity and cancer, which are involved in alterations of immunological tolerance and maintenance of immunological tolerance, respectively. Thus it is easy to understand that immunological tolerance in cancer and autoimmune disease has opposite effects in the patient: in cancer patients it stimulates the growth of the cancer, but in patients with autoimmune disease immunological tolerance may stop the attack by autoantibodies and thereby benefit the patient. In fact, cancer cells are able to employ a pseudo-autoimmune status (cancer associated autoimmune disease) and induce immunological tolerance by producing autoantibodies to tumour antigens derived from impaired clearance of apoptotic cells, resulting in an increase of regulatory T cells, thus increasing tolerance toward tumour cells.

However, further investigations are needed to better define new therapeutic strategies controlling inflammatory components, responsible of both autoimmunity and cancer progression.

11. References

Abu-Shakra, M.; Buskila, D.; Ehrenfeld, M. et al. (2001) Cancer and autoimmunity: autoimmune and rheumatic features in patients with malignancies, *Ann Rheum Dis*, Vol.60,pp.433-440

Adachi, M.; Suematsu, S.; Kondo, T. et al. (1995). Targeted mutation in the Fas gene causes hyperplasia in peripheral lymphoid organs and liver. *Nature Genet*, Vol.11, pp. 294–300

Afzali, B.; Lombardi, G.; Lechler, R.I. et al. (2007) The role of T helper 17 (Th17) and regulatory T cells (Treg) in human organ transplantation and autoimmune disease, *Clin Exp Immunol*, Vol. 148,pp. 32–46

Amoura, Z.; Piette, J.C.; Bach, J.F. et al. (1999) The key role of nucleosomes in Lupus. *Arthritis Rheum*, Vol. 42, pp833-843

Andrai, C.; Csiki, Z.; Ponyi, A. et al. (2006) Paraneoplastic rheumatic syndromes. *Rheumatol Int.* Vol. 26, pp.376–82.

Anthoney, D.A.; McIlwrath, A.J.; Gallagher, W.M. et al. (1996). Microsatellite Instability, Apoptosis, and Loss of p53 Function in Drug-resistant Tumour Cells. *Cancer Res,* Vol.56, pp. 1374- 1381

Askling, J.; Fored, C.M.; Brandt, L. et al. (2005a) Risks of solid cancers in patients with rheumatoid arthritis and after treatment with tumour necrosis factor antagonists, *Ann Rheum Dis,* Vol. 64, pp.1421-6

Askling, J.; Fored, S.M.; Baecklund, E. et al. (2005b) Haematopoietic malignancies in rheumatoid arthritis: lymphoma risk and characteristics after exposure to tumour necrosis factor antagonists, *Ann Rheum Dis,* Vol.64, pp. 1414-20.

Attardi, L.D. & Jacks, T. (1999). The role of p53 in tumour suppression: lessons from mouse models. *Cell Mol. Life Sci.,* Vol.55, pp.48–63

Baechler, E.C.; Batliwalla, F.M.; Karypis, G. et al. (2003). Interferon-inducible gene expression signature in peripheral blood cells of patients with severe lupus. *Proc. Natl. Acad. Sci.* USA, Vol.100, pp. 2610–2615

Bardeesy, N.; Beckwith, J.B. & Pelletier, J. (1995) Clonal expansion and attenuated apoptosis in Wilms' tumours are associated with p53 gene mutations. *Cancer Res.,* Vol.55, pp.215–219

Bazzoni, F. & Beutler, B. (1996) The tumor necrosis factor ligand and receptor families. *N Engl J Med,* Vol.334, pp. 1717-1725

Becker, J.C.; Winkler, B.; Klingert, S. et al. (1994) Antiphospholipid syndrome associated with immunotherapy for patients with melanoma, *Cancer,* Vol.73, No. (6), pp.1621–4

Bei, R.; Masuelli, L.; Palumbo, C. et al. (2009) A common repertoire of autoantibodies is shared by cancer and autoimmune disease patients: inflammation in their induction and impact on tumour growth. *Cancer Lett,* Vol. 281, pp.8–23

Bernatsky, S.; Clarke, A. & Ramsey-Goldman, R. (2002) Malignancy and systemic lupus erythematosus. *Curr Rheumatol Rep,* Vol.4, No. (4), pp.351–8

Bernatsky, S.; Ramsey-Goldman, R. & Clarke, A. (2006) Malignancy and autoimmunity, *Curr Opin Rheumatol,* Vol.18, pp.129–34

Bernatsky, S.; Lee, J.L. & Rahme, E. (2007) Non-Hodgkin's lymphoma—meta-analyses of the effects of corticosteroids and non-steroidal anti-inflammatories. *Rheumatology;* Vol. 46, pp.690–4

Biancone, L.; Orlando, A.; Kohn, A. et al. (2006) Infliximab and newly diagnosed neoplasia in Crohn's disease: a multicentre matched pair study. *Gut,* Vol.55, pp.228-33

Bickston, S.J.; Lichtenstein, G.R.; Arseneau K.O. et al. (1999) The Relationship Between Infliximab Treatment and Lymphoma in Crohn's Disease. *Gastroenterology,* Vol. 117, pp.1433–1437

Boldin, M.P.; Goncharov, T.M.; Goltsev, Y.V. et al. (1996). Involvement of MACH, a novel MORT1/FADD-interacting protease, in Fas/APO-1- and TNF receptor-induced cell death. *Cell,* Vol.85, pp. 803-815

Bolstad, A.I.; Wargelius, A.; Nakken, B. et al. (2000). Fas and Fas ligand gene polymorphisms in primary Sjögren's syndrome. *J Rheumatol,* Vol.27, pp.2397–2405

Bongartz, T.; Sutton, A.J.; Sweeting, M.J. et al. (2006) Anti-TNF antibody therapy in rheumatoid arthritis and the risk of serious infections and malignancies: systematic review and meta-analysis of rare harmful effects in randomized controlled trials, *JAMA*, Vol. 295, pp.2275-85

Briani, C.; Doria, A.; Sarzi-Puttini, P. et al. (2006) Update on idiopathic inflammatory myopathies. *Autoimmunity*, Vol. 39, pp.161–70

Brown, C.J.; Lain, S.; Verma, C.S. et al. (2009). Awakening guardian angels: drugging the p53 pathway. *Nat Rev Cancer*, Vol.9, No.12, pp. 862-873

Brown, E.R.; Charles, K.A. ; Hoare, S.A. et al. (2008) A clinical study assessing the tolerability and biological effects of infliximab, a TNF-alpha inhibitor, in patients with advanced cancer, *Ann Oncol*, Vol. 19,pp.1340-6

Brown, S.L.; Greene, M.H.; Gershon, S.K. et al. (2002) Tumour necrosis factor antagonist therapy and lymphoma development, *Arthritis Rheum*, Vol.46, pp.3151-8

Brunner, T.; Mogil, R.J.; La Face, D. et al. (1995). Cell-autonomous Fas (CD95)/Fas-ligand interaction mediates activation-induced apoptosis in T-cell hybridomas. *Nature*, Vol.373, pp. 441–444.

Buchbinder, R.; Forbes, A.; Hall, S. et al. (2001) Incidence of malignant disease in biopsy-proven inflammatory myopathy. A population-based cohort study. *Ann Intern Med*, Vol. 134, pp.1087–95.

Burge, D. (2003) Etanercept and squamous cell carcinoma. *J Am Acad Dermatol*, Vol. 49,pp.358-9.

Burnet, F.M. (1988). 'The Clonal Selection Theory of Acquired Immunity', In: *Milestones in Immunology: A Historical Exploration,* Debra Jan Bibel (Ed.), 185-187, Science Tech, London

Cao, D.; Malmström, V.; Baecher-Allan, C. et al. (2003) Isolation and functional characterization of regulatory CD25bright CD4+ T cells from the target organ of patients with rheumatoid arthritis, *Eur J Immunol*; Vol. 33, No. (1), pp. 215–223.

Casciola-Rosen, L.; Nagaraju, K.; Plots, P. et al. (2005) Enhanced autoantigen expression in regenerating muscle cells in idiopathic inflammatory myopathy. *J Exp Med*, Vol.4, pp.591–601

Catrina, A.I.; Ulfgren, A.K.; Lindblad, S. et al. (2002). Low levels of apoptosis and high FLIP expression in early rheumatoid arthritis synovium. *Ann Rheum Dis,* Vol.61, pp.934-936

Cellier, C.; Delabesse, E.; Helmer, C. et al. (2000) Refractory sprue, coeliac disease, and enteropathy associated T-cell lymphoma. *Lancet*, Vol.356, pp.203–8

Cepika, A.M.; Marinic, I.; Morovic-Vergles, J. et al. (2007) Effect of steroids on the frequency of regulatory T cells and expression of FOXP3 in a patient with systemic lupus erythematosus: A two-year follow-up, *Lupus*, Vol. 16, No.(5), pp.374–377

Chakravarty, E. & Genovese, M.C. (2003) Rheumatic syndromes associated with malignancy. *Curr Opin Rheumatol*, Vol. 15, No. , pp.35–43

Chang, J.; Clark, G.M.; Allred, D.C. et al. (2003). Survival of patients with metastatic breast carcinoma: importance of prognostic markers of the primary tumour. *Cancer*, Vol.97, No.3, pp. 545-553

Chen, M.L.; Pittet, M.J.; Gorelik, L. et al. (2005) Regulatory T cells suppress tumour-specific CD8 T cell cytotoxicity through TGF-beta signals *in vivo*, *Proc Natl Acad Sci U S A*, Vol. 102, pp. 419-424

Chinnaiyan, A.M.; O'Rourke, K.; Tewari, M. et al. (1995). FADD, a novel death domain-containing protein interacts with the death domain of Fas and initiates apoptosis. *Cell*, Vol.81, pp. 505-512

Ciric, B.; El-behi, M.; Cabrera, R. et al. (2009) IL-23 drives pathogenic IL-17- producing CD8+ T cells, *J Immunol*, Vol.182, pp.5296–5305.

Conrad, K. (2000) Autoantibodies in cancer patients and in persons with a higher risk of cancer development. In: *Cancer and autoimmunity*, Shoenfeld, Y. & Gershwin, M.F. (Eds.), 159-74, Elsevier, The Netherlands.

Coussens, L.M. & Werb, Z. (2002) Inflammation and cancer, *Nature*, Vol.420, pp.860–7

Curiel,T.J.; Coukos, G.; Zou, L. et al (2004) Specific recruitment of regulatory T cells in ovarian carcinoma fosters immune privilege and predicts reduced survival, *Nat Med*, Vol. 10, pp. 942-949

Dewan, P.; Jawad, A.; Goldsmith, P. et al. (2009) Melanoma in patients with rheumatoid arthritis treated with antitumour necrosis factor: cause or coincidence? Report of two cases, *British Journal of Dermatology, Vol.* 161, pp1399–1424

Dighiero, G. (1998) Autoimmunity and B-cell malignancies *Hematol Cell Ther*, Vol.40, pp.1–9

Eisenlohr, L.C. & Rothstein, J.L. (2006) Oncogenic inflammation and autoimmune disease, *Autoimmun Rev*, Vol. 6, pp.*107–14*

Emlen, W.; Niebur, J., & Kadera, R. (1994). Accelerated in vitro apoptosis of lymphocytes from patients with systemic lupus erythematosus. *J Immunol*, Vol.152, pp. 3685-3692

Engels, E.A. (2007) Infectious agents as causes of non-Hodgkin lymphoma. *Cancer Epidemiol Biomarkers Prev*, Vol.16, pp.401–4

Erickson, S.L.; de Sauvage, F.J.; Kikly, K. et al. (1994) Decreased sensitivity to tumour-necrosis factor but normal T-cell development in TNF receptor-2–deficient mice, *Nature*, Vol.372, pp. 560–563

Eskes, R.; Desagher, S.; Antonsson, B. et al. (2000). Bid induces the oligomerization and insertion of Bax into the outer mitochondrial membrane. *Mol Cell Biol*, Vol.20, pp. 929-935

Feldmann, M.; Elliott, M.J.; Woody, J. et al. (1997) Anti-tumour necrosis factor alpha therapy of RA, *Adv Immunol*, Vol.64, pp.283–350

Fernandes, R.S.; Kirszberg, C.; Rumjanek, V.M. et al. (2006) On the molecular mechanisms for the highly procoagulant pattern of C6 glioma cells, *J Thromb Haemost*, Vol.4, pp.1546–52

Finazzi, G. (1997) The Italian registry of antiphospholipid antibodies, *Haematologica*, Vol. 82, No. (1), pp.101–5

Firestein, G.S.; Nguyen, K.; Aupperle, K.R. et al. (1996). Apoptosis in rheumatoid arthritis: p53 overexpression in rheumatoid arthritis synovium. *Am J Pathol*, Vol.149, pp. 2143-2151

Gascoyne, R.D.; Adomat, S.A.; Krajewski, S. et al. (1997). Prognostic significance of Bcl-2 protein expression and Bcl-2 gene rearrangement in diffuse aggressive non-Hodgkin's lymphoma. *Blood*, Vol.90, No.1, pp. 244-251

Goodnow, C.C. (2007) Multistep pathogenesis of autoimmune disease, *Cell*; Vol.130,pp. 25–35

Hill, C.L.; Zhang, Y.; Sigurgeirsson, B. et al. (2001) Frequency of specific cancer types in dermatomyositis and polymyositis: a population-based study. *Lancet*, Vol. 357, pp.96–100.

Holzelova, E.; Vonarbourg, C.; Stolzenberg, M.C. et al. (2004) Autoimmune lymphoproliferative syndrome with somatic Fas mutations, *N Engl J Med*, Vol.351, pp.1409–18

Hori, S.; Nomura, T. & Sakaguchi, S. (2003) Control of regulatory T cell development by the transcription factor Foxp3, *Science*, Vol.299, No.(5609), pp.1057–1061

Hsu, H.; Shu, H.B.; Pan, M.G. et al. (1996). TRADD-TRAF2 and TRADD-FADD interactions define two distinct TNF Receptor 1 signal transduction pathways. *Cell*, Vol.84, pp. 299–308

Humphreys-Beher, M.G.; Peck, A.B.; Dang, H. et al. (1999). The role of apoptosis in the initiation of the autoimmune response in Sjögren's syndrome. *Clin Exp Immunol*, Vol.116, pp.383-387

Illes, A.; Varoczy, L.; Papp, G. et al. (2009) Aspects of B-cell non- Hodgkin's lymphoma development: a transition from immune-reactivity to malignancy, *Scand J Immunol*, Vol.69, No.(5), pp.387–400

Irmler, M.; Thome, M.; Hahne, M. et al. (1997). Inhibition of death receptor signals by cellular FLIP. *Nature*, Vol.388, pp. 190-195

Itoh, N. & Nagata, S. (1993). A novel protein domain required for apoptosis: mutational analysis of human Fas antigen. *J Biol Chem.*, Vol.268, pp. 10932-10937

Janicke, R.U.; Ng, P.; Sprengart, M.L. et al. (1998). Caspase-3 is required for a-fodrin cleavage but dispensable for cleavage of other death substrates in apoptosis. *J Biol Chem*, Vol.273, pp.15540-15545

Kalden, J.R.; Winkler, T.H.; Herrmann, M. et al. (1991). Pathogenesis of SLE: Immunopathology in man. *Rheumatol Int*, Vol.11, pp. 95–100

Kawakami, A.; Nakashima, T.; Sakai, H. et al. (1999). Regulation of synovial cell apoptosis by proteasome inhibitor. *Arthritis Rheum*, Vol.42, pp. 2440-2448

Kelliher, M.A.; Grimm, S.; Ishida, Y. et al. (1998). The death domain kinase RIP mediates the TNF-induced NF-kB signal. *Immunity*, Vol.8, pp. 297–303

Kim, R.; Emi, M. & Tanabe, K. (2005). Cancer cell immune escape and tumour progression by exploitation of anti-inflammatory and pro inflammatory responses. *Cancer Biol Ther*, Vol.4, pp.924-933

Kischkel, F.C.; Hellbardt, S.; Behrmann, I. et al. (1995). Cytotoxicity-dependent APO-1 (Fas/CD95)-associated proteins form a death-inducing signaling complex (DISC) with the receptor. *EMBO J*, Vol.14, pp. 5579-5588

Kiss, E.; Kovacs, L. & Szodoray, P. (2010) Malignancies in systemic lupus erythematosus, *Autoimmun Rev*, Vol.9, pp.195–9

Kolls, J.K. & Linden, A. (2004) Interleukin-17 family members and inflammation, *Immunity*,Vol. 21, p.467–476

Kormeyer, S.J. (1995) Regulators of cell death. *Trends Genet* , Vol.11, pp.101-105

Kovács, L.; Szodoray,P. & Kiss, E. (2010) Secondary tumours in Sjögren's syndrome, *Autoimmunity Reviews*, Vol.9, pp.203–206

Kryczek, I.; Banerjee, M.; Cheng, P. et al. (2009) Phenotype, distribution, generation, functional and clinical relevance of Th17 cells in the human tumour environments, *Blood*, Vol. 114, pp.1141–9

Kuhn, A.; Beissert, S. & Krammer, P.H. (2009) CD4+ CD25+ regulatory T cells in human lupus erythematosus, *Arch Dermatol Res*, Vol.301, No.(1), pp.71–81

La Cava, A. (2008) T-regulatory cells in systemic lupus erythematosus, *Lupus*, Vol.17, No.(5), pp.421–425

Landgren, O.; Engels, E.A., Pfeiffer, R.M. et al. (2006) Autoimmunity and susceptibility to Hodgkin lymphoma: a population based case–control study in Scandinavia. *J Natl Cancer Inst*,Vol. 98, pp.1321–30

Lang, K.S.; Recher, M.; Junt, T. et al. (2005). Toll-like receptor engagement converts T-cell autoreactivity into overt autoimmune disease. *Nat Med*, Vol.1, pp.138-145

Langier, S.; Sade, K. & Kivity, S. (2010) Regulatory T cells: The suppressor arm of the immune system. *Autoimmunity Reviews*, Vol.10, pp.112-115

Lawson, C.A.; Brown, A.K., Bejarano, V. et al. (2006) Early rheumatoid arthritis is associated with a deficit in the CD4+ CD25high regulatory T cell population in peripheral blood, *Rheumatology*, Vol.45, No. (10), pp.1210–1217

Lee, J.H.; Wang, L.C.; Lin, Y.T. et al. (2006) Inverse correlation between CD4+ regulatory T-cell population and autoantibody levels in paediatric patients with systemic lupus erythematosus, *Immunology*, Vol.117, No.(2),pp. 280–286

Linden, A.; Laan, M. & Anderson, G.P. (2005) Neutrophils, interleukin-17A and lung disease, *Eur Respir J*, Vol. 25, pp.159–172

Lorenz, H.M.; Herrmann, M.; Winkler, T. et al (2000). Role of apoptosis in autoimmunity. *Apoptosis*, Vol.5, pp. 443–449

Love, L.A. (1994). New environmental agents associated with lupus-like disorders. *Lupus*, Vol.3, pp. 467–471

Lovell, D.J.; Giannini, E.H.; Reiff, A. et al.. (2000) Etanercept in children with polyarticular juvenile rheumatoid arthritis. Pediatric Rheumatology Collaborative Study Group. *N Engl J Med, Vol.* 342, pp.763-9

Lowe, S.W.; Schmitt, E.M.; Smith, S.W. et al. (1993). p53 is required for radiation-induced apoptosis in mouse thymocytes. *Nature*, Vol.362, pp. 847-849

Lu, L. & Osmond, D.G. (1997). Apoptosis during B lymphopoiesis in mouse bone marrow. *J Immunol*, Vol.158, pp. 5136–5145

Maas, K.; Chan, S.; Parker, J. et al. (2002). Cutting edge: molecular portrait of human autoimmune disease. *J Immunol*, Vol.169, pp.5-9

Malaguarnera, L.; Cristaldi, E. & Malaguarnera, M. (2010) The role of immunità in elderly cancer, *Critical Reviews in Oncology/Hematology*, Vol. 74, pp. 40–60

Martin-Orozco, N. & Dong, C. (2009a) The IL-17/IL-23 axis of inflammation in cancer: Friend or foe? *Current Opinion in Investigational Drugs*, Vol.10, No.6, pp.543-9.

Martin-Orozco, N.; Muranski, P.; Chung, Y. et al. (2009b) Th17 cells promote cytotoxic T cell activation in tumour immunity, *Immunity*, Vol. 31, No (5), pp.787–798

Mc Arthur, C.; Wang, Y.; Veno, P. et al. (2002). Intracellular trafficking and surface expression of SS-A (Ro), SS-B (La), poly(ADP-ribose) polymerase and α-fodrin autoantigens during apoptosis in human salivary gland cells induced by tumour necrosis factor-α. *Arch Oral Biol*, Vol.47, pp.443-448

Mc Cubrey, J.A.; May, W.S.; Duronio, V. et al. (2000). Serine/threonine phosphorylation in cytokine signal transduction. *Leukemia*, Vol.14, pp. 9-21

Mease, P.J.; Goffe, B.S.; Metz, J. et al. (2000) Etanercept in the treatment of psoriatic arthritis and psoriasis: a randomised trial, *Lancet*, Vol.356,pp.385-90

Medh, R.D. & Thompson, E.B. (2000). Hormonal regulation of physiological cell turnover and apoptosis. *Cell Tissue Res*, Vol.301, pp. 101-124

Meenan, J.; Hommes, D.W.; van Dulleman, H. et al. (1997) The influence of TNF mAB, cA2, on circulating lymphocyte populations (abstr). *Gastroenterology*, Vol.122:A1039

Melichar, B.; Bures˘, J. & De˘dic˘, K. (2006) Anorectal Carcinoma After Infliximab Therapy in Crohn's Disease: Report of a Case, *Dis Colon Rectum,* Vol. 49,pp. 1228–1233

Mevorach, D.; Zhou, J.L.; Song, X. et al (1998). Systemic exposure to irradiated apoptotic cells induces autoantibody production. *J. Exp. Med.,* Vol.188, pp. 387-392

Miyara, M.; Amoura, Z.; Parizot, C. et al. (2005) Global natural regulatory T cell depletion in active systemic lupus erythematosus, *J Immunol*,Vol.175, No.(12), pp. 8392–8400

Morgan, M.E.; Flierman, R.; van Duivenvoorde, L.M. et al. (2005) Effective treatment of collagen-induced arthritis by adoptive transfer of CD25+ regulatory T cells. *Arthritis Rheum*, Vol. 52, No.(7), pp.2212–2221.

Moriishi, K.; Huang, D.C.; Cory, S. et al. (1999). Bcl-2 family members do not inhibit apoptosis by binding the caspase activator Apaf-1. *Proc Natl Acad Sci* USA, Vol.96, pp. 9683-9688

Mountz, J.D.; Wu, J.; Cheng, J. et al (1994). Autoimmune disease: a problem of defective apoptosis. *Arthritis Rheum*, Vol.37, pp. 1415-1420

Moutsopoulos, H.M.; Chused, T.M.; Mann, D.L. et al. (1980). SjÖgren's syndrome (sicca syndrome): current issues. *Ann Intern Med*, Vol.92, pp. 212-226

Muzio, M.; Salvesen, G.S. & Dixit, V.M. (1997). FLICE induced apoptosis in a cell free system. *J Biol Chem,* Vol.272, pp. 2952-2956

Mysler, E.; Bini, P.; Drappa, J. et al. (1994). The apoptosis-1/Fas protein in human systemic lupus erythematosus. *J Clin Invest*, Vol.93, pp. 1029–1034

Nagamine, K.; Peterson, P.; Scott, H.S. et al. (1997) Positional cloning of the APECED gene. *Nat Genet*, Vol.17, pp.393–8

Naschitz, J.E. (2001) Rheumatic syndromes: clues to occult neoplasia, *Curr Opin Rheumatol,*Vol. 13, pp.62–6

Newton, K.; Harris, A.W.; Bath, M.L. et al. (1998).Smith KGC, Strasser A. A dominant interfering mutant of Fadd/Mort1 enhances deletion of autoreactive thymocytes and inhibits proliferation of mature T lymphocytes. *EMBO J*, Vol.17, pp. 706–718

Nossal, G.; Pike, B. & Boyd, A. (1982). Clonal anergy: the universally anergic B lymphocyte. *Proc Natl Acad Sci,* USA, Vol.79, No 6, pp. 2013-2017

O'Reilly, L.A.; Harris, A.W.; Tarlinton, D.M. et al. (1997). Expression of a bcl-2 transgene reduces proliferation and slows turnover of developing B lymphocytes in vivo. *J Immunol*, Vol.159, pp.2301-2311

Ohmura, Y.; Yoshikawa, K.; Saga, S. et al. (2008) Combinations of tumour-specific $CD8^+$ CTLs and anti-CD25 mAb provide improved immunotherapy, *Oncol Rep,* Vol.19, pp. 1265-1270

Pap, T.; Muller-Ladner, U.; Gay, R. E. et al. (2000). Fibroblast biology: role of synovial fibroblasts in the pathogenesis of rheumatoid arthritis. *Arthritis Res.*, Vol.2, pp. 361–367

Patel, Y.I. & McHugh, N.J. (2000). Apoptosis–new clues to the pathogenesis of Sjögren's syndrome?. *Rheumatology,* Vol.39, pp. 119-121

Pérez, P.; Goicovich, E.; Alliende, C. et al. (2000). Differential expression of matrix metalloproteinases in labial salivary glands of patients with primary Sjögren's syndrome. Mechanisms of exocrine parenchyma destruction. *Arthritis Rheum,* Vol.43, pp. 2807-2817

Perlman, H.; Liu, H.; Georganas, C. et al. (2001). Differential expression pattern of the anti apoptotic proteins, Bcl-2 and FLIP, in experimental arthritis. *Arthritis Rheum,* Vol.44, pp. 2899-2908

Pope, R.M. & Perlman, H. (2000). Rheumatoid Arthritis, In: *Principles of Molecular Rheumatology,* G.C. Tsokas, (Ed.), pp. 325-361, Totowa, New Jersey

Pusterla, S.; Previstali, S.; Marziali, S. et al. (2004) Antiphospholipid antibodies in lymphoma: prevalence and clinical significance. *Hematol J,* Vol.5, No.(4), pp.341-6

Racanelli, V.; Prete, M.; Minoia, C. et al. (2008) Rheumatic disorders as paraneoplastic syndromes, *Autoimmunity Rev,* Vol.7, pp.352-8

Ramsey-Goldman, R.; Mattai, S.A.; Schilling, E. et al. (1998) Increased risk of malignancy in patients with systemic lupus erythematosus. *J Invest Med* Vol. 46, pp.217-22

Ran, S.; Downes, A. & Thorpe, P.E. (2002) Increased exposure of anionic phospholipids on the surface of tumour blood vessels. *Cancer Res,* Vol.62, pp.6132-40

Ranger, A.M.; Zha, J.; Harada, H. et al. (2003). Bad-deficient mice develop diffuse large B cell lymphoma. *Proc Natl Acad Sci,* USA, Vol.100, No.16, pp.9324-9329

Rayet, B. & Gelinas, C. (1999). Aberrant rel/nfkb genes and activity in human cancer. *Oncogene,* Vol.18, pp. 6938-6947

Reed, J. (1999). Dysregulation of Apoptosis in Cancer. *J. Clin. Oncol,* Vol.17, No. 9 (September) p. 2941

Reinstein, E. & Shoenfeld, Y. (2007) Antiphospholipid syndrome and cancer, *Clin Rev Allergy Immunol,* Vol.32, No.(2), pp.184-7

Rieux-Laucat, F.; Le Deist, F.; Hivroz, C. et al. (1995). Mutations in Fas associated with human lymphoproliferative syndrome and autoimmunity. *Science,* Vol.268, pp. 1347-1349

Rosenquist, R. (2008) Introduction: the role of inflammation, autoimmune disease and infectious agents in development of leukaemia and lymphoma. *J Intern Med,* Vol.264, pp. 512-3

Russell, J.H. & Ley, T.J. (2002). Lymphocyte-mediated cytotoxicity. *Annu Rev Immunol,* Vol.20, pp. 323-70

Sakaguchi, S. (2004) Naturally arising CD4_ regulatory T cells for immunologic self-tolerance and negative control of immune responses. *Annu Rev Immunol,* Vol. 22, pp.531-562

Sawamura, M.; Yamaguchi, S.; Murakami, H. et al. (1994) Multiple autoantibody production in a patient with splenic lymphoma, *Ann Hematol,* Vol. 68, No. (5), pp251-4

Scaffidi, C.; Schmitz, I.; Zha, J. et al. (1999). Differential modulation of apoptosis sensitivity in CD95 type I and type II cells. *J Biol Chem,* Vol.274, pp. 22532-22538

Schuetz, C.; Niehues, T.; Friedrich, W. et al. (2010) Autoimmunity, autoinflammation and lymphoma in combined immunodeficiency (CID). *Autoimmunity Reviews,* Vol.9, pp. 477-482

Schuler, M.; Bossy-Wetzel, E.; Goldstein, J.C. et al. (2000). p53 induces apoptosis by caspase activation through mitochondrial cytochrome c release. *J Biol Chem,* Vol.275, No.10, pp. 7337-7342

Scott, R.S.; McMahon, E.J.; Pop, S.M. et al. (2001). Phagocytosis and clearance of apoptotic cells is mediated by MER. *Nature,* Vol.411, pp. 207-211

Sekine, C.; Yagita, H.; Kobata, T. et al. (1996). Fas-mediated stimulation induces IL-8 sercretion by rheumatoid arthritis synoviocytes independently of CPP32-mediated apoptosis. *Biochem Biophys Res Commun*, Vol.228, pp. 14-20

Sentman, C.L.; Shutter, J.R.; Hockenbery, D. et al. (1991). bcl-2 inhibits multiple forms of apoptosis but not negative selection in thymocytes. *Cell*, Vol.67, pp. 879–88

Silink, M. (2002) Childhood diabetes: a global perspective, *Horm Res*, Vol.57, pp.1–5

Skarstein, K.; Nerland, A.H.; Eidsheim, M. et al. (1997). Lymphoid cell accumulation in salivary glands of autoimmune MRL mice can be due to impaired apoptosis. *Scand J Immunol*, Vol.46, pp.373–378

Skopouli, F.N.; Fox, P.C.; Galanopoulou, V. et al. (1991). T cell subpopulations in the labial minor salivary gland histopathologic lesion of SjÖgren's syndrome. *J Rheumatol*, Vol.18, pp.210-214

SLEGEN; Harley, J.B.; Alarcon-Riquelme, M.E.; et al. (2008). Genome-wide association scan in women with systemic lupus erythematosus identifies susceptibility variants in ITGAM, PXK, KIAA1542 and other loci. *Nat Genet*, Vol 40, pp. 204–209

Soengas, M.S.; Alarcon, R.M.; Yoshida, H. et al. (1999). apaf-1 and caspase-9 in p53-dependent apoptosis and tumour inhibition. *Science*, Vol.284, pp.156-159

Strasser, A.; Harris, A.W.; Huang, D.C.S. et al. (1995). Bcl- 2 and Fas/APO-1 regulate distinct pathways to lymphocyte apoptosis. *EMBO J*, Vol.14, pp. 6136–6147

Straus, S.E.; Sneller, M.; Lenardo, M.J.; et al. (1999) An inherited disorder of lymphocyte apoptosis: the autoimmune lymphoproliferative syndrome. Ann Intern Med, Vol. 130, No.7, pp. 591-601.

Suarez, F.; Lortholary, O.; Hermine, O. et al. (2006) Infection-associated lymphomas derived from marginal zone B cells: a model of antigen-driven lymphoproliferation. *Blood*, Vol.107, pp3034–44

Szekanecz, E.; András, C.; Sándor, Z. et al. (2006) Malignancies and soluble tumour antigens in rheumatic diseases, *Autoimmun Rev*, Vol. 6, pp.42–7

Tartaglia, L.A.; Ayres, T.M.; Wong, G.H.W. et al. (1993). A novel domain within the 55 kd TNF receptor signals cell death. *Cell*, Vol.74, pp. 845-853

Tincani, A.; Taraborelli, M. & Cattaneo, R. (2010) Antiphospholipid antibodies and malignancies. *Autoimmunity Reviews*, Vol.9, pp.200-202

Tsimberidou, A.M. & Giles, F.J. (2002) TNF-alpha targeted therapeutic approaches in patients with hematologic malignancies. *Expert Rev Anticancer Ther*, Vol.2, pp.277-86

Tsimberidou, A.M.; Giles, F.J.; Duvic, M. et al. (2004) Pilot study of etanercept in patients with relapsed cutaneous T-cell lymphomas, *J Am Acad Dermatol*, Vol.51, pp.200-4

Turbyville, J.C. & Rao, V.K. (2010) The autoimmune lymphoproliferative syndrome: a rare disorder providing clues about normal tolerance. *Autoimmun Rev*, Vol.9, pp.488–93

Ueda, H.; Howson, J.M.; Esposito, L. et al. (2003). Association of the T-cell regulatory gene CTLA4 with susceptibility to autoimmune disease. *Nature*, Vol. 423, pp. 506-511

Ulbricht, K.U.; Schmidt, R.E. & Witte T. (2003). Antibodies against alpha- fodrin in Sjögren's syndrome. *Autoimmunity Rev*, Vol.2, pp. 109-113

Utz, P.J. & Anderson, P. (1998). Posttranslational protein modifications, apoptosis and the bypass of tolerance to autoantigens. *Arthritis Rheum*, Vol.41, pp. 1152-1160

Van Parijs, L.; Peterson, D.A. & Abbas, A.K. (1998). The Fas/Fas ligand pathway and Bcl-2 regulate T cell responses to model self and foreign antigens. *Immunity*, Vol.8, pp. 265–274

Vidalino, L.; Doria, A.; Quarta, S. et al. (2009) SERPINB3, apoptosis and autoimmunity. *Autoimmunity Reviews, Vol.* 9, pp. 108–112

Vogt, E.; Ng, A.K. & Rote, N.S. (1997) Antiphosphatidylserine antibody removes annexin-V and facilitates the binding of prothrombin at the surface of a choriocarcinoma model of trophoblast differentiation, *Am J Obstet Gynecol*, Vol. 177, No.(4), pp.964–72

Von Muhlen, C.A. & Tan, E.M. (1995). Autoantibodies in the diagnosis of syotemic rheumatic diseases. *Semin Arthritis Rheum*, Vol.24, pp. 323-358

Wakata, N.; Kurihara, T.; Saito, E. et al. (2002) Polymyositis and dermatomyositis associated with malignancy: a 30-year retrospective study, *Int J Dermatol*, Vol.41, pp. 729–34

Wallach, D. (1997). Cell death induction by TNF: a matter of self control. *Trends Biochem Sci*, Vol.22, pp. 107–109

Wan, Y.Y. & Flavell, R.A. (2007) Regulatory T-cell functions are subverted and converted owing to attenuated Foxp3 expression. *Nature* , Vol. 15, No.445(7129), pp. 766-70

Ward, J.M.; Nikolov, N.P.; Tschetter, J.R. et al. (2004). Progressive glomerulonephritis and histiocytic sarcoma associated with macrophage functional defects in CYP1B1-deficient mice. *Toxicol Pathol*, Vol.32, pp.710-718

Watson, M.L.; Rao, J.K.; Gilkeson, G.S. et al. (1992). Genetic analysis of MRL-lpr mice: Relationship of the Fas apoptosis gene to disease manifestations and renal disease-modifying loci. *J Exp Med*, Vol.176, pp. 1645–1656

Weaver, C.T.; Hatton, R.D.; Mangan, P.R. et al. (2007) IL-17 family cytokines and the expanding diversity of effector T cell lineages. *Annu Rev Immunol*, Vol. 25, pp.821–852

Weiner, H.L. (2001) Induction and mechanism of action of transforming growth factor-b-secreting Th3 regulatory cells. *Immunol Rev*, Vol. 182, pp.207–214

Williams, G.M. (2008) Antitumour necrosis factor-alpha therapy and potential cancer inhibition, *Eur J Cancer Prev*, Vol.17, pp.169-77

Yamaguchi, Y.; Seta, N.; Kaburaki, J. et al. (2007) Excessive exposure to anionic surfaces maintains autoantibody response to beta(2)-glycoprotein I in patients with antiphospholipid syndrome, *Blood*, Vol. 110, pp.4312–8

Yang, X.O.; Nurieva, R.; Martinez, G.J. et al. (2008) Molecular antagonism and plasticity of regulatory and inflammatory T cell programs, *Immunity*, Vol.29, pp.44–56

Ye, P.; Garvey, P.B.; Zhang, P. et al. (2001) Interleukin-17 and lung host defence against Klebsiella pneumoniae infection, *Am J Respir Cell Mol Biol* Vol. 25, pp.335–340

Yeh, W.C.; Shahinian, A.; Speiser, D. et al. (1997). Early lethality, functional NF-kB activation, and increased sensitivity to TNF-induced cell death in TRAF2- deficient mice. *Immunity*, Vol.7, pp. 715-725

Zampieri, S.; Valente, M.; Adami, N. et al. (2010) Polymyositis, dermatomyositis and malignancy: a further intringuing link, *Autoimmun Rev*, Vol 9, pp.449–53

Zhang, J.; Cado, D.; Chen, A. et al. (1998). Fas-mediated apoptosis and activation-induced T-cell proliferation are defective in mice lacking FADD/Mort1. *Nature*, Vol.392, pp. 296–299

Zheng, S.G., Wang, J.H.; Gray, J.D. et al. (2004) Natural and induced $CD4^{+}CD25^{+}$ cells educate $CD4^{+}CD25^{-}$ cells to develop suppressive activity: the role of IL-2, TGF-beta, and IL-10, *J Immunol*, Vol.172, pp. 5213-5221

Zinkel, S.S.; Hurov, K.E.; Ong, C. et al. (2005). A role for proapoptotic BID in the DNA-damage response. *Cell*, Vol.122, No.4, pp.579-591

Zintzaras, E.; Voulgarelis, M. & Moutsopoulos, H.M. (2005) The risk of lymphoma development in autoimmune diseases: a meta-analysis. *Arch Intern Med*, Vol. 165, No.(20), pp. 2337–44

Zou, W. (2005). Immunosuppressive networks in the tumour environment and their therapeutic relevance. *Nat Rev Cancer, Vol.* 5, pp.263–267

Zuckerman, E.; Toubi, E.; Golan, T.D. et al. (1995) Increased thromboembolic incidence in anti-cardiolipin-positive patients with malignancy. *Br J Cancer*, Vol. 72, No. (2), pp.447–51.

Part 4

Immunology of Pregnancy

20

Mechanism of Autoimmunity in Pregnancy - The Good and the Bad

Lotti Tajouri[1,2], Ekua W. Brenu[1,2],
Donald R. Staines[1,3] and Sonya M. Marshall-Gradisnik[1,2]
[1]*Population Health and Neuroimmunology Unit, Faculty of Health Science and Medicine, Bond University, Robina,*
[2]*Faculty of Health Science and Medicine, Bond University, Robina,*
[3]*Queensland Health, Gold Coast Population Health Unit, Southport, Australia*

1. Introduction

In humans, female's humoral and cellular immunity are actually stronger than men (Nalbandian & Kovats, 2005) and present a higher antibody serum titration than men (Giron-Gonzalez et al., 2000) which could logically and possibly explain their gender predisposition and susceptibility to autoimmunity. Holding an autoimmune disease and becoming pregnant is a serious matter for a woman and knowledge of the course of the condition during pregnancy is essential. Relational variations exist between types of autoimmuny during pregnancy and consequently proper advices from physicians are provided accordingly. In Systemic lupus erythematosus, all advices provided to the patients are meant to dissuade women from getting pregnant while being in a relapse stage of the disease and better wait for the end of the flare pathological course. As for Rheumatoid arthritis and multiple sclerosis, no real dangers are encountered while being pregnant and while the disease symptoms are expressed it still does not present life threatening risks to the gestation. In Myasthenia gravis, during gestation the risks are variable and retrospective studies show increase complications.

Logically, the baby carrying semi-allogenic antigens should prompt an autoimmune reaction from the mother. However a plethora of tolerance measures is put into action by both the mother and the foetus. Pre implantation immunological events are in place to best prepare the nidation of the foetus into the mother endometrium. There is large paucity of published scientific research studies that have attempted to understand the entire pregnancy immune profile due to low power studies, limiting longitudinal samplings and narrow immune component analysis. However, a recent study has shown a Th1 toTh2 shift with increase interleukin 10 synthesis and a decrease responses to pro-inflammatory cytokines such as TNFα, Il-1β and Il-6 during pregnancy (Denney et al., 2011). Immunological adaptations occur early in gestation and are mediated by the uterine epithelium including the fallopian tube secretion of granulocyte macrophage colony stimulating factors (GM-CSF) (Rosendaal, 1975). In addition, the trophoblast that is derived from the fertilized egg secretes GM-CSF to prepare best for the next step of implantation and formation of the placenta (Burgess et al., 1977). Post implantation, the placenta is formed to accommodate, protect and feed with key nutrients the growing foetus. The placenta is formed of different layers with the basal plate or deciduas basalis, a structure in direct contact with the endometrium, the intermediate layer being the lacunar system and finally the chorionic plate made of two leaflets, the chorionic plate and the amniotic plate. Interestingly, the content of the decidua is composed of different key factors aiming at inducing tolerance and include cells such as maternal Natural killers and regulatory T-cells. Natural killer cells are secreting lots of cytokines with immunoregulation purposes and are non cytotoxic (Chantakru et al., 2002). As for the regulatory T-cells, data showed that human chorionic gonadotropin hormone is responsible for the attraction of such cells in the placenta (Schumacher et al., 2009). It has also been proved that Treg are key determinants in murine pregnancy (Zenclussen et al., 2005) with possibly the mediation of interleukin 10 (Taylor et al., 2006 & Akdis et al., 2001). The relative proportion of immune cells found in the deciduas are as follows, 70% of natural killers (Moffet et al., 2004), 20% of macrophages (Lessin et al., 1988), around 2% of T lymphocytes (Lessin et al., 1988), 1% of dendritic cells (Gardner et al., 2003) and very minute B cell lymphocytes (Veenstra Van Nieuwenhoven et al., 2003). In addition, regulatory proteins decreasing complement action are found in the decidua basalis more precisely on the syncyciotrophoblast T-cells along with cellular membranar Fas ligands and MHC molecules. MHC molecules consist of class III MHC molecules but lack of particular HLAI and HLA II molecules including HLA-A and -B as well as HLA-DP, -DQ and –DR is noticed (Landek-Salgado et al., 2010). Interestingly the placenta is maintaining a tied tolerance status mediated by each of its functional molecular and cellular components playing a major role in this process. Mostly, any activated T-cells that would reach this mother-foetus interface border would be bound to Fas ligand on their Fas receptor condemning them to enter apoptosis (Pongcharoen et al., 2004). This apoptotic process is mediated by Fas pathway through the activation of the death induce signaling complex that ultimately activates the caspase apoptotic cascade. More importantly, regulatory T-cells accumulating in the decidua during pregnancy, dampen any pro-inflammatory that harm the foetus (Tilburgs et al., 2008).

Along with this immunosuppressive function, an immune tolerance is strongly put in place. Transient gestational lowering reactivity is set to prevent potent T-cells from reacting against the semi-allogenic foetus and previously demonstrated in animal studies (Tafuri et al., 1995). Immuno tolerance features that directly play roles on pro-inflammatory immune cells are relying on particular cells called T regulatory cells or Tregs (Kuniyasu et al., 2000). Tregs can be Th4 lymphocytes or T8 lymphocytes and are mostly found to act as immunomodulators in regions of inflammation (Gavin et al., 2002). The action is mediated by contact inhibition of non Treg cells such include subsets of T 4 and T8 lymphocytic cells. Specific markers are differentiating these subsets from regulatory to non regulatory effective T-cells (Teff) and include CD25 markers (α chain of IL-2 receptor) with the so called CD4+ CD25+ and CD8+CD25+ cells. Additional markers are also found in Tregs such as FoxP3+ marker, a repressor activator of activated T-cells such as CD4+CD25+FoxP3+ Treg cells or Cd8+ CD25+ CDFoxP3+ Treg cells. Another Treg marker is CXCR3+ seen in CD8+ CXCR3+ Treg cells. The Treg mediation in tolerance restoration can be undertaken through different mechanisms. Tolerance could be undertaken by contact interaction such as Fas- Fas ligand interaction dictating an apoptotic faith to the Teff cells (Watanabe et al, 2002). The other way Tregs are promoting tolerance to Teff cells is to inhibit Teff cytokine synthesis and subsequently their Teff cytolytic activation as well as diminishing their proliferation (Duthoit et al., 2005). Teff cells can be CD8+ or CD4+ cells with the latter being classified into two types, TH1 and TH2 both differing in action as pro-inflammatory and anti-inflammatory actions respectively. Briefly, the Th1 activation pathway consists in interferon γ inducing activation of its cell surface receptor on T cells and subsequent intracellular cascade activation. Such cascade leads to the activation of the transcription factor T-bet which function is to bind DNA responsive elements of genes within the nucleus. The main responsive elements controlled and activated belong to the genes interferon γ and IL-12 receptor β2 chain. Upon activation, further expression of these genes is undertaken and IL-12 receptor becomes widely available at higher amounts in the cellular T-cell membranar surface and therefore can be prompted to activation due to the presence of local IL-12 cytokine. IL-12 receptor actiavtion induces a second cascade that is Stat 4 dependent, with the ultimate goal to produce furthermore T-bet transcription factor. Relation between Tregs and pro-inflammatory TH1 and CD8+ T-cells demonstrate an interesting phenomenon that is build around the competition for Interleukin 2 binding. In sites of inflammation, binding of IL-2 by Tregs diminishes the availability of IL-2 to Teffs and therefore limiting their growth, function and even at early stage turning Teffs to be anergic towards antigens (Piccirillo et al., 2001). Briefly, T-cells are activated through the contact of antigen with T-cell receptor under the restriction of MHC class molecules. Such binding activates p56lck tyrosine kinase with subsequent downstream phosphorylation of proteins and activation of phospholipase C. Such phospholipase generates from phosphatidyl inositol diphosphate, two compounds; the diacyl glycerol and inositol tri-phosphate, IP3. The endoplasmic reticulum IP3 receptor is therefore activated with release of calcium in the cytosol. Such Ca2++ induces a membranar activation of the cell membrane calcium release activated calcium channel named CRAC and subsequently increases highly the intracellular Ca2++ concentration. High levels of Ca2++ activate caclineurin, a phosphatase that dephosphorylates the transcriptional factor NFAT (nuclear factor of activated T-cells). Such dephosphorylated NFAT translocates into the nucleus to reach responsive elements of Il-2, AP1 and NFKB enabling their expression and future function. Beside the roles of Tregs as pro-apoptotic cytolytic Teff cells inducers and Teff cells expansion inhibitors, Tregs are capable to modulate the inflammatory 'soup' and pattern observed in inflammation sites. Such action of Tregs is mediated by their synthesis and secretion of both TGFβ and interleukin 10. A higher content of Il-10 is maintained due to Teffs response to TGFβ action and secondly by Il-10 action on dictating Teffs to respond with higher affinity to TGFβ. In addition, the constant increase of progesterone in gestation, which is peaking at the third trimester, is responsible for the activation of particular subsets of T-cells called γδ T-cells. Upon binding to its receptor, progesterone activates γδ T-cells to secrete Il-10 and progesterone induced blocking factor (PIBF) that result in the inhibition of natural killer cells (Barakonyi et al., 1999). In addition, these cells synthesise TGFβ that enhances the mother's T-cell tolerance for the foetus (Mincheva-Nilsson et al., 1992).

2. Autoimmunity and pregnancy

Women are more prevalent to autoimmunity and 3 to 5% will be affected by such disorders. During pregnancy, clinical course of several autoimmune disease are expressed with variable degrees. Some range from higher remission of signs and symptoms while others are being increased in exacerbations. These influences observed in Pregnancy denote a complex interaction between the pathophysiological course of the disease and the physiological adaptations during pregnancy. Presence of a wide spectrum of auto-antibodies correlates with the parturient pathophysiological course. In some autoimmune diseases, the risk of transient neonatal illness could be observed and can range from low risk as in myasthenia gravis to relatively higher as in Lupus. Self tolerance mechanisms at the cellular and genetic levels are modulated during pregnancy by these autoimmune diseases. Such modulation might reside at different levels and include, allelic variation with the HLA loci and expression, physiological adaptations during pregnancy (hormones) and alteration towards the host immunity or the foetal antigens (paternal HLAs), cytokine profile during pregnancy, HLA from foetus (HLA-G), structural interface integrity between foetus and mother, status of intrinsic and extrinsic controls preventing autoimmunity. We aim in this review at discussing the immunological events that surround pregnancy and autoimmunity especially by focusing on Systemic lupus erythematosus, Rheumatoid arthritis, Myasthenia gravis and Multiple sclerosis.

2.1 Systemic Lupus Erythematosus

2.1.1 Pathophysiology of SLE

Systemic lupus erythematosus (SLE) is an autoimmune disease mainly affecting the connective tissue that consequently demonstrating a plethora of systemic effects mostly observed in individuals of African-Asian origin. A staggering 9:1 ratio females to males is noted with a peak age of onset in young woman between 25 and 35 years of age. More than 98% of SLE patients are positive for the antinuclear auto-antibody (ANA), a marker of the disease. Other auto-antibodies are used to better refine the diagnosis of SLE and include anti cytoplasmic and anti DNA antibodies. The pathology shows a diverse range of symptoms affecting several organs ranging from common cutaneous lesions, serous membrane alteration and intermittent joints debilitations. More precisely, facial malar rashes, arthralagia, polyathritis, pleurisy, pericarditis are experienced along with other symptoms like Raynand's phenomenon and fever. The etiology of this complex disease is unknown but several hypotheses have been raised. Cellular release of antigens from apoptotic and necrotic cells is raised that will trigger macrophage phagocytosis and subsequent antigen presentation, under MHC class II, of such autoantigens to both T and B-cells. Intracellular and extracellular signaling are thought to be dysregulated such as the so called interferon signature, a cytokine profile under scrutiny as links with IRF5 has been shown to be associated with SLE (Graham et al., 2006). CD19 positive B-cells are of high attention in research as several auto-antibodies are pathogenic in the disease such as the anti nuclear antibodies (Madaio et al., 2003).

The genetics of SLE has pinpointed several chromosomal loci with interestingly the 1q23-24 region also called the pentraxin locus, a region harboring some key candidates including the CRP4 allele gene and the PDCD1 gene. A single nucleotide polymorphism in the PDCD1 gene was found to disrupt an intronic enhancer that prevents the gene from further activation with subsequent apoptotic process alterations. Other hypotheses have been investigated such as the possible occupational exposure or environmental effects but with no direct significant links to the disease. An interesting phenomenon though is well documented with the attention on precipitating factors. Such precipitating factors seen in SLE are the intake of oral estrogen contraceptives and hormonal replacement therapies (HRT) (Sanchez-Guerrero et al., 1997). Several studies including a nurse health study for oral contraceptive use have shown an increase of 1.9 time SLE manifestations compared to non users (Sanchez-Guerrero et al., 1995) and similar effect have been demonstrated with HRT (Cooper et al., 2002). In addition a lot of evidence is showing that the SLE manifestations are correlated with ovarian cycle alterations (Shabanova et al., 2008). A clear link is seen between hormonal changes and SLE therefore higher vigilance is sought for SLE women willing to become pregnant.

2.1.2 Modulation effects of pregnancy in SLE mothers

Pregnancy presents as a life experience where mother's hormonal levels are evolutionally and physiologically adapting to host the baby. Careful monitoring is undertaken as different gestational outcome scenarios are observed, with some being unpredictable, due to recurrence of flares and possible life threatening issues affecting both the mother and the child. Such dangers ranges from intra-uterine growth retardations in 30% of cases (Meyer Oliver, 2003), preterm birth with 25-30% of cases to miscarriages and foetal death. Co-morbidity is most likely to be observed in SLE patients with increase manifestation of the disease in the third trimester of gestation. Lots of evidence show detrimental effects to the kidney such as lupus nephritis, and atheroslcerotic pathophysiological establishments (Roman et al., 2003 and Asanuma et al., 2003) all to which can be further aggravated with other common pregnancy experienced problems like seen with preeclampsia occurrence. Death of the mother can be observed with common SLE risks due to high elevations of pulmonary hypertension. In 37% of SLE pregnant patients, mild increased of pulmonary arterial hypertension can be seen (Johnson et al., 2004). Such monitoring requires the use of several tests, serum antibodies, choice of specific medication, compliance with hydroxychloroquine, as well as the monitoring of SLE disease activity index (SLEDAI) measuring the flaring panel observed in SLE patients. Interestingly, SLE patients would have positive benefits and gains to start their gestation in period of remission before conception. An otherwise preconception with active disease otherwise shows increased flares with particularly renal disease associated problems (Moroni et al., 2002). In addition, lower birth weigths and high number of caesarian deliveries are encountered in proliferative nephritis cohorts. Foetal loss in SLE is a major problem with several studies attempting to link this fatal outcome to molecular triggering factors. The Hughes syndrome is a phospholipid induced pregnancy syndrome commonly named the antiphospholipid syndrome. Such syndrome is part of the coagulopathy diseases and SLE pregnant women are commonly tested for the presence of lupus anticoagulant factor, an anti phospholipid factor named anti-cardiolipin. This immunoglobulin G anti-cardiolipin antibody targets the apoprotein H or beta 2 glycoprotein 1. Such antibody prevents the glycoprotein from undertaking its possible known function as an inhibitor of the intrinsic coagulation cascade, an inhibition required and mediated by the release of complement molecules, C3 and C5 from the liver. As a consequence, SLE mothers with increase anti-ApoH denote a procoagulant pattern with detrimental foetal loss as an outcome. Interestingly, with treatment regimens of aspirin and heparin intakes, levels of live birth rates from SLE pregnant patients is now around 80% (Clark et al., 2007 and Girardi et al., 2004). Several markers for the disease have been found to better classify and understand the pathological course.

Efforts of the research community have helped in the discovery of a series of serum markers for SLE such as adipokine, a cell to cell signaling protein secreted by the adipose tissue (De Sanctis et al., 2009), CD40L or CD154 found in T-cell surface (De Sanctis et al., 2009 b) and the poly-reactive immunoglobulin M from B-cells (Zhang et al., 2009). All these markers denote an intense cell to cell communication and intense modulatory involvement of the immune system. Both arms of the immunity system are involved in SLE and particular attentions are drawn to further unravel the pathophysiological mechanism in SLE patient's immunity. SLE immune dysregulation involves a role to T-cell activation (Fernandez et al., 2009), B-cell signaling (Liu et al., 2009 and Peng, 2009) along with altered chemokine patterns (Youinou et al., 2009 and Wittmann et al., 2009) with IL-6 playing a role in polyarthritis and joint damage (Fonseca et al., 2009) and as mentioned previously an interferon signature (Finke et al., 2009).

The complex cascade of T-cell activation from the T-cell receptor (TCR) the consequently increase in intracellular content of $Ca2++$ and NFAT mediated IL-2 Transcriptional activation is an important immune component in SLE. In SLE, such pathway of activation is altered and seems to be associated with the calcium processing. ER calcium content not being an issue, a lot of attention was given to CRAC and studies have shown altered efficiency in this $Ca2+$ channel. Evidence has also shown that in SLE patients a $Ca+$ alteration was observed and linked to an upstream mitochondrial dysregulation. Evidence of high membrane hyperpolarisation (MHP) of the inner membrane of the mitochondrial has been pinpointed in SLE T-cells with subsequent ATP decreasing synthesis and failure to regenerate glutathione reduced forms, a anti oxidant molecule. Such dysregulation seems to be as well the cause of the unbalance fate observed in SLE T-cells deaths. Instead of progressing to a program cell death, with the common FAS pathway and death inducing signaling complex cascade, SLE T-cells instead enter necrosis. As both ATP and reduced glutathione pools are low, apoptosis is prevented and as such unbalance of quality cell death tends to develop into two main consequences. First, necrosis is favored and induces inflammation whereas apoptotic bodies do not. Secondly, in SLE, such overall dysregulation of calcium (katsiari et al., 2002), ATP formation (Perl et al., 2004) and low antioxidant capacity profile (Wang et al., 2010) is in favor to auto-reactive T-cells.

A strong correlation has been found between CXCL10 and SLE disease (Kong et al., 2009). CXCL10 is the interferon inducible factor, chemokine (C-X-C motif) ligand 10 also known as IP10 that acts on the receptor CXCR3. Interestingly, the gene coding for such receptor is the unique chemokine receptor found in chromosome X. This is in clear contrast to all other chemokine receptor genes, suggesting unique functions for CXCR3 and the ligand CXCL10 in possibly the role in SLE immunity. In sites of inflammation, a subset of B-cells with high expression of the marker CD19, a co-receptor of the B-cell receptor and known to be implicated in auto-immuniy, shows elevated CXCR3 levels (Nicholas et al., 2007). More challenges are met during pregnancy where placental tissues and the new born semi-allogenic foetal cells are brought together along with SLE (Doria et al., 2008). High consequences were recently tabulated in pregnant women with SLE with approximately 25% of women presenting with disease exacerbations (Lockshin et al., 1989).

2.2 Myasthenia and pregnancy

2.2.1 Pathophysiology of myasthenia gravis

Besides T-cells, breakdown of self tolerance in autoimmune diseases can be associated with humoral B-cell mediated immunity producing pathological auto-antibodies contributing to tissue damage as seen in myasthenia gravis (MG). MG is an autoimmune disease affecting predominantly women with clinical muscle fatigability with patients suffering from degrees of weakness at various body systems. Under approximately 40 years of age, women are prevalent but after 50 years of age, incidence is then lesser in women than men. (Grob et al., 2008). The disease is categorised into two clinical presentations with on one hand, the ocular MG affecting of the levator and extra ocular palpebrae skeletal muscles with common diplopia and ptosis and in the other hand, generalised MG affecting other skeletal muscles. Interestingly, the disease can occur as relapsing remitting and the onset of symptomatology is varying from acute to subacute. Auto-antibodies target different antigens including the acetylcholine receptor (AchR) and, in most intense disease presentation, target the muscle specific muscle protein named MuSK (Padua et al., 2006). AchR and MusK seropositivity lead to neuromuscular dysfunctions. In the case of anti AChR, the antibodies trigger neutralisation of AChR function (Drachman et al., 1982), as well as antibody dependent complement activation with membrane attack complex formation (Engel et al., 1987) and finally antibody cross link with the ACHR leading to the destruction of AChR. The early onset MG is also associated with the possible occurrence of other autoimmune insults most commonly against the thyroid (Christensen, 1995). In early onset MG, the thymus gland is enlarged and patients present with multiple auto-antibodies. However, late onset MG is not associated with enlarged thymus. Association of HLA markers with individual type of MG onset has been undertaken and data showed that the early onset MG is associated with HLA-B8 and DR3 (Compston et al., 1980) whereas late onset MG is associated with HLA B7 and DR2 (Maggi et al., 1991). Immunologically the thymus is a primary lymphoid organ with a highly responsible function to maturate T-cells. T-cells that were produced in the bone marrow enter the thymus to become thymocytes to undergo a subsequent series of selection. The whole thymus is built to this process with a well vascularised content, clusters of different types of cells including antigen presenting cells such as macrophages, dendritic cells and parenchymal epithelial cells. When maturation of thymocytes is terminated, an efferent drainage successfully drains these cells into mediastinal lymph nodes. This selection is aiming at positively selecting immature T-cells which T-cell receptor would recognise MHC molecules. In the other hand, the negative selection aims at discarding the T-cells that would react to autoantigens presented by APCs. A failure in undertaking the removal of autoimmune T-cells is thought to be the problem occurring in MG disease. Certain T-cells, Th4 or CD4 + were investigated for their possible cell mediated autoimmune dysregulations. Interestingly though, both patients and free of disease normal individuals do have autoimmune T-cells targeting AChR (Schluep et al., 1987). Using experimental autoimmune **myasthenia** gravis (EAMG) animal models with Th1 deficient cells, researchers have shown actually that such animals have susceptibility to autoimmunity (Balasa et al., 1997). In this latter study, the focus was to distinguish between wild type and EAMG interferon gamma knockout mice. Result showed that EAMG knockout mice had no weakness to their muscles and were resistance to MG. However, the level of proliferation of AChR primed lymph nodes was still proliferating as normally observed in wild type mice. As interferon gamma is the primary pro-inflammatory stimulator of TH1 cells with downstream activation of the T-bet transcription factor inducing further interferon gamma transcription, MG autoimmunity induced solely with Th1 cannot be explaining the entire course of the disease. Even other types of autoimmunity such as in multiple sclerosis experimental allergic encephalomyelitis animals, observation of both interferon gamma deficient mice and T-bet knockout mice did not protect these autoimmunity disorders (Ferber et al., 1996). In Balasa et al. study, lymphogenic changes using mice with intact thymus were investigated but researchers focus is also turned into directly thymectomized animals. The thymic tissue is also harboring regulatory T-cells CD4+ CD25+ cells or Tregs that are anergic to antigen presentation (Crispin et al., 2003). These cells act as suppressors of effective autoimmune T-cells as demonstrated in Tregs deficient animal studies showing increase signs of autoimmunity disorders (Sakaguchi et al., 1995). Particular markers on the surface of Tregs are responsible for the immunological self tolerance function of Treg and include CD80, CD28, CD40 and CTLA4 with the later being a strong negative regulator of T-cell activity. Other subsets of cells called CD4+ CD25+ CD103+ are showing furthermore potentials in self tolerance and suppressive functional features in comparison to CD4+ CD25+ T-cells.

2.2.2 Modulation effects of pregnancy in Myasthenia gravis mothers

T-cells detain estrogen receptors on their membrane and studies have shown a high correlation between estrogens and disease detrimental activity. Interestingly, estrogens induce an expansion of specific Th1 effector cells with subsequent MG autoimmunity and increase of anti AChR antibodies (Delpy et al., 2005). In normal pregnancy, Tregs mediate immune tolerance (Guerin et al., 2009) and data previous data show that in early pregnancy estrogens do act on these CD4+ CD25+ T-cells to mediate indeed immunosuppression and higher immune tolerance. Such effect is relayed by progesterone during the rest of the gestation (Mao et al., 2010). Such positive effect might resign in the difference between CD4+ CD25+ and CD4+ CD25- T-cells. Differential gene expression of these two subsets showed higher expression levels of CTLA4, galactin, CD103, TNFRSF18, TNFRSF4 and the glucocorticoid induced TNF receptor called GITR (McHugh et al., 2002) in CD4+ CD25+ cells. Interestingly, inhibition of GITR abrogates regulatory T-cell activity precipitating autoimmunity. In addition, GITR can be activated by progesterone receptor (Nelson et al., 1999 and Kanamaru et al., 2004) and possibly progesterone acts on Treg cells by upregulating GITR among other effects. Interestingly, in studies experimenting EAMG animals, the treatment of analogs of myasthenogenic peptides notably demonstrated a decrease in lymph node proliferation as well as a decrease of INFγ involving the action of CD8+ Tregs (Ben-David et al., 2007).
Newborn can develop neonatal MG and is observed in around 10 % of mother holding the burden of the disease (Beekman etal., 1997). This acquisition is mediated by the passage from the mother to the foetus of immunoglobulin G anti acetylcholine receptors. In large majority, babies do not pursue the course of neonatal MG and few weeks following their birth, neonatal MG naturally undergo full resolution.

2.3 Rheumatoid arthritis and pregnancy

2.3.1 Pathophysiology of rheumatoid arthritis

Rheumatoid arthritis is a severe chronic inflammatory disease of relatively high prevalence that primarily affects the joints via a systemic autoimmune reaction. While its aetiology remains unknown, many cell populations contribute to the inflammatory response in the synovium, leading to joint erosions, joint deformation and loss of function. Histological features often include proliferation of synovial cells, plasma and lymphoid cell infiltration, neovascularisation, macrophage accumulation and typical palisading structure of the cell lining hyperblasting synovial membranes. One particular hallmark used in diagnosis of RA is the rheumatoid factor (RF) and the particular association with HLA-DR4. Common cytokine abnormalities in RA include an increase in tumor necrosis factor alpha (TNFα) and interleukin-1β (IL-1β) with subsequent induction of metalloproteinases (MMPs) degrading the synovial matrix (Dayer et al., 2001). Gene expression studies sampling synovial tissue have highlighted the heterogeneous nature of the disease and suggest the existence and contribution of multiple pathogenic pathways (van der Pouw Kraan et al. 2003). As tissue biopsies are invasive, alternative and clinically more practical studies of gene expression changes in peripheral blood mononuclear cells (PBMC) from patients with RA have been reported (Olsen et al., 2004 & Edwards et al., 2007), with a recent study highlighting that 10 differentially regulated transcripts in RA patient PBMC mapped to chromosome region 6p21.3, the major histocompatibility (MHC) locus III (Edwards et al., 2007). In addition to the cellular involvement, Rheumatoid arthritis is an auto-antibody disorder that will ultimately affect the joints. Antibodies like IgM and IgA are known to target the Fc fragments of IgG but in addition targeted citrullinated antigens are found in RA patients but are not exclusive to these patients. The autoimmune attack mainly is associated with elevated amounts of Tumor necrosis factor (Feldmann et al., 1996) and elevation of specific joint cells (found in both cartilage and synovium). The synovium contains macrophage like synovial cells and fibroblast like synovial cells. In RA, the joint macrophage like cells are known to secrete a large panel of pro-inflammatory cytokines whereas the fibroblast like cells are showing invasive the cartilage (Muller-Ladner et al., 1996) and are responsible, at some extent, to joint destruction with osteoclastic activity (Tolboom et al., 2005). Interestingly, inhibiting and preventing osteoclast induce destruction of the joints is not associated cessation of the overall localised pro-inflammatory profile (Cohen et al., 2008). Common therapeutic agents used in treating RA include disease-modifying anti-rheumatic drugs (DMARDs), such as methotrexate, non steroidal anti-inflammatory drugs (NSAIDs), corticosteroids and Tumor Necrosis Factor (TNF) inhibitors which inhibit the pro-inflammatory activity of TNF, identified as a key mediator in the inflammatory response. Despite the improvement of joint function in 60-80% of patients with TNF inhibitors and methotrexate combination therapy, a remaining 20-40% of patients do not respond to this treatment (Baton et al., 2000 & Keystone et al., 2004 & Maini et al., 2004).

2.3.2 Modulation effects of pregnancy in Rheumatoid Arthritis mothers

In pregnancy, RA signs are improved in more than 76% of cases (Pope et al., 1983) but beneficial signs disappear postpartum for approximately 6 to 8 months post delivery. These gestational ameliorations seem to be independent of cortisol rises in pregnancy and independent to administration of different exogenous estrogen levels (Van den Brink et al., 1992). Of note, twenty five percent of RA pregnant women have continuing active arthritis. Interestingly two reports reported that pregnancy decreases by two fold in RA when compared to nulliparous RA women (Spector et al., 1990 & Hazes et al., 1990). During pregnancy, important tolerance occurs in RA. Auto-reactive B cells in RA are somewhat down-regulated since serum levels of alloantibodies remain the same while improvement in the severity is observed (Elenkov et al., 1997). Autoantibodies such as ANA have been reported to decrease in RA pregnancy (Ostensen et al., 1983) as well as the rheumatoic factor, RF (Pope et al., 1983). Interstingly, the disparity between the foetus and the mother seems to be positive for the pregnancy course in RA (Nelson et al, 1993). The impact of the disease on pregnancy and outcomes of RA to gestation seem to show no adverse effects with RA women falling pregnant and giving birth with no life threatening consequences. However, postpartum flares are high and possibly aggravated due to high correlated levels of prolactin postpartum (Zrour et al., 2010). The influence of pregnancy on RA disease is still unknown and no explannations to date are given for the reasons for observing either remission or none of RA during pregnancy. As for the remissions, attention is dedicated to the maternofetal HLA incompatibility but investigations is generating contrasting reports (Brennan et al., 2000). As for what is possibly occuring in RA and pregancy, a hormonal conditioning mediated by estradiol and progesterone contribute to a shift from TH1 to Th2 immune profile (Ekerfelt et al., 1997) and suppression of both autoreactive T cells and NK cells (Otensen & Villiger, 2002).

2.4 Multiple Sclerosis and pregnancy

2.4.1 Pathophysiology of Multiple Sclerosis

MS is a neurological debilitating disorder that affects particularly Caucasians in their second to fourth decades of their life (Weinshenker BG, 1998). MS was characterised for the first time, by Dr Jean Martin Charcot in 1868 from the hospital "Salpêtrière", in Paris who reported the presence of multiple plaques in the central nervous system (CNS) of a deceased patient. Despite the progress of research in the last 150 years the aetiology of MS remains still unknown.

The disorder is well documented for its neuroinflammatory course and symptoms. The disease has particular hallmarks and is more prevalent in women, and symptoms appear typically between 20 and 40 years of age (Weinshenker BG, 1998). Females account for approximately 60% of MS cases (Weinshenker BG et al., 1994). There are several forms of MS, characterised by the degree of symptomatic debilitation over time: Benign MS (B-MS), Relapsing Remitting MS (RR-MS), Secondary Progressive (SP-MS), Progressive-Relapsing MS (PR-MS), Primary Progressive MS (PP-MS). MS plaques appear as lesions in the normal white matter (NWM) and occasionally in the gray matter (Peterson et al., 2001). Lesions are restricted to the CNS and are not present in the peripheral nervous system (PNS). Plaques are classified into three main types: acute (A), chronic active (CA) and chronic silent (CS) MS lesions. Acute MS lesions are not well-demarcated (oedematous) and are filled with macrophages commonly containing myelin debris. Additionally, these lesions contain hypertrophic astrocytes but no fibrous astrogliosis with an abundance of demyelinated axons. This plaque-type is characterised by the presence of perivascular lymphocytic infiltration and damaged of the blood brain barrier (BBB) (Gay et al., 1991). Chronic active MS lesions, are the second type and do contain a well-demarcated margin. In this case the centre of the plaque is lacking in lymphocyte activity. Instead macrophages reside in a margin which contains the debris of myelin degeneration. These macrophages are microglia in origin. The centre of a CA plaque is astrogliotic, with a generally absence of myelin. However, in this case the centre of CA lesions is characterised by signs of remyelination.

In contrast to both CA and A lesions, CS MS lesions have a highly demarcated margin with a fibrous centre with no inflammatory component. Remyelination can occur in the centre and within the margin. These plaques appear circular and differ from other forms of demyelination (eg. Balo's syndrome). Balo's syndrome, is characterised by alternate rings of degeneration and regeneration (or intact myelin)(Moore et al., 1985). MS also has an autoimmune component, characterised by infiltration in the CNS of activated T-cells that are auto-reactive to myelin white matter proteins. MS is also more prevalent at higher latitudes of the globe (Hernan et al., 1999), suggesting a strong environmental influence; while disease susceptibility has a strong genetic link, as evidenced by numerous twin studies (Mumford et al., 1994). Symptoms include limb weakness, sensory loss, visual alterations and bladder dysfunction, and the appearance of lesions or plaques that are disseminated in time and space. Multiple sclerosis is an autoimmune disease of the central nervous system, characterized by zones of demyelination and inflammatory plaques.

The genetic of MS has been extensively researched and a major focus in comparison to other autoimmune diseases. Studies appreciating the concordance of twins have shown a six time increase in risk in monozygoting than among dizogotic twins (Sadovnick et al, 1993).

2.4.1.1 The Major Histocompatibility Complex (MHC) and Multiple Sclerosis

The MHC Locus on Chromosome 6p has been linked to the pathogenenesis of MS with the fundamental basis of this association being established as a strong association with HLA-DRB1*15 of the class II gene *HLA-DRB1*(Fogdell et al., 1995). In addition to the problem in exploring possible etiological reasons behind MS, epistatic interaction across alleles are taking place that even are mors of a risky as seen with *HLA-DRB1*08,* on interaction with *HLA-DRB1*15.* A number of genes have been implicated in MS pathophysiology and were discovered throughout both immunological and genetic studies. One of the most consistent findings has been an association of specific major histocompatibility class II haplotypes in MS (Kellar-Wood et al., 1995). The MHC region in 6p21.3, includes MHC I, II and III. As all evidences are supporting an autoimmune basis for MS, the MHC locus is the focus of a lot of research attention as the genes in this locus are involved in antigen presentation. Class I and class II are involved in antigen presentation to CD8 and CD4 lymphocytes respectively. Class I has a region containing HLA loci (HLA A, B, C, E, F, G) known to be altered in normal pregnancy especially at the placental border between the foetus and the mother. Association between MS and molecules on the chromosome 6p21 is variable to the type of population studied. Northern European populations affected with MS do show an association with Class II DR15 and DQ6 phenotypes in (Hillert, 1994). In the other hand, Asians with MS are associated with DPB1 (Ito et al., 1998).

The MHC Class II locus is composed of genes coding for proteins LMP2 (proteasome subunit, beta type, 9) and LMP7 (proteasome subunit, beta type, 7), two protein being integrative of the proteasome complex. Normally, viral proteins or cellular proteins are turned into small peptides by the proteasome. These fragmented petides are then entering the reticulum endoplasmic (RE) binding with new synthesised MHC class I molecules. Both molecules are then deposited to the surface cell where the peptide is then presented to vigilant immune cells. The translocation into the RE is facilitated by the transporter 1, ATP-binding cassette (TAP) 1 and 2 which are coded by genes in the MHC Class II region. Studies attempted to demonstrate a probable association between TAP1 and TAP2 locus polymorphisms but data showed no association with MS (Vandevyver et al., 1994). However, the same study revealed though a differential level of gene expression of these two genes between affected and non-affected tissues. Interestingly, a lot of attention was brought into a region 100kb telomeric to HLA F. This locus harbors the myelin oligodendrocyte glycoprotein (MOG), another potential candidate gene in multiple sclerosis as it plays an important role in myelin sheath maintenance and immunogenicity. Experiments using antisera raised against MOG would activate a downstream signaling pathway resulting in the degradation of microtubules and disruption of myelin basic protein (MBP) (Johns et al., 1999). This pathway is also triggered by antibodies of a marker of myelin-producing cells, the galactolipid galactocerebroside, that was illustrated in glioma cells (Joshi et al., 1992), with possibly engaging a second messenger (most likely Inositol Phosphate 3) activating a voltage Ca^{2+} channel (Joshi et al., 1998) that ultimately results into in an increase of intracellular calcium and microtubule disruption.

In the Class III MHC region, candidate genes possibly implicated in MS pathology include the steroid enzyme 21-hydroxylase gene (CYP21A2) and heat shock proteins (HSP): HSP70-1 and HSP70-2. In addition, MHC class III region contains genes coding for complement molecules of the immune system and interestingly the tumour necrosis factor genes (TNFα and TNFβ). In Multiple sclerosis, TNFα has been shown to be toxic to oligodendrocytes and myelin (Wingerchuk et al., 1997). In MS plaques, TNFβ is present and is at the origin of tissue repair (De Groot et al., 1999). Some studies have investigated TNFα polymorphisms (Wingerchuk et al., 1997) however no association was found with MS except in HLA-DR2+ MS patients compared with HLA-DR2- individuals (Oturai et al., 1999). Studies investigating Caucasians of European descent have shown that class II HLA alleles are more strongly associated with the HLA-DR2 haplotype in MS (Haines et al., 1998).
Noteworthy a predominant immunological hallmark of multiple sclerosis is the important clonal expansion of class I MHC T8 lymphocytes observed in MS (Gay et al., 1997).

2.4.1.2 Immunological mechanism involved in MS

The immune system response is comprised of two immune systems: humoral and cellular. In the case of MS, both systems apply resulting in CNS inflammation coupled with degeneration in myelin sheath. A plethora of cells may be involved in this disorder including microglial cells (macrophages of the CNS), B and T lymphocytes, natural killer cells and peripheral macrophages (Li et al., 1993). Their activities are coupled with the secretion of activating signals such as cytokines and interleukines that upon production affect surrounding cells. It has been reported that auto-reactive T-cells exist in the peripheral blood from both MS affected and healthy individuals (Lindert et al., 1999). In order to reach the CNS, the immune cells have to cross through the BBB but only activated T-cells can penetrate this fence. However, it has been reported that in MS the BBB undergoes a breakdown resulting in facilitated passage of immune cells (McDonald et al., 1992). The activation of T-cells is supposed to be due to a misguided immune response secondary to cross recognition of epitopes shared between a microbial pathogen and a putative antigen in the CNS (Wucherpfennig et al., 1995). These CNS-antigen specific T-cells transmigrate through the endothelial BBB by secreting and expressing adhesion molecules such as selectins and integrins (Monteyne et al., 1997). The T-cells occupy the CNS in regions where further events take place. Furthermore, once they have occupied the CNS, the T-cells stimulate the entry of further immune cells such as peripheral macrophages. Passage of macrophages in the CNS is facilitated by the T-cell induced BBB disruption due to secretion of activated matrix metalloproteases (MMPs). In the cerebrospinal fluid of MS patients, a high gelatinase (MMP9) concentration has been found (Rosenberg et al., 1996). Gelatinase B breaks down the BBB and its inhibition, by serine protease inhibitors, shows a protective effect on the MS animal model, EAE Lewis rats (Brosnan et al., 1980). In the parenchymal of the CNS, T-cells are reactivated with the myelin antigen proximity and secrete a vast group of pro-inflammatory agents such as interferon gamma (INFγ), tumour necrosing factor alpha and beta (TNFα and TNFβ), interleukin 2 (IL-2) (Olsson et al., 1995). IL-2 is an autocrine interleukin triggering a T-cell auto-activation loop process. On both astrocytes and microglial cells, those inflammatory mediators trigger an up-regulation of MHC class II molecules. The increase of MHC class II molecules at the surface of these cells improves the amount of antigen presenting cells. Moreover, microglia as well as T lymphocytes are developing a proliferating process in response of INFγ action (Martino et al., 1995 & Grau et al., 1997). Interestingly, T-bet knockout mice show resistance to autoimmunity (Bettelli et al., 2004).

Activated astrocytes trigger an up-regulation of adhesion molecules at the surface of the BBB (Weiss et al., 1998). Chemo-attractants are produced such as the monocyte chemo-attractant protein 1 (MCP-1) (Van Der Voon et al., 1999) that chemically orientate peripheral phagocytes towards the BBB. The BBB endothelium is thus facilitated for further influx of inflammatory cells such as macrophages. Even macrophages disrupt the BBB with the secretion of neurotoxins (Brosnan et al., 1981). Secondly, activated astrocytes are able to excrete more pro-inflammatory molecules that turn the local CNS microglia (CNS resident macrophages) into ameboid microglia, a more active macrophage state. The activated astrocytes excrete factors such as GM-CSF (granulocyte monocyte-colony stimulating factor) whose role is to induce the proliferation of the ameboid cells.

The local microglia plays an important role in local antigen presentation in the CNS of EAE animals (Bauer et al., 1994) allowing an immune response. The microglia is expressing B7 (Dangond et al., 1997) and vascular cell adhesion molecule (VCAM-1). These two molecules bind CD28 and the very late antigen 4 (VLA4) respectively, on the surface of T-cells (Chabot et al., 1997) and these molecular interactions affect T-cell activation. Complement receptors (CR1 and CR2) are also found and are molecules that allow the binding of complement coated targets to phagocytosis. Complement activation constitutes the major component mechanism of humoral immunity. Contact with complement permits a better activation of the microglia but also the release of TNFα and interleukins (IL-1 and IL-6) (Rajan et al., 1996). Microglia express receptors for Fc fragments of immunoglobulins (Ulvestad et al., 1994) and completes an association action with B-lymphocytes. Those B-lymphocytes, fewer in numbers, can pass the damaged BBB and produce antibodies against myelin proteins (Gerritse et al., 1994). The antibodies are observed, after a lumbo-puncture, in CSF from MS patients appearing as oligoclonal bands in agarose gel electrophoresis. T-cell infiltration in the CNS not only induces microglial activation but also triggers the recruitment of high numbers of macrophages (Hulkower et al., 1993).

Besides inflammation, demyelination is the second most characteristic feature of MS pathology. Both microglia and macrophages are capable of ingesting myelin in EAE animals (Rinner et al., 1995). However, oligodendrocytes do not express MHC calls II molecules so CD4+T-cells cannot have a direct effect. Studies have shown that both complement and immunoglobulins are detected on oligodendrocytes and microglia in MS brain but none of the studies have ever shown the complement system alone (Fabry et al., 1994). Oligodendrocytes are damaged via antibody cell mediated cytotoxicity (ADCC) triggered by microglia, macrophages with the help of T4+, B-cells and complements molecules (Ozawa et al., 1994). The macrophages act as APCs via the major histocompatibility molecule class II. Their activities are indicators of ongoing demyelination activity (Li et al., 1993). Furthermore, the interaction of B-cells with T4 cells (CD40-CD40L) turns the B-lymphocytes into APCs, which in consequence increase the myelinotoxic activity. Antibodies to CD 40 ligand (CD 40L) can prevent the MS like disease in EAE animals (Boon et al., 2001). MBP-specific CD8+ T-cells are detected in MS plaques and have been shown to be cytotoxic in vitro on HLA-A2 not HLA-A3 transfected oligodendrocyte cell lines in the presence of MBP peptide 110-118 (Jurewicz et al., 1998).

2.4.2 Modulation effects of pregnancy in Multiple Sclerosis mothers

A first and remarkable large prospective study was undertaken to monitor MS and pregnancy relation and finally counseling MS pregnant women for their venture into pregnancy (Confavreux et al, 1998). MS disease does not affect the outcome of pregnancy and interestingly from the first to the successive trimesters of gestation, a decrease in exacerbation rates is observed with at the third trimester a decrease of 87.5% of relapse rates (Confavreux et al., 1998). This gestational decrease in symptomatology is directly observed with a decrease of MS MRI abnormalities in the CNS in MS pregnant women (Van Walderveen et al., 1994). Most interestingly MS patients entering pregnancy even show a reduced MS progressive course and severity in comparison to controls (Runmarker et al., 1995 & Verdru et al., 1994). No differences in rates of caesarians are seen in MS (Mueller et al., 2002). A lot of attention is driven towards obvious gestational steroids such as estrogens and progesterone. Previous studies have shown the autoimmune protection of estrogens which action decrease TNF-α secretion from microglial cells (Dimayuga et al., 2005) and the neurosteroid enhancement effects of progesterone on myelin formation (Jung-Testas et al., 1999). Progesterone has been shown to act on myelination in the peripheral nervous system with marked remyelination following cryo-lesions in mouse sciatic nerves (Koenig et al., 2000). Progesterone acts on its receptor, progesterone receptor (PGR), a receptor localized in Chromosome 11q12, a locus with denotes slight association in MS susceptibility in Australia (Ban et al, 2003). In animals, progesterone shows remarkable actions as a neuro-protector agent (Singh et al., 2008). Activation of the PR by progesterone exerts immunosuppressive roles by directly inhibiting a subunit of NF-κB, a well known intermediate of the pro-inflammatory molecule TNF alpha action (Kalkhoven et al., 1996). In addition, it has been demonstrated that progesterone exerts a protective role on damage brain tissues (Cutler et al., 2007) especially in Traumatic Brain Injuries (TBI) (VanLandingham et al., 2007).

A very interesting study has been undertaken to assess the immunogenic activity occurring in MS pregnancy (Saraste et al., 2007). Natural killer cells and B and T-cells populations with both CD4+ and CD8 + T-cells were all assessed during pregnancy in MS with staggering results showing a decrease from first to third trimester of nearly 40% of NK count in blood of MS patients to then increase by 53% by three months postpartum. In healthy pregnant women a same trend of decrease in NK population is observed (Saraste et al., 2007). This fluctuation of such important innate immunity cellular component is obviously strongly altered by pregnancy and accomplished seen in MS women. Steroids such as progesterone were investigated to establish their roles on NK cells and it has been shown that progesterone induces apoptosis of mature peripheral blood natural killers CD16+ CD56 dim (Arruvito et al., 2008). In Saraste et al. study, an important hallmark demonstrated though a grand difference in CD4+/CD8+ ratios in MS pregnant women versus healthy pregnant women. In From the first to third trimester, MS pregnant women have a CD4+/CD8+ ratio of 1.9 that increase to 2.7 in the third trimester whereas healthy pregnant women showed an inverse trend from 2.4 to 1.6. Authors attempted to give an explanation by seeing such trend as either an increase in T regulatory T-cells or the act that T-cells were prevented from reaching the CNS in pregnancy.

In contrary to gestational time, post partum MS condition is associated with an increase of relapse rate (Bernardi et al., 1991) to resume back to baseline values approximately three months post partum (Roullet et al.,1993). Breast feeding is not affecting the postpartum relapse rate frequency and could be encouraged by the physician except if particular drug treatments are in use (Nelson et al., 1988).

3. Conclusion

The following review was aimed at understanding the interactive relation of the physiological gestational adaptations in coexistence with particular autoimmune diseases. Discussion focused on four diseases that include SLE, MS, MG and RA. Such relation is of no doubt a very complicating process that progressively starts to unravel. Thanks to the overall international research on both the pathogenic mechanism of autoimmunity and enhancement of gestational immunity understanding, new hypothesises and more importantly more insights are found. A powerful physiological protective process occurs in pregnancy, a process strong enough to demonstrate decrease symptomatology in MS, RA and MG pregnancies. In the other hand, SLE pregnancies do not follow such trend and even is showing further aggravation. Mothers are facing a double challenge by undertaking all physiological adaptations of their pregnancy and going through these autoimmune diseases. Steroid hormones play an important role and attempt to orchestrate the foeto-maternal immunological cross communication. In addition regulatory T cells are the direct biological 'diplomats' that taking act on immune-modulating this complex biological enigma.

4. References

Akdis CA, Blaser K. Mechanisms of interleukin-10-mediated immune suppression. Immunology. 2001 Jun;103(2):131-6. Review.

Asanuma Y, Oeser A, Shintani AK, Turner E, Olsen N, Fazio S, Linton MF, Raggi P, Stein CM. Premature coronary-artery atherosclerosis in systemic lupus erythematosus. N Engl J Med. 2003 Dec 18;349(25):2407-15.

Ashley Moffett, Lesley Regan, Peter Braude. Natural killer cells, miscarriage, and infertility. BMJ. 2004 NOV;329.

Balasa B, Deng C, Lee J, Bradley LM, Dalton DK, Christadoss P, Sarvetnick N. Interferon gamma (IFN-gamma) is necessary for the genesis of acetylcholine receptor-induced clinical experimental autoimmune myasthenia gravis in mice. J Exp Med. 1997 Aug 4;186(3):385-91.

Ban M, Sawcer SJ, Heard RN, Bennetts BH, Adams S, Booth D, Perich V, Setakis E, Compston A, Stewart GJ. A genome-wide screen for linkage disequilibrium in Australian HLA-DRB1*1501 positive multiple sclerosis patients. J Neuroimmunol. 2003;143(1-2):60-4.

Barakonyi A, Polgar B, Szekeres-Bartho J. The role of gamma/delta T-cell receptor-positive cells in pregnancy: part II. Am J Reprod Immunol. 1999 Aug;42(2):83-7.

Barcellos LF, Thomson G, Carrington M, Schafer J, Begovich AB, Lin P, Xu XH, Min BQ, Marti D, Klitz W. Chromosome 19 single-locus and multilocus haplotype associations with multiple sclerosis. Evidence of a new susceptibility locus in Caucasian and Chinese patients. JAMA. 1997;278(15):1256-61.

Bauer J, Sminia T, Wouterlood FG, Dijkstra CD. Phagocytic activity of macrophages and microglial cells during the course of acute and chronic relapsing experimental autoimmune encephalomyelitis. J Neurosci Res. 1994;38(4):365-75.

Beekman R, Kuks JB, Oosterhuis HJ. Myasthenia gravis: diagnosis and follow-up of 100 consecutive patients. J Neurol. 1997 Feb;244(2):112-8.

Ben-David H, Sharabi A, Dayan M, Sela M, Mozes E.The role of CD8+CD28 regulatory cells in suppressing myasthenia gravis-associated responses by a dual altered peptide ligand. Proc Natl Acad Sci U S A. 2007 Oct 30;104(44):17459-64.

Bernardi S, Grasso MG, Bertollini R, Orzi F, Fieschi C. The influence of pregnancy on relapses in multiple sclerosis: a cohort study. Acta Neurol Scand. 1991 Nov;84(5):403-6.

Bettelli E, Sullivan B, Szabo SJ, Sobel RA, Glimcher LH, Kuchroo VK. Loss of T-bet, but not STAT1, prevents the development of experimental autoimmune encephalomyelitis. J Exp Med. 2004 Jul 5;200(1):79-87.

Mueller BA, Zhang J, Critchlow CW. Birth outcomes and need for hospitalization after delivery among women with multiple sclerosis.. Am J Obstet Gynecol. 2002 Mar;186(3):446-52.

Boon L, Brok HP, Bauer J, Ortiz-Buijsse A, Schellekens MM, Ramdien-Murli S, Blezer E, van Meurs M, Ceuppens J, de Boer M, Hart BA, Laman JD. Prevention of experimental autoimmune encephalomyelitis in the common marmoset (Callithrix jacchus) using a chimeric antagonist monoclonal antibody against human CD40 is associated with altered B cell responses. J Immunol. 2001;167(5):2942-9.

Brennan P, Barrett J, Fiddler M, et al. Maternal-fetal HLA incompatibility and the course of inflammatory arthritis during pregnancy. J Rheumatol 2000;27:2843–8

Brosnan CF, Bornstein MB, Bloom BR. The effects of macrophage depletion on the clinical and pathologic expression of experimental allergic encephalomyelitis. J Immunol. 1981;126(2):614-20.

Brosnan CF, Cammer W, Norton WT, Bloom BR. Proteinase inhibitors suppress the development of experimental allergic encephalomyelitis. Nature. 1980;285(5762):235-7.

Burgess AW, Wilson EM, Metcalf D. Stimulation by human placental conditioned medium of hemopoietic colony formation by human marrow cells. Blood. 1977 Apr;49(4):573-83.

Chabot S, Williams G, Yong VW. Microglial production of TNF-alpha is induced by activated T lymphocytes. Involvement of VLA-4 and inhibition by interferonbeta-1b. J Clin Invest. 1997;100(3):604-12.

Chantakru S, Miller C, Roach LE, Kuziel WA, Maeda N, Wang WC, Evans SS, Croy BA. Contributions from self-renewal and trafficking to the uterine NK cell population of early pregnancy. J Immunol. 2002 Jan 1;168(1):22-8.

Christensen PB, Jensen TS, Tsiropoulos I, Sørensen T, Kjaer M, Højer-Pedersen E, Rasmussen MJ, Lehfeldt E. Associated autoimmune diseases in myasthenia gravis. A population-based study. Acta Neurol Scand. 1995 Mar;91(3):192-5.

Clark CA, Spitzer KA, Crowther MA, Nadler JN, Laskin MD, Waks JA, Laskin CA. Incidence of postpartum thrombosis and preterm delivery in women with antiphospholipid antibodies and recurrent pregnancy loss. J Rheumatol. 2007 May;34(5):992-6.

Cohen SB, Cohen MD, Cush JJ, Fleischmann RM, Mease PJ, Schiff MH, Simon LS, Weaver AL. Unresolved issues in identifying and overcoming inadequate response in rheumatoid arthritis: weighing the evidence. J Rheumatol Suppl. 2008 Feb;81:4-30; quiz 31-4. Review.

Compston DA, Vincent A, Newsom-Davis J, Batchelor JR. Clinical, pathological, HLA antigen and immunological evidence for disease heterogeneity in myasthenia gravis. Brain. 1980 Sep;103(3):579-601.

Confavreux C, Hutchinson M, Hours MM, Cortinovis-Tourniaire P, Moreau T. Rate of pregnancy-related relapse in multiple sclerosis. Pregnancy in Multiple Sclerosis Group. N Engl J Med. 1998 Jul 30;339(5):285-91.

Cooper GS, Dooley MA, Treadwell EL, St Clair EW, Gilkeson GS. Hormonal and reproductive risk factors for development of systemic lupus erythematosus: results of a population-based, case-control study. Arthritis Rheum. 2002 Jul;46(7):1830-9.

Crispin JC, Martínez A, Alcocer-Varela J. Quantification of regulatory T cells in patients with systemic lupus erythematosus. J Autoimmun. 2003 Nov;21(3):273-6.

Culton DA, Nicholas MW, Bunch DO, Zhen QL, Kepler TB, Dooley MA, Mohan C, Nachman PH, Clarke SH. Similar CD19 dys-regulation in two autoantibody-associated autoimmune diseases suggests a shared mechanism of B-cell tolerance loss. J Clin Immunol. 2007 Jan;27(1):53-68.

Cutler SM, Cekic M, Miller DM, Wali B, VanLandingham JW, Stein DG. Progesterone improves acute recovery after traumatic brain injury in the aged rat. J Neurotrauma. 2007 Sep;24(9):1475-86.

Dangond F, Windhagen A, Groves CJ, Hafler DA. Constitutive expression of costimulatory molecules by human microglia and its relevance to CNS autoimmunity. J Neuroimmunol. 1997;76(1-2):132-8.

Dayer JM, Feige U, Edwards CK 3rd, Burger D. Anti-interleukin-1 therapy in rheumatic diseases. Curr Opin Rheumatol. 2001 May;13(3):170-6. Review.

De Groot CJ, Montagne L, Barten AD, Sminia P, Van Der Valk P. Expression of transforming growth factor (TGF)-beta1, -beta2, and -beta3 isoforms and TGF-beta type I and type II receptors in multiple sclerosis lesions and human adult astrocyte cultures. J Neuropathol Exp Neurol. 1999;58(2):174-87.

De Sanctis JB, Garmendia JV, Chaurio R, Zabaleta M, Rivas L. Total and biologically active CD154 in patients with SLE. Autoimmunity. 2009 May;42(4):263-5.

De Sanctis JB, Zabaleta M, Bianco NE, Garmendia JV, Rivas L. Serum adipokine levels in patients with systemic lupus erythematosus. Autoimmunity. 2009 May;42(4):272-4.

Delpy L, Douin-Echinard V, Garidou L, Bruand C, Saoudi A, Guéry JC. Estrogen enhances susceptibility to experimental autoimmune myasthenia gravis by promoting type 1-polarized immune responses. J Immunol. 2005 Oct 15;175(8):5050-7.

Denney JM, Nelson EL, Wadhwa PD, Waters TP, Mathew L, Chung EK, Goldenberg RL, Culhane JF. Longitudinal modulation of immune system cytokine profile during pregnancy. Cytokine. 2011 Feb;53(2):170-7.

Dimayuga FO, Reed JL, Carnero GA, Wang C, Dimayuga ER, Dimayuga VM, Perger A, Wilson ME, Keller JN, Bruce-Keller AJ. Estrogen and brain inflammation: effects on microglial expression of MHC, costimulatory molecules and cytokines. J Neuroimmunol. 2005 Apr;161(1-2):123-36.

Doria A, Tincani A, Lockshin M. Challenges of lupus pregnancies. Rheumatology (Oxford). 2008 Jun;47 Suppl 3:iii9-12. Review.

Drachman DB, Adams RN, Josifek LF, Self SG. Functional activities of autoantibodies to acetylcholine receptors and the clinical severity of myasthenia gravis. N Engl J Med. 1982 Sep 23;307(13):769-75.

Duthoit CT, Mekala DJ, Alli RS, Geiger TL. Uncoupling of IL-2 signaling from cell cycle progression in naive CD4+ T cells by regulatory CD4+CD25+ T lymphocytes. J Immunol. 2005 Jan 1;174(1):155-63.

Dyer CA, Benjamins JA. The structure and function of myelin oligodendrocyte glycoprotein. J Neurochem. 1992;72(1):1-9.

Edwards CJ, Feldman JL, Beech J, Shields KM, Stover JA, Trepicchio WL, Larsen G, Foxwell BM, Brennan FM, Feldmann M, Pittman DD. Molecular profile of peripheral blood mononuclear cells from patients with rheumatoid arthritis. Mol Med. 2007 Jan-Feb;13(1-2):40-58.

Ekerfelt C, Matthiesen L, Berg G, Ernerudh J. Paternal leukocytes selectively increase secretion of Il-4 in peripheral blood during normal pregnancies: Demonstrated by a novel one-way MLC measuring cytokine secretion. Am J Reprod Immunol 1997;38:320 -326.

Elenkov IJ, Hoffman J, Wilder RL. Does differential neuroendocrine control of cytokine production govern the expression of autoimmune diseases in pregnancy and the postpartum period? Mol Med Today. 1997 Sep;3(9):379-83.

Engel AG, Arahata K. The membrane attack complex of complement at the endplate in myasthenia gravis. Ann N Y Acad Sci. 1987;505:326-32.

Fabry Z, Raine CS, Hart MN. Nervous tissue as an immune compartment: the dialect of the immune response in the CNS. Immunol Today. 1994;15(5):218-24.

Feldmann M. What is the mechanism of action of anti-tumour necrosis factor-alpha antibody in rheumatoid arthritis? Int Arch Allergy Immunol. 1996 Dec;111(4):362-5. Review.

Ferber IA, Brocke S, Taylor-Edwards C, Ridgway W, Dinisco C, Steinman L, Dalton D, Fathman CG. Mice with a disrupted IFN-gamma gene are susceptible to the induction of experimental autoimmune encephalomyelitis (EAE). J Immunol. 1996 Jan 1;156(1):5-7.

Fernandez D, Bonilla E, Phillips P, Perl A. Signaling abnormalities in systemic lupus erythematosus as potential drug targets. Endocr Metab Immune Disord Drug Targets. 2006 Dec;6(4):305-11. Review.

Finke D, Eloranta ML, Rönnblom L. Endogenous type I interferon inducers in autoimmune diseases. Autoimmunity. 2009 May;42(4):349-52. Review.

Fogdell-Hahn A, Ligers A, Gronning M, Hillert J, Olerup O. Multiple sclerosis: a modifying influence of HLA class I genes in an HLA class II associated autoimmune disease. Tissue Antigens. 2000;55(2):140-8.

Fonseca JE, Santos MJ, Canhão H, Choy E. Interleukin-6 as a key player in systemic inflammation and joint destruction. Autoimmun Rev. 2009 Jun;8(7):538-42. Review.

Gardner L, Moffett A. Dendritic cells in the human decidua. Biol Reprod. 2003 Oct;69(4):1438-46.

Gay D, Esiri M. Blood-brain barrier damage in acute multiple sclerosis plaques. An immunocytological study. Brain. 1991;114(Pt 1B):557-72.

Gay FW, Drye TJ, Dick GW, Esiri MM. The application of multifactorial cluster analysis in the staging of plaques in early multiple sclerosis. Identification and characterization of the primary demyelinating lesion. Brain. 1997;120 (Pt 8):1461-83.

Gerritse K, Deen C, Fasbender M, Ravid R, Boersma W, Claassen E. The involvement of specific anti myelin basic protein antibody-forming cells in multiple sclerosis immunopathology. J Neuroimmunol. 1994;49(1-2):153-9.

Girardi G, Redecha P, Salmon JE. Heparin prevents antiphospholipid antibody-induced fetal loss by inhibiting complement activation. Nat Med. 2004 Nov;10(11):1222-6.

Girón-González JA, Moral FJ, Elvira J, García-Gil D, Guerrero F, Gavilán I, Escobar L. Consistent production of a higher TH1:TH2 cytokine ratio by stimulated T cells in men compared with women. Eur J Endocrinol. 2000 Jul;143(1):31-6.

Graham RR, Kozyrev SV, Baechler EC, Reddy MV, Plenge RM, Bauer JW, Ortmann WA, Koeuth T, González Escribano MF; Argentine and Spanish Collaborative Groups, Pons-Estel B, Petri M, Daly M, Gregersen PK, Martín J, Altshuler D, Behrens TW, Alarcón-Riquelme ME. A common haplotype of interferon regulatory factor 5 (IRF5) regulates splicing and expression and is associated with increased risk of systemic lupus erythematosus. Nat Genet. 2006 May;38(5):550-5.

Grau V, Herbst B, van der Meide PH, Steiniger B. Activation of microglial and endothelial cells in the rat brain after treatment with interferon-gamma in vivo. Glia. 1997;19(3):181-9.

Guerin LR, Prins JR, Robertson SA. Regulatory T-cells and immune tolerance in pregnancy: a new target for infertility treatment? Hum Reprod Update. 2009 Sep-Oct;15(5):517-35.

Haines JL, Terwedow HA, Burgess K, Pericak-Vance MA, Rimmler JB, Martin ER, Oksenberg JR, Lincoln R, Hazes JM, Dijkmans BA, Vandenbroucke JP, de Vries RR, Cats A. Pregnancy and the risk of developing rheumatoid arthritis. Arthritis Rheum. 1990 Dec;33(12):1770-5.

Hernan MA, Olek MJ, Ascherio A. Geographic variation of MS incidence in two prospective studies of US women. Neurology. 1999;53(8):1711-8.

Hillert J. Human leukocyte antigen studies in multiple sclerosis. Ann Neurol. 1994;36(l):15-7.

Hulkower K, Brosnan CF, Aquino DA, Cammer W, Kulshrestha S, Guida MP, Rapoport DA, Berman JW. Expression of CSF-1, c-fms, and MCP-1 in the central nervous system of rats with experimental allergic encephalomyelitis. J Immunol. 1993;150(6):2525-33.

Ito H, Yamasaki K, Kawano Y, Horiuchi I, Yun C, Nishimura Y, Kira J. HLA-DP-associated susceptibility to the optico-spinal form of multiple sclerosis in the Japanese. Tissue Antigens. 1998 Aug;52(2):179-82.

Johns TG, Bernard CC. The structure and function of myelin oligodendrocyte glycoprotein. J Neurochem. 1999;72(1): 1-9.

Johnson SR, Gladman DD, Urowitz MB, Ibañez D, Granton JT. Pulmonary hypertension in systemic lupus. Lupus. 2004;13(7):506-9.

Joshi PG, Mishra S. A novel type of Ca^{2+} channel in U-87 MG cells activated by anti-galactocerebroside. Life Sci. 1998;62(5): 469-77.

Joshi PG, Mishra S. Galactocerebroside mediates Ca^{2+} signaling in cultured glioma cells. Brain Res. 1992;597(1):108-13.

Jung-Testas I, Do Thi A, Koenig H, Désarnaud F, Shazand K, Schumacher M, Baulieu EE. Progesterone as a neurosteroid: synthesis and actions in rat glial cells. J Steroid Biochem Mol Biol. 1999 Apr-Jun;69(1-6):97-107. Review.

Jurewicz A, Biddison WE, Antel JP. MHC class I-restricted lysis of human oligodendrocytes by myelin basic protein peptide-specific CD8 T lymphocytes. J Immunol. 1998;160(6):3056-9.

Kalkhoven E, Wissink S, van der Saag PT, van der Burg B. Negative interaction between the RelA(p65) subunit of NF-kappaB and the progesterone receptor. J Biol Chem. 1996 Mar 15;271(11):6217-24.

Kanamaru F, Youngnak P, Hashiguchi M, Nishioka T, Takahashi T, Sakaguchi S, Ishikawa I, Azuma M. Costimulation via glucocorticoid-induced TNF receptor in both conventional and CD25+ regulatory CD4+ T cells. J Immunol. 2004 Jun 15;172(12):7306-14.

Kariuki SN, Kirou KA, MacDermott EJ, Barillas-Arias L, Crow MK, Niewold TB. Cutting edge: autoimmune disease risk variant of STAT4 confers increased sensitivity to IFN-alpha in lupus patients in vivo. J. Immunol. 2009;182:34–38.

Katsiari CG, Liossis SN, Dimopoulos AM, Charalambopoulo DV, Mavrikakis M, Sfikakis PP. CD40L overexpression on T cells and monocytes from patients with systemic lupus erythematosus is resistant to calcineurin inhibition. Lupus. 2002;11(6):370-8.

Kellar-Wood HF, Wood NW, Holmans P, Clayton D, Robertson N, Compston DA. Multiple sclerosis and the HLA-D region: linkage and association studies. J Neuroimmunol. 1995;58(2):183-90.

Keystone EC, Kavanaugh AF, Sharp JT, Tannenbaum H, Hua Y, Teoh LS, Fischkoff SA, Chartash EK. Radiographic, clinical, and functional outcomes of treatment with adalimumab (a human anti-tumor necrosis factor monoclonal antibody) in patients with active rheumatoid arthritis receiving concomitant methotrexate therapy: a randomized, placebo-controlled, 52-week trial. Arthritis Rheum. 2004 May;50(5):1400-11.

Koenig HL, Gong WH, Pelissier P. Role of progesterone in peripheral nerve repair. Rev Reprod. 2000 Sep;5(3):189-99. Review.

Kong KO, Tan AW, Thong BY, Lian TY, Cheng YK, Teh CL, Koh ET, Chng HH, Law WG, Lau TC, Leong KP, Leung BP, Howe HS. Enhanced expression of interferon-inducible protein-10 correlates with disease activity and clinical manifestations in systemic lupus erythematosus. Clin Exp Immunol. 2009 Apr;156(1):134-40.

Kozyrev SV, Alarcon-Riquelme ME. The genetics and biology of Irf5-mediated signaling in lupus. Autoimmunity. 2007;40:591–601.

Kuniyasu Y, Takahashi T, Itoh M, Shimizu J, Toda G, Sakaguchi S. Naturally anergic and suppressive CD25(+)CD4(+) T cells as a functionally and phenotypically distinct immunoregulatory T cell subpopulation. Int Immunol. 2000 Aug;12(8):1145-55.

Landek-Salgado MA, Gutenberg A, Lupi I, Kimura H, Mariotti S, Rose NR, Caturegli P. Pregnancy, postpartum autoimmune thyroiditis, and autoimmune hypophysitis: intimate relationships. Autoimmun Rev. 2010 Jan;9(3):153-7. Review.

Lessin DL, Hunt JS, King CR, Wood GW. Antigen expression by cells near the maternal-fetal interface. Am J Reprod Immunol Microbiol. 1988 Jan;16(1):1-7.

Li H, Newcombe J, Groome NP, Cuzner ML. Characterization and distribution of phagocytic macrophages in multiple sclerosis plaques. Neuropathol Appl Neurobiol. 1993;19(3):214-23.

Lifetime course of myasthenia gravis. Grob D, Brunner N, Namba T, Pagala M. Muscle Nerve. 2008 Feb;37(2):141-9. Review.

Lindert RB, Haase CG, Brehm U, Linington C, Wekerle H, Hohlfeld R. Multiple sclerosis: B- and T-cell responses to the extracellular domain of the myelin oligodendrocyte glycoprotein. Brain. 1999;122 (Pt 11):2089-100.

Liu K, Mohan C. Altered B-cell signaling in lupus. Autoimmun Rev. 2009 Jan;8(3):214-8. Review.

Lockshin MD, Qamar T, Levy RA, Druzin ML. Pregnancy in systemic lupus erythematosus. Clin Exp Rheumatol. 1989 Sep-Oct;7 Suppl 3:S195-7. Review.

Maggi G, Casadio C, Cavallo A, Cianci R, Molinatti M, Ruffini E. Thymoma: results of 241 operated cases. Ann Thorac Surg. 1991 Jan;51(1):152-6.

Mao G, Wang J, Kang Y, Tai P, Wen J, Zou Q, Li G, Ouyang H, Xia G, Wang B. Progesterone increases systemic and local uterine proportions of CD4+CD25+ Treg cells during midterm pregnancy in mice. Endocrinology. 2010 Nov;151(11):5477-88.

Martino G, Moiola L, Brambilla E, Clementi E, Comi G, Grimaldi LM. Interferon-gamma induces T lymphocyte proliferation in multiple sclerosis via a Ca(2+)-dependent mechanism. J Neuroimmunol. 1995;62(2):169-76.

McDonald WI, Miller DH, Barnes D. The pathological evolution of multiple sclerosis. Neuropathol Appl Neurobiol. 1992;18(4):319-34.

McHugh RS, Whitters MJ, Piccirillo CA, Young DA, Shevach EM, Collins M, Byrne MC. CD4(+)CD25(+) immunoregulatory T cells: gene expression analysis reveals a functional role for the glucocorticoid-induced TNF receptor. Immunity. 2002 Feb;16(2):311-23.

Meyer O. Neonatal cutaneous lupus and congenital heart block: it's not all antibodies. Lancet. 2003 Nov 15;362(9396):1596-7.

Mincheva-Nilsson L, Hammarström S, Hammarström ML. Human decidual leukocytes from early pregnancy contain high numbers of gamma delta+ cells and show selective down-regulation of alloreactivity. J Immunol. 1992 Sep 15;149(6):2203-11.

Monteyne P, Van Laere V, Marichal R, Sindic CJ. Cytokine mRNA expression in CSF and peripheral blood mononuclear cells in multiple sclerosis: detection by RT-PCR without in vitro stimulation. J Neuroimmunol. 1997;80(1-2):137-42.

Moore GR, Neumann PE, Suzuki K, Lijtmaer HN, Traugott U, Raine CS. Balo's concentric sclerosis: new observations on lesion development. Ann Neurol. 1985;17(6):604-11.

Moroni G, Quaglini S, Banfi G, Caloni M, Finazzi S, Ambroso G, Como G, Ponticelli C. Pregnancy in lupus nephritis. Am J Kidney Dis. 2002 Oct;40(4):713-20.

Müller-Ladner U, Kriegsmann J, Franklin BN, Matsumoto S, Geiler T, Gay RE, Gay S. Synovial fibroblasts of patients with rheumatoid arthritis attach to and invade normal human cartilage when engrafted into SCID mice. Am J Pathol. 1996 Nov;149(5):1607-15.

Mumford, C J; Wood, N W; Kellar-Wood, H; Thorpe, J W; Miller, D H; Compston, D A. The British Isles survey of multiple sclerosis in twins. Neurology. 1994;44:11–15.

Nalbandian G, Kovats S. Understanding sex biases in immunity: effects of estrogen on the differentiation and function of antigen-presenting cell. Immunol Res. 2005;31(2):91-106. Review

Nelson CC, Hendy SC, Shukin RJ, Cheng H, Bruchovsky N, Koop BF, Rennie PS. Determinants of DNA sequence specificity of the androgen, progesterone, and glucocorticoid receptors: evidence for differential steroid receptor response elements. Mol Endocrinol. 1999 Dec;13(12):2090-107.

Nelson JL, Hughes KA, Smith AG, Nisperos BB, Branchaud AM, Hansen JA. Maternal-fetal disparity in HLA class II alloantigens and the pregnancy-induced amelioration of rheumatoid arthritis. N Engl J Med. 1993 Aug 12;329(7):466-71.

Nelson LM, Franklin GM, Jones MC. Risk of multiple sclerosis exacerbation during pregnancy and breast-feeding. JAMA. 1988 Jun 17;259(23):3441-3.

Arruvito L, Giulianelli S, Flores AC, Paladino N, Barboza M, Lanari C, Fainboim L. NK cells expressing a progesterone receptor are susceptible to progesterone-induced apoptosis.. J Immunol. 2008 Apr 15;180(8):5746-53.

Olsen N, Sokka T, Seehorn CL, Kraft B, Maas K, Moore J, Aune TM. A gene expression signature for recent onset rheumatoid arthritis in peripheral blood mononuclear cells. Ann Rheum Dis. 2004 Nov;63(11):1387-92.

Olsson T. Critical influences of the cytokine orchestration on the outcome of myelin antigen-specific T-cell autoimmunity in experimental autoimmune encephalomyelitis and multiple sclerosis. Immunol Rev. 1995;144:245-68.

Østensen M, Peter M Villiger PM. Immunology of pregnancy - pregnancy as a remission inducing agent in rheumatoid arthritis. Transplant Immunology 2002;9(2-4):155-160.

Ostensen M, Lundgren R, Husby G, Rekvig OP. Studies on humoral immunity in pregnancy: immunoglobulins, alloantibodies and autoantibodies in healthy pregnant women and in pregnant women with rheumatoid disease. J Clin Lab Immunol. 1983 Jul;11(3):143-7.

Oturai A, Larsen F, Ryder LP, Madsen HO, Hillert J, Fredrikson S, Sandberg-Wollheim M, Laaksonen M, Koch-Henriksen N, Sawcer S, Fugger L, Sorensen PS, Svejgaard A. Linkage and association analysis of susceptibility regions on chromosomes 5 and 6 in 106 Scandinavian sibling pair families with multiple sclerosis. Ann Neurol. 1999;46(4):612-6.

Ozawa K, Suchanek G, Breitschopf H, Bruck W, Budka H, Jellinger K, Lassmann H. Patterns of oligodendroglia pathology in multiple sclerosis. Brain. 1994;117(Pt 6):1311-22.

Padua L, Tonali P, Aprile I, Caliandro P, Bartoccioni E, Evoli A. Seronegative myasthenia gravis: comparison of neurophysiological picture in MuSK+ and MuSK- patients. Eur J Neurol. 2006 Mar;13(3):273-6.

Peng SL. Altered T and B lymphocyte signaling pathways in lupus. Autoimmun Rev. 2009 Jan;8(3):179-83. Review.

Perl A, Nagy G, Gergely P, Puskas F, Qian Y, Banki K. Apoptosis and mitochondrial dysfunction in lymphocytes of patients with systemic lupus erythematosus. Methods Mol Med. 2004;102:87-114.

Peterson JW, Bo L, Mork S, Chang A, Trapp BD. Transected neurites, apoptotic neurons, and reduced inflammation in cortical multiple sclerosis lesions.Ann Neurol. 2001;50(3):389-400.

Pongcharoen S, Searle RF, Bulmer JN. Placental Fas and Fas ligand expression in normal early, term and molar pregnancy. Placenta. 2004 Apr;25(4):321-30.

Pope RM, Yoshinoya S, Rutstein J, Persellin RH. Effect of pregnancy on immune complexes and rheumatoid factors in patients with rheumatoid arthritis. Am J Med. 1983 Jun;74(6):973-9.

Rajan AJ, Gao YL, Raine CS, Brosnan CF. A pathogenic role for gamma delta T cells in relapsing-remitting experimental allergic encephalomyelitis in the SJL mouse. J Immunol. 1996;157(2):941-9.

Rinner WA, Bauer J, Schmidts M, Lassmann H, Hickey WF. Resident microglia and hematogenous macrophages as phagocytes in adoptively transferred experimental autoimmune encephalomyelitis: an investigation using rat radiation bone marrow chimeras. Glia. 1995;14(4):257-66.

Roman MJ, Shanker BA, Davis A, Lockshin MD, Sammaritano L, Simantov R, Crow MK, Schwartz JE, Paget SA, Devereux RB, Salmon JE. Prevalence and correlates of accelerated atherosclerosis in systemic lupus erythematosus. N Engl J Med. 2003 Dec 18;349(25):2399-406. Erratum in: N Engl J Med. 2006 Oct 19;355(16):1746.

Rosenberg GA, Dencoff JE, Correa N Jr, Reiners M, Ford CC. Effect of steroids on CSF matrix metalloproteinases in multiple sclerosis: relation to blood-brain barrier injury. Neurology. 1996;46(6):1626-32.

Rosendaal M. Colony-stimulating factor (CSF) in the uterus of the pregnant mouse. J Cell Sci. 1975 Nov;19(2):411-23.

Roullet E, Verdier-Taillefer MH, Amarenco P, Gharbi G, Alperovitch A, Marteau R. Pregnancy and multiple sclerosis: a longitudinal study of 125 remittent patients. J Neurol Neurosurg Psychiatry. 1993 Oct;56(10):1062-5.

Runmarker B, Andersen O. Pregnancy is associated with a lower risk of onset and a better prognosis in multiple sclerosis. Brain. 1995 Feb;118 (Pt 1):253-61.

Sadovnick AD, Amstrong H, Rice GP, Bulman D, Hashimoto L, Paty DW, Hashimoto SA, Warren S, Hader W, Murray TJ, et al. A population-based study of multiple sclerosis in twins: update. Ann Neurol. 1993;33(3):281-5.

Sakaguchi Y, Nakamura Y, Sutani T, Tsuchihashi M, Yamano S, Hashimoto T, Dohi K, Hiasa Y, Kawai S, Okada R. Immunohistochemical study of the endomyocardial biopsy of systemic lupus erythematosus. J Cardiol. 1995 Apr;25(4):181-8.

Sanchez-Guerrero J, Karlson EW, Liang MH, Hunter DJ, Speizer FE, Colditz GA. Past use of oral contraceptives and the risk of developing systemic lupus erythematosus. Arthritis Rheum. 1997 May;40(5):804-8.

Sánchez-Guerrero J, Liang MH, Karlson EW, Hunter DJ, Colditz GA. Postmenopausal estrogen therapy and the risk for developing systemic lupus erythematosus. Ann Intern Med. 1995 Mar 15;122(6):430-3.

Saraste M, Väisänen S, Alanen A, Airas L; Finnish Multiple Sclerosis And Pregnancy Study Group. Clinical and immunologic evaluation of women with multiple sclerosis during and after pregnancy. Gend Med. 2007 Mar;4(1):45-55

Schluep M, Willcox N, Vincent A, Dhoot GK, Newsom-Davis J. Acetylcholine receptors in human thymic myoid cells in situ: an immunohistological study. Ann Neurol. 1987 Aug;22(2):212-22.

Schumacher A, Brachwitz N, Sohr S, Engeland K, Langwisch S, Dolaptchieva M, Alexander T, Taran A, Malfertheiner SF, Costa SD, Zimmermann G, Nitschke C, Volk HD, Alexander H, Gunzer M, Zenclussen AC. Human chorionic gonadotropin attracts regulatory T cells into the fetal-maternal interface during early human pregnancy. J Immunol. 2009 May 1;182(9):5488-97.

Shabanova SS, Ananieva LP, Alekberova ZS, Guzov II. Ovarian function and disease activity in patients with systemic lupus erythematosus. Clin Exp Rheumatol. 2008 May-Jun;26(3):436-41.

Shlomchik MJ, Madaio MP. Springer Semin Immunopathol. The role of antibodies and B cells in the pathogenesis of lupus nephritis. 2003 May;24(4):363-75. Review.

Spector TD. Rheumatoid arthritis. Rheum Dis Clin North Am. 1990 Aug;16(3):513-37. Review.

Tafuri A, Alferink J, Möller P, Hämmerling GJ, Arnold B. Science. T cell awareness of paternal alloantigens during pregnancy.1995 Oct 27;270(5236):630-3.

Taylor A, Verhagen J, Blaser K, Akdis M, Akdis CA. Mechanisms of immune suppression by interleukin-10 and transforming growth factor-beta: the role of T regulatory cells. Immunology. 2006 Apr;117(4):433-42. Review.

Tilburgs T, Roelen DL, van der Mast BJ, de Groot-Swings GM, Kleijburg C, Scherjon SA, Claas FH. Evidence for a selective migration of fetus-specific CD4+CD25bright regulatory T cells from the peripheral blood to the decidua in human pregnancy. J Immunol. 2008 Apr 15;180(8):5737-45.

Tolboom TC, van der Helm-Van Mil AH, Nelissen RG, Breedveld FC, Toes RE, Huizinga TW, Ulvestad E, Williams K, Vedeler C, Antel J, Nyland H, Mork S, Matre R. Reactive microglia in multiple sclerosis lesions have an increased expression of receptors for the Fc part of IgG. J Neurol Sci. 1994;121(2):125-31.

Van den Brink HR, van Wijk MJ, Bijlsma JW. Influence of steroid hormones on proliferation of peripheral blood mononuclear cells in patients with rheumatoid arthritis. Br J Rheumatol. 1992 Oct;31(10):663-7.

Van der Pouw Kraan TC, van Gaalen FA, Huizinga TW, Pieterman E, Breedveld FC, Verweij CL. Discovery of distinctive gene expression profiles in rheumatoid synovium using cDNA microarray technology: evidence for the existence of multiple pathways of tissue destruction and repair. Genes Immun. 2003 Apr;4(3):187-96.

Van Der Voorn P, Tekstra J, Beelen RH, Tensen CP, Van Der Valk P, De Groot CJ. Expression of MCP-1 by reactive astrocytes in demyelinating multiple sclerosis lesions. Am J Pathol. 1999;154(1):45-51.

Van Walderveen MA, Tas MW, Barkhof F, Polman CH, Frequin ST, Hommes OR, Valk J. Magnetic resonance evaluation of disease activity during pregnancy in multiple sclerosis. Neurology. 1994 Feb;44(2):327-9.

Vandevyver C, Raus P, Stinissen P, Philippaerts L, Cassiman JJ, Raus J. Polymorphism of the tumour necrosis factor beta gene in multiple sclerosis and rheumatoid arthritis. Eur J Immunogenet. 1994;21(5):377-82.

Veenstra van Nieuwenhoven AL, Heineman MJ, Faas MM. The immunology of successful pregnancy. Hum Reprod Update. 2003 Jul-Aug;9(4):347-57. Review.

Verdru P, Theys P, D'Hooghe MB, Carton H. Pregnancy and multiple sclerosis: the influence on long term disability. Clin Neurol Neurosurg. 1994 Feb;96(1):38-41.

Walters E, Rider V, Abdou NI, Greenwell C, Svojanovsky S, Smith P, Kimler BF. Estradiol targets T cell signaling pathways in human systemic lupus. Clin Immunol. 2009 Dec;133(3):428-36.

Wang G, Pierangeli SS, Papalardo E, Ansari GA, Khan MF. Markers of oxidative and nitrosative stress in systemic lupus erythematosus: correlation with disease activity. Arthritis Rheum. 2010 Jul;62(7):2064-72.

Watanabe T, Yoshida M, Shirai Y, Yamori M, Yagita H, Itoh T, Chiba T, Kita T, Wakatsuki Y. Administration of an antigen at a high dose generates regulatory CD4+ T cells expressing CD95 ligand and secreting IL-4 in the liver. J Immunol. 2002 Mar 1;168(5):2188-99.

Weinshenker BG, Santrach P, Bissonet AS, McDonnell SK, Schaid D, Moore SB, Rodriguez M. Major histocompatibility complex class II alleles and the course and outcome of MS: a population-based study Neurology 1998;51(3):742-7.

Weinshenker BG. Natural history of multiple sclerosis. Ann Neurol. 1994;36 Suppl:S6-11.

Weiss JM, Downie SA, Lyman WD, Berman JW. Astrocyte-derived monocyte-chemoattractant protein-1 directs the transmigration of leukocytes across a model of the human blood-brain barrier. J Immunol. 1998;161(12):6896-903.

Wingerchuk D, Liu Q, Sobell J, Sommer S, Weinshenker BG. A population-based case-control study of the tumour necrosis factor alpha-308 polymorphism in multiple sclerosis. Neurology. 1997;49(2): 626-8.

Wittmann L, Sensky T, Meder L, Michel B, Stoll T, Büchi S. Suffering and posttraumatic growth in women with systemic lupus erythematosus (SLE): a qualitative/ quantitative case study. Psychosomatics. 2009 Jul-Aug;50(4):362-74.

Wucherpfennig KW, Strominger JL. Molecular mimicry in T cell-mediated autoimmunity: viral peptides activate human T cell clones specific for myelin basic protein. Cell. 1995;80(5):695-705.

Youinou P, Taher TE, Pers JO, Mageed RA, Renaudineau Y. B lymphocyte cytokines and rheumatic autoimmune disease. Arthritis Rheum. 2009 Jul;60(7):1873-80. Review.

Zenclussen AC, Gerlof K, Zenclussen ML, Ritschel S, Zambon Bertoja A, Fest S, Hontsu S, Ueha S, Matsushima K, Leber J, Volk HD. Regulatory T cells induce a privileged tolerant microenvironment at the fetal-maternal interface. Eur J Immunol. 2006 Jan;36(1):82-94.

Zhang DY, Banatao DR, Gatto N, Goodkin DE, Hauser SL. Linkage of the MHC to familial multiple sclerosis suggests genetic heterogeneity. Hum. Mol. Genet. 1998;7(8):1229–1234.

Zhang J, Jacobi AM, Wang T, Berlin R, Volpe BT, Diamond B. Polyreactive autoantibodies in systemic lupus erythematosus have pathogenic potential. J Autoimmun. 2009 Nov-Dec;33(3-4):270-4.

Zrour SH, Boumiza R, Sakly N, Mannai R, Korbaa W, Younes M, Bejia I, Touzi M, Bergaoui N. The impact of pregnancy on rheumatoid arthritis outcome: the role of maternofetal HLA class II disparity. Joint Bone Spine. 2010 Jan;77(1):36-40.

21

T Lymphocyte Characteristics and Immune Tolerance During Human Pregnancy

Gergely Toldi, András Treszl and Barna Vásárhelyi
Research Group of Pediatrics and Nephrology, Hungarian Academy of Sciences
Hungary

1. Introduction

To ensure a fruitful and healthy pregnancy, every maternal organ system needs to adapt to the novel physiological needs raised by the developing fetus. The maternal immune system is no exception. Since the conceptus is half of foreign origins, presenting paternal antigens, it is considered a semi-allograft to maternal immunity. Therefore, an immune tolerance must develop to avoid immunological rejection of the fetus. In the normal course of pregnancy, the mother extends her 'definition of self' for 40 weeks on the foreign antigens of the fetus, and the conceptus is accepted by the mother's immune system. The impairment of this tolerance and the development of an abnormal immune response directed at the fetus play a major role in adverse pregnancy outcomes, including spontaneous abortion, preterm labour and preeclampsia. In recurrent abortion and preeclampsia, abnormal maternal immune reactions have an autoimmune character, and the disorders resemble many features typically seen in autoimmune diseases, or in association with autoimmune reactions. Although this does not mean that recurrent abortion or preeclampsia should be considered autoimmune conditions, it still suggests that abnormal autoimmune processes play an important role in their pathogenesis. In this regard, preeclampsia mimics autoimmune responses observed in both allograft rejection and graft-versus-host disease.

Several aspects of the development of the pregnancy-specific immune tolerance have been described recently. Initially, the contact between maternal and fetal cells is taking place on a local level and is restricted to the decidua, but during the second trimester of pregnancy, it is extended to the entire body of the mother. Both the innate and adaptive arms of immunity are involved in these events. In this chapter we will focus on the role of T lymphocytes, the adaptive cellular elements of the immune system. We will discuss the characteristic alterations of T lymphocyte subsets in prevalence and functionality in healthy and pathologic development of the immune tolerance in human pregnancy.

2. Th1 and Th2 cells

T helper (Th) lymphocytes are traditionally classified into the Th1 and Th2 subsets based on their cytokine production pattern (Romagnani, 1991). The most important cytokines produced by Th1 cells are interleukin-2 (IL-2), tumor necrosis factor-α (TNF-α) and interferon-γ (IFN-γ). Considered to be the main effectors of phagocyte-induced host defense, these cells are highly protective against infections sustained by intracellular agents. On the other hand, Th2 cells produce IL-4, which stimulates IgE and IgG1 antibody production, IL-5, which promotes the growth and differentiation of eosinophils, and IL-10 and IL-13, which together with IL-4 inhibit macrophage functions. The Th2 subset is mainly responsible for phagocyte-independent host defense, for example against helminthic infections.

For many years, it was hypothesized that normal pregnancy induces a shift from Th1 immunity towards Th2 immunity. However, it has been demonstrated recently that the levels of particular Th1 cytokines are raised, instead of lowered in normal pregnancy compared with the non-pregnant state (Challis et al., 2009). Current findings indicate that gravidity is both a pro-inflammatory and an anti-inflammatory condition, depending upon the stage of gestation. Grossly, pregnancy has three distinct immunological phases. The events of implantation and the first trimester require a strong inflammatory response to ensure the adequate remodelling of the uterine epithelium and the removal of cellular debris following the implantation of the blastocyst. Therefore, healthy pregnancy cannot be regarded as merely a state of relative immunosuppression, as once thought. On the contrary, by means of various cytokines, successful implantation is dependent upon the active contribution of the maternal immune system to stimulate adequate invasion of the trophoblastic tissue into the maternal uterine wall. Thus, the first trimester of pregnancy is hallmarked by pro-inflammatory events. The second immunological phase of gravidity consists of the second and third trimesters. This is the period of fetal growth and development, when an anti-inflammatory state is established. Finally, delivery represents the third immunological phase of pregnancy, when pro-inflammatory events dominate again and promote uterinal contractions to deliver the fetus and the placenta (Mor & Cardenas, 2010).

IFN-γ appears to be a key cytokine in the regulation of pregnancy related inflammatory events. Under pathologic conditions with insufficient immune tolerance such as in preeclampsia, IFN-γ production is significantly increased compared with healthy pregnancy (Piccinni, 2010). In mice, it was reported that IL-4, IL-5 and IL-10 are detectable at the fetomaternal interface during all periods of gestation, whereas the presence of IFN-γ is transient, being detectable only in the first period (Lin et al., 1993; Wegmann et al., 1993). Although decidual NK cells are able to produce IFN-γ (Ashkar et al., 1998), they do not have a central role in fetal allograft rejection, since they do not express receptors specific for antigens and thus are not sensitive for the presence of paternal alloantigens. The significance of local Th2-type cytokine production in the decidua has been observed in humans as well. Piccinni et al. measured cytokine production in decidual CD4 cells isolated from women with recurrent spontaneous abortions. Compared with women with a normal pregnancy, the decidual CD4 cells from women with abortion show a defect in IL-4 and IL-10 production (Piccinni et al., 1998).

The antigens of the developing fetus are present at two interfaces as pregnancy progresses. The first interface is found between the invasive extravillous cytotrophoblast and maternal immune cells in the decidua. This local, tissue interface is of importance for immune adaptation during implantation. The second interface is that between the syncytiotrophoblast and the immune cells in maternal blood. This systemic interface is established at about the 10th gestational week and becomes increasingly important in the second half of pregnancy (Sargent et al., 2006a). Two contrary requirements influence the extent of invasion by fetal extravillous cytotrophoblast cells in the maternal decidua: the anchorage of the placenta to ensure fetal nutrition and the protection of the uterine wall against over-invasion (von Rango, 2008). If, due to excessive immunological tolerance and acceptance of trophoblast cells, the uterine wall is over-invaded, pathologic conditions, such as placenta accreta, increta or percreta might develop (Bulmer, 1992). If the adequate invasion of the uterinal spiral arterioles by extravillous cytotrophoblasts does not occur, this sets up the conditions for placental hypoxia and oxidative stress that eventually triggers a maternal systemic inflammatory response, leading to clinical manifestations of preeclampsia (von Rango, 2008).

This disorder is characterized by hypertension, proteinuria, edema and endothelial dysfunction generally evolving in the third trimester of pregnancy; however, it may also occur earlier. Although preeclampsia is quite common (i.e. it affects about 5-8% of all pregnancies globally), its clear cause and the mechanisms leading to immune dysfunction remain to be elucidated. Preeclampsia is estimated to be responsible for about 70,000 maternal deaths each year worldwide (Walker, 2000). HELLP syndrome (consisting of hemolysis, elevated liver enzymes, low platelet count) and eclampsia are other manifestations of the same disorder. Although these conditions are generally coupled with a number of other symptoms (including headaches, abdominal pain, nausea, vomiting, abnormal vision, dyspnoe, anxiety, mental confusion, seizures), these manifestations are not necessarily more serious than preeclampsia. Besides a maternal systemic inflammatory response, signs of systemic vasoconstriction may also be observed in the mother in these pregnancy-associated disorders (Baumwell & Karumanchi, 2007).

In preeclampsia, the anti-inflammatory state during the second and third trimesters develops insufficiently (Saito et al., 2007). An excessive maternal systemic inflammation is considered to be a dominant component in the pathogenesis of this pregnancy-specific disorder, since its important feature is the absence of Th2 skewness and thus the predominance of pro-inflammatory cytokines. Saito et al. reported on their observations regarding higher prevalence of IFN-γ and lower prevalence of IL-4-producing CD4 lymphocytes among peripheral blood mononuclear cells (PBMCs) of preeclamptic women compared with healthy pregnant women. Furthermore, the percentage of Th1 and Th2 cells and the Th1/Th2 ratio correlated with IFN-γ and IL-4 secretion levels (Saito et al., 1999a). In another study, this group observed increased production of IL-2, IFN-γ and TNF-α by PBMCs in preeclampsia and, interestingly, a positive correlation between mean blood pressure and Th1 cytokines (Saito et al., 1999b). The shift to a predominant Th1-type immunity in preeclampsia is reinforced by other experiments on intracellular cytokine measurements in T and NK cells, as well as by the assessment of cytokine secretion levels of PBMCs isolated from preeclamptic patients. (Azizieh et al., 2005; Darmochwal-Kolarz et al., 2002; Rein et al., 2002).

3. The influence of galectin-1 on the Th1/Th2 cell ratio

Previous studies demonstrated that soluble factors may also play a role in the development of the Th2 shift characteristic for healthy pregnancy. Such a factor is galectin-1, also produced by peripheral lymphocytes. Galectin-1, a 14 kDa protein, is a β-galactoside-binding mammalian lectin. Within the immune system, it is expressed by activated T, B and NK cells as well as macrophages (Blaser et al., 1998; Koopman et al., 2003; Rabinovich et al., 1998; Zuniga et al., 2001). Galectin-1 exerts immunoregulatory effects through various mechanisms. By binding to the cell surface glycoproteins, it inhibits T cell proliferation and induces apoptosis of activated Th1, Th17 and CD8 cells (Blaser et al., 1998; Perillo et al., 1995; Toscano et al., 2007). Galectin-1 has been demonstrated in vitro to inhibit T cell adhesion to the extracellular matrix and to abrogate the secretion of proinflammatory cytokines (Rabinovich et al., 1999a). Furthermore, in vivo administration of galectin-1 in experimental models of autoimmunity skewed the balance toward a Th2-dominant cytokine profile (Rabinovich et al., 1999b; Toscano et al., 2006). Recent data show that galectin-1 promotes fetomaternal tolerance, since treatment with recombinant galectin-1 prevented fetal loss in an abortion-prone mouse model. The protective effect of galectin-1 was abrogated in regulatory T cell (Treg) depleted mice (Blois et al., 2007). Garin et al. showed that Tregs selectively up-regulate galectin-1 expression (Garin et al., 2007). Experiments using galectin-1 homozygous null mutant mice showed a reduced regulatory activity in Tregs and the blockage of galectin-1 binding diminished the inhibitory effects of human and mouse Treg cells (Rabinovich et al., 1998). These findings suggest that Tregs expressing galectin-1 may also support the acceptance of the fetus by maternal immune cells.

In a recent study, we measured circulating galectin-1 and anti-galectin-1 autoantibody levels, as well as intracellular galectin-1 expression of unstimulated peripheral blood T and NK cells in healthy pregnancy and preeclampsia (Molvarec et al., 2011). Our findings indicate that the majority of CD4+ and CD8+ T cells and NK cells express intracellular galectin-1 in healthy pregnant women, while only a small fraction of them do so in healthy non-pregnant women. In preeclampsia, the proportion of galectin-1-expressing peripheral T and NK cells was markedly decreased compared with healthy pregnancy. However, circulating levels of galectin-1 and anti-galectin-1 autoantibodies were not altered in preeclamptic patients as compared to healthy pregnant women, nor were related to the proportions of galectin-1-expressing peripheral blood lymphocytes in any of the study groups.

While Th1 and Th17 cells are susceptible to galectin-1-induced cell death, Th2 cells are protected from galectin-1 due to the differential sialylation of their cell surface glycoproteins. Indeed, galectin-1-deficient mice were shown to develop greater Th1 and Th17 responses (Toscano et al., 2007). Therefore, it is tempting to speculate that decreased production of galectin-1 by circulating T and NK cells might contribute to the development of the pro-inflammatory Th1 and Th17 immune responses, which are characteristic features of preeclampsia (Saito et al., 1999b; Toldi et al., 2011a).

4. Regulatory T cells

The recent discovery of a distinct T helper lymphocyte subset, referred to as Th17 cells, led to the transformation of the Th1/Th2 paradigm of immunity into a four-component model. This novel viewpoint incorporates Th1, Th2, Th17 and regulatory T cells (Tregs) as elements of a complex and mutually interacting network in the establishment of pregnancy-specific immune tolerance. Indeed, besides the imbalance of Th1 and Th2 cells, alterations of the prevalence of Th17 and Treg cells have been suggested to be of importance in the pathogenesis of adverse pregnancy outcomes (Saito, 2010).

Tregs are important regulators of tolerance induction. During pregnancy, a systemic expansion of Tregs specific for paternally derived cells can be observed already at very early stages, indicating that their function is to protect paternally derived cells from immune rejection (Mjösberg et al., 2007). The prevalence of Tregs expands in the periphery and these cells are also present at significant numbers at the fetomaternal interface, preferentially in the maternal decidua. Sasaki et al. were the first to describe an increase in the CD4+ CD25+ Treg cell prevalence in decidual tissue in early human pregnancy (Sasaki et al., 2004). This was supported by the works of Heikkinen et al. and Somerset et al. who observed an increase in the population of CD4+ CD25+ circulating Treg cells in early pregnancy and described a peak of this population during the second trimester and a subsequent gradual decrease to levels slightly higher than non-pregnant levels during the postpartum period (Heikkinen et al., 2004; Somerset et al., 2004). The tolerogenic impact of Tregs needs permanent antigen presentation without inflammatory co-stimulation. This explains the transient nature of the fetal tolerance and the fact that, especially during the first weeks of pregnancy, inflammatory infection of the mother may compromise pregnancy outcome. An expansion of Tregs in the decidua in healthy pregnant women accompanied by a low occurrence of Th17 cells was recently confirmed by Mjösberg et al. (Mjösberg et al., 2009). Furthermore, these authors propose that Tregs may be in charge of controlling the Th1 activity found locally in healthy early pregnancy.

Decreased Treg cell numbers during pregnancy are associated with immunological rejection of the fetus (Zenclussen, 2006). Sasaki et al. reported that spontaneous abortion cases are associated with lower systemic Treg levels when compared to normally developing pregnancies (Sasaki et al., 2004). A number of groups including ours demonstrated that the prevalence of peripheral Tregs is lower in preeclampsia compared with healthy pregnancy (Darmochwal-Kolarz et al., 2007; Sasaki et al., 2007; Steinborn et al., 2008; Toldi et al., 2008). Furthermore, Sasaki et al. reported that the prevalence of Tregs is lower not only in peripheral blood samples but also in deciduas of preeclamptic patients compared with healthy pregnant women (Sasaki et al., 2007).

Tregs function in a delicate cellular network that includes inducer (myeloid and lymphoid dendritic cells) and target cells (CD4 and CD8 cells, NK cells and NKT cells) of Tregs (Fig. 1). Besides the peripheral prevalence of Tregs, we also characterized the prevalence of inducers and cellular targets of this T cell subset in preeclampsia and healthy pregnancy in the third trimester. We made efforts to find out whether the alteration of the number of Treg inducers is associated with the decreased number of Tregs. According to a previous study, the ratio of these cells is skewed toward the myeloid dendritic cells in the third trimester of preeclamptic pregnancy (Darmochwal-Kolarz et al., 2003). Theoretically, this may contribute to low Treg prevalence due to the lower Treg inducer capacity of myeloid dendritic cells than that of lymphoid dendritic cells (Ito et al., 2007). In our patients, however, the prevalence and ratio of myeloid and lymphoid dendritic cells did not differ, possibly indicating that dendritic cells are not responsible for low Treg numbers, at least in this stage of pregnancy. The lack of association may support the contribution of non-cellular factors, including pro-inflammatory cytokines such as TNF-α which has a direct inhibitory effect on suppressive Treg function in vitro (Valencia et al., 2006). TNF-α and other pro-inflammatory cytokine levels (such as IFN-γ, IL-6 and IL-12) are reportedly increased in PE (Rusterholz et al., 2007). Lower Treg numbers are not reflected in the proportion of NK, NK-T and activated CD4 and CD8 cells, at least at this stage of pregnancy. This does not exclude, however, that the function (such as the cytokine production pattern) of these cells is modified due to altered Treg numbers.

Steinborn et al. further analyzed the prevalence of Tregs using various markers to identify this subset. Their analysis revealed two distinct Treg subsets that differed with regard to their FoxP3 and CD25 expression: CD4+ CD25+ FoxP3high+ and CD4+ CD25high+ FoxP3+ cells. When monitoring the two populations during healthy pregnancy and preeclampsia, they found a strong increase in the percentage of the CD4+ CD25+ FoxP3high+ Treg

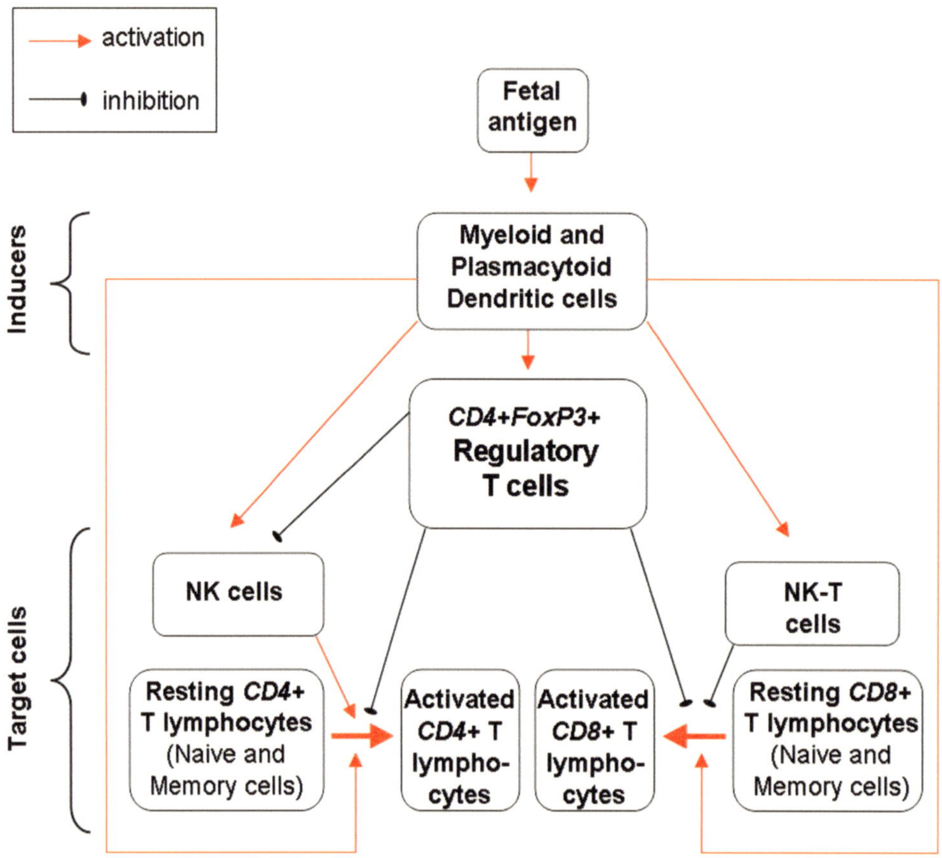

(Based on Toldi et al., 2008.)

Fig. 1. The cellular network of regulatory T cells (Tregs). Tregs are in connection with inducer and target cells through various mechanisms of activation and inhibition.

population during the first and second trimesters, while in the third trimester, this Treg subset decreased gradually until term. The prevalence of CD4+ CD25+ FoxP3high+ Tregs correlated with suppressive capacity: Treg cells obtained from healthy pregnant women during the first and second trimester showed a two-fold higher suppressive activity than cells obtained in the third trimester or at term. The same correlation was true for patients affected by preeclampsia. The significantly diminished percentage of CD4+ CD25+ FoxP3high+ Tregs correlated with low suppressive capacity. In contrast to healthy pregnancy, the percentage of CD4+ CD25high+ FoxP3+ Treg cells was found to be increased in the circulation of preeclamptic women. In healthy pregnant women these cells expanded during the first trimester and reached maximum levels in the second trimester. Therefore, in preeclamptic women the population of CD4+ CD25high+ FoxP3+ Treg cells was particularly apparent, while the population of CD4+ CD25+ FoxP3high+ Tregs was significantly decreased. The authors proposed that CD4+ CD25+ FoxP3high+ and CD4+ CD25high+ FoxP3+ cell populations represent distinct Treg subsets, and that abnormalities in the balance of these subsets are associated with the presence of preeclampsia (Steinborn et al., 2008).

5. The role of regulatory T cells in the process of tolerance induction

Preeclampsia occurs more frequently in the first conception (Dekker & Sibai, 1998). However, preeclampsia appears to be a problem of primipaternity rather than primigravidity, since epidemiological data indicate that when the conception is with a new partner in multiparous mothers, the risk increases to the level seen in the first pregnancy (Robillard et al., 1993; Trupin et al., 1996). The symptoms of preeclampsia regress rapidly after delivery, suggesting that the exposure of the maternal immune system to the fetus and placenta, expressing paternal alloantigens, are of central importance in the pathogenesis.

In donated spermatozoa, semen exposure does not occur and the fetus is a semi-allograft to the mother. The risk of preeclampsia in donated spermatozoa is very high (18.2%) (Salha et al., 1999), suggesting that semen exposure reduces the risk of preeclampsia. Soluble MHC class I antigens in the seminal fluid are taken up by vaginal and uterine epithelial cells, and these antigens might induce tolerance to cells expressing paternally derived MHC class I antigens. Indeed, semen triggers an influx of antigen-presenting cells into the female reproductive tract (Robertson et al., 2003). Usually, the fetus is a semi-allograft to the maternal host. The risk of preeclampsia is also increased in complete allograft-pregnant cases. In ovum donation, the antigens of the fetus are derived from the husband and the donor woman. Exposure to the husband's semen is appropriately present. The risk of preeclampsia in ovum donation cases is high (16%), suggesting that the allografted fetus is a greater challenge for the maternal immune system, and is a risk factor for preeclampsia (Salha et al., 1999). In donated embryo transfer cases, the fetus is an allograft and semen exposure is not present. In this case, this risk of preeclampsia is even higher (33%), probably due to an additive effect of the allografted fetus and the absence of sperm exposure.

Regulatory T cells, which induce tolerance to paternal antigens, may explain these epidemiological findings. Darmochwal-Kolarz et al. demonstrated that the levels of CD4+ CD45RO+ and CD8+ CD25+ cells are increased in preeclampsia, suggesting the activation of CD4+ and CD8+ T lymphocytes. It seems possible that the activation of T lymphocytes is associated with the deficiency of Tregs (Darmochwal-Kolarz etal., 2007). Before the first pregnancy, Treg cell numbers may increase due to seminal priming. Koelman et al. reported that soluble MHC class I antigens are present in the seminal fluid. It is well known that continuous oral exposure to antigens induces tolerance, called 'oral tolerance'. Similarly, a continuous vaginal exposure to paternal soluble MHC class I antigens may induce tolerance to these antigens (Koelman et al., 2000). Robertson et al. suggest that insemination activates the maternal immune system and leads to hypo-responsiveness in T cells reactive with paternal alloantigens in mice (Robertson et al., 2003). This idea is supported by the epidemiological finding that condom users have a high risk for preeclampsia (Klonoff-Cohen et al., 1989).

The prevalence of Tregs is low in the mother before pregnancy (Fig. 2). This minor population of T cells, which reacts to paternal antigens and induces tolerance to them, expands after conception. When a threshold of prevalence is reached, sufficient immune tolerance to paternal antigens is achieved to ensure a healthy development of pregnancy. If the prevalence of Tregs does not reach the threshold, the risk for the development of preeclampsia is high. Subsequently, Tregs increase to a maximum in the second trimester of pregnancy and gradually decrease in the third trimester (Somerset et al., 2004). This finding is related to the clinical observation that the symptoms of preeclampsia generally appear in the third trimester, after 24 weeks of gestation. After delivery, the prevalence of Tregs may

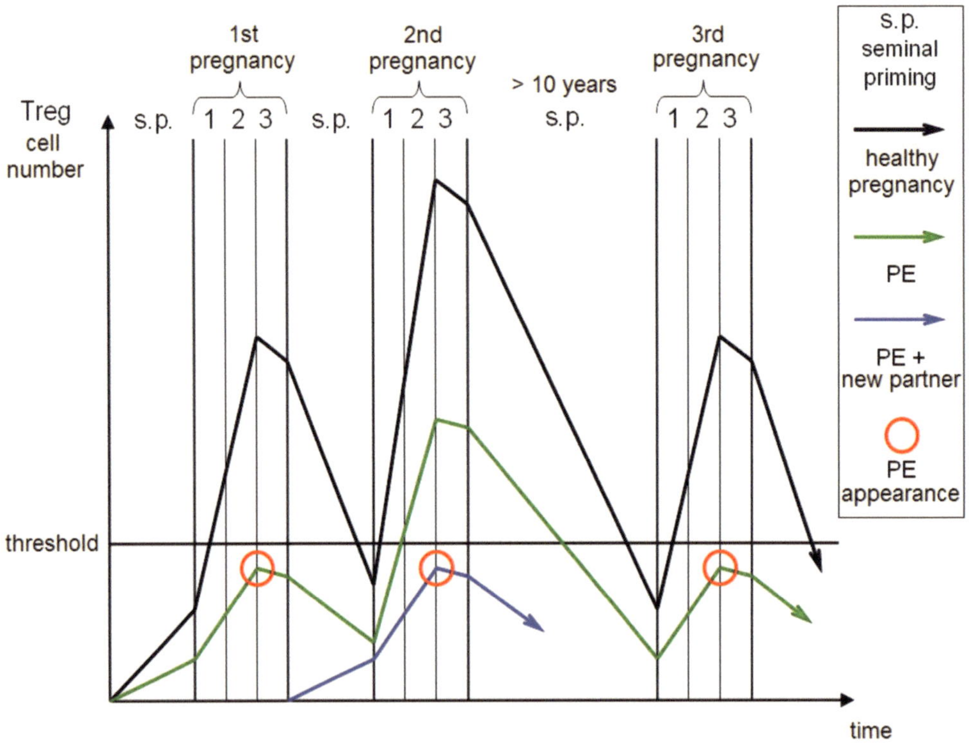

Fig. 2. Alterations of maternal regulatory T cell (Treg) numbers during pregnancy. The prevalence of Tregs is low before pregnancy. When a threshold of Treg prevalence is reached during healthy pregnancy (black curve), the symptoms of preeclampsia do not develop. This is aided by seminal priming. If the prevalence of Tregs does not reach the threshold, the risk of preeclampsia is high (green curve). After the conception of a second pregnancy with the same partner, the number of Tregs increases more rapidly compared with the first pregnancy, independently from the initial prevalence of Tregs during the first pregnancy. However, in a second pregnancy with a new partner, the risk for developing preeclampsia is similar to that in the first pregnancy (blue curve). An increasing interval (> 10 years) between the second and third deliveries was associated with an increasing risk of preeclampsia, and a lower prevalence of Tregs.

rapidly decrease and at the beginning of a second pregnancy, there may be only a low number of Tregs present. Seminal priming may keep the number of these cells to a certain level (Fig. 2). After the conception of a second pregnancy with the same partner, the number of Tregs increases more rapidly compared with the first pregnancy, independently from the initial prevalence of Tregs (and the presence or lack of preeclampsia) during the first pregnancy. However, in a second pregnancy with a new partner, Tregs which induce tolerance to the new partner's antigens may be very rare. Therefore, the risk for developing preeclampsia is similar to that in the first pregnancy.

Skjaerven et al. reported that preeclampsia occurred in 3.9% of first pregnancies, 1.7% of second pregnancies, and 1.8% of third pregnancies when mothers had the same partner. Furthermore, an increasing interval between the second and third deliveries was associated with an increasing risk of preeclampsia. When more than 10 years had passed after the previous delivery, the frequency rose to 3.0%. They also showed that a paternal change was not associated with an increased risk of preeclampsia after adjustment for the interval between births (Skjaerven et al., 2002). These findings might be explained by the population of Tregs. Tregs may gradually decrease and reach very low levels when more than 10 years have passed after the last delivery. A low level of these tolerance-inducing T cells may be maintained by seminal priming. However, in a subsequent pregnancy, some pregnant women may not be able to achieve adequate tolerance, resulting in an increased risk of preeclampsia.

6. Th17 cells

CD4+ IL-17+ (Th17) cells, this recently identified subpopulation of CD4 lymphocytes, originate from a developmental lineage that is distinct from both Th1 and Th2 cells. Th17 cells produce IL-17 and other pro-inflammatory cytokines. IL-17 has an important role in the development of autoimmune disorders and in the induction and maintenance of chronic inflammation (Basso et al., 2009). The effect of Th17 cells on the inflammatory balance is opposed by Tregs. Th17 cells and Tregs originate from the same developmental lineage, distinct from both Th1 and Th2 cells. An exclusive dichotomy was observed in their generation: either Th17 or Treg cells develop from the ancestor cells depending on whether they are activated in the presence of transforming growth factor-β (TGF-β) or TGF-β plus inflammatory cytokines (Basso et al., 2009).

In addition to their distinct role in the regulation of the inflammatory status, Th1, Th2, Th17 and Treg cells mutually influence one another through the production of different cytokines. For instance, an increase in the Th17/Treg cell ratio may contribute to a shift towards the Th1 direction because IL-17 induces the production of other pro-inflammatory cytokines, such as that of IFN-γ (Afzali et al., 2007), while the inhibitory effect of Tregs on Th1 cells is decreased at the same time.

In a previous study, Santner-Nanan et al. found that, besides a higher prevalence of Tregs, the percentage of Th17 cells is significantly decreased in the third trimester of healthy pregnancy compared with non-pregnant controls and preeclamptic patients. Consequently, the Th17/Treg cell ratio was significantly decreased in healthy but not in preeclamptic pregnancies. Thus, preeclampsia is associated with the absence of normal systemic skewing away from IL-17 production towards FoxP3 expression. Additionally, preeclamptic women had significantly higher levels of soluble endoglin, an inhibitor of TGF-β receptor signaling, which may bias towards IL-17 production (Santner-Nanan et al., 2009).

In accordance with the above data, we also found that simultaneously with higher than normal Th17 numbers, the prevalence of Tregs is lower in PE, resulting in an elevated Th17/Treg ratio compared with uncomplicated pregnancy. The altered ratio of Th17/Treg cells may contribute to the shift towards the Th1 direction in preeclampsia. However, we could not detect a correlation between the prevalence of Th17 and Th1 cells (using the cell surface marker, CXCR3 for the identification of the latter subset). Thus, the effect of Th17 cells and IL-17 on the inflammatory status is more likely to be exerted in a direct manner rather than through the modulation of the Th1/Th2 balance in preeclampsia (Toldi et al., 2011a).

The alterations of Th17 cells have been observed in other pregnancy-related disorders as well, suggesting that the balance of Th17 cells and Tregs and not only that of Th1 and Th2 cells has crucial effects on the inflammatory status in human pregnancy. Ito et al. recently demonstrated the importance of IL-17-producing cells in the pathomechanism of preterm labour (Ito et al., 2010). Nakashima et al. found that the prevalence of decidual IL-17-producing cells is significantly higher in inevitable abortion cases (but not in missed abortion) than in normal pregnancy, indicating that these cells might be involved in the induction of inflammation in the late stage of abortion, but not in the early stage (Nakashima et al., 2010). In another study, Wang et al. showed that the prevalence of Th17 cells in the peripheral blood and decidua is increased in unexplained recurrent spontaneous abortion patients (Wang et al., 2010). They observed that the expression of a Th17-associated factor, RAR-related orphan receptor gamma (ROR-γ or RORc), is also higher in peripheral blood lymphocytes and decidua of these patients. In a recent study, Jianjun et al. found that the mRNA level of this factor in PBMCs and decidua is elevated in preeclamptic patients when compared with healthy pregnant women (Jianjun et al., 2010). Therefore, the increased expression of this transcription factor may partly be responsible for the increased prevalence of Th17 cells in peripheral blood of preeclamptic patients.

7. IL-17-producing CD8 and NK cells

Although IL-17 was first identified in CD4 cells, later on other immune cells, including CD8 and NK cells, were also shown to produce this cytokine (Passos et al., 2010; Shin et al., 1999). Emerging evidence suggests that these IL-17-producing lymphocyte subsets, especially NK cells, largely contribute to the inflammatory status during pregnancy. Sargent et al. proposed that the innate rather than the adaptive immune system controls immune regulation during human pregnancy, and that NK cells are of central importance to this process (Sargent et al., 2006b; Sargent et al., 2007). The aberrant activation of NK cells both systematically and locally in the placenta may be of major interest in the malfunction of immune tolerance and the pathogenesis of pregnancy-associated disorders.

In our previously unpublished investigation, we measured the peripheral prevalence of IL-17-producing cells in the CD4, CD8 and NK subsets and that of the IL-17 producing CD4, CD8 and NK cells in the overall lymphocyte population. We took peripheral blood samples from 24 healthy non-pregnant and 23 healthy pregnant age-matched women (with a median of 32 and 33 years, respectively), in the third trimester of pregnancy (with a median of 31 weeks of gestation). Non-pregnant women were in the early follicular phase of the menstrual cycle (between cycle days 3 and 5), and none of them received hormonal contraception. Informed consent was obtained from all participating subjects. We separated the mononuclear cells from the samples and performed cell surface marker and intracellular cytokine staining. Finally, samples were measured on a flow cytometer.

The prevalence of Th17 cells was lower among healthy pregnant compared with healthy non-pregnant women (2.8 [2.4-3.1] % vs. 3.2 [2.9-3.5] %). The prevalence of CD8+ IL-17+ (Tc17) cells among CD8 lymphocytes was higher in healthy pregnant than in healthy non-pregnant samples (4.8 [3.6-6.2] % vs. 2.4 [1.7-3.7] %). The frequency of CD56+ IL-17+ (IL-17-producing NK) cells was lower in healthy pregnant than in healthy non-pregnant samples (1.0 [0.6-1.2] % vs. 1.6 [1.1-2.5] %).

We further analyzed the frequency of IL-17-producing CD4, CD8 and NK lymphocytes. After the initial assessment of the Th17, Tc17 and IL-17-producing NK cell prevalence among CD4, CD8 and NK cells, respectively (Fig. 3, graphs a-c), we also determined the prevalence of these subsets among the overall lymphocyte population (Fig. 3, graphs d-f) along with the frequency of CD4+ IL-17-, CD8+ IL-17- and CD56+ IL-17- cells among the overall lymphocyte population (Fig. 3, graphs g-i).

Our findings revealed two different mechanisms explaining the differing alterations observed in the prevalence of Th17 and Tc17 cells in the study groups. The alteration of CD4+ IL-17+ cell prevalence in the overall lymphocyte subset (Fig. 3, graph d) followed that seen among CD4 cells (Fig. 3, graph a), as the frequency of CD4+ IL-17- cells was comparable in both study groups (Fig. 3, graph g). Therefore, the prevalence of Th17 (CD4+ IL-17+) cells show absolute alterations, since Th17 cell numbers are altered not only in the CD4 subset, but also in the overall lymphocyte population. In contrast, Tc17 cell frequencies do not show significant difference if assessed among the overall lymphocyte population (Fig. 3, graph e); only the prevalence of CD8+ IL-17- cells differs between the study groups

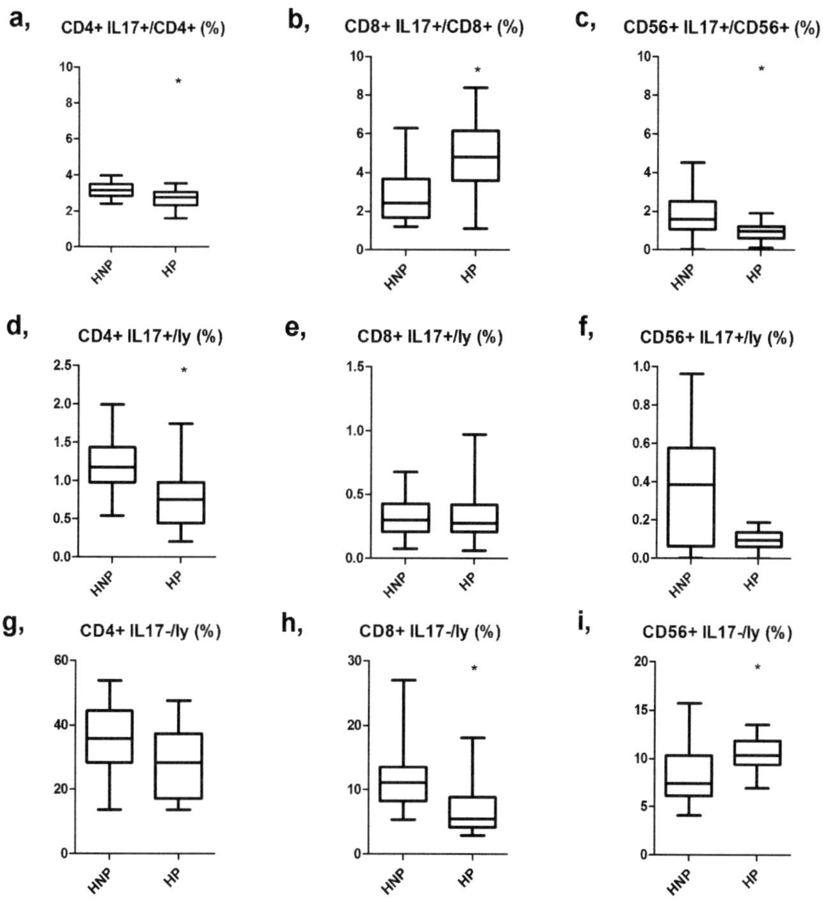

Fig. 3. Box-plots representing the prevalence of IL-17+ cells among CD4, CD8 and NK (CD56+) cells (graphs a-c) and in the overall lymphocyte population (ly) (graphs d-f), as well as the prevalence of IL-17- cells in the overall lymphocyte population (ly) (graphs g-i) in healthy non-pregnant (HNP) and healthy pregnant (HP) women. Horizontal line: median, box: interquartile range, whisker: range. * p values less than 0.05 were regarded significant.

(Fig. 3, graph h) and the direction of IL-17- cell alteration is the opposite of that seen at Tc17 cell prevalence in the CD8 subset (Fig. 3, graph b). Therefore, the prevalence of Tc17 cells does not show absolute alterations, only relative ones, as a consequence of different CD8+ IL-17- cell frequencies in the study groups. The alteration of IL-17-producing NK cell prevalences among parent populations showed similar tendencies to that observed in case of CD4 cells.

Of note, existing data are not consistent concerning the alterations of CD4 and CD8 cell frequencies during pregnancy. Tallon et al. found that CD4 cell numbers decrease in the second and third trimesters, while CD8 cells decrease during the third trimester (Tallon et al., 1984). Another study demonstrated that peripheral blood CD8 cells decreased during the first trimester, while CD4 cells decreased in the third trimester, with both populations increasing to non-pregnant values four months postpartum (Watanabe et al., 1997). The investigations by Kühnert et al. found no significant changes in the percentage CD4 and CD8 lymphocytes, nor in the CD4/CD8 ratio at any stage of pregnancy or postpartum.

Based on our results, the apparent increase in Tc17 cell prevalence in healthy pregnancy compared with non-pregnant controls appears to be the consequence of decreased CD8+ IL-17- cell frequency in this group, resulting in a higher proportion of Tc17 cells in the CD8 subset. Since Tc17 cells have been described to have a lower cytotoxic activity in comparison with CD8+ IL-17- cells (Huber et al., 2009), the decrease in the latter subset and a relative increase in Tc17 prevalence may be regarded as part of the immunosuppressive mechanisms characterizing healthy pregnancy.

In preeclampsia, our results show that in addition to CD4 cells, the prevalence of CD8 and NK cells that express IL-17 is also higher compared with healthy pregnant women. IL-17 production by these lymphocyte subsets might contribute to the development of a systemic pro-inflammatory environment in PE (Toldi et al., 2011a).

8. Lymphocyte activation kinetics

Previous studies demonstrated that not only the prevalence of T lymphocyte subsets, but also their functionality is altered during pregnancy. For instance, calcium handling of T cells differs in healthy pregnancy and in the non-pregnant state. Previous reports indicate a sustained increase of basal intracellular calcium level in lymphocytes of healthy pregnant and preeclamptic women compared with non-pregnant women, with the highest levels in preeclampsia (Hojo et al., 1999; Thway et al., 2004; von Dadelszen et al., 1999). The availability of cytoplasmic free calcium has an important role in controlling the level of lymphocyte activation. We hypothesized that the elements of calcium handling of activated T lymphocytes, including lymphocyte potassium channels, may be affected in healthy pregnancy and preeclampsia compared to the non-pregnant state. Voltage-gated Kv1.3 channels along with calcium-dependent IKCa1 channels play a key role in the regulation of intracellular calcium homeostasis as they counterbalance the increase of cytoplasmic free calcium content in the course of lymphocyte activation. These channels grant the efflux of potassium from the cytoplasm, thus maintaining an electrochemical potential gradient needed for further calcium entry. Specific inhibition of these channels results in a diminished calcium influx into lymphocytes and a lower level of lymphocyte activation (Panyi et al., 2006). Our group characterized the activation-elicited calcium influx in the Th1, Th2, CD4 and CD8 lymphocyte subsets in healthy pregnant, preeclamptic and non-pregnant women and tested its alteration upon the inhibition of Kv1.3 and IKCa1 potassium channels (Toldi et al., 2011b).

Until recently, primarily single-cell techniques were applied to study the process of lymphocyte activation, and no reliable high-throughput method was available to investigate lymphocyte activation kinetics in more than one lymphocyte subsets simultaneously. The use of single-cell techniques are limited by the fact that they are not suitable for the description of kinetic processes in a complex cellular milieu that contains different types of interacting immune cells. For this purpose, we developed a novel, flow cytometry-based approach that enabled us to monitor lymphocyte activation simultaneously in different lymphocyte subtypes.

For our measurements, we collected peripheral blood samples from healthy pregnant, preeclamptic and non-pregnant women. PBMCs were separated by a standard density gradient centrifugation. PBMCs were then incubated with conjugated anti-human surface marker monoclonal antibodies (CD4, CD8, CXCR3 for Th1 cells, CCR4 for Th2 cells) to identify lymphocyte subsets and were loaded with calcium sensitive Fluo-3 and Fura Red dyes to monitor alterations of the cytoplasmic free calcium level. PBMCs were divided into three vials. One vial was treated with margatoxin (MGTX), a selective blocker of the Kv1.3 channel. Another vial was treated with a triarylmethane compound (TRAM), a specific inhibitor of the IKCa1 channel. The third vial was used as control. Measurements were initiated directly after the addition of 20 µg of phytohemagglutinin (PHA) as an unspecific activating stimulus. Cell fluorescence data were measured and recorded for 10 minutes in a kinetic manner on flow cytometer.

Data acquired from the measurements were evaluated by fitting a double-logistic function for each recording (Kaposi et al., 2008). This function is used to describe measurements that have an increasing and a decreasing intensity as time passes. The software also calculates parameter values describing each function, such as the Maximum value (Max), the Time to reach maximum value (t_{max}), and the Area Under the Curve (AUC). These parameters represent different characteristics of lymphocyte calcium influx kinetics. The Maximum value represents the peak value of the calcium influx curve upon lymphocyte activation, thus it reflects the maximal amount of cytoplasmic free calcium in the course of activation. The Time to reach maximum value describes how soon the peak value of the calcium influx curve is reached. The Area Under the Curve describes the full amount of cytoplasmic free calcium during the whole period of lymphocyte activation and thus the magnitude of the elicited calcium response in general.

Our results indicate that calcium influx kinetics in activated T lymphocytes markedly differs in healthy pregnancy compared with the non-pregnant state: AUC values of the calcium response are lower in healthy pregnancy in the Th1, CD4 and CD8 lymphocyte subsets (Fig. 4). Based on this observation, it is reasonable to assume that the physiological immune tolerance towards fetal antigens in pregnancy is partly attributed to a lower calcium response. This hypothesis is further supported by the particular role of the impaired function of Th1 and CD8 lymphocyte subsets in maternal immune tolerance. On contrary to Th1 cells, the activation induced calcium response of the Th2 subset is not decreased compared with the non-pregnant state. The decreased activation of the Th1 subset (reflected by low AUC values in our study) and the lack of decrease in Th2 cells may partly be responsible for the well established Th2 skewness in healthy pregnancy.

Unlike in healthy pregnancy, we could not detect a difference in the AUC values of calcium influx kinetics of Th1 and CD8 cells in preeclampsia compared to non-pregnant women (Fig. 4). The absence of calcium influx characteristics specific for healthy pregnancy suggests that

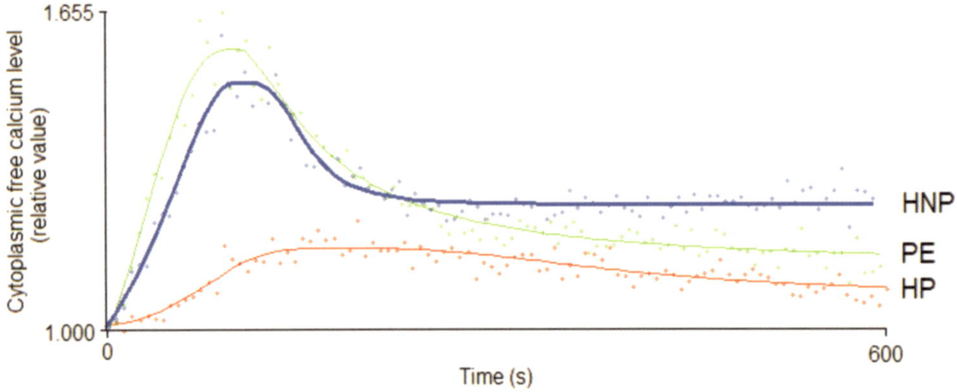

Fig. 4. Calcium influx kinetics of peripheral Th1 lymphocytes isolated from healthy non-pregnant (HNP), healthy pregnant (HP) and preeclamptic (PE) women (without lymphocyte potassium channel inhibitor treatment). Calcium influx is lower in healthy pregnancy compared with the non-pregnant state and preeclampsia.

this element may associate with the impaired maternal immune tolerance present in preeclampsia, since the calcium influx kinetics is comparable to that seen in non-pregnant samples. Indeed, the maintained activation properties of Th1 lymphocytes in preeclamptic patients may contribute to the lack of Th2 dominance associated with normal pregnancy. Similarly to the Th1 subset, CD8 cells in preeclampsia are also characterized by the lack of suppressed activation kinetics. Thus the decrease of cytotoxic activity observed in healthy pregnancy (Malinowski et al., 1994) is not present in preeclampsia. Interestingly, t_{max} values were decreased in Th2 and CD4 cells in preeclampsia compared with healthy pregnancy. This finding may indicate an increased reactivity of lymphocytes in preeclampsia, possibly reflecting an elevated responsiveness of T lymphocytes due to the ongoing maternal systemic inflammation.

Since Kv1.3 and IKCa1 potassium channels significantly influence the calcium response elicited upon lymphocyte activation, we tested their expression and function in healthy pregnancy and preeclampsia. According to comparable fluorescence values of the samples stained with specific antibodies against Kv1.3 channels, their expression is not altered in any of the investigated T lymphocyte subsets. Therefore, the differences detected between calcium influx of non-pregnant, healthy pregnant and preeclamptic lymphocytes upon treatment with specific inhibitors of the potassium channels is probably due to the altered function, and not to the altered expression of these channels.

Our results suggest that the overall lymphocyte population and particularly the CD4 subset are sensitive to MGTX and TRAM inhibition in each investigated study group, indicating that both Kv1.3 and IKCa1 channels play an important regulatory role in calcium influx. This is reflected by the decrease of the AUC and Max values compared with the respective samples where no inhibitors were applied. However, the sensitivity of calcium influx measured in other lymphocyte subsets shows clear variability. It is of particular interest that calcium influx of Th2 lymphocytes in healthy pregnancy was insensitive to potassium channel inhibition, while calcium influx decreased significantly in non-pregnant samples upon treatment with the specific channel blockers. Of note, Th2 lymphocytes in preeclampsia presented with non-pregnant-like characteristics, and were also sensitive to MGTX and TRAM treatment. Since the regulatory function of Kv1.3 and IKCa1 channels on calcium influx appears to be limited in healthy pregnant samples (as the inhibition of these channels did not result in a decrease of the AUC and Max values), it is tempting to speculate that this may be an element contributing to the Th2 shift present in healthy pregnancy, but absent in preeclampsia. This hypothesis may be supported by reports suggesting that the shape of calcium influx influenced by potassium channel functions may determine the cytokine production profile of helper T lymphocytes (Dolmetsch et al., 1998; Fanger et al., 2000).

Interestingly, other differences were also observed between healthy pregnancy and preeclampsia. While calcium influx in CD8 and Th1 lymphocytes was resistant to potassium channel inhibition in preeclamptic samples, that of healthy pregnant lymphocytes was sensitive. Similarly to Th2 cells, while it is unclear whether the resistance of Th1 lymphocytes to potassium channel inhibition is reflected in their function, the insensitivity of the Th1 subset to the inhibition of regulatory lymphocyte potassium channels in preeclampsia may be linked to the Th1 skewness.

Our findings suggest that there is a characteristic pattern of calcium influx in T lymphocytes and its sensitivity to potassium channel inhibition in normal pregnancy that is missing in preeclampsia. This raises the notion that T lymphocyte calcium handling may have a role in the development of the pregnancy-specific immune tolerance.

9. The association between preeclampsia and autoimmunity

Considering the immunological alterations described in preeclampsia, one may notice characteristic similarities in the etiology shared with autoimmune disorders. As a result of the impaired immune tolerance, preeclampsia is distinguished by many features typically seen in autoimmune diseases, or in association with autoimmune reactions. This does not mean that preeclampsia should be considered an autoimmune condition. However, it does suggest that abnormal autoimmune processes play an important part in the pathogenesis of preeclampsia. An interpretation of preeclampsia can be found in analogies to organ rejection after allograft transplantation and in graft-versus-host disease (GVHD); like preeclampsia, these conditions are also characterized by a multitude of systemic symptoms. The similarities with acute organ rejection and GVHD are paralleled by the notion that if a 100% allograft can elicit autoimmune responses during organ transplantation, one should not be surprised that a 50:50 autograft-allograft can do the same thing. This recognition may lead to better clinical approaches to preeclampsia and thereby to better diagnosis and treatment (Gleicher, 2007).

The clinical relationship between autoimmune diseases and pregnancy is unique. No other diseases are characterized by an exacerbation pattern that is particularly pronounced in the peripartum and postpartum periods (Gleicher et al., 1993). A recently recognized example is peripartum cardiomyopathy, with disease flares from late pregnancy up to approximately three months postpartum (Ansari et al., 2002). Preeclampsia is also characterized by a peripartal exacerbation pattern, with the majority of cases developing after 36 weeks of gestation.

Besides the cellular abnormalities already discussed, autoantibody abnormalities have also been reported in association with preeclampsia. So far, a number of autoantibodies have been implicated in the pathogenesis (Branch et al., 1994; Milliez et al., 1990; Rappaport et al.,

1990; Yamamoto et al., 1993). The most important one of them appears to be an agonistic autoantibody against the angiotensin II type 1 receptor (Wallukat et al., 1999). Moreover, as in classical autoimmune diseases, more severe preeclampsia appears to result in more autoantibody abnormalities (El-Roeiy et al., 1991). Evidence suggests that classical, nonorgan-specific autoantibodies, such as antiphospholipid antibodies, are characteristic of preeclampsia, and especially in its more severe clinical expression (El-Roeiy et al., 1991; Yamamoto et al., 1993). Dekker et al. therefore recommended active laboratory surveillance for patients at risk (Dekker et al., 1995).

Both GVHD-related and classical autoimmune conditions often improve upon treatments that have been found successful also in preeclampsia and HELLP syndrome. Three examples are the treatment with corticosteroids, removal of autoantibody abnormalities via plasmapheresis, and the competitive binding of autoantibodies with intravenous immunoglobulin (Katz et al., 1990; Martin et al., 1990; Martin et al., 2006).

Considering the significant degree of bidirectional cell traffic during pregnancy, one can speculate that, in analogy to GVHD, the autoimmune phenomena, seen in association with preeclampsia, may be immune responses by fetal lymphocytes to epitopes shared by mother and fetus. Alternatively, the autoimmune response in preeclampsia could be distinct from that in GVHD, and purely autoimmune in nature. This would then represent an immune response solely against maternal self-epitopes on fetal cells that have entered the maternal circulation. A number of observations indicate that the paternal genotype is of importance in that regard. For instance, the more similar the paternal histocompatibility complex is to that of the mother, the more likely a miscarriage will occur due to increased autoantigenity (Kishore et al., 1996). The fetus is not only an allograft but also an autograft. Since one half of the fetus is maternally derived in its antigenicity, the maternal immune system also faces an unprecedented autoimmune load. At no other period in life needs the maternal immune system to be prepared for autoimmune challenges of this extent. The immunological adjustment to pregnancy, therefore, does not only involve the development of tolerance to the paternal allogenic, but also to the maternal autoimmunogenic components of the fetus.

Autoimmune phenomena are mostly seen in two periods of pregnancy: during early conception and the peripartum period. In early conception, abnormal immune activation may be coupled with pregnancy loss. Later stage presentation appears to be associated with preeclampsia. Indeed, women with early autoimmune activation, who (with treatment) do not miscarry, demonstrate a greatly increased risk for preeclampsia (Gleicher et al., 1993). This observation supports the idea of a common alloimmune or autoimmune etiology for both of these conditions. It has also been suggested that an analogy might exist not only between chronic graft rejection and preeclampsia, but also between acute graft rejection and recurrent abortion (Wilczyński, 2006).

Accepting the concept that preeclampsia is characterized by autoimmune phenomena may have benefits for better diagnosis and treatment. For example, autoimmune phenomena usually go through pre- or subclinical stages before their clinical manifestation. Laboratory markers are often already detectable at those early stages (Davidson & Diamond, 2001). If the autoimmune phenomena of preeclampsia were to follow a similar pattern, earlier diagnosis and specific treatment might become possible.

10. Conclusion

T lymphocytes play a central role in the development of the maternal immune tolerance during pregnancy. Pathologic alterations of T cells in prevalence and functionality

contribute to the onset of pregnancy-related disorders, and might represent a possible future target for therapeutic intervention.
It has been recognized for many years that the prevalence of distinct T cell subpopulations are subject to a characteristic adjustment during pregnancy in order to facilitate the specific needs raised by the developing fetus. The course of this adjustment may be insufficient in pregnancy-related disorders. Recently, it has been demonstrated that not only cell numbers, but also the functionality of cells needs to go through specific alterations to help the maternal immune system in acquisition of the pregnancy-specific tolerance. As an example, we have demonstrated that there is a characteristic pattern of calcium influx in T lymphocytes and its sensitivity to lymphocyte potassium channel inhibition in healthy pregnancy that is missing in preeclampsia, raising the notion that T lymphocyte calcium handling may have a role in the distinctive immune status of uncomplicated pregnancy. Further research needs to be carried out applying different methods to identify additional factors involved in these alterations. This approach might lead to better strategies for the prevention and treatment of adverse pregnancy outcomes, facilitating the development and maintenance of immune tolerance needed for healthy pregnancy.

11. Acknowledgement

The preparation of this chapter was supported by grants OTKA 76316 and ETT 05-180/2009.

12. References

Afzali, B., Lombardi, G., Lechler, R.I., Lord, G.M. (2007). The role of T helper 17 (Th17) and regulatory T cells (Treg) in human organ transplantation and autoimmune disease. *Clin Exp Immunol,* Vol.148, No.1, (April 2007), pp. 32-46

Ansari, A.A., Fett, J.D., Carraway, R.E., Mayne, A.E., Onlamoon, N., Sundstrom, J.B. (2002). Autoimmune mechanisms as the basis of human peripartum cardiomyopathy. *Clin Rev Allergy Immunol,* Vol.23, No.3, (December 2002), pp. 301-324

Ashkar, A.A., Di Santo, J.P., Croy, B.A. (1998). Interferon gamma contributes to initiation of uterine vascular modification, decidual integrity, and uterine natural killer cell maturation during normal murine pregnancy. *J Exp Med,* Vol.192, No.2, (July 2000), pp. 259-270

Azizieh, F., Raghupathy, R., Makhseed, M. (2005). Maternal cytokine production patterns in women with pre-eclampsia. *Am J Reprod Immunol,* Vol.54, No.1, (July 2005), pp. 30-37

Basso, A.S., Cheroutre, H., Mucida, D. (2009). More stories on Th17 cells. *Cell Res,* Vol.19, No.4, (April 2009), 399-411

Baumwell, S., Karumanchi, S.A. (2007). Pre-eclampsia: clinical manifestations and molecular mechanisms. *Nephron Clin Pract,* Vol.106, No.2, (June 2007), pp. c72-81

Blaser, C., Kaufmann, M., Müller, C., Zimmermann, C., Wells, V., Mallucci, L., Pircher, H. (1998). Beta-galactoside-binding protein secreted by activated T cells inhibits antigen-induced proliferation of T cells. *Eur J Immunol,* Vol.28, No.8, (August 1998), pp. 2311-2319

Blois, S.M., Ilarregui J.M., Tometten, M., Garcia, M., Orsal, A.S., Cordo-Russo, R., Toscano, M.A., Bianco, G.A., Kobelt, P., Handjiski, B., Tirado, I., Markert, U.R., Klapp, B.F., Poirier, F., Szekeres-Bartho, J., Rabinovich, G.A., Arck, P.C. (2007). A pivotal role for galectin-1 in fetomaternal tolerance. *Nat Med,* Vol.13, No.12, (December 2007), pp. 1450-1457

Branch, D.W., Mitchell, M.D., Miller, E., Palinski, W., Witztum, J.L. (1994). Pre-eclampsia and serum antibodies to oxidised low-density lipoprotein. *Lancet,* Vol.343, No.8898, (March 1994), pp. 645-646

Bulmer, J.N. (1992). Immune aspects of pathology of the placental bed contributing to pregnancy pathology. *Baillieres Clin Obstet Gynaecol,* Vol.6, No.3, (September 1992), pp. 461-488

Challis, J.R., Lockwood, C.J., Myatt, L., Norman, J.E., Strauss, J.F. 3rd, Petraglia, F. (2009). Inflammation and pregnancy. *Reprod Sci,* Vol.16, No.2, (February 2009), pp. 206-215

Darmochwal-Kolarz, D., Rolinski, J., Leszczynska-Goarzelak, B., Oleszczuk, J. (2002). The expressions of intracellular cytokines in the lymphocytes of preeclamptic patients. *Am J Reprod Immunol,* Vol.48, No.6, (December 2002), pp. 381-386

Darmochwal-Kolarz, D., Rolinski, J., Tabarkiewicz, J., Leszczynska-Gorzelak, B., Buczkowski, J., Wojas, K., Oleszczuk, J. (2003). Myeloid and lymphoid dendritic cells in normal pregnancy and preeclampsia. *Clin Exp Immunol,* Vol.132, No.2, (May 2003), pp. 339-344

Darmochwal-Kolarz, D., Saito, S., Rolinski, J., Tabarkiewicz, J., Kolarz, B., Leszczynska-Gorzelak, B., Oleszczuk, J. (2007). Activated T lymphocytes in pre-eclampsia. *Am J Reprod Immunol,* Vol.58, No.1, (July 2007), pp. 39-45

Davidson, A., Diamond, B. (2001). Autoimmune diseases. *N Engl J Med,* Vol.345, No.5, (August 2001), pp. 340-350

Dekker, G.A., de Vries, J.I., Doelitzsch, P.M., Huijgens, P.C., von Blomberg, B.M., Jakobs, C., van Geijn, H.P. (1995). Underlying disorders associated with severe early-onset preeclampsia. *Am J Obstet Gynecol,* Vol.173, No.4, (October 1995), pp. 1042-1048

Dekker, G.A., Sibai, B.M., (1998). Etiology and pathogenesis of preeclampsia: current concepts. *Am J Obstet Gynecol,* Vol.179, No.5, (November 1998), pp. 1359-1375

Dolmetsch, R.E., Xu, K., Lewis, R.S. (1998). Calcium oscillations increase the efficiency and specificity of gene expression. *Nature,* Vol.392, No.6679, (April 1998), pp. 933-936

El-Roeiy, A., Myers, S.A., Gleicher, N. (1991). The relationship between autoantibodies and intrauterine growth retardation in hypertensive disorders of pregnancy. *Am J Obstet Gynecol,* Vol.164, No.5 Pt 1, (May 1991), pp. 1253-1261

Fanger, C.M., Neben, A.L., Cahalan, M.D. (2000). Differential Ca2+ influx, KCa channel activity, and Ca2+ clearance distinguish Th1 and Th2 lymphocytes. *J Immunol,* Vol.164, No.3, (February 2000), pp. 1153-1160

Garin, M.I., Chu, C.C., Golshayan, D., Cernuda-Morollón, E., Wait, R., Lechler, R.I. (2007). Galectin-1: a key effector of regulation mediated by CD4+CD25+ T cells. *Blood,* Vol.109, No.5, (March 2007), pp. 2058-2065

Gleicher, N., Pratt, D., Dudkiewicz, A. (1993). What do we really know about autoantibody abnormalities and reproductive failure: a critical review. *Autoimmunity,* Vol.16, No.2, (February 1993), pp. 115-140

Gleicher, N. (2007). Why much of the pathophysiology of preeclampsia-eclampsia must be of an autoimmune nature. *Am J Obstet Gynecol,* Vol.196, No.1, (January 2007), pp. 5.e1-7

Heikkinen, J., Möttönen, M., Alanen, A., Lassila, O. (2004). Phenotypic characterization of regulatory T cells in the human decidua. *Clin Exp Immunol,* Vol.136, No.2, (May 2004), pp. 373-378

Hojo, M., Suthanthiran, M., Helseth, G., August, P. (1999). Lymphocyte intracellular free calcium concentration is increased in preeclampsia. *Am J Obstet Gynecol,* Vol.180, No.5, (May 1999), 209-214

Huber, M., Heink, S., Grothe, H., Guralnik, A., Reinhard, K., Elflein, K., Hünig, T., Mittrücker, H.W., Brüstle, A., Kamradt, T., Lohoff, M. (2009). A Th17-like developmental process leads to CD8(+) Tc17 cells with reduced cytotoxic activity. *Eur J Immunol,* Vol.39, No.7, (July 2009), pp. 1716-1725

Ito, T., Yang, M., Wang, Y.H., Lande, R., Gregorio, J., Perng, O.A., Qin, X.F., Liu, Y.J., Gilliet, M. (2007). Plasmacytoid dendritic cells prime IL-10-producing T regulatory cells by inducible costimulator ligand. *J Exp Med,* Vol.204, No.1, (January 2007), pp. 105-115

Ito, M., Nakashima, A., Hidaka, T., Okabe, M., Bac, N.D., Ina, S., Yoneda, S., Shiozaki, A., Sumi, S., Tsuneyama, K., Nikaido, T., Saito, S. (2010). A role for IL-17 in induction of an inflammation at the fetomaternal interface in preterm labour. *J Reprod Immunol,* Vol.84, No.1, (January 2010), pp. 75-85

Jianjun, Z., Yali, H., Zhiqun, W., Mingming, Z., Xia, Z. (2010). Imbalance of T-cell transcription factors contributes to the Th1 type immunity predominant in pre-eclampsia. *Am J Reprod Immunol,* Vol.63, No.1, (January 2010), pp. 38-45

Kaposi, A.S., Veress, G., Vásárhelyi, B., Macardle, P., Bailey, S., Tulassay, T., Treszl, A. (2008). Cytometry-acquired calcium-flux data analysis in activated lymphocytes. *Cytometry A,* Vol.73, No.3, (March 2008), pp. 246-253

Katz, V.L., Thorp, J.M. Jr, Watson, W.J., Fowler, L., Heine, R.P. (1990). Human immunoglobulin therapy for preeclampsia associated with lupus anticoagulant and anticardiolipin antibody. *Obstet Gynecol,* Vol.76, No.5 Pt 2, (November 1990), pp. 986-988

Kishore, R., Agarwal, S., Halder, A., Das, V., Shukla, B.R., Agarwal, S.S. (1996). HLA sharing, anti-paternal cytotoxic antibodies and MLR blocking factors in women with recurrent spontaneous abortion. *J Obstet Gynaecol Res,* Vol.22, No.2, (April 1996), pp. 177-183

Klonoff-Cohen, H.S., Savitz, D.A., Cefalo, R.C., McCann, M.F. (1989). An epidemiologic study of contraception and preeclampsia. *JAMA,* Vol.262, No.22, (December 1989), pp. 3143-3147

Koelman, C.A., Coumans, A.B., Nijman, H.W., Doxiadis, I.I., Dekker, G.A., Claas, F.H. (2000). Correlation between oral sex and a low incidence of preeclampsia: a role for soluble HLA in seminal fluid? *J Reprod Immunol,* Vol.46, No.2, (March 2000), pp. 155-166

Koopman, L.A., Kopcow, H.D., Rybalov, B., Boyson, J.E., Orange, J.S., Schatz, F., Masch, R., Lockwood, C.J., Schachter, A.D., Park, P.J., Strominger, J.L. (2003). Human decidual natural killer cells are a unique NK cell subset with immunomodulatory potential. *J Exp Med,* Vol.198, No.8, (October 2003), pp. 1201-1212

Kühnert, M., Strohmeier, R., Stegmüller, M., Halberstadt, E. (1998). Changes in lymphocyte subsets during normal pregnancy. *Eur J Obstet Gynecol Reprod Biol,* Vol.76, No.2, (February 1998), pp. 147-151

Lin, H., Mosmann, T.R., Guilbert, L., Tuntipopipat, S., Wegmann, T.G. (1993). Synthesis of T helper 2-type cytokines at maternal-fetal interface. *J Immunol,* Vol.151, No.9, (November 1993), pp. 4562-4573

Malinowski, A., Szpakowski, M., Tchórzewski, H., Zeman, K., Pawlowicz, P., Wozniak, P. (1994). T lymphocyte subpopulations and lymphocyte proliferative activity in normal and pre-eclamptic pregnancy. *Eur J Obstet Gynecol Reprod Biol,* Vol.53, No.1, (January 1994), pp. 27-31

Martin, J.N. Jr, Files, J.C., Blake, P.G., Norman, P.H., Martin, R.W., Hess, L.W., Morrison, J.C., Wiser, W.L. (1990). Plasma exchange for preeclampsia. I. Postpartum use for persistently severe preeclampsia-eclampsia with HELLP syndrome. *Am J Obstet Gynecol,* Vol.162, No.1, (January 1990), pp. 126-137

Martin, J.N. Jr, Rose, C.H., Briery, C.M. (2006). Understanding and managing HELLP syndrome: the integral role of aggressive glucocorticosteroids for mother and child. *Am J Obstet Gynecol,* Vol.195, No.4, (October 2006), pp. 914-934

Milliez, J., Lelong, F., Bayani, N., Jannet, D., El Medjadji, M., Latrous, H., Hammami, M., Paniel, B.J. (1991). The prevalence of autoantibodies during third trimester pregnancy complicated by hypertension or idiopathic fetal growth retardation. *Am J Obstet Gynecol,* Vol.165, No.1, (July 1991), pp. 51-56

Mjösberg, J., Berg, G., Ernerudh, J., Ekerfelt, C. (2007). CD4+ CD25+ regulatory T cells in human pregnancy: development of a Treg-MLC-ELISPOT suppression assay and indications of paternal specific Tregs. *Immunology,* Vol.120, No.4, (April 2007), pp. 456-466

Mjösberg, J., Berg, G., Jenmalm, M.C., Ernerudh, J. (2010). FOXP3+ regulatory T cells and T helper 1, T helper 2, and T helper 17 cells in human early pregnancy decidua. *Biol Reprod,* Vol.82, No.4, (April 2010), pp. 698-705

Molvarec, A., Blois, S.M., Stenczer, B., Toldi, G., Tirado-Gonzalez, I., Ito, M., Shima, T., Yoneda, S., Vásárhelyi, B., Rigó, J. Jr, Saito, S. (2011). Peripheral blood galectin-1-expressing T and natural killer cells in normal pregnancy and preeclampsia. *Clin Immunol,* (February 2011), in press

Mor, G., Cardenas, I. (2010). The immune system in pregnancy: a unique complexity. *Am J Reprod Immunol,* Vol.63, No.6, (June 2010), pp. 425-433

Nakashima, A., Ito, M., Shima, T., Bac, N.D., Hidaka, T., Saito, S. (2010). Accumulation of IL-17-positive cells in decidua of inevitable abortion cases. *Am J Reprod Immunol,* Vol.64, No.1, (July 2010), pp. 4-11

Panyi, G., Possani, L.D., Rodríguez de la Vega, R.C., Gáspár, R., Varga, Z. (2006). K+ channel blockers: novel tools to inhibit T cell activation leading to specific immunosuppression. *Curr Pharm Des,* Vol.12, No.18, (December 2006), pp. 2199-2220

Passos, S.T., Silver, J.S., O'Hara, A.C., Sehy, D., Stumhofer, J.S., Hunter, C.A. (2010). IL-6 promotes NK cell production of IL-17 during toxoplasmosis. *J Immunol,* Vol.184, No.4, (February 2010), pp. 1776-1783

Perillo, N.L., Pace, K.E., Seilhamer, J.J., Baum, L.G. (1995). Apoptosis of T cells mediated by galectin-1. *Nature,* Vol.378, No.6558, (December 1995), pp. 736-739

Piccinni, M.P., Beloni, L., Livi, C., Maggi, E., Scarselli, G.F., Romagnani, S., (1998). Defective production of both leukemia inhibitory factor and type 2 T-helper cytokines by decidual T cells in unexplained recurrent abortions. *Nat Med,* Vol.4, No.9, (September 1998), pp. 1020-1024

Piccinni, M.P. (2010). T cell tolerance towards the fetal allograft. *J Reprod Immunol,* Vol.85, No.1, (May 2010), pp. 71-75

Rabinovich, G.A., Iglesias, M.M., Modesti, N.M., Castagna, L.F., Wolfenstein-Todel, C., Riera, C.M., Sotomayor, C.E. (1998). Activated rat macrophages produce a galectin-1-like protein that induces apoptosis of T cells: biochemical and functional characterization. *J Immunol,* Vol.160, No.10, (May 1998), pp. 4831-4840

Rabinovich, G.A., Ariel, A., Hershkoviz, R., Hirabayashi, J., Kasai, K.I., Lider, O. (1999a). Specific inhibition of T-cell adhesion to extracellular matrix and proinflammatory cytokine secretion by human recombinant galectin-1. *Immunology,* Vol.97, No.1, (May 1999), pp. 100-106

Rabinovich, G.A., Daly, G., Dreja, H., Tailor, H., Riera, C.M., Hirabayashi, J., Chernajovsky, Y. (1999b). Recombinant galectin-1 and its genetic delivery suppress collagen-induced arthritis via T cell apoptosis. *J Exp Med,* Vol.190, No.3, (August 1999), pp. 385-398

Rappaport, V.J., Hirata, G., Yap, H.K., Jordan, S.C. (1990). Anti-vascular endothelial cell antibodies in severe preeclampsia. *Am J Obstet Gynecol,* Vol.162, No.1, (January 1990), pp. 138-146

Rein, D.T., Schondorf, T., Gohring, U.J., Kurbacher, C.M., Pinto, I., Breidenbach, M., Mallmann, P., Kolhagen, H., Engel, H. (2002). Cytokine expression in peripheral blood lymphocytes indicates a switch to T(HELPER) cells in patients with preeclampsia. *J Reprod Immunol,* Vol.54, No.1-2, (March 2002), pp. 133-142

Robillard, P.Y., Hulsey, T.C., Alexander, G.R., Keenan, A., de Caunes, F., Papiernik, E. (1993). Paternity patterns and risk of preeclampsia in the last pregnancy in multiparae. *J Reprod Immunol,* Vol.24, No.1, (May 1993), pp. 1-12

Robertson, S.A., Bromfield, J.J., Tremellen, K.P. (2003). Seminal 'priming' for protection from pre-eclampsia - a unifying hypothesis. *J Reprod Immunol,* Vol.59, No.2, (August 2003), pp. 253-265

Romagnani, S. (1991). Human Th1 and Th2: doubt no more. *Immunol Today,* Vol.12, No.8, (August 1991), pp. 256-257

Rusterholz, C., Hahn, S., Holzgreve, W. (2007). Role of placentally produced inflammatory and regulatory cytokines in pregnancy and the etiology of preeclampsia. *Semin Immunopathol,* Vol.29, No.2, (June 2007), pp. 151-162

Saito, S., Sakai, M., Sasaki, Y., Tanebe, K., Tsuda, H., Michimata, T. (1999a). Quantitative analysis of peripheral blood Th0, Th1, Th2 and the Th1:Th2 cell ratio during normal human pregnancy and preeclampsia. *Clin Exp Immunol,* Vol.117, No.3, (September 1999), pp. 550-555

Saito, S., Umekage, H., Sakamoto, Y., Sakai, M., Tanebe, K., Sasaki, Y., Morikawa, H. (1999b). Increased T-helper-1-type immunity and decreased T-helper-2-type immunity in patients with preeclampsia. *Am J Reprod Immunol,* Vol.41, No.5, (May 1999), pp. 297-306

Saito, S., Shiozaki, A., Nakashima, A., Sakai, M., Sasaki, Y. (2007). The role of the immune system in preeclampsia. *Mol Aspects Med,* Vol.28, No.2, (April 2007), pp. 192-209

Saito, S. (2010). Th17 cells and regulatory T cells: new light on pathophysiology of preeclampsia. *Immunol Cell Biol,* Vol.88, No.6, (August 2010), pp. 615-617

Salha, O., Sharma, V., Dada, T., Nugent, D., Rutherford, A.J., Tomlinson, A.J., Philips, S., Allgar, V., Walker, J.J. (1999). The influence of donated gametes on the incidence of hypertensive disorders of pregnancy. *Hum Reprod,* Vol.14, No.9, (September 1999), pp. 2268-2273

Santner-Nanan, B., Peek, M.J., Khanam, R., Richarts, L., Zhu, E., Fazekas de St Groth, B., Nanan, R. (2009). Systemic increase in the ratio between Foxp3+ and IL-17-producing CD4+ T cells in healthy pregnancy but not in preeclampsia. *J Immunol,* Vol.183, No.11, (December 2009), pp. 7023-7030

Sargent, I.L., Borzychowski, A.M., Redman, C.W. (2006a). Immunoregulation in normal pregnancy and pre-eclampsia: an overview. *Reprod Biomed Online,* Vol.13, No.5, (November 2006), pp. 680-686

Sargent, I.L., Borzychowski, A.M., Redman, C.W. (2006b). NK cells and human pregnancy--an inflammatory view. *Trends Immunol,* Vol.27, No.9, (September 2006), pp. 399-404

Sargent, I.L., Borzychowski, A.M., Redman, C.W. (2007). NK cells and preeclampsia. *J Reprod Immunol,* Vol.76, No.1-2, (December 2007), pp. 40-44

Sasaki, Y., Sakai, M., Miyazaki, S., Higuma, S., Shiozaki, A., Saito, S. (2004). Decidual and peripheral blood CD4+CD25+ regulatory T cells in early pregnancy subjects and spontaneous abortion cases. *Mol Hum Reprod,* Vol.10, No.5, (May 2004), pp. 347-353

Sasaki, Y., Darmochwal-Kolarz, D., Suzuki, D., Sakai, M., Ito, M., Shima, T., Shiozaki, A., Rolinski, J., Saito, S. (2007). Proportion of peripheral blood and decidual CD4(+) CD25(bright) regulatory T cells in preeclampsia. *Clin Exp Immunol,* Vol.149, No.1, (July 2007), pp. 139-145

Shin, H.C., Benbernou, N., Esnault, S., Guenounou, M. (1999). Expression of IL-17 in human memory CD45RO+ T lymphocytes and its regulation by protein kinase A pathway. *Cytokine,* Vol.11, No.4, (April 1999), pp. 257-266

Skjaerven, R., Wilcox, A.J., Lie, R.T. (2002). The interval between pregnancies and the risk of preeclampsia. *N Engl J Med,* Vol.346, No.1, (January 2002), pp. 33-38

Somerset, D.A., Zheng, Y., Kilby, M.D., Sansom, D.M., Drayson, M.T. (2004). Normal human pregnancy is associated with an elevation in the immune suppressive CD25+ CD4+ regulatory T-cell subset. *Immunology,* Vol.112, No.1, (May 2004), pp. 38-43

Steinborn, A., Haensch, G.M., Mahnke, K., Schmitt, E., Toermer, A., Meuer, S., Sohn, C. (2008). Distinct subsets of regulatory T cells during pregnancy: is the imbalance of these subsets involved in the pathogenesis of preeclampsia? *Clin Immunol,* Vol.129, No.3, (December 2008), pp. 401-412

Tallon, D.F., Corcoran, D.J., O'Dwyer, E.M., Greally, J.F. (1984). Circulating lymphocyte subpopulations in pregnancy: a longitudinal study. *J Immunol,* Vol.132, No.4, (April 1984), pp. 1784-1787

Thway, T.M., Shlykov, S.G., Day, M.C., Sanborn, B.M., Gilstrap, L.C. 3rd, Xia, Y., Kellems, R.E. (2004). Antibodies from preeclamptic patients stimulate increased intracellular Ca2+ mobilization through angiotensin receptor activation. *Circulation,* Vol.110, No.12, (September 2004), pp. 1612-1619

Toldi, G., Svec, P., Vásárhelyi, B., Mészáros, G., Rigó, J., Tulassay, T., Treszl, A. (2008). Decreased number of FoxP3+ regulatory T cells in preeclampsia. *Acta Obstet Gynecol Scand,* Vol.87, No.11, (November 2008), pp. 1229-1233

Toldi, G., Rigó, J. Jr, Stenczer, B., Vásárhelyi, B., Molvarec, A. (2011a). Increased prevalence of IL-17-producing peripheral blood lymphocytes in preeclampsia. *Am J Reprod Immunol,* (February 2011), in press

Toldi, G., Stenczer, B., Treszl, A., Kollár, S., Molvarec, A., Tulassay, T., Rigó, J., Vásárhelyi, B. (2011b). Lymphocyte calcium influx characteristics and their modulation by Kv1.3 and IKCa1 channel inhibitors in healthy pregnancy and preeclampsia. *Am J Reprod Immunol,* Vol.65, No.2, (February 2011), pp. 154-163

Toscano, M.A., Commodaro, A.G., Ilarregui, J.M., Bianco, G.A., Liberman, A., Serra, H.M., Hirabayashi, J., Rizzo, L.V., Rabinovich, G.A. (2006). Galectin-1 suppresses autoimmune retinal disease by promoting concomitant Th2- and T regulatory-mediated anti-inflammatory responses. *J Immunol,* Vol.176, No.10, (May 2006), pp. 6323-6332

Toscano, M.A., Bianco, G.A., Ilarregui, J.M., Croci, D.O., Correale, J., Hernandez, J.D., Zwirner, N.W., Poirier, F., Riley, E.M., Baum, L.G., Rabinovich, G.A. (2007). Differential glycosylation of TH1, TH2 and TH-17 effector cells selectively regulates susceptibility to cell death. *Nat Immunol,* Vol.8, No.8, (August 2007), pp. 825-834

Trupin, L.S., Simon, L.P., Eskenazi, B. (1996). Change in paternity: a risk factor for preeclampsia in multiparas. *Epidemiology,* Vol.7, No.3, (May 1996), pp. 240-244

Valencia, X., Stephens, G., Goldbach-Mansky, R., Wilson, M., Shevach, E.M., Lipsky, P.E. (2006). TNF downmodulates the function of human CD4+CD25hi T-regulatory cells. *Blood,* Vol.108, No.1, (July 2006), pp. 253-261

von Dadelszen, P., Wilkins, T., Redman, C.W. (1999). Maternal peripheral blood leukocytes in normal and pre-eclamptic pregnancies. *Br J Obstet Gynaecol,* Vol.106, No.6, (June 1999), pp. 576-581

von Rango, U. (2008). Fetal tolerance in human pregnancy--a crucial balance between acceptance and limitation of trophoblast invasion. *Immunol Lett,* Vol.115, No.1, (January 2008), pp. 21-32

Walker, J.J. (2000). Pre-eclampsia. *Lancet,* Vol.356, No.9237, (October 2000), pp. 1260-1265

Wallukat, G., Homuth, V., Fischer, T., Lindschau, C., Horstkamp, B., Jupner, A., Baur, E., Nissen, E., Vetter, K., Neichel, D., Dudenhausen, J.W., Haller, H., Luft, F.C. (1999). Patients with preeclampsia develop agonistic autoantibodies against the angiotensin AT1 receptor. *J Clin Invest,* Vol.103, No.7, (April 1999), pp. 945-952

Wang, W.J., Hao, C.F., Lin, Y., Yin, G.J., Bao, S.H., Qiu, L.H., Lin, Q.D. (2010). Increased prevalence of T helper 17 (Th17) cells in peripheral blood and decidua in unexplained recurrent spontaneous abortion patients. *J Reprod Immunol,* Vol.84 No.2, (March 2010), pp. 164-170

Watanabe, M., Iwatani, Y., Kaneda, T., Hidaka, Y., Mitsuda, N., Morimoto, Y., Amino, N. (1997). Changes in T, B, and NK lymphocyte subsets during and after normal pregnancy. *Am J Reprod Immunol,* Vol.37, No.5, (May 1997), pp. 368-377

Wegmann, T.G., Lin, H., Guilbert, L., Mossmann, T.R. (1993). Bidirectional cytokine interactions in the maternal-fetal relationship: is successful pregnancy a Th2 phenomenon? *Immunol Today,* Vol.14, No.7, (July 1993), pp. 353-356

Wilczyński, J.R. (2006). Immunological analogy between allograft rejection, recurrent abortion and pre-eclampsia - the same basic mechanism? *Hum Immunol,* Vol.67, No.7, (July 2006), pp. 492-511

Yamamoto, T., Yoshimura, S., Geshi, Y., Sasamori, Y., Okinaga, S., Kobayashi, T., Mori, H. (1993). Measurement of antiphospholipid antibody by ELISA using purified beta 2-glycoprotein I in preeclampsia. *Clin Exp Immunol,* Vol.94, No.1, (October 1993), pp. 196-200

Zenclussen, A.C. (2006). Regulatory T cells in pregnancy. *Springer Semin Immunopathol,* Vol.28, No.1, (August 2006), pp. 31-39

Zuniga, E., Rabinovich, G.A., Iglesias, M.M., Gruppi, A. (2001). Regulated expression of galectin-1 during B-cell activation and implications for T-cell apoptosis. *J Leukoc Biol,* Vol.70, No.1, (July 2001), pp. 73-79

Part 5

Osteoimmunology

22

Osteoimmunology and Cancer - Clinical Implications

Evangelos Terpos, Maria Gkotzamanidou,
Dimitrios Christoulas and Meletios A. Dimopoulos
Department of Clinical Therapeutics, University of Athens School of Medicine, Athens, Greece

1. Introduction

The skeletal and immune systems are interconnected in normal (physiologic) and pathologic conditions. Both systems are intimately coupled, as osteoclastogenesis and hematopoiesis occur in the bone marrow. Osteoclasts, macrophages, and dendritic cells also share common precursors. Furthermore, the skeletal and immune systems share various cytokines, receptors, adaptor proteins, signaling molecules, and transcription factors, thereby allowing crosstalk to occur between the various cells and their respective signal transduction pathways involved in osteoclastogenesis and hematopoiesis.

Hematopoietic stem cells are maintained in the bone marrow. Adjacent osteoblast precursors produce signals that control hematopoietic stem cell replication and differentiation. Hematopoietic stem cells may either maintain their pluripotency or differentiate into multipotential progenitor cells, which have the capacity to form common lymphoid progenitor or common myeloid precursor cells. Common lymphoid progenitor cells undergo additional differentiation to form T lymphocytes, B lymphocytes, or natural killer cells, whereas common myeloid precursor cells form all other myeloid lineages and preosteoclasts. Activated osteoclasts are formed from the fusion of preosteoclasts and multinucleated osteoclasts, the regulation of which is complex and affected by multiple factors. Multipotential stem cells differentiate into chondrocytes, adipocytes, and mesenchyme precursors; the latter undergo differentiation to form preosteoblasts and, eventually, mature matrix-producing osteoblasts. Osteoblasts may remain on the bone surface as lining cells or undergo terminal differentiation to form osteocytes, which become encased in the mineralized bone matrix [1]. The shared lineages and paracrine signaling between osteoclasts and hematopoietic cells highlight the potential for bone-targeted agents to influence the immune system.

2. Transduction signaling pathways between skeletal and immune system

The skeletal and immune systems share various signal transduction pathways, thereby allowing a complex interplay to occur between bone metabolism and immunology. Furthermore, immune system components, such as T cells, cytokines, and chemokines, can exert substantial effects on osteoclastogenesis.

2.1 Osteoclastogenesis and immune system

Osteoclastogenesis is primarily regulated via interactions between c-FMS and macrophage colony-stimulating factor, receptor activator of nuclear factor (NF)-kappaB (RANK) and RANK ligand (RANKL), and immunoglobulin (Ig)-like receptors and their ligands [2]. The role of RANK signaling in osteoclastogenesis has also been reviewed elsewhere [2-16]. Other key regulatory pathways are described below.

RANK/RANKL/osteoprotegerin signaling

Receptor activator of NF-κB ligand is a member of the tumor necrosis factor (TNF) cytokine superfamily that is expressed by osteoblasts, monocytes, neutrophils, dendritic cells, B lymphocytes, and T lymphocytes [3]. Secretion of RANKL by osteoclastogenesis-supporting cells (osteoblasts and synovial fibroblasts) occurs in response to osteoclastogenic factors such as 1,25-dihydroxyvitamin D3, prostaglandin E2, and parathyroid hormone [2]. T cells express RANKL as a type-2 membrane-bound protein and also release it in soluble form, although the function of the soluble form remains unknown [16]. Inflammatory cytokines, such as interleukin (IL)-1, IL-6, and TNF-α, also potently induce RANKL expression on osteoblasts and synovial fibroblasts, thereby stimulating RANKL signaling [2].
Receptor activator of NF-κB, the RANKL receptor, shares high homology with CD40, which is expressed on lymphocytes and, similar to RANKL, is reported to play a role in atherosclerosis and coronary artery disease [17-19]. Interaction of RANK with RANKL is inhibited by osteoprotegerin (OPG), a soluble competitor (decoy) receptor that binds to RANKL [12, 13]. Receptor activator of NF-κB lacks intrinsic enzymatic activity in its intracellular domain and transduces signals by recruiting adaptor molecules such as the TNF-receptor–associated factor (TRAF) family of proteins, especially TRAF6 [4, 5, 15]. By an unknown mechanism, RANKL binding to RANK induces trimerization of RANK and TRAF6, leading to activation of NF-κB and of mitogen-activated protein kinases such as Jun N-terminal kinase and p38 [6]. Activated RANK can also lead to stimulation of Ig-like receptor signaling.

Nuclear factor of activated t cells cytoplasmic (NFATc)-1 pathway

Expression of NFATc-1, the master regulator of osteoclast differentiation, depends on induction of the TRAF6–NF-κB and c-FOS pathways, in addition to activation of calcium signaling [20]. Nuclear factor of activated T cells cytoplasmic-1 is initially induced by TRAF6-activated NF-κB and NFATc-2. After translocation into the nucleus, NFATc-1 autoregulates its own expression by binding to the NFAT-binding site of its promoter, enabling robust induction of NFATc-1 expression [21]. Activator protein 1 and continuous activation of calcium signaling by calcineurin are crucial for NFATc-1 autoamplification [20]. Nuclear factor of activated T cells cytoplasmic-1 cooperates with other transcription factors, such as AP1, PU.1, microphthalmia-associated transcription factor, and cyclic AMP responsive-element-binding protein, to regulate various osteoclast-specific genes, including tartrate-resistant acid phosphatase, cathepsin K, calcitonin receptor, osteoclast-associated receptor, and β3-integrin [2, 20, 22-24].

2.2 Cytokines, chemokines and osteoclastogenesis

Immune cells produce a variety of proinflammatory cytokines that contribute to bone damage [25]. Tumor necrosis factor-alpha and IL-1, -3, -6, -7, -11, -15, and -17 potentiate bone loss by inducing RANKL expression on osteoblasts or by increasing osteoclast differentiation and activation. In contrast, IL-4, -5, -10, -12, -13, and -18, and interferon (IFN)-α, -β, and -γ, inhibit osteoclastogenesis by directly or indirectly blocking RANKL signaling

(Table 1). Interleukin-1 stimulates TRAF6 expression, thereby potentiating the RANKL-RANK signaling cascade and inducing mature osteoclasts to perform bone-resorbing activity. Interferon gamma down-regulates TRAF6 expression via proteosomal degradation,

Cytokine	Main producer cells	Primary target in osteoclastogenesis	Effect on osteoclastogenesis	Role in osteoimmunology
RANKL	T-cells; Osteoblasts	Osteoclast precursor cells	Activation	Induction of osteoclast differentiation
TNF-α	Macrophages; Th1 cells	Osteoclast precursor cells; mesenchymal cells	Activation	RANKL induction on mesenchymal cells, RANKL synergy, inflammation
IL-6	Th2 cells; dendritic cells	Mesenchymal cells; T cells	Activation	RANKL induction on mesenchymal cells, Th17-cell differentiation, inflammation
IL-17	Th17 cells; memory T cells	Mesenchymal cells	Activation	RANKL induction on mesenchymal cells, inflammation
IFN-γ	Th1 cells; natural killer cells	Osteoclast precursor cells	Inhibition	RANKL signaling inhibition, cellular immunity
IL-4	Th2 cells; natural killer T cells	Osteoclast precursor cells	Inhibition	RANKL signaling inhibition, humoral immunity
IL-10	Th2 cells	Osteoclast precursor cells	Inhibition	RANKL signaling inhibition, anti-inflammatory
IL-12	Macrophages; dendritic cells	T cells	Inhibition	Th1-cell differentiation, IFN-γ and GM-CSF induction
IL-18	Macrophages; dendritic cells	T cells	Inhibition	Th1-cell differentiation, IFN-γ induction
GM-CSF	Th1 cells	Osteoclast precursor cells	Inhibition	RANKL signaling inhibition, granulocyte differentiation

Abbreviations: GM-CSF, granulocyte-macrophage colony-stimulating factor; IFN, interferon; IL, interleukin; RANKL, receptor activator of nuclear factor-κB ligand; Th, T-helper; TNF, tumor necrosis factor.

Table 1. Cytokines Involved in Osteoclastogenesis

resulting in termination of osteoclast formation [26, 27]. Receptor activator of NF-κB induces expression of IFN-β in osteoclast precursor cells, and IFN-β functions as a negative-feedback regulator of osteoclast differentiation by interfering with RANKL-induced c-FOS expression [28]. Tumor necrosis factor-alpha stimulates NF-κB activation primarily via interacting with TRAF2. Although TNF-α alone cannot induce osteoclastogenesis and TNF-α overexpression cannot rescue RANKL deficiency, TNF-α combined with transforming growth factor (TGF)-β induces osteoclastogenesis even in the absence of RANK or TRAF6 [29-31]. These results suggest that TNF-α plays a pivotal role in the pathologic activation of osteoclasts associated with inflammation [2]. Osteoblast-mediated bone formation is also affected by various soluble cytokines such as TNF-α, IL-1, and IL-4 [32]. The molecular mechanisms involved in osteoblast regulation by the immune system and the pathologic significance of such regulation are less understood than in osteoclasts.

2.3 T cells and osteoclastogenesis

In general, activated T cells exert an inhibitory effect on osteoclastogenesis. The $CD4^+$ T helper (Th) cells have traditionally been divided into 2 main subtypes—Th1 and Th2—based on their associated cytokine profiles. The Th1 cells mainly produce IFN-γ and IL-2, and mediate cellular immunity. In contrast, Th2 cells mainly produce IL-4, IL-5, and IL-10, and mediate humoral immunity. Although T cells express RANKL, most Th1 cytokines, as well as certain Th2 cytokines (eg, IL-4 and IL-10), exert an inhibitory effect on osteoclastogenesis. However, the Th-cell subset involved in producing IL-17 (Th17 cells) is considered to be the typical osteoclastogenic Th subset. The Th17 cells express RANKL at higher levels than Th1 or Th2 cells and, as a result, may directly participate in osteoclastogenesis. In addition, Th17 cells do not produce large amounts of IFN-γ, an inhibitor of osteoclastogenesis. Furthermore, Th17 cells activate local inflammation, triggering release of proinflammatory cytokines that potentiate RANKL expression on osteoclastogenesis-supporting cells and RANKL-RANK signal transduction in osteoclast precursor cells [33]. Interleukin-17, produced by Th17 cells, induces the synthesis of matrix-degrading enzymes, such as matrix metalloproteinases, that mediate bone and cartilage degradation [34]. The effects of Th17 cells on osteoclastogenesis are balanced by regulatory T cells, which suppress osteoclast formation via a cytokine-dependent mechanism mediated by TGF-β, IFN-γ, IL-4, and IL-10 [35-37]. Therefore, the effects of T cells on osteoclastogenesis depend on the balance between positive and negative factors expressed by these cells under pathologic conditions.

3. Disruption of the skeletal and immune systems in cancer

Tumorigenesis can disrupt the skeletal and immune systems. Tumor growth and metastasis necessitate evasion of the immune system, especially phosphoantigen-targeted gamma delta T cells (γδ T cells), which can detect and destroy cancer cells. Immune system components also play other key roles in tumor development and progression. For example, tumor-associated macrophages (TAMs) are abundant in the bone microenvironment and influence multiple steps in tumor development, including growth, survival, invasion, and metastasis, as well as angiogenesis and lymphangiogenesis [38, 39]. During early metastasis of solid tumors, disseminated tumor cells (DTCs) survive in the bone marrow of patients with various tumor types. Cancers for which DTCs have been detected in patients who have not developed overt metastases include breast, colon, gastric, lung, and prostate cancers [40-46]. The hematopoietic niche in the bone marrow also provides a "harbor" for DTCs to survive despite anticancer therapies. Whether this niche also harbors cancer cells against anticancer immune defenses is unknown. However, the shared signal transduction pathways among the bone remodeling and immune system machineries in this common microenvironment suggest that activation of this vicious cycle of tumor growth and osteolytic bone destruction could also lead to localized immunosuppression or recruitment of metastasis-supporting TAMs, an unfortunate juxtaposition of osteoimmunology effects. Later in the disease course, interactions between malignant cells and bone may result in a vicious cycle of bone destruction and cancer growth (the "seed and soil theory") [47]. The effects of cancer on bone can result in skeletal-related events (SREs) that include pathologic fracture, spinal cord compression, hypercalcemia of malignancy, and the need for radiotherapy. Furthermore, some cancers such as myeloma can exert additional deleterious effects on bone metabolism via inducing osteolysis, systemic bone loss, and suppression of new bone formation throughout the skeleton [48, 49].

3.1 Osteoclastogenesis and cancer cell growth and metastases

Osteoclast-mediated osteolysis results in release of growth factors in the bone microenvironment that facilitate cancer growth and metastases. Bone-derived cytokines provide a chemotactic stimulus for directed tumor cell migration [50]. Recent studies established that RANKL is a chemoattractant that increases migration and invasion of RANK-positive cancer cells (bone tropism) [51, 52]. In preclinical models, bone resorption by bone cell cultures stimulated proliferation of various tumor cell types, including breast cancer that possessed bone-metastasizing properties [53]. In animal models, cancer cells located immediately adjacent to bone surfaces had significantly greater proliferation rates compared with those distant from bone, suggesting a mitogenic effect within the bone microenvironment [54]. Furthermore, in an animal model wherein bone resorption was stimulated by tumor cells, the proliferation rate of metastatic cancer cells was increased in bone but not in other tissues [55].

3.2 Cancer cell biology and bone resorption

Cancer cells stimulate osteoclast-mediated osteolysis via several mechanisms. Cancer cells may express RANKL and RANK, up-regulate RANKL expression by other osteoimmune cell types, down-regulate OPG expression, and stimulate release of factors that activate RANKL-RANK signaling in osteoclasts [56]. Expression of RANKL has been detected in prostate cancer cells [57] and multiple myeloma (MM) cells [58, 59], and RANKL expression by MM cells correlated with the propensity to cause bone destruction [58]. Although breast cancer cells do not typically express RANKL [60, 61], they can up-regulate RANKL expression by osteoblasts [60, 61] and bone marrow stromal cells [61, 62]. Prostate cancer cells can up-regulate RANKL expression in osteoblasts [63], and MM cells up-regulate RANKL expression in bone marrow stromal cells [64], endothelial cells [65], and T cells [66]. Several studies also reported expression of functional RANK by breast cancer, prostate, and melanoma cell lines [51, 52]. Breast cancer cells and MM cells down-regulate OPG production by osteoblasts and bone marrow stromal cells [60, 64]. Multiple myeloma cells express the heparin sulfate proteoglycan, syndecan, on their surface, which sequesters and degrades heparin-binding proteins including OPG [67]. Notably, the RANKL-OPG balance is disturbed in severe osteolytic pathologies in favor of RANKL, with large quantities of OPG being released within the tumor microenvironment to counterbalance high RANKL concentrations [64, 68].

Bisphosphonate	Cancer type	Patients, N	Reduction of SREs	Reduction of pain	Acute-phase reaction	Survival benefit
Clodronate [70]	Multiple myeloma	350	Yes	Yes	No	NE
Clodronate [72]	Multiple myeloma	536	Yes	Yes	No	+/–[a]
Clodronate [74]	Breast cancer	173	Yes	Yes	No	No
Clodronate [75]	Prostate cancer	819	NR	NR	No	Yes
Pamidronate [76]	Multiple myeloma	392	Yes	Yes	Yes	+/–[b]
Ibandronate [77]	Multiple myeloma	198	No	No	+/–	No
Zoledronic acid [78]	Multiple myeloma or breast cancer	1,648	Yes	Yes	Yes	Yes
Zoledronic acid [79]	Breast cancer	228	Yes	Yes	Yes	NE
Zoledronic acid [80]	Lung cancer and other solid tumors	773	Yes	NE	Yes	No
Zoledronic acid [81]	Hormone-refractory prostate cancer	122	Yes	Yes	Yes	NE
Denosumab [82]	Breast cancer	2,046	Yes	NE	Yes	NE

Abbreviations: NE, not evaluated; NR, not reported; SREs, skeletal-related events.
[a]In a post hoc analysis, patients without vertebral fracture at study entry survived significantly longer on clodronate therapy (median survival was 23 months longer compared with patients receiving placebo).
[b]Survival of patients with more advanced disease was significantly increased in the pamidronate group (median survival of 21 vs 14 months, P = .041).

Table 2. Efficacy of Bone-Targeted Agents in Patients With Bone Metastases

4. Bone-targeted therapies and immune system in cancer

4.1 Early generation bisphosphonates

In general, early generation bisphosphonates do not appear to activate the immune system against cancer cells. However, clodronate combined with IL-2 stimulated proliferation of γδ T cells in the absence of other cellular components in peripheral blood mononuclear cell (PBMC) cultures (wherein nitrogen-containing bisphosphonates have been tested), and clodronate-treated γδ T cells exhibited higher cytotoxic activity against neuroblastoma cells compared with untreated control cells [69]. There are currently no data on whether these effects can result in meaningful anticancer activities in in vivo models. Clodronate has shown efficacy in preventing SREs in patients with bone metastases from MM [70-73] and breast cancer [74], and was recently reported to significantly prolong survival in men with bone metastases from prostate cancer [75] (Table 2) [70, 72, 74-82]. Results from trials in the adjuvant breast cancer setting were inconsistent, and provided some evidence to suggest that clodronate can delay not only metastasis to bone but also to visceral sites.

4.2 Nitrogen-containing bisphosphonates

Nitrogen-containing bisphosphonates, such as zoledronic acid (ZOL) and pamidronate, cause immune system activation against cancer cells via activating γδ T cells [83, 84]. By blocking G-protein signaling, these agents prevent differentiation of monocytes into osteoclasts, inhibit osteoclast recruitment and maturation, induce osteoclast apoptosis, and inhibit adhesion of osteoclasts to bone [85].

Pamidronate therapy is associated with SRE reductions in patients with bone metastases from MM [76]. Although there was no overall difference in survival between pamidronate- and placebo-treated patients, pamidronate prolonged survival among patients who had received more than 1 previous antimyeloma regimen (14 vs 21 months; $P = .041$; N = 392) [86]. Although evidence is limited, pamidronate has demonstrated effects on the immune system that may result in anticancer activity. Treatment with pamidronate induced expansion of γδ T cells in PBMC cultures from healthy donors, and pamidronate-activated γδ T cells produced immunostimulatory cytokines and exhibited specific cytotoxicity against lymphoma and myeloma cell lines. Furthermore, pamidronate-treated bone marrow cultures from patients with MM exhibited reduced plasma cell survival compared with untreated cultures, especially in pamidronate-treated cultures, in which activation of bone marrow γδ T cells was evident (14 of 24 patients) [87].

Administration of ibandronate to patients with advanced MM failed to reduce bone morbidity or prolong survival [77]. Ibandronate also produced a lesser reduction in markers of bone resorption and disease activity, including N-telopeptide of type I collagen (NTX), IL-6, and β_2-microglobulin, compared with pamidronate [88]. However, ibandronate has demonstrated efficacy in the reduction of skeletal complications in other tumor types such as breast cancer [89].

Numerous studies established that zoledronic acid (ZOL) exhibits consistent efficacy in delaying and preventing SREs in patients with malignant bone disease from MM [78, 90, 91] and various solid tumors including breast [79], lung [80, 92], and prostate cancers [81]. In a 25-month randomized trial comparing ZOL with pamidronate in patients with bone lesions from MM or breast cancer (N = 1,648), a 15-minute infusion of 4 mg ZOL was at least as effective as a 2-hour infusion of 90 mg pamidronate at reducing the risk of SRE complications in the overall population [78]. Similarly, treating patients with lung cancer and other solid tumors with ZOL resulted in fewer patients developing SREs (ZOL 8 mg reduced to 4 mg = 36%, placebo = 46%; *P* = .023; N = 773) [80]. Administration of ZOL to men with hormone-refractory metastatic prostate cancer also reduced the proportion of patients with SREs (38% vs 49%; *P* = .028 vs placebo; N = 122) [81].

A recent study also demonstrated that ZOL may elicit anticancer effects associated with immune system stimulation. Zoledronic acid activated γδ T cells in vitro, and administration of ZOL to patients with prostate cancer resulted in the activation of γδ T cells in peripheral blood after the first infusion. Moreover, after the first ZOL infusion, serum prostate-specific antigen (PSA) levels were reduced in 3 of 11 evaluable patients, and PSA velocity was reduced in 5 of 10 evaluable patients [93]. These results suggest that ZOL-activated γδ T cells may be associated with the induction of an anticancer response in patients with prostate cancer.

Numerous in vitro studies established that ZOL directly and indirectly inhibits multiple steps involved in the processes of cancer development and progression. In addition, ZOL stimulates cancer cell apoptosis and expansion of γδ T cells, which play an important role in immune surveillance against neoplasia [94]. Preclinical studies reported that ZOL elicits anticancer activity in various cancer types and exhibits synergy with cytotoxic agents [95-100]. Four separate studies reported that ZOL reduced the persistence of DTCs in the bone marrow of patients with breast cancer [101-104]. In the clinical setting, adding ZOL to standard anticancer therapy improved clinical outcomes in early breast cancer. Administration of ZOL combined with adjuvant endocrine therapy to premenopausal women improved disease-free survival (hazard ratio [HR] = 0.64; *P* = .01) compared with endocrine therapy alone in the ABCSG-12 trial (N = 1,803) [105]. Similarly, ZOL plus neoadjuvant chemotherapy reduced residual invasive tumor size by 44% compared with chemotherapy in an exploratory subgroup from the AZURE trial (*P* = .006; n = 205) [106]. A multivariate analysis adjusted for potential prognostic factors in addition to neoadjuvant treatment group demonstrated that patients treated with ZOL plus neoadjuvant chemotherapy had a 2-fold greater complete pathologic response rate (breast and axilla) compared with patients treated with chemotherapy alone (odds ratio = 2.2; *P* = .1457). In the ZO-FAST (N = 1,065; median follow-up = 48 months; HR = 0.59; *P* = .0176) and Z-FAST (N = 602; median follow-up = 61 months; *P* = .6283) studies in postmenopausal women receiving adjuvant letrozole, immediate addition of ZOL reduced disease recurrence [107, 108]. In contrast with ABCSG-12, which had disease-free survival as a primary endpoint, ZO-FAST and Z-FAST were not designed or powered to evaluate disease recurrence (primary endpoints were bone loss); however, these studies demonstrated that upfront administration of ZOL resulted in improved disease-free survival among women with breast cancer. Subset analyses of the phase III clinical studies revealed that ZOL significantly prolonged survival compared with placebo among patients with high baseline NTX levels. Benefits were independent of SRE prevention, and multiple anticancer mechanisms, some of which involved immune system activation, may have contributed [109, 110]. Additionally, ZOL elicited anticancer responses in patients with MM, bladder cancer, lung cancer, or advanced solid tumors [111-114]. The Medical Research Council (MRC) Myeloma IX trial demonstrated that, after median follow-up of 3.7 years, ZOL significantly improved overall survival (by 5.5 months; 16% reduction in risk of death; *P* = .0118) and progression-free survival (by 2 months; 12% reduction in risk of disease progression; *P* = .0179) versus clodronate in patients with newly diagnosed MM (N = 1,960 evaluable patients) [111]. The survival benefit associated with ZOL was maintained in analyses adjusting for the potential effects of SREs on survival (*P* = .0178 vs clodronate), again supporting anticancer mechanisms for ZOL, which may involve positive effects on anticancer immune responses [111].

4.3 Anti-RANKL agents

Denosumab is a fully human IgG2 monoclonal antibody that binds to RANKL with high affinity and specificity, thereby inhibiting osteoclastogenesis. The effects of denosumab on bone remodeling have been evaluated in patients with postmenopausal osteoporosis, rheumatoid arthritis, and various cancers [115-118]. Limited safety data from the advanced cancer setting have been released. However, results from phase III studies in bone-loss settings suggested that adverse immunologic effects might occur. The FREEDOM trial, a phase III clinical study of 7,868 healthy postmenopausal women with osteoporosis, demonstrated that denosumab reduced the risk of new vertebral fractures by 68% compared with placebo ($P < .001$) [117]. A number of recent studies also demonstrated that denosumab can prevent SREs among patients with bone metastases from breast cancer, prostate cancer, other solid tumors, or MM. Denosumab was superior to ZOL in delaying time to first on-study SRE (HR = 0.82; $P = .01$ superiority), and time to first and subsequent on-study SREs (rate ratio = 0.77; $P = .001$) in 2,046 patients with advanced breast cancer [82], and in delaying time to first on-study SRE in patients with advanced castration-resistant prostate cancer (CRPC) (HR = 0.82; $P = .008$ superiority; N = 1,901) [119]. Median time to first on-study SRE was 20.7 months for denosumab versus 17.1 months for ZOL [119]. However, a significantly greater proportion of denosumab-treated patients experienced increased PSA levels compared with ZOL-treated patients (3.8% vs 2.0%, respectively; $P < .05$) [119]. Based on these results, it is possible that RANKL inhibition may impair immunosurveillance. Denosumab was non-inferior to ZOL in delaying time to first SRE in 1,776 patients with other advanced solid tumors or MM (HR = 0.84; $P = .0007$) [115]. Denosumab demonstrated antitumor activity in a phase II trial in 37 patients with benign giant-cell tumor (GCT) of bone, a tumor type that overexpresses RANKL and is associated with increased osteoclastic activity [120]. Given the low metastatic potential of GCT, the results observed in this patient population may not translate to patients with malignancies wherein the pathophysiology is distinct from that of GCT. Anticancer activity of blocking RANKL has been recently described in mouse models. RANKL inhibition was acting directly on hormone-induced mammary epithelium at early stages in tumorigenesis, and the permissive contribution of progesterone to increased mammary cancer incidence was due to RANKL-dependent proliferative changes in the mammary epithelium [121]. Based on these data, we assume that denosumab may have an anticancer activity; however, this has not yet been demonstrated in the clinical setting. Signaling via the RANKL-RANK pathway is involved in B-cell and T-cell differentiation and in survival of dendritic cells. As a result, concerns have been raised regarding possible immunosuppression with RANKL inhibitors. Recent clinical studies suggest that increased infection risk may be associated with denosumab therapy. The incidence of skin infections requiring hospitalization (cellulitis: 0.3% vs < 0.1% for placebo; $P = .002$) and endocarditis (3 patients vs 0 for placebo) was increased among postmenopausal women with osteoporosis who received denosumab therapy (FREEDOM) [115, 117]. A meta-analysis of 10,329 patients with osteopenia or osteoporosis also reported an increased risk of serious infections (odds ratio = 4.54 for denosumab vs placebo; $P = .03$) [122]. Serious infections were reported in 2.3% of denosumab-treated patients with early stage breast cancer compared with 0.8% of placebo-treated patients (P = not reported [NR];

N = 249; HALT-BC trial) [123]. Similarly, serious infections occurred at a higher incidence among denosumab-treated patients with androgen-dependent prostate cancer (5.9% vs 4.6% for placebo; *P* = NR; N = 1,468; HALT-PC trial) [124]. Urinary-tract infections also occurred more frequently among denosumab-treated patients with prostate cancer-related bone metastases (15% vs 6% for bisphosphonates; *P* = NR; N = 49) [125].

Denosumab is specific for human and certain nonhuman primate RANKL, and fails to inactivate rodent RANKL. Consequently, no carcinogenicity studies have been performed with denosumab because of the absence of an appropriate animal model. However, safety analyses from clinical trials of denosumab to prevent bone loss in patients receiving hormone-ablation therapy (HALT) for early stage breast or prostate cancer suggest that the potential for cancer progression may be increased with denosumab therapy. Among 1,456 patients with androgen-dependent prostate cancer in HALT-PC, 8.2% (n = 60) of denosumab-treated patients and 5.5% (n = 40) of placebo-treated patients experienced metastatic events (*P* = NR) [115]. Similarly, metastatic events were reported in 7% (n = 9) of denosumab-treated patients compared with 4.2% (n = 5) of placebo-treated patients with breast cancer in HALT-BC (*P* = NR; N = 249) [115]. Indeed, given the significantly increased rates of PSA progression in patients with CRPC and the significantly reduced survival in patients with MM treated with denosumab versus ZOL in the phase III clinical trials program (HR = 2.26) [126], further investigations on the potential effects of RANKL inhibition on cancer immunosurveillance and response are warranted.

5. Conclusions

The skeletal and immune systems have a complex relationship under normal (physiologic) and pathologic conditions. The RANKL-RANK-OPG signal transduction pathway plays a key role in regulating osteoclastogenesis. However, the effects of RANKL signaling are not limited to the skeletal system; RANKL is also expressed in other regulatory systems including the immune, cardiovascular, endocrine, and nervous systems. Expression of RANKL in the immune system regulates antigen-specific T-cell and B-cell responses, as well as the ability of T cells to interact with dendritic cells. Furthermore, RANKL directly affects the survival of antigen-presenting dendritic cells, which help other cells in the immune system to recognize and destroy abnormal cells and foreign antigens. Because of the systemic nature of RANKL expression, RANKL inhibition to prevent bone destruction may result in unintended consequences outside of the bone, including immune suppression with resulting possible increases in risk of infection or new malignancies. The long-term safety profiles of agents targeting this pathway are not yet known.

Currently available therapies designed to reduce pathologic osteolysis may also result in modulation of the immune system. Nitrogen-containing bisphosphonates such as ZOL exert beneficial effects on the immune system, resulting in activation of anticancer responses, as demonstrated in several clinical studies in various malignancies. Careful consideration should be paid to the shared pathways in bone immunology to maximize beneficial and minimize potentially negative effects in the clinical setting.

6. References

[1] Lorenzo J, Horowitz M, Choi Y (2008) Osteoimmunology: interactions of the bone and immune system. Endocr Rev 29:403-440

[2] Takayanagi H (2007) Osteoimmunology: shared mechanisms and crosstalk between the immune and bone systems. Nat Rev Immunol 7:292-304

[3] Caetano-Lopes J, Canhao H, Fonseca JE (2009) Osteoimmunology—the hidden immune regulation of bone. Autoimmun Rev 8:250-255

[4] Gohda J, Akiyama T, Koga T, Takayanagi H, Tanaka S, Inoue J (2005) RANK-mediated amplification of TRAF6 signaling leads to NFATc1 induction during osteoclastogenesis. EMBO J 24:790-799

[5] Kadono Y, Okada F, Perchonock C, Jang HD, Lee SY, Kim N, Choi Y (2005) Strength of TRAF6 signalling determines osteoclastogenesis. EMBO Rep 6:171-176

[6] Kobayashi N, Kadono Y, Naito A, Matsumoto K, Yamamoto T, Tanaka S, Inoue J (2001) Segregation of TRAF6-mediated signaling pathways clarifies its role in osteoclastogenesis. EMBO J 20:1271-1280

[7] Koga T, Inui M, Inoue K, Kim S, Suematsu A, Kobayashi E, Iwata T, Ohnishi H, Matozaki T, Kodama T, Taniguchi T, Takayanagi H, Takai T (2004) Costimulatory signals mediated by the ITAM motif cooperate with RANKL for bone homeostasis. Nature 428:758-763

[8] Mao D, Epple H, Uthgenannt B, Novack DV, Faccio R (2006) PLCgamma2 regulates osteoclastogenesis via its interaction with ITAM proteins and GAB2. J Clin Invest 116:2869-2879

[9] Mocsai A, Humphrey MB, Van Ziffle JA, Hu Y, Burghardt A, Spusta SC, Majumdar S, Lanier LL, Lowell CA, Nakamura MC (2004) The immunomodulatory adapter proteins DAP12 and Fc receptor gamma-chain (FcRgamma) regulate development of functional osteoclasts through the Syk tyrosine kinase. Proc Natl Acad Sci U S A 101:6158-6163

[10] Ross FP, Teitelbaum SL (2005) alphavbeta3 and macrophage colony-stimulating factor: partners in osteoclast biology. Immunol Rev 208:88-105

[11] Sato K, Suematsu A, Nakashima T, Takemoto-Kimura S, Aoki K, Morishita Y, Asahara H, Ohya K, Yamaguchi A, Takai T, Kodama T, Chatila TA, Bito H, Takayanagi H (2006) Regulation of osteoclast differentiation and function by the CaMK-CREB pathway. Nat Med 12:1410-1416

[12] Simonet WS, Lacey DL, Dunstan CR, Kelley M, Chang MS, Luthy R, Nguyen HQ, Wooden S, Bennett L, Boone T, Shimamoto G, DeRose M, Elliott R, Colombero A, Tan HL, Trail G, Sullivan J, Davy E, Bucay N, Renshaw-Gegg L, Hughes TM, Hill D, Pattison W, Campbell P, Sander S, Van G, Tarpley J, Derby P, Lee R, Boyle WJ (1997) Osteoprotegerin: a novel secreted protein involved in the regulation of bone density. Cell 89:309-319

[13] Tsuda E, Goto M, Mochizuki S, Yano K, Kobayashi F, Morinaga T, Higashio K (1997) Isolation of a novel cytokine from human fibroblasts that specifically inhibits osteoclastogenesis. Biochem Biophys Res Commun 234:137-142

[14] Wagner EF, Eferl R (2005) Fos/AP-1 proteins in bone and the immune system. Immunol Rev 208:126-140

[15] Wong BR, Josien R, Lee SY, Vologodskaia M, Steinman RM, Choi Y (1998) The TRAF family of signal transducers mediates NF-kappaB activation by the TRANCE receptor. J Biol Chem 273:28355-28359

[16] Wong BR, Rho J, Arron J, Robinson E, Orlinick J, Chao M, Kalachikov S, Cayani E, Bartlett FS, 3rd, Frankel WN, Lee SY, Choi Y (1997) TRANCE is a novel ligand of

the tumor necrosis factor receptor family that activates c-Jun N-terminal kinase in T cells. J Biol Chem 272:25190-25194
[17] Gururajan P, Gurumurthy P, Nayar P, Babu S, Sarasabharati A, Victor D, Cherian KM (2009) Increased serum concentrations of soluble CD40 ligand as a prognostic marker in patients with acute coronary syndrome. Indian J Clin Biochem 24:229-233
[18] Montecucco F, Steffens S, Mach F (2007) The immune response is involved in atherosclerotic plaque calcification: could the RANKL/RANK/OPG system be a marker of plaque instability? Clin Dev Immunol 2007:75805
[19] Chakraborty S, Cheek J, Sakthivel B, Aronow BJ, Yutzey KE (2008) Shared gene expression profiles in developing heart valves and osteoblast progenitor cells. Physiol Genomics 35:75-85
[20] Takayanagi H, Kim S, Koga T, Nishina H, Isshiki M, Yoshida H, Saiura A, Isobe M, Yokochi T, Inoue J, Wagner EF, Mak TW, Kodama T, Taniguchi T (2002) Induction and activation of the transcription factor NFATc1 (NFAT2) integrate RANKL signaling in terminal differentiation of osteoclasts. Dev Cell 3:889-901
[21] Asagiri M, Sato K, Usami T, Ochi S, Nishina H, Yoshida H, Morita I, Wagner EF, Mak TW, Serfling E, Takayanagi H (2005) Autoamplification of NFATc1 expression determines its essential role in bone homeostasis. J Exp Med 202:1261-1269
[22] Crotti TN, Flannery M, Walsh NC, Fleming JD, Goldring SR, McHugh KP (2006) NFATc1 regulation of the human beta3 integrin promoter in osteoclast differentiation. Gene 372:92-102
[23] Kim Y, Sato K, Asagiri M, Morita I, Soma K, Takayanagi H (2005) Contribution of nuclear factor of activated T cells c1 to the transcriptional control of immunoreceptor osteoclast-associated receptor but not triggering receptor expressed by myeloid cells-2 during osteoclastogenesis. J Biol Chem 280:32905-32913
[24] Matsumoto M, Kogawa M, Wada S, Takayanagi H, Tsujimoto M, Katayama S, Hisatake K, Nogi Y (2004) Essential role of p38 mitogen-activated protein kinase in cathepsin K gene expression during osteoclastogenesis through association of NFATc1 and PU.1. J Biol Chem 279:45969-45979
[25] Herman S, Kronke G, Schett G (2008) Molecular mechanisms of inflammatory bone damage: emerging targets for therapy. Trends Mol Med 14:245-253
[26] Datta HK, Ng WF, Walker JA, Tuck SP, Varanasi SS (2008) The cell biology of bone metabolism. J Clin Pathol 61:577-587
[27] Takayanagi H, Ogasawara K, Hida S, Chiba T, Murata S, Sato K, Takaoka A, Yokochi T, Oda H, Tanaka K, Nakamura K, Taniguchi T (2000) T-cell-mediated regulation of osteoclastogenesis by signalling cross-talk between RANKL and IFN-gamma. Nature 408:600-605
[28] Takayanagi H, Kim S, Matsuo K, Suzuki H, Suzuki T, Sato K, Yokochi T, Oda H, Nakamura K, Ida N, Wagner EF, Taniguchi T (2002) RANKL maintains bone homeostasis through c-Fos-dependent induction of interferon-beta. Nature 416:744-749
[29] Lam J, Takeshita S, Barker JE, Kanagawa O, Ross FP, Teitelbaum SL (2000) TNF-alpha induces osteoclastogenesis by direct stimulation of macrophages exposed to permissive levels of RANK ligand. J Clin Invest 106:1481-1488

[30] Li P, Schwarz EM, O'Keefe RJ, Ma L, Boyce BF, Xing L (2004) RANK signaling is not required for TNFalpha-mediated increase in CD11(hi) osteoclast precursors but is essential for mature osteoclast formation in TNFalpha-mediated inflammatory arthritis. J Bone Miner Res 19:207-213
[31] Kim N, Kadono Y, Takami M, Lee J, Lee SH, Okada F, Kim JH, Kobayashi T, Odgren PR, Nakano H, Yeh WC, Lee SK, Lorenzo JA, Choi Y (2005) Osteoclast differentiation independent of the TRANCE-RANK-TRAF6 axis. J Exp Med 202:589-595
[32] Walsh MC, Kim N, Kadono Y, Rho J, Lee SY, Lorenzo J, Choi Y (2006) Osteoimmunology: interplay between the immune system and bone metabolism. Annu Rev Immunol 24:33-63
[33] Sato K, Suematsu A, Okamoto K, Yamaguchi A, Morishita Y, Kadono Y, Tanaka S, Kodama T, Akira S, Iwakura Y, Cua DJ, Takayanagi H (2006) Th17 functions as an osteoclastogenic helper T cell subset that links T cell activation and bone destruction. J Exp Med 203:2673-2682
[34] David JP (2007) Osteoimmunology: a view from the bone. Adv Immunol 95:149-165
[35] Askenasy N, Kaminitz A, Yarkoni S (2008) Mechanisms of T regulatory cell function. Autoimmun Rev 7:370-375
[36] Kim YG, Lee CK, Nah SS, Mun SH, Yoo B, Moon HB (2007) Human CD4+CD25+ regulatory T cells inhibit the differentiation of osteoclasts from peripheral blood mononuclear cells. Biochem Biophys Res Commun 357:1046-1052
[37] Kelchtermans H, Geboes L, Mitera T, Huskens D, Leclercq G, Matthys P (2009) Activated CD4+CD25+ regulatory T cells inhibit osteoclastogenesis and collagen-induced arthritis. Ann Rheum Dis 68:744-750
[38] Biswas SK, Lewis CE (2010) NF-κB as a central regulator of macrophage function in tumors. J Leukoc Biol 88:877-884
[39] Hagemann T, Biswas SK, Lawrence T, Sica A, Lewis CE (2009) Regulation of macrophage function in tumors: the multifaceted role of NF-kappaB. Blood 113:3139-3146
[40] Pantel K, Alix-Panabieres C, Riethdorf S (2009) Cancer micrometastases. Nat Rev Clin Oncol 6:339-351
[41] Raimondi C, Gradilone A, Gandini O, Petracca A, Nicolazzo C, Palazzo A, Naso G, Cortesi E, Gazzaniga P (2010) Circulating tumor cells in breast cancer: are currently available detection methods enough? (abstract 170PD). In: Presented at the 35th ESMO Congress; 8-12 October 2010, Milan, Italy
[42] De Giorgi U, Mego M, Scarpi E, Handy BC, Jackson SA, Reuben J, Valero V, Hortobagyi GN, Ueno N, Cristofanilli M (2010) Relationship between lymphopenia and circulating tumor cells as prognostic factors for overall survival in metastatic breast cancer (abstract 171PD). In: Presented at the 35th ESMO Congress; 8-12 October 2010, Milan, Italy
[43] Sastre J, Maestro ML, Gomez MA, Rivera Herrero F, Valladares M, Massuti B, Gallen M, Benavides M, Diaz Rubio E, Aranda E (2010) Enumeration circulating tumor cells (CTCs) is a prognostic and predictive factor for progression-free survival (PFS) and overall survival (OS) in colon cancer patients receiving first-line chemotherapy plus bevacizumab. A TTD Spanish Group Cooperative Study (abstract 173PD). In: Presented at the 35th ESMO Congress; 8-12 October 2010, Milan, Italy

[44] Seeliger H, Spatz H, Jauch KW (2003) Minimal residual disease in gastric cancer. Recent Results Cancer Res 162:79-87

[45] Passlick B (2001) Micrometastases in non-small cell lung cancer (NSCLC). Lung Cancer 34(suppl 3):S25-S29

[46] Morgan TM, Lange PH, Porter MP, Lin DW, Ellis WJ, Gallaher IS, Vessella RL (2009) Disseminated tumor cells in prostate cancer patients after radical prostatectomy and without evidence of disease predicts biochemical recurrence. Clin Cancer Res 15:677-683

[47] Roodman GD, Dougall WC (2008) RANK ligand as a therapeutic target for bone metastases and multiple myeloma. Cancer Treat Rev 34:92-101

[48] Kyle RA, Gertz MA, Witzig TE, Lust JA, Lacy MQ, Dispenzieri A, Fonseca R, Rajkumar SV, Offord JR, Larson DR, Plevak ME, Therneau TM, Greipp PR (2003) Review of 1027 patients with newly diagnosed multiple myeloma. Mayo Clin Proc 78:21-33

[49] Hjorth-Hansen H, Seifert MF, Borset M, Aarset H, Ostlie A, Sundan A, Waage A (1999) Marked osteoblastopenia and reduced bone formation in a model of multiple myeloma bone disease in severe combined immunodeficiency mice. J Bone Miner Res 14:256-263

[50] Orr W, Varani J, Gondex MK, Ward PA, Mundy GR (1979) Chemotactic responses of tumor cells to products of resorbing bone. Science 203:176-179

[51] Mori K, Le Goff B, Charrier C, Battaglia S, Heymann D, Redini F (2007) DU145 human prostate cancer cells express functional receptor activator of NFkappaB: new insights in the prostate cancer bone metastasis process. Bone 40:981-990

[52] Jones DH, Nakashima T, Sanchez OH, Kozieradzki I, Komarova SV, Sarosi I, Morony S, Rubin E, Sarao R, Hojilla CV, Komnenovic V, Kong YY, Schreiber M, Dixon SJ, Sims SM, Khokha R, Wada T, Penninger JM (2006) Regulation of cancer cell migration and bone metastasis by RANKL. Nature 440:692-696

[53] Manishen WJ, Sivananthan K, Orr FW (1986) Resorbing bone stimulates tumor cell growth. A role for the host microenvironment in bone metastasis. Am J Pathol 123:39-45

[54] Kostenuik PJ, Singh G, Suyama KL, Orr FW (1992) A quantitative model for spontaneous bone metastasis: evidence for a mitogenic effect of bone on Walker 256 cancer cells. Clin Exp Metastasis 10:403-410

[55] Kostenuik PJ, Singh G, Suyama KL, Orr FW (1992) Stimulation of bone resorption results in a selective increase in the growth rate of spontaneously metastatic Walker 256 cancer cells in bone. Clin Exp Metastasis 10:411-418

[56] Kearns AE, Khosla S, Kostenuik PJ (2008) Receptor activator of nuclear factor kappaB ligand and osteoprotegerin regulation of bone remodeling in health and disease. Endocr Rev 29:155-192

[57] Brown JM, Corey E, Lee ZD, True LD, Yun TJ, Tondravi M, Vessella RL (2001) Osteoprotegerin and rank ligand expression in prostate cancer. Urology 57:611-616

[58] Farrugia AN, Atkins GJ, To LB, Pan B, Horvath N, Kostakis P, Findlay DM, Bardy P, Zannettino AC (2003) Receptor activator of nuclear factor-kappaB ligand expression by human myeloma cells mediates osteoclast formation in vitro and correlates with bone destruction in vivo. Cancer Res 63:5438-5445

[59] Sezer O, Heider U, Zavrski I, Kuhne CA, Hofbauer LC (2003) RANK ligand and osteoprotegerin in myeloma bone disease. Blood 101:2094-2098

[60] Thomas RJ, Guise TA, Yin JJ, Elliott J, Horwood NJ, Martin TJ, Gillespie MT (1999) Breast cancer cells interact with osteoblasts to support osteoclast formation. Endocrinology 140:4451-4458
[61] Kitazawa S, Kitazawa R (2002) RANK ligand is a prerequisite for cancer-associated osteolytic lesions. J Pathol 198:228-236
[62] Mancino AT, Klimberg VS, Yamamoto M, Manolagas SC, Abe E (2001) Breast cancer increases osteoclastogenesis by secreting M-CSF and upregulating RANKL in stromal cells. J Surg Res 100:18-24
[63] Fizazi K, Yang J, Peleg S, Sikes CR, Kreimann EL, Daliani D, Olive M, Raymond KA, Janus TJ, Logothetis CJ, Karsenty G, Navone NM (2003) Prostate cancer cells-osteoblast interaction shifts expression of growth/survival-related genes in prostate cancer and reduces expression of osteoprotegerin in osteoblasts. Clin Cancer Res 9:2587-2597
[64] Giuliani N, Bataille R, Mancini C, Lazzaretti M, Barille S (2001) Myeloma cells induce imbalance in the osteoprotegerin/osteoprotegerin ligand system in the human bone marrow environment. Blood 98:3527-3533
[65] Okada T, Akikusa S, Okuno H, Kodaka M (2003) Bone marrow metastatic myeloma cells promote osteoclastogenesis through RANKL on endothelial cells. Clin Exp Metastasis 20:639-646
[66] Giuliani N, Colla S, Sala R, Moroni M, Lazzaretti M, La Monica S, Bonomini S, Hojden M, Sammarelli G, Barille S, Bataille R, Rizzoli V (2002) Human myeloma cells stimulate the receptor activator of nuclear factor-kappa B ligand (RANKL) in T lymphocytes: a potential role in multiple myeloma bone disease. Blood 100:4615-4621
[67] Standal T, Seidel C, Hjertner O, Plesner T, Sanderson RD, Waage A, Borset M, Sundan A (2002) Osteoprotegerin is bound, internalized, and degraded by multiple myeloma cells. Blood 100:3002-3007
[68] Grimaud E, Soubigou L, Couillaud S, Coipeau P, Moreau A, Passuti N, Gouin F, Redini F, Heymann D (2003) Receptor activator of nuclear factor kappaB ligand (RANKL)/osteoprotegerin (OPG) ratio is increased in severe osteolysis. Am J Pathol 163:2021-2031
[69] Schilbach K, Geiselhart A, Handgretinger R (2001) Induction of proliferation and augmented cytotoxicity of gammadelta T lymphocytes by bisphosphonate clodronate. Blood 97:2917-2918
[70] Lahtinen R, Laakso M, Palva I, Virkkunen P, Elomaa I (1992) Randomised, placebo-controlled multicentre trial of clodronate in multiple myeloma. Finnish Leukaemia Group. Lancet 340:1049-1052
[71] Laakso M, Lahtinen R, Virkkunen P, Elomaa I (1994) Subgroup and cost-benefit analysis of the Finnish multicentre trial of clodronate in multiple myeloma. Finnish Leukaemia Group. Br J Haematol 87:725-729
[72] McCloskey EV, MacLennan IC, Drayson MT, Chapman C, Dunn J, Kanis JA (1998) A randomized trial of the effect of clodronate on skeletal morbidity in multiple myeloma. MRC Working Party on Leukaemia in Adults. Br J Haematol 100:317-325
[73] McCloskey EV, Dunn JA, Kanis JA, MacLennan IC, Drayson MT (2001) Long-term follow-up of a prospective, double-blind, placebo-controlled randomized trial of clodronate in multiple myeloma. Br J Haematol 113:1035-1043

[74] Paterson AHG, Powles TJ, Kanis JA, McCloskey E, Hanson J, Ashley S (1993) Double-blind controlled trial of oral clodronate in patients with bone metastases from breast cancer. J Clin Oncol 11:59-65
[75] Dearnaley DP, Mason MD, Parmar MKB, Sanders K, Sydes MR (2009) Adjuvant therapy with oral sodium clodronate in locally advanced and metastatic prostate cancer: long-term overall survival results from the MRC PR04 and PR05 randomised controlled trials. Lancet Oncol 10:872-876
[76] Berenson JR, Lichtenstein A, Porter L, Dimopoulos MA, Bordoni R, George S, Lipton A, Keller A, Ballester O, Kovacs MJ, Blacklock HA, Bell R, Simeone J, Reitsma DJ, Heffernan M, Seaman J, Knight RD (1996) Efficacy of pamidronate in reducing skeletal events in patients with advanced multiple myeloma. Myeloma Aredia Study Group. N Engl J Med 334:488-493
[77] Menssen HD, Sakalova A, Fontana A, Herrmann Z, Boewer C, Facon T, Lichinitser MR, Singer CR, Euller-Ziegler L, Wetterwald M, Fiere D, Hrubisko M, Thiel E, Delmas PD (2002) Effects of long-term intravenous ibandronate therapy on skeletal-related events, survival, and bone resorption markers in patients with advanced multiple myeloma. J Clin Oncol 20:2353-2359
[78] Rosen LS, Gordon D, Kaminski M, Howell A, Belch A, Mackey J, Apffelstaedt J, Hussein M, Coleman RE, Reitsma DJ, Seaman JJ, Chen BL, Ambros Y (2001) Zoledronic acid versus pamidronate in the treatment of skeletal metastases in patients with breast cancer or osteolytic lesions of multiple myeloma: a phase III, double-blind, comparative trial. Cancer J 7:377-387
[79] Kohno N, Aogi K, Minami H, Nakamura S, Asaga T, Iino Y, Watanabe T, Goessl C, Ohashi Y, Takashima S (2005) Zoledronic acid significantly reduces skeletal complications compared with placebo in Japanese women with bone metastases from breast cancer: a randomized, placebo-controlled trial. J Clin Oncol 23:3314-3321
[80] Rosen LS, Gordon D, Tchekmedyian NS, Yanagihara R, Hirsh V, Krzakowski M, Pawlicki M, De Souza P, Zheng M, Urbanowitz G, Reitsma D, Seaman J (2004) Long-term efficacy and safety of zoledronic acid in the treatment of skeletal metastases in patients with nonsmall cell lung carcinoma and other solid tumors: a randomized, phase III, double-blind, placebo-controlled trial. Cancer 100:2613-2621
[81] Saad F, Gleason DM, Murray R, Tchekmedyian S, Venner P, Lacombe L, Chin JL, Vinholes JJ, Goas JA, Zheng M (2004) Long-term efficacy of zoledronic acid for the prevention of skeletal complications in patients with metastatic hormone-refractory prostate cancer. J Natl Cancer Inst 96:879-882
[82] Stopeck AT, Lipton A, Body JJ, Steger GG, Tonkin K, de Boer RH, Lichinitser M, Fujiwara Y, Yardley DA, Viniegra M, Fan M, Jiang Q, Dansey R, Jun S, Braun A (2010) Denosumab compared with zoledronic acid for the treatment of bone metastases in patients with advanced breast cancer: a randomized, double-blind study. J Clin Oncol Epub ahead of print
[83] Coxon FP, Thompson K, Rogers MJ (2006) Recent advances in understanding the mechanism of action of bisphosphonates. Curr Opin Pharmacol 6:307-312
[84] Thompson K, Roelofs AJ, Jauhiainen M, Monkkonen H, Monkkonen J, Rogers MJ (2010) Activation of gammadelta T cells by bisphosphonates. Adv Exp Med Biol 658:11-20

[85] Terpos E, Dimopoulos MA (2005) Myeloma bone disease: pathophysiology and management. Ann Oncol 16:1223-1231
[86] Berenson JR, Lichtenstein A, Porter L, Dimopoulos MA, Bordoni R, George S, Lipton A, Keller A, Ballester O, Kovacs M, Blacklock H, Bell R, Simeone JF, Reitsma DJ, Heffernan M, Seaman J, Knight RD (1998) Long-term pamidronate treatment of advanced multiple myeloma patients reduces skeletal events. Myeloma Aredia Study Group. J Clin Oncol 16:593-602
[87] Kunzmann V, Bauer E, Feurle J, Weissinger F, Tony HP, Wilhelm M (2000) Stimulation of gammadelta T cells by aminobisphosphonates and induction of antiplasma cell activity in multiple myeloma. Blood 96:384-392
[88] Terpos E, Viniou N, de la Fuente J, Meletis J, Voskaridou E, Karkantaris C, Vaiopoulos G, Palermos J, Yataganas X, Goldman JM, Rahemtulla A (2003) Pamidronate is superior to ibandronate in decreasing bone resorption, interleukin-6 and beta 2-microglobulin in multiple myeloma. Eur J Haematol 70:34-42
[89] Devitt B, McLachlan SA (2008) Use of ibandronate in the prevention of skeletal events in metastatic breast cancer. Ther Clin Risk Manag 4:453-458
[90] Berenson JR, Rosen LS, Howell A, Porter L, Coleman RE, Morley W, Dreicer R, Kuross SA, Lipton A, Seaman JJ (2001) Zoledronic acid reduces skeletal-related events in patients with osteolytic metastases. Cancer 91:1191-1200
[91] Rosen LS, Gordon D, Kaminski M, Howell A, Belch A, Mackey J, Apffelstaedt J, Hussein MA, Coleman RE, Reitsma DJ, Chen BL, Seaman JJ (2003) Long-term efficacy and safety of zoledronic acid compared with pamidronate disodium in the treatment of skeletal complications in patients with advanced multiple myeloma or breast carcinoma: a randomized, double-blind, multicenter, comparative trial. Cancer 98:1735-1744
[92] Rosen LS, Gordon D, Tchekmedyian S, Yanagihara R, Hirsh V, Krzakowski M, Pawlicki M, de Souza P, Zheng M, Urbanowitz G, Reitsma D, Seaman JJ (2003) Zoledronic acid versus placebo in the treatment of skeletal metastases in patients with lung cancer and other solid tumors: a phase III, double-blind, randomized trial—the Zoledronic Acid Lung Cancer and Other Solid Tumors Study Group. J Clin Oncol 21:3150-3157
[93] Naoe M, Ogawa Y, Takeshita K, Morita J, Shichijo T, Fuji K, Fukagai T, Iwamoto S, Terao S (2010) Zoledronate stimulates gamma delta T cells in prostate cancer patients. Oncol Res 18:493-501
[94] Lipton A (2008) Emerging role of bisphosphonates in the clinic—antitumor activity and prevention of metastasis to bone. Cancer Treat Rev 34(suppl 1):S25-S30
[95] Senaratne SG, Pirianov G, Mansi JL, Arnett TR, Colston KW (2000) Bisphosphonates induce apoptosis in human breast cancer cell lines. Br J Cancer 82:1459-1468
[96] Santini D, Martini F, Fratto ME, Galluzzo S, Vincenzi B, Agrati C, Turchi F, Piacentini P, Rocci L, Manavalan JS, Tonini G, Poccia F (2009) In vivo effects of zoledronic acid on peripheral gammadelta T lymphocytes in early breast cancer patients. Cancer Immunol Immunother 58:31-38
[97] Ferretti G, Fabi A, Carlini P, Papaldo P, Cordiali Fei P, Di Cosimo S, Salesi N, Giannarelli D, Alimonti A, Di Cocco B, D'Agosto G, Bordignon V, Trento E, Cognetti F (2005) Zoledronic-acid-induced circulating level modifications of

angiogenic factors, metalloproteinases and proinflammatory cytokines in metastatic breast cancer patients. Oncology 69:35-43

[98] Santini D, Vincenzi B, Galluzzo S, Battistoni F, Rocci L, Venditti O, Schiavon G, Angeletti S, Uzzalli F, Caraglia M, Dicuonzo G, Tonini G (2007) Repeated intermittent low-dose therapy with zoledronic acid induces an early, sustained, and long-lasting decrease of peripheral vascular endothelial growth factor levels in cancer patients. Clin Cancer Res 13:4482-4486

[99] Ottewell PD, Monkkonen H, Jones M, Lefley DV, Coleman RE, Holen I (2008) Antitumor effects of doxorubicin followed by zoledronic acid in a mouse model of breast cancer. J Natl Cancer Inst 100:1167-1178

[100] Neville-Webbe HL, Rostami-Hodjegan A, Evans CA, Coleman RE, Holen I (2005) Sequence- and schedule-dependent enhancement of zoledronic acid induced apoptosis by doxorubicin in breast and prostate cancer cells. Int J Cancer 113:364-371

[101] Rack B, Schindlbeck C, Strobl B, Sommer H, Friese K, Janni W (2008) [Efficacy of zoledronate in treating persisting isolated tumor cells in bone marrow in patients with breast cancer. A phase II pilot study]. Dtsch Med Wochenschr 133:285-289

[102] Solomayer E, Gebauer G, Hirnle P, Janni W, Lück H-J, Becker S, Huober J, Kraemer B, Fehm T (2009) Influence of zoledronic acid on disseminated tumor cells (DTC) in primary breast cancer patients (abstract 2048). Cancer Res 69(suppl):170s-171s

[103] Aft R, Naughton M, Ylagen L, Watson M, Chavez-MacGregor M, Trinkaus K, Zhai J, Weilbaecher K (2008) Effect of zoledronic acid on bone marrow micrometastases in women undergoing neoadjuvant chemotherapy for breast cancer (abstract 1021). In: Presented at the 44th Annual Meeting of the American Society of Clinical Oncology, 30 May-3 June 2008, Chicago, IL, USA

[104] Lin AY, Park JW, Scott J, Melisko M, Goga A, Moasser MM, Moore DH, Rugo HS (2008) Zoledronic acid as adjuvant therapy for women with early-stage breast cancer and disseminated tumor cells in bone marrow (abstract 559). In: Presented at the 44th Annual Meeting of the American Society of Clinical Oncology, 30 May-3 June 2008, Chicago, IL, USA

[105] Gnant M, Mlineritsch B, Schippinger W, Luschin-Ebengreuth G, Postlberger S, Menzel C, Jakesz R, Seifert M, Hubalek M, Bjelic-Radisic V, Samonigg H, Tausch C, Eidtmann H, Steger G, Kwasny W, Dubsky P, Fridrik M, Fitzal F, Stierer M, Rucklinger E, Greil R, Marth C (2009) Endocrine therapy plus zoledronic acid in premenopausal breast cancer. N Engl J Med 360:679-691

[106] Coleman RE, Winter MC, Cameron D, Bell R, Dodwell D, Keane MM, Gil M, Ritchie D, Passos-Coelho JL, Wheatley D, Burkinshaw R, Marshall SJ, Thorpe H (2010) The effects of adding zoledronic acid to neoadjuvant chemotherapy on tumour response: exploratory evidence for direct anti-tumour activity in breast cancer. Br J Cancer 102:1099-1105

[107] Coleman R, Bundred N, De Boer R, Llombarto A, Campbell I, Neven P, Barrios C, Dias R, Miller J, Brufsky A (2009) Impact of zoledronic acid in postmenopausal women with early breast cancer receiving adjuvant letrozole: Z-FAST, ZO-FAST, and E-ZO-FAST (abstract 4082). Cancer Res 69(suppl):733s

[108] Brufsky A, Graydon Harker W, Beck JT, Carroll R, Jin L, Warsi G, Argonza-Aviles E, Ericson S, Perez EA (2009) The effect of zoledronic acid on aromatase inhibitor-

associated bone loss in postmenopausal women with early breast cancer receiving adjuvant letrozole: the Z-FAST study 5-year final follow-up (abstract 4083). In: Presented at the 32nd Annual San Antonio Breast Cancer Symposium, 9-13 December 2009, San Antonio, TX, USA

[109] Costa L, Cook R, Body J-J, Brown J, Terpos E, Saad F, Lipton A, Coleman R (2009) Zoledronic acid treatment delays disease progression and improves survival in patients with bone metastases from solid tumors and elevated levels of bone resorption (abstract 50) In: Presented at the IX International Meeting on Cancer Induced Bone Disease, 28-31 October 2009, Arlington, VA, USA

[110] Body J-J, Cook R, Costa L, Brown J, Terpos E, Saad F, Lipton A, Coleman R (2009) Possible survival benefits from zoledronic acid treatment in patients with bone metastases from solid tumors and poor prognostic features (abstract 71). In: Presented at the IX International Meeting on Cancer Induced Bone Disease, 28-31 October 2009, Arlington, VA, USA

[111] Morgan GJ, Davies FE, Gregory WM, Cocks K, Bell SE, Szubert AJ, Navarro-Coy N, Drayson MT, Owen RG, Feyler S, Ashcroft AJ, Ross F, Byrne J, Roddie H, Rudin C, Cook G, Jackson GH, Child JA; National Cancer Research Institute Haematological Oncology Clinical Study Group (2010) First-line treatment with zoledronic acid as compared with clodronic acid in multiple myeloma (MRC Myeloma IX): a randomised controlled trial. Lancet 376:1989-1999

[112] Zaghloul MS, Boutrus R, El-Hosieny H, A-Kader Y, El-Attar I, Nazmy M (2008) A controlled prospective randomized placebo-controlled trial of zoledronic acid in bony metastatic bladder cancer patients (abstract 5033). J Clin Oncol 26(suppl):257s

[113] Zarogoulidis K, Boutsikou E, Zarogoulidis P, Eleftheriadou E, Kontakiotis T, Lithoxopoulou H, Tzanakakis G, Kanakis I, Karamanos NK (2009) The impact of zoledronic acid therapy in survival of lung cancer patients with bone metastasis. Int J Cancer 125:1705-1709

[114] Mystakidou K, Katsouda E, Parpa E, Kelekis A, Galanos A, Vlahos L (2005) Randomized, open label, prospective study on the effect of zoledronic acid on the prevention of bone metastases in patients with recurrent solid tumors that did not present with bone metastases at baseline. Med Oncol 22:195-201

[115] United States Food and Drug Administration. Background document for meeting of Advisory Committee for Reproductive Health Drugs (August 13, 2009). Available from: http://www.fda.gov/downloads/AdvisoryCommittees/CommitteesMeetingMaterials/Drugs/ReproductiveHealthDrugsAdvisoryCommittee/UCM176605.pdf [Accessed April 21, 2010].

[116] Anastasilakis AD, Toulis KA, Polyzos SA, Terpos E (2009) RANKL inhibition for the management of patients with benign metabolic bone disorders. Expert Opin Investig Drugs 18:1085-1102

[117] Cummings SR, San Martin J, McClung MR, Siris ES, Eastell R, Reid IR, Delmas P, Zoog HB, Austin M, Wang A, Kutilek S, Adami S, Zanchetta J, Libanati C, Siddhanti S, Christiansen C (2009) Denosumab for prevention of fractures in postmenopausal women with osteoporosis. N Engl J Med 361:756-765

[118] Stopeck A, Body JJ, Fujiwara Y, Lipton A, Steger GG, Viniegra M, Fan M, Braun A, Dansey R, Jun S (2009) Denosumab versus zoledronic acid for the treatment of

breast cancer patients with bone metastases: results of a randomized phase 3 study (abstract 2LBA). Eur J Cancer Suppl 7:2

[119] Fizazi K, Carducci M, Smith M, Damiao R, Brown J, Karsh L, Milecki P, Rader M, Shore N, Tadros S, Wang H, Jiang Q, Dansey R, Goessl C (2010) Denosumab compared with zoledronic acid for the treatment of bone metastases in patients with castration-resistant prostate cancer (abstract LBA4507). In: Presented at the 46th Annual Meeting of the Americal Society of Clinical Oncology, 4-8 June 2010, Chicago, IL, USA

[120] Thomas D, Henshaw R, Skubitz K, Chawla S, Staddon A, Blay JY, Roudier M, Smith J, Ye Z, Sohn W, Dansey R, Jun S (2010) Denosumab in patients with giant-cell tumour of bone: an open-label, phase 2 study. Lancet Oncol 11:275-280

[121] Gonzalez-Suarez E, Jacob AP, Jones J, Miller R, Roudier-Meyer MP, Erwert R, Pinkas J, Branstetter D, Dougall WC (2010) RANK ligand mediates progestin-induced mammary epithelial proliferation and carcinogenesis. Nature 468:103-107

[122] Anastasilakis AD, Toulis KA, Goulis DG, Polyzos SA, Delaroudis S, Giomisi A, Terpos E (2009) Efficacy and safety of denosumab in postmenopausal women with osteopenia or osteoporosis: a systematic review and a meta-analysis. Horm Metab Res 41:721-729

[123] Ellis GK, Bone HG, Chlebowski R, Paul D, Spadafora S, Smith J, Fan M, Jun S (2008) Randomized trial of denosumab in patients receiving adjuvant aromatase inhibitors for nonmetastatic breast cancer. J Clin Oncol 26:4875-4882

[124] Smith MR, Egerdie B, Hernandez Toriz N, Feldman R, Tammela TL, Saad F, Heracek J, Szwedowski M, Ke C, Kupic A, Leder BZ, Goessl C (2009) Denosumab in men receiving androgen-deprivation therapy for prostate cancer. N Engl J Med 361:745-755

[125] Fizazi K, Bosserman L, Gao G, Skacel T, Markus R (2009) Denosumab treatment of prostate cancer with bone metastases and increased urine N-telopeptide levels after therapy with intravenous bisphosphonates: results of a randomized phase II trial. J Urol 182:509-515; discussion follows

[126] Xgeva (denosumab) injection [prescribing information]. Amgen; Thousand Oaks, CA, USA; 2010.